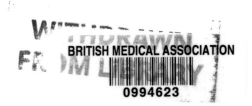

Successful Training in Gastrointestinal Endoscopy

Companion DVD-ROM

This book is accompanied by a companion DVD with:

- Over 130 annotated teaching videos of both actual procedures and ex-vivo animal model simulations.

- A search feature

- All videos are referenced in the text where you see this logo

Successful Training in Gastrointestinal Endoscopy

EDITED BY

Jonathan Cohen, MD
Clinical Professor of Medicine
New York University School of Medicine
New York, NY, USA

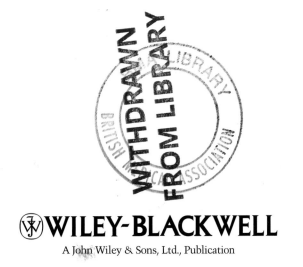

⟨W⟩WILEY-BLACKWELL

A John Wiley & Sons, Ltd., Publication

Library of Congress Cataloging-in-Publication Data

Successful training in gastrointestinal endoscopy / edited by Jonathan Cohen.
　　　p. ; cm.
　　Includes bibliographical references and index.
　　ISBN 978-1-4051-9663-5 (hardcover : alk. paper)　1. Gastroscopy–Study and teaching.　2. Gastrointestinal system–Endoscopic surgery–Study and teaching.　I. Cohen, Jonathan, 1964–
　　[DNLM: 1. Endoscopy, Gastrointestinal.　2. Endoscopy–education.　WI 141]
　　RC804.G3S83 2011
　　617.4′30597–dc22

2010047391

A catalogue record for this book is available from the British Library.

This book is published in the following electronic formats: ePDF 9781444397758; Wiley Online Library 9781444397772; ePub 9781444397765

Set in 9.25/11.5pt Minion by Aptara® Inc., New Delhi, India
Printed and bound in Singapore by Markono Print Media Pte Ltd

1　2011

Contents

Part IV Challenges for the Future

List of Contributors

Douglas G. Adler, MD, FACG, FASGE
Associate Professor of Medicine
Director of Therapeutic Endoscopy
Division of Gastroenterology and Hepatology
University of Utah School of Medicine
Huntsman Cancer Center
Salt Lake City, UT, USA

Alan Barkun, MD,CM, FRCP(C), FACP, MSc
Chairholder
The Douglas G. Kinnear Chair in Gastrology
Professor of Medicine
Division of Gastroenterology
McGill University
McGill University Health Centre
Montreal, QC, Canada

Todd H. Baron, MD, FASGE
Professor of Medicine
Director Pancreaticobiliary Endoscopy
Division of Gastroenterology & Hepatology
Mayo Clinic
Rochester, MN, USA

Anna M. Buchner, MD, PhD
Instructor of Medicine
Division of Gastroenterology
Department of Medicine
University of Pennsylvania School of Medicine
Philadelphia, PA, USA

Karl-Friedrich Buerrig, MD, PhD
Department of Medicine III—Gastroenterology, Interventional Endoscopy
St. Bernward Academic Teaching Hospital
Hildesheim, Germany

Jonathan M. Buscaglia, MD
Director, Center for Advanced Endoscopy
Assistant Professor of Medicine
Division of Gastroenterology and Hepatology
State University of New York
Stony Brook, NY, USA

David L. Carr-Locke, MB, FRCP, FASGE
Chief, Division of Digestive Diseases;
Co-Director, Center for Digestive Health;
Director, GI Services
Continuum Cancer Centers of NY
Beth Israel Medical Center
New York, NY, USA

Jonathan Cohen, MD
Clinical Professor of Medicine
New York University School of Medicine
New York, NY, USA

Gregory A. Coté, MD, MS
Assistant Professor of Clinical Medicine
Indiana University School of Medicine
Indianapolis, IN, USA

Peter B. Cotton, MD, FRCP, FRCS
Professor of Medicine
Digestive Disease Center
Medical University of South Carolina
Charleston, SC, USA

SongSa Dammer, CN
Department of Medicine III—Gastroenterology, Interventional Endoscopy
St. Bernward Academic Teaching Hospital
Hildesheim, Germany

John Day, BBA
Vice-President, Marketing
ERBE USA Inc.
Marietta, GA, USA

James A. DiSario, MD, FASGE
Monterey Bay Gastroenterology Consultants
Monterey, CA, USA;
Adjunct Professor of Medicine
University of Utah Health Sciences Center
Salt Lake City, UT, USA

John A. Dumot, DO
Digestive Health Institute
University Hospitals
Cleveland, OH, USA

Brian J. Dunkin, MD, FACS
Professor of Clinical Surgery
Weill Cornell Medical College;
Head, Section of Endoscopic Surgery;
Medical Director, The Methodist Institute for Technology, Innovation,
    and Education
The Methodist Hospital
Houston, TX, USA

Steven A. Edmundowicz, MD
Professor of Medicine
Director of Endoscopy
Washington University School of Medicine
St. Louis, MO, USA

Douglas O. Faigel, MD
Professor of Medicine
Mayo Clinic
Scottsdale, AZ, USA

Syed M. Abbas Fehmi, MD, MSc
Assistant Professor
Division of Gastroenterology
Department of Medicine
University of California San Diego
San Diego, CA, USA

David E. Fleischer, MD
Professor of Medicine
Mayo School of Medicine
Mayo Clinic
Scottsdale, AZ, USA

Evan L. Fogel, MD, FRCP(C)
Professor of Clinical Medicine
Indiana University School of Medicine
Indianapolis, IN, USA

Martin L. Freeman, MD
Professor of Medicine
Interim Director, Division of Gastroenterology, Hepatology, and Nutrition
Director of Pancreaticobiliary Endoscopy Fellowship
University of Minnesota
Minneapolis, MN, USA

Gerald M. Fried, MD
Professor of Surgery and Adair Family Chair of Surgical Education
McGill University;
Steinberg—Bernstein Chair of Minimally Invasive Surgery and Innovation
McGill University Health Centre;
Montreal General Hospital
Montreal, QC, Canada

Shai Friedland, MD
Assistant Professor of Medicine
Division of Gastroenterology and Hepatology
Stanford University School of Medicine
Stanford, CA, USA

Lauren B. Gerson, MD, MSc
Associate Professor of Medicine
Division of Gastroenterology and Hepatology
Stanford University School of Medicine
Stanford, CA, USA

Sahar Ghassemi, MD
Director of EUS
Santa Rosa Community Hospital
Santa Rosa, OR, USA

Christopher J. Gostout, MD, FASGE
Professor of Medicine
Mayo Clinic
Rochester, MN, USA

Bruce D. Greenwald, MD
Professor of Medicine
University of Maryland
School of Medicine and Greenebaum Cancer Center
Baltimore, MD, USA

David A. Greenwald, MD
Gastroenterology Fellowship Process Director
Associate Division Director
Montefiore Medical Center;
Associate Professor of Clinical Medicine
Albert Einstein College of Medicine
New York, NY, USA

Frank G. Gress, MD, FACP, FACG
Professor of Medicine
Chief, Division of Gastroenterology and Hepatology
State University of New York (SUNY)
Downstate Medical Center
New York, NY, USA

Mark A. Gromski, BA
Research Fellow in Developmental Endoscopy
Beth Israel Deaconess Medical Center
Harvard Medical School
Boston, MA, USA

Gregory B. Haber, MD, FRCP(C)
Director, Division of Gastroenterology
Director, Center for Advanced Therapeutic Endoscopy
Lenox Hill Hospital
New York, NY, USA

Robert Hawes, MD
Professor of Medicine
Peter Cotton Chair for Endoscopic Innovation
Division of Gastroenterology and Hepatology
Medical University of South Carolina
Charleston, SC, USA

Juergen Hochberger, MD, PhD
Professor of Medicine and Chairman
Department of Medicine III—Gastroenterology, Interventional Endoscopy
St. Bernward Academic Teaching Hospital
Hildesheim, Germany

Douglas A. Howell, MD, FASGE
Associate Clinical Professor of Medicine
University of Vermont College of Medicine
Burlington, VT, USA;
Director, Advanced Training Fellowship
Director, Pancreaticobiliary Center
Maine Medical Center
Portland, ME, USA

Dennis M. Jensen, MD
Professor of Medicine
David Geffen School of Medicine at UCLA
Los Angeles, CA, USA

Sreenivasa S. Jonnalagadda, MD, FASGE
Professor of Medicine
Director of Biliary and Pancreatic Endoscopy
Division of Gastroenterology
Washington University School of Medicine
St. Louis, MO, USA

Nithin Karanth, MD
Center for Advanced Therapeutic Endoscopy
Lenox Hill Hospital
New York, NY, USA

Peter Kelsey, MD
Associate Director of Endoscopic Services
Massachusetts General Hospital;
Assistant Professor of Medicine
Harvard Medical School
Boston, MA, USA

Michael L. Kochman, MD, FACP
Willmott Family Professor of Medicine
Vice-Chair of Medicine for Clinical Services
Center for Endoscopic Innovation, Research, and Training
Gastroenterology Division
University of Pennsylvania Health System
Philadelphia, PA, USA

Peter Koehler, PhD
Federal Research Institute for Animal Health (FLI)
Mariensee, Neustadt, Germany

Elena Kruse, MD
Department of Medicine III—Gastroenterology, Interventional Endoscopy
St. Bernward Academic Teaching Hospital
Hildesheim, Germany

Jeffrey H. Lee, MD, FACG, FASGE
Professor
Director of Advanced Endoscopy Fellowship and Training
Department of Gastroenterology, Hepatology, and Nutrition
MD Anderson Cancer Center
Houston, TX, USA

Glen A. Lehman, MD
Professor of Medicine and Radiology
Indiana University School of Medicine
Indianapolis, IN, USA

Joseph Leung, MD, FRCP, FACP, FACG, FASGE
Mr. & Mrs. C.W. Law Professor of Medicine
University of California, Davis School of Medicine
Sacramento, CA, USA;
Chief of Gastroenterology
VA Northern California Health Care System
Mather, CA, USA

Michael J. Levy, MD
Division of Gastroenterology and Hepatology
Mayo Clinic
Rochester, MN, USA

Jenifer R. Lightdale, MD, MPH
Assistant Professor of Pediatrics
Harvard Medical School;
Associate in Medicine, Gastroenterology and Nutrition
Children's Hospital Boston
Boston, MA, USA

Brian S. Lim, MD, MCR
Staff Gastroenterologist
Department of Gastroenterology
Kaiser Permanente
Riverside Medical Center
Riverside, CA, USA

Michael A. Manfredi, MD
Instructor in Pediatrics
Harvard Medical School
Boston, MA, USA;
Associate Director of Endoscopy
Children's Hospital Boston
Boston, MA, USA

John A. Martin, MD
Associate Professor of Medicine and Surgery
Director of Endoscopy
Division of Gastroenterology
Northwestern University Feinberg School of Medicine
Chicago, IL, USA

Kai Matthes, MD, PhD
Director
Developmental Endoscopy
Department of Gastroenterology
Beth Israel Deaconess Medical Center
Harvard Medical School
Boston, MA, USA

Detlev Menke, MD
Department of Medicine III—Gastroenterology, Interventional Endoscopy
St. Bernward Academic Teaching Hospital
Hildesheim, Germany

Girish Mishra, MD, MSc, FACG, FACP
Vice-Chief & Associate Professor
Director, Endoscopy & GI Fellowship Program
Section on Gastroenterology
Wake Forest University School of Medicine
Winston-Salem, NC, USA

Patrick I. Okolo, MD, MPH
Chief of Endoscopy
Division of Gastroenterology
Johns Hopkins University School of Medicine
Baltimore, MD, USA

John L. Petrini, MD, FASGE
Chairman
Department of Gastroenterology
Sansum Clinic
Santa Barbara, CA, USA

Gottumukkla S. Raju, MD, FRCP, FACG, FASGE
Professor of Medicine
Department of Gastroenterology, Hepatology, and Nutrition
University of Texas, MD Anderson Cancer Center
Houston, TX, USA

Marvin Ryou, MD
Advanced Endoscopy Fellow
Brigham and Women's Hospital
Massachusetts General Hospital
Boston, MA, USA

Yasushi Sano, MD, PhD
Director
Gastrointestinal Center
Sano Hospital
Tarumi-ku, Kobe, Hyogo, Japan

Thomas J. Savides, MD
Professor of Clinical Medicine
Division of Gastroenterology
University of California
San Diego, CA, USA

Felice Schnoll-Sussman, MD, FACG
Weill Medical College
Cornell University
New York, NY, USA

Robert E. Sedlack, MD, MHPE
Division of Gastroenterology and Hepatology
Mayo Clinic
Rochester, MN, USA

Sohail N. Shaikh, MD
Developmental and Bariatric Endoscopy Research Fellow
Division of Gastroenterology
Brigham and Women's Hospital;
Post-Doctoral Fellow
Harvard Medical School
Boston, MA, USA

Prateek Sharma, MD
Professor of Medicine
Division of Gastroenterology and Hepatology
Veterans Affairs Medical Center
University of Kansas School of Medicine
Kansas City, KS, USA

Virender K. Sharma, MD, FASGE, FACG, AGAF
Director
Arizona Center for Digestive Health
Gilbert, AZ, USA

Stuart Sherman, MD
Professor of Medicine
Indiana University School of Medicine
Indianapolis, IN, USA

Peter D. Siersema, MD, PhD
Professor of Gastroenterology
Director, Department of Gastroenterology and Hepatology
University Medical Center Utrecht
Utrecht, The Netherlands

Christopher C. Thompson, MD, MHES, FACG, FACGE
Director of Developmental and Bariatric Endoscopy
Brigham and Women's Hospital;
Assistant Professor of Medicine
Harvard Medical School
Boston, MA, USA

Roland M. Valori, MD, FRCP, MSc
Gloucestershire Hospitals NHS Foundation Trust
Gloucestershire, UK

Michael B. Wallace, MD, MPH
Professor and Vice-Chairman of Medicine
Department of Gastroenterology and Hepatology
Mayo Clinic
Jacksonville, FL, USA

Kevin A. Waschke, MD, CM, FRCPC, CPSQ
Director of Therapeutic Endoscopy and Endosonography
McGill University Health Centre
McGill University
Montreal, QC, Canada

Jerome D. Waye, MD
Director of Endoscopic Education
Mt. Sinai Hospital
New York, NY, USA

Edris Wedi, MD
Department of Medicine III—Gastroenterology, Interventional Endoscopy
St. Bernward Academic Teaching Hospital
Hildesheim, Germany

Foreword

Throughout the years, it is evident that the best practitioners of endoscopy are not necessarily the best teachers and, parenthetically, the best teachers may not be the best practitioners of this discipline. Teaching is a skill that can be learned, but in the field of gastrointestinal endoscopy, most teachers acquire their ability to impart their knowledge to others by watching their teachers over years of schooling and incorporating the best parts of several educators into their personal style of educational communication. In the field of endoscopy, all who become teachers have an enormous responsibility, not only to share their knowledge completely and selflessly with the student, but to watch over the patient at all times to ensure their safety and that the teaching aspect of the procedure does not infringe upon the ability to provide the best endoscopic examination possible. The information that is given must become a part of the student's approach to the entire endoscopic experience including such aspects as informed consent, the preparation of the patient, the discussion of the procedure both before and after the instrumentation takes place and, of course, the careful and repetitive steps needed for the effortless and practiced performance of the examination itself. The endoscopic approach, learned by the side of the instructor, will be used for the rest of the professional lives of the students and are skills that will be further enhanced as the student becomes more familiar with the myriad procedures that are possible and seemingly impossible but that can be built upon by a solid foundation to cope with emerging technology. It is not possible in this book to present all the facets of learning all aspects of endoscopy, but Dr. Cohen has made it a priority to present all facets of teaching the procedural aspect of gastrointestinal endoscopy, and has done it well.

Prior to assigning chapters to write, Dr. Cohen identified three attributes that had to be realized in each of the authors whom he invited to participate in this unique teaching endeavor. Each author had to be a superb endoscopic technician who also is currently engaged in formally teaching endoscopy to students as well as other endoscopists, and has demonstrated skill in writing and putting their thoughts on paper in an organized fashion. Having written a multiauthored book on narrow band imaging (*Comprehensive Atlas of High Resolution Endoscopy and Narrowband Imaging*), Dr. Cohen used his networking ability to find the right endoscopy colleagues for each chapter of the present book. In spite of its title "*Successful Gastrointestinal Endoscopy*", this book is not just a teaching manual, but is actually a "how I do it" textbook developed from the standpoint of an endoscopic expert who also teaches. The accumulated mass of knowledge from these teachers of endoscopy are spread evenly throughout each chapter, which showcases their techniques developed over years of teaching fellows while standing by their side, giving verbal instructions, sharing tips, discussing the approach to problems, and being mentors in their training.

In addition to the wisdom imparted through the transfer of knowledge via the written page, there is an extensive video section contained on the enclosed DVD, which demonstrates the techniques that are written about. The videos complement the book and walk the student through the process to increase the understanding of the training set.

The World Endoscopy Organization (WEO) is pleased to endorse this book since its goals are clear and well defined: that to perform endoscopy one needs to have proper training. This training is best accomplished under the watchful tutelage of a person who is dedicated, expert, and facile not only in the performance of the procedure but also in the ability to transfer skills to the next generation of endoscopists. The WEO promotes excellence in endoscopy throughout all parts of the world and focuses on bringing endoscopy to underserved areas where endoscopy is underutilized.

This book will serve as a valuable resource for those who are in training, those accomplished endoscopists who want to increase their knowledge of techniques, and all the endoscopists who train others in this rapidly growing and exciting field.

Jerome D. Waye, MD
President, World Endoscopy Organization

Preface

The field of gastrointestinal endoscopy today faces a frenetic intersection of change. Many new technologies are emerging to expand the diagnostic and therapeutic capabilities of endoscopists. Innovative investigators are also devising new therapeutic applications of existing equipment. A heightened focus on optimizing quality performance in our procedures necessarily has required a renewed attention on how to ensure that the individuals asked to practice endoscopy are fully trained to achieve the highest possible outcomes. Competing diagnostic and therapeutic modalities threaten to make some of the standard procedures obsolete and challenge the individuals who spend most of their time performing them to adapt. For many individuals caught in this crossroads mid-career, finding the time and opportunities to retool can be very challenging, irrespective of the personal economic concerns involved in making the commitment to upgrade skills in response to the changing conditions.

At the same time, practitioners from specialties previously not involved with endoscopy have been drawn by various forces to learn endoscopy. Resources for training in major GI endoscopy procedures and in specific advanced techniques are limited. For many procedures, the trainers and trainees are hindered by the lack of sufficient case volume in the given technique to be taught. The availability of expert mentors to teach required skills can be another major impediment to training opportunities.

The increased demand for high-quality training and the supply limitations due to the costs and time required for this labor intensive process have driven the development of novel teaching tools which aim to increase the efficiency of training, and where possible increase the potential for independent learning.

The purpose of this book is to provide a comprehensive examination of the principles and specific components of training in endoscopy. The first section explores the important concepts of training and describes the range of tools that have been utilized in this regard. The next two sections provide in-depth discussion of the major current endoscopic procedure categories as well as most specialized diagnostic and therapeutic techniques. For each of these chapters, the authors have considered prerequisite skills for training, skill sets to be mastered, step-by-step components that must be taught and assessed by trainers, typical learning curve for trainees, and objective measures of competency which

trainees must strive to attain. For some of these topics, there has been scant literature to define these parameters. Accordingly, the authors have drawn from their extensive experience in training and performing these procedures to provide their recommendations where data is lacking. The material presented will identify important questions about training that warrant future investigation. The accompanying edited and annotated video clips on the DVD highlight key teaching points for instructors to emphasize. The final section looks to the future of training and retraining in gastrointestinal endoscopy. Key logistical hurdles to this process are examined and the importance of keeping track of outcomes, the ultimate indicator of successful training, is emphasized.

This combined textbook with DVD provides a comprehensive guide for trainees and trainers in gastrointestinal endoscopy of all aspects of the process of acquiring expertise in the techniques that are currently performed. For each procedure, the focus is to cover what needs to be learned, how best to learn it, and how to ensure that sufficient training has taken place to ensure competency.

The chapters examine the specific skills sets and procedure-related tasks that must be mastered in learning a particular technique. They contain specific descriptions of accessories required, standard training methods for the particular procedure, and optimal utilization of novel learning modalities such as simulators. Quality measures and objective parameters for competency for each procedure are considered when available, along with available tools for assessing competency once training has been completed.

The accompanying DVD included with the text contains over 130 annotated video clips of both actual procedures and ex vivo animal model simulations to illustrate proper techniques in a step-by-step fashion and demonstrates common mistakes and improper technique.

The purpose of this volume is to help endoscopists realize optimal levels of skill as they perform the procedures they aspire to learn.

Though the focus of this textbook/DVD remains on how to learn and how to teach each technique, because doing so requires delineation and illustration of all skill sets to master, the textbook chapters and particularly the video unavoidably serve as learning tools for the proper performance of endoscopic techniques in addition to an authoritative primer on training.

Jonathan Cohen, MD

Acknowledgements

I wish to thank the many authors who contributed text and video for this volume for their great efforts and willingness in many cases to take on topics that have not been fully explored before. Beyond that, I want to extend my gratitude to the individuals who have been my teachers in endoscopy. Despite all advances in tools and methods of training detailed in this book, the importance of having wonderful mentors remains paramount to successful training in endoscopy. I have been particularly fortunate in this regard. Besides imparting their wisdom and expertise, they have given me a strong appreciation for the importance of training and of ongoing learning in this ever changing and exciting field.

Thanks also to Cori, Juliette, and Ben for their tremendous understanding, encouragement, and support.

This book is dedicated to JJC for his lifelong inspiration and for giving me the idea for this project. AELCFIS!

The Evolution of Basic Principles and Practice

1 Training in Endoscopy: A Historical Background

Jonathan Cohen[1] & David A. Greenwald[2,3]

[1] New York University School of Medicine, New York, NY, USA
[2] Montefiore Medical Center, New York, NY, USA
[3] Albert Einstein College of Medicine, New York, NY, USA

Introduction

Gastrointestinal endoscopy has grown increasingly more complex as the field has evolved over the past several decades, now requiring the practitioner to become proficient at many techniques. To perform high-quality care, endoscopists often have had to devote time to learn new techniques as well as take care to continually maintain existing skills. As the technology and applications have progressed, so too have the methods by which individuals have learned to perform these procedures. In this chapter, we will trace the evolution in training from the self-taught pioneers of the early days to the advent of formal proctored tutelage that remains the mainstay of training in this field. The chapter will also relate the emergence of numerous innovative learning tools that have already served to further transform training in gastrointestinal endoscopy. In particular, we will describe the development of simulator-based instruction from the creation of realistic models to their validation and growing importance in endoscopic training. Lastly, we will address a number of novel principles of education in endoscopy that have paralleled the growing availability of these new teaching tools.

Standard training in endoscopy: then and now

Self-training for gastrointestinal procedures was the mode by which many of the early endoscopists progressed, largely because devices and equipment became available for which there was no "expert" instruction. In general, this method is not appropriate any longer for training in standard procedures (i.e., colonoscopy, upper endoscopy) where sufficient proctoring is readily available. However, as newer techniques are introduced (i.e., endoscopic suturing, endoscopic mucosal resection (EMR), endoscopic submucosal dissection (ESD), stent placement, transluminal surgery), the question of how to satisfactorily teach these new skills becomes relevant [1]. In fact, "short courses" have been developed to review the cognitive and technical aspects associated with such procedures. American Society for Gastrointestinal Endoscopy (ASGE) guidelines concerning such "short courses" exist, and suggest them as a possible way for experienced endoscopists to acquire new skills, but reject such methods for initial training for "standard" endoscopic techniques such as colonoscopy, upper endoscopy, ERCP, and EUS [2].

The need to impart the wisdom from the growing expertise with endoscopes was readily apparent to the pioneer generation of flexible fiberoptic endoscopy. As early as 1962, the then recently renamed ASGE conducted a symposium entitled "Teaching Methods in Gastrointestinal Endoscopy" in New York City [3]. Two years later, the ASGE formed a committee to examine the requirements for training endoscopists; the conclusions established training as a priority and created a framework that guided formal endoscopy training for many years to follow. Three items were required: (1) full training in medicine or surgery, (2) special training specifically in GI endoscopy under the supervision of an appropriately skilled teacher, and (3) performance of an adequate number of procedures. Soon to follow was the first annual postgraduate training course.

These efforts at a national level have been complemented by a proliferation of local and regional efforts to promote training with local courses and lectures aimed to supplement the one-on-one supervised instruction of trainees in the endoscopy laboratory as well as keep practicing endoscopists up on all of the latest techniques and advances. In 1973, Jim Eddy, Jerry Waye, Hiromi Shinya, Sid Winawer, Paul Sherlock, Henry Colcher, David Zimmon, and Richard Mc Cray met at the Yale Club to discuss how they might disseminate their knowledge and excitement about colonoscopy and polypectomy to practicing gastroenterologists. The result was the formation of the New York Society for Gastrointestinal Endoscopy (NYSGE) and shortly thereafter, an annual endoscopy course initially designated "A Day in the Colon." In this case, a regional society was founded for the sole purpose of promoting training. The evolving role of societies in training is the subject of a subsequent chapter in this book. However, it is important to recognize that from the national to the local level, the endoscopic societies have provided the dedication, organization, and resources to innovate and advance the field of training.

Successful Training in Gastrointestinal Endoscopy, First Edition. Edited by Jonathan Cohen.
© 2011 Blackwell Publishing Ltd. Published 2011 by Blackwell Publishing Ltd.

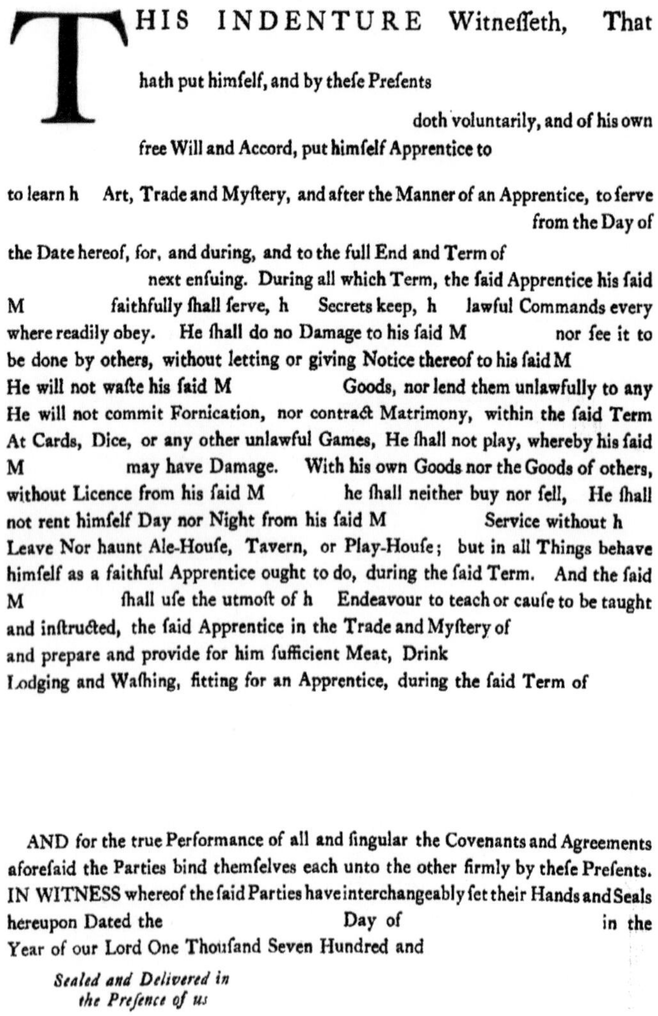

T HIS INDENTURE Witneſſeth, That

hath put himſelf, and by theſe Preſents

doth voluntarily, and of his own

free Will and Accord, put himſelf Apprentice to

to learn h   Art, Trade and Myſtery, and after the Manner of an Apprentice, to ſerve
from the Day of
the Date hereof, for, and during, and to the full End and Term of
next enſuing. During all which Term, the ſaid Apprentice his ſaid
M   faithfully ſhall ſerve, h   Secrets keep, h   lawful Commands every
where readily obey.   He ſhall do no Damage to his ſaid M   nor ſee it to
be done by others, without letting or giving Notice thereof to his ſaid M
He will not waſte his ſaid M   Goods, nor lend them unlawfully to any
He will not commit Fornication, nor contract Matrimony, within the ſaid Term
At Cards, Dice, or any other unlawful Games, He ſhall not play, whereby his ſaid
M   may have Damage.   With his own Goods nor the Goods of others,
without Licence from his ſaid M   he ſhall neither buy nor ſell, He ſhall
not rent himſelf Day nor Night from his ſaid M   Service without h
Leave Nor haunt Ale-Houſe, Tavern, or Play-Houſe; but in all Things behave
himſelf as a faithful Apprentice ought to do, during the ſaid Term.   And the ſaid
M   ſhall uſe the utmoſt of h   Endeavour to teach or cauſe to be taught
and inſtructed, the ſaid Apprentice in the Trade and Myſtery of
and prepare and provide for him ſufficient Meat, Drink
Lodging and Waſhing, fitting for an Apprentice, during the ſaid Term of

AND for the true Performance of all and ſingular the Covenants and Agreements
aforeſaid the Parties bind themſelves each unto the other firmly by theſe Preſents.
IN WITNESS whereof the ſaid Parties have interchangeably ſet their Hands and Seals
hereupon Dated the   Day of   in the
Year of our Lord One Thouſand Seven Hundred and

*Sealed and Delivered in
the Preſence of us*

Figure 1.1 An example of a typical apprenticeship contract in colonial America, circa 1750.

Supervised performance of actual endoscopies remains the predominant mode of endoscopy education today. Such apprenticeship-type relationships between mentor and mentee have evolved greatly from the autocratic and unidirectional flow of information characteristic of similar learning environments dating back to the Middle Ages (Figure 1.1). Recognition and adoption of key concepts such as the benefits of learning in a reduced stress environment, the need for constructive feedback and interactive dialog, and the importance of gradually increasing autonomy of the trainee as skills progress are among the concepts that would make current trainee learning environments quite foreign to medical apprentices of earlier eras.

In the United States today, most instruction in the techniques of gastrointestinal endoscopy are accomplished in the setting of formalized training programs of 3 years duration, with additional training available for selected "advanced" procedures such as ERCP and EUS. Proctored teaching of endoscopic techniques within such highly structured environments has been the "traditional" training method in gastrointestinal endoscopy. Endoscopic skills are developed concurrently with the immersion of the trainee in a complete curriculum that encompasses the range of normal and abnormal functioning of the digestive system, GI anatomy, and pathology. Trainees learn the indications for endoscopy, diagnostic and therapeutic capabilities of endoscopy, technical endoscopic skills, and application of therapeutic endoscopic intervention all in the context of intensive active supervised participation in consultative gastroenterology, for both outpatients and hospitalized individuals. While many physical aspects of endoscope manipulation and even lesion recognition can be taught to individuals not versed in the science and art of caring for patients with gastrointestinal complaints and disorders, to date, patients and practitioners alike have recognized the value and requirement that endoscopy be performed by individuals trained in such a comprehensive fashion, something that in this day can only be achieved in formal gastroenterology and surgical training programs. For this reason, this remains a first principle of published ASGE training guidelines [4,5].

Within these training programs, didactic information about endoscopy is included in the curriculum to an extent, but much of the actual endoscopic training remains directly imparted from instructor to student in the course of the performance of actual procedures on actual patients. Such hands-on supervision allows for increasing independence on the part of the trainee, as the teacher constantly assesses both technical and cognitive progress [6,7]. In this process, the endoscopy teacher must give the trainee sufficient time to develop skills while protecting the patient's safety at all times, and must be able to give appropriate feedback [8,9]. This process is both time and labor intensive. Additionally, sufficient case volume is necessary to allow for development of necessary skills through repetition, and enough variation in pathology needs to be present to allow the development of cognitive skills to go along with advances in technical expertise [10,11]. Mere possession of clinical judgment and endoscopic proficiency do not guarantee that an individual is qualified to be a good endoscopy teacher. The importance of having instructors who know how to teach and the constraints that limit the time such mentors have to devote to teaching can pose significant challenges for this "traditional method" of endoscopy training–challenges which some of the newer complementary teaching tools discussed later in this chapter were developed to address. While many of the chapters in this book refer to the importance and characteristics of good mentors, very little investigation has yet been conducted to understand how to best train the trainers to teach endoscopy.

What must be learned?

Guidelines for training in gastrointestinal endoscopy have been published and widely disseminated [4,5]. Skill sets that trainees must acquire to successfully perform endoscopic procedures have been outlined [12–16] and include the following:

1 Understanding of the indications and contraindications for endoscopic procedures and risk factors for complications.

2 Knowledge of the endoscopic equipment and accessories and how to set up this equipment for use.

3 Familiarity with the endoscope control dials and buttons.

4 Dexterity in controlling the scope range of motion using the dials and torque applied to the endoscope shaft.

5 Hand–eye coordination to produce deliberate, precise manipulation of the endoscope within the lumen and of accessories.

6 Communication with nursing and technical staff regarding required assistance during the procedure.

7 Knowledge of normal anatomic landmarks and possible abnormal pathologies that might be encountered.

8 Interpretive skills to correctly identify abnormalities that are detected.

9 Judgment of how to manage appropriately those lesions that are encountered.

10 Familiarity with patient monitoring and the administration of conscious sedation.

11 Awareness of how to recognize and manage adverse events.

12 Understanding of risks and benefits of intended procedures and the ability to obtain informed consent.

13 Documentation of findings.

14 Communication of results to patients and other physicians.

Standards and endpoints of current endoscopic training

Since the early establishment that training in endoscopy was a high-priority activity among academic endoscopy centers and GI societies, a great deal of effort has been devoted to assess the efficacy of training, determine learning curves for various procedures, and explore new methods for imparting proficiency. A number of important guidelines on the subject have incorporated much of this data and expert opinion on the subject [5]. One large recent review delves into the data for each procedure in great detail [16]. Specific chapters in this volume address training as it relates to quality in endoscopy and to specific standards for each of the major endoscopic procedures that are performed. Apart from the specific recommendations about learning particular procedures, a number of themes have emerged throughout all current guidelines, which reflect the evolution of the concepts of optimal training in endoscopy. Key principles include the following:

• *Specificity of training and privileging*: Individuals must be trained for each particular procedure they wish to perform.

• *Threshold numbers for competency*: Guidelines have steered away from earlier emphasis that trainees gain competence after independently performing a certain minimum number of procedures. It has been increasingly accepted that numbers do not guarantee competency; individuals develop proficiency at different rates; and accordingly, the best way to assess competency is to do so on the basis of some objective measures. Threshold numbers have been derived from evidence-based studies in which objective competency for a particular procedure is achieved after a particular amount of training; however, these numbers are now viewed merely as a minimum amount of training that must be performed before competency can even be assessed. The endpoint of successful endoscopic training should be objective demonstration of competency.

Emergence of complementary teaching modalities

Why use simulators?

Simulators have been proposed as a way to facilitate endoscopic training from the time of the earliest development of the field. In fact, Rudolf Schindler described using a model stomach for practice in orientation [17]. Many of the items in the "skill sets" listed above, and particularly those that involve dexterity, hand–eye coordination, and recognition of normal anatomy and abnormal pathology, can be addressed through the use of various endoscopic simulators.

Endoscopy simulators, including *ex vivo* artificial tissue, animal tissue, and virtual reality computer-based models, provide a unique method for endoscopic teaching. These devices allow for teaching which is free from the possibility of patient discomfort or injury. This factor alone confers several benefits to the learning process. First, the stress of the learning environment is reduced for the trainee and the trainer alike. There is more time for questions and feedback than available when an actual patient is involved. The issue of reduced trainee endoscope time due to critical clinical exigencies is eliminated, and there is ample opportunity for repetition. In fact, the sequence of demonstration of proper technique, repetitive practice of skills with expert feedback, and assessment of skill are all possible in this environment. Creative teaching exercises such as demonstrating common errors and what constitute poor technique are also uniquely possible using such alternative means of instruction to the traditional proctored human endoscopy setting for instruction (Video 1.1). In this way, simulators can confer excellent opportunities for "standard" techniques to be practiced by trainees and allow for new procedures to be taught to experienced clinicians [1]. To the extent that certain models might be used independently by trainees without real-time instructor feedback, and to the extent that simulator work might hasten the time in which trainees can perform unsupervised procedures on their own, simulators also have the potential to address the time constraints facing endoscopy instructors with substantial nonteaching clinical responsibilities of their own to fulfill. However, as we will relate below, much of the actual effective learning using endoscopy simulators does require fairly labor-intensive expert instruction, and to date, the potential for freeing up time spent mentoring trainees has not yet been realized.

Evolution and types of endoscopy simulators

Static models

The initial attempts to complement endoscope training with simulators utilized static models. Such "phantoms" were intended to teach basic hand–eye coordination, the use of the endoscope dials, and even the recognition of basic pathology. In the 1970s, as upper endoscopy and colonoscopy were becoming established as important modalities, other models were developed. These included the Heinkel hemispheric anatomical model [18] and the upper GI plastic dummy introduced by Classen [19].

In the early 1970s, homemade demonstration models of the colon, featuring a mobile transverse colon and the ability to demonstrate an "N" or alpha loop, were devised (Figure 1.2). In 1972, a colonoscopy model fashioned from the spiral metal-reinforced tubing of a hair dryer was introduced, with the ability to demonstrate corkscrewing movements (Figure 1.3). This early simulator featured the ability for the colonoscope to "become stuck" and then to be "straightened out." Christopher Williams' St. Marks/KeyMed colonoscopy model of 1975, shown in Figure 1.4, had an improved feeling of realism and was made commercially available. Twisting movements were required to negotiate the lumen, and endoscopists found it challenging [20].

Simultaneously, hand–eye coordination models were developed. These included an electronic targeting model (Figure 1.5), which had a photocell at the center, tested two-handed coordination, and allowed for "scoring" of results. An endoscopic version of

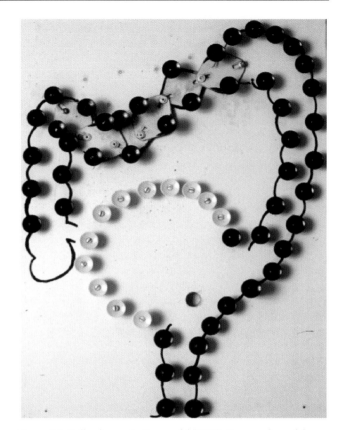

Figure 1.2 Roller demonstration model (1971): Homemade model showing alpha loop and mobile transverse colon. (Courtesy: Dr Christopher Williams.)

the popular game "Pong" was even developed in 1977 (Figure 1.6), allowing for reinforcement of left/right coordination maneuvers in an enjoyable and motivating "game."

The Imperial College/St Mark's College Simulator was introduced in 1980 (Figure 1.7) and allowed for insertion of a limited

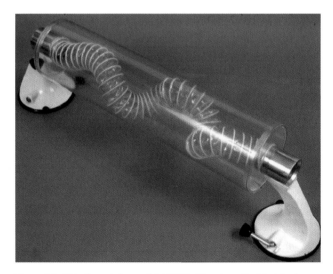

Figure 1.3 Hair dryer tube model (1972). (Courtesy: Dr. Christopher Williams.)

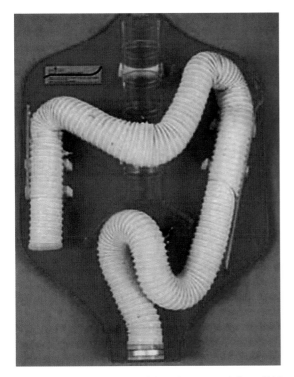

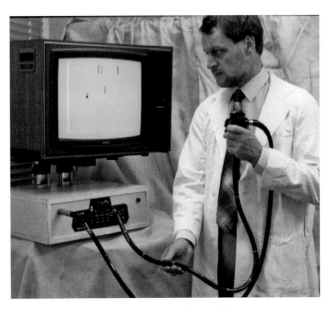

Figure 1.6 Endoscopic Pong Game (1977): Tested hand–eye coordination. (Courtesy: Dr. Christopher Williams.)

Figure 1.4 St Mark's/KeyMed model (1975): Commercially available with semirealistic feel. (Courtesy: Dr. Christopher Williams.)

amount of the shaft of an endoscope into the computer model, with real-time video feedback. This model demonstrated that such devices were feasible, although the particular model was limited by the fragility of the microswitches. Improvements were made over the ensuing 5 years, and by 1985, an updated and substantially more robust version of that simulator existed. The MK2 simulator allowed full "shaft" insertion, a sensation of resistance during looping, and audio tracks to simulate patient "complaints" (Figure 1.8). The computer allowed for a database and record

keeping. Still, the simulator was felt to be crude and somewhat unrealistic.

In 1992, Leung and Chung developed a static model and described its use in teaching ERCP [21]. Unfortunately, the utility of each of these models has been limited by their inability to truly simulate realistic conditions. To date, while these static learning devices can be useful in instruction and learning of appropriate manipulation of the endoscope within the bowel lumen, they offer little in the way of simulated pathology. The lack of motility, the "feel" of actual compliant tissue, and the inability to practice

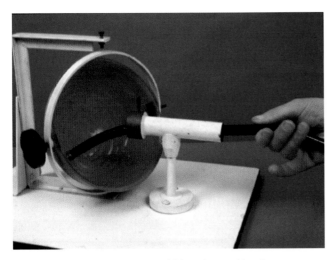

Figure 1.5 Electronic targeting model (1975): Tested hand–eye coordination. (Courtesy: Dr. Christopher Williams.)

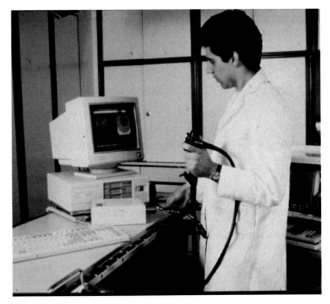

Figure 1.7 Imperial College/St Mark's simulator (1980): Limited shaft insertion, but feasibility of simulator demonstrated. (Courtesy: Dr. Christopher Williams.)

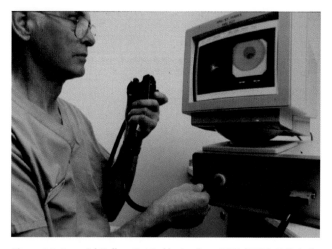

Figure 1.8 Imperial College/St Mark's simulator MK2 (1985): Full shaft insertion and audible "complaints." (Courtesy: Dr. Christopher Williams.)

therapeutic maneuvers have largely limited the use of static models to introductory training.

Perhaps the most comprehensive application of static models in endoscopic teaching was described by Lucero et al. in 1995 [22]. This group designed a psychomotor training program called SimPrac-EDF y VEE (simulator for the practice of fiberoptic digestive endoscopy and electronic video endoscopy). Moreover, they described a series of courses in which they included static models and superimposed painted pictures to recreate frequently seen endoscopic abnormalities. These courses featured didactic lessons, slides, tapes, and supervised hands-on training on models. In addition to the Lucero model, those of Classen and Heinkel were also used. A specific Billroth II model was designed to demonstrate the unique features of this altered anatomy. Participants were offered sessions with increasingly challenging manual and cognitive tasks; faculty at the course assessed objective skills of the participants [22].

In Lucero's courses, 8–25 individuals were included in each particular workshop, and trainees had a mean duration of hands-on practice of 28 hours. In all, 422 trainees in over 22 such courses were described, and the authors noted that 95% of trainees demonstrated an "acceptable level of skill" by the end of the training [22]. However, the authors failed to describe other details of the possible benefits of such training. Such courses would appear to be difficult logistically to conduct and hugely labor intensive. Perhaps the most important contribution of this work was the concept of intergrating various hands-on training tools into a comprehensive training program that combined didactic lesions, cognitive training, and specific hands-on exercise geared to develop particular skill sets. Lucero's use of a patterned lesson plan integrated into multimodality workshops using expert faculty, a blend of manual training and cognitive skills, and immediate feedback and evaluation served as a model for subsequent efforts using more realistic and sophisticated simulators. As such, it remains an important example for future endeavors in endoscopic training.

Ex vivo artificial tissue models: the "Phantom" Tübingen models

A further advance in endoscopic simulation was developed by Grund et al. at the University of Tübingen in Germany [23]. In this "Interphant" or "Phantom" model, artificial electrically conductive tissue called Artitex is used to fashion abnormalities such as polyps and strictures and incorporate this into static models. These "pathologies" are in place of the painted-on abnormalities used in some of the pure static models mentioned above. Grund's "Artitex" abnormalities are sewn directly into a three-dimensional latex anatomical model (Figure 1.9a). While these models generally lack a realistic representation of bowel wall compliance and motility, the integrated pathology appears realistic and allows practice in electrosurgical techniques.

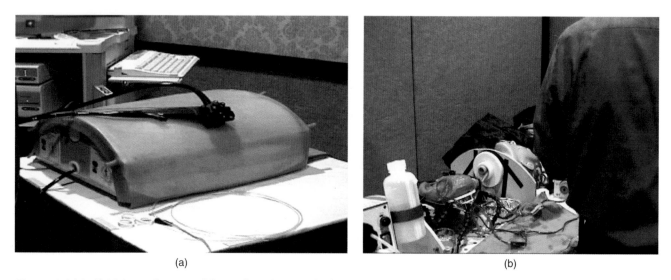

(a)   (b)

Figure 1.9 (a) Artificial tissue colonoscopy "Phantom" simulator, U. of Tübingen. (b) Combined artificial tissue "Phantom" upper GI simulator with integrated chicken heart tissue papilla for ERCP simulation.

In order to simulate the resistance to endoscope passage in an actual procedure, this colon model uses a semiflexible series of coils. In addition, to allow for a still wider possibility of simulated techniques, Grund's model can incorporate real animal tissue into the existing framework. For example, using a chicken heart, they can fashion an ampulla of Vater replete with separate pancreatic and biliary orifices and insert this into their upper endoscopy simulator (Figure 1.9b). The advantage of using this type of system is that several "polyp-laden" colons and "chicken-heart papillae" can be prepared in advance and quickly inserted into the chassis of the model during a training session, after the initially prepared material has been depleted.

The Tübingen simulators made possible the teaching of polypectomy and provided an excellent means of teaching therapeutic procedures such as argon plasma coagulation and simple therapeutic ERCP. In particular, the orientation of the man-made papilla more closely resembled that of humans than the porcine papilla found in the Erlangen models described below. Pancreatic cannulation and endotherapy was possible, in contrast to the porcine tissue models in which the pancreatic orifice was not readily accessible. However, procedures that required submucosal injection were still not feasible.

While this model represented a technological advance over prior static models and added many new capabilities, there remained several limitations that hindered its more widespread use in training. The main drawbacks were that the pathology remained hand-prepared and that the models were not mass-produced. Therefore, the "Phantoms" have not been readily available and have required the presence of the Tübingen team if the device was to be used at a training course. The trade-off for increased realism and the ability to start practicing therapeutic manipulations were significant increases in the logistical and cost obstacles to widespread use. Furthermore, models combining the real tissue abnormalities of the Tübingen model with the more accessible ex vivo animal tissue simulators described below now exist.

Ex vivo animal tissue simulators: Erlanger and EASIE models

In 1996, Hochberger and Neuman created an innovative simulator using pig organs obtained from a slaughterhouse and fastened to a plastic platform [24,25]. In order to create a model that would allow training and practice in therapeutic techniques, Hochberger then created a highly realistic simulation of pulsatile arterial bleeding (Figures 1.10a,b). This was accomplished by inserting tubes through the stomach, and sewing real arteries attached to a roller pump capable of pulsatile perfusion with a cherry-colored saline solution. Following this, Hochberger developed representations of other pathologies for this model, including polyps, varices, and strictures [26,27].

Currently, there are two basic model types based on these principles. The original Erlanger model features pig organs inserted into a dummy mannequin. This model has been used in the simulation of various laparoscopic surgical procedures [28]. Hochberger then created the compact-EASIE model, a smaller portable, lightweight version using a tabletop platform. There are now several commercially available versions of this type of simulator in which only the organs needed for endoscopy simulation are secured to the platform plastic tray (Figures 1.10a,b). For example, only the esophagus to the duodenal bulb may be needed for a specific training session, but the model has the flexibility to allow the liver and hepatobiliary tree for an ERCP simulation involving fluoroscopy. Multiple therapeutic procedures may be demonstrated, taught, and evaluated on both of these animal tissue-based simulators. With the advent of portable, compact tabletop *ex vivo* models that can easily be shipped to a location along with pre-prepared frozen organ packages, some of the obstacles to simulator availability have diminished.

While the most common application of the Hochberger model has been for hemostasis training, this group has conducted a number of training courses using the EASIE model in other areas, including EMR, stricture management, vital staining,

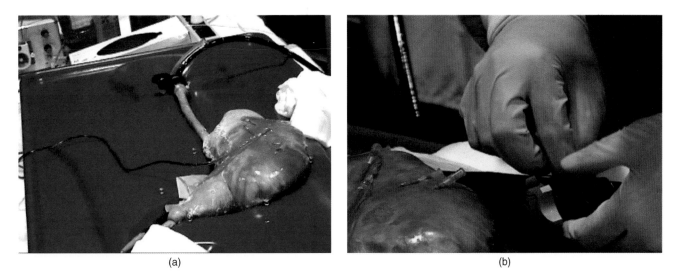

(a)   (b)

Figure 1.10 (a) Compact-EASIE porcine model hemostasis simulator. (b) Close-up view of porcine stomach with arteries sutured in attached to catheters for hook-up to tubing connecting vessels to pump. The trainee puts together a band ligation device for varices treatment simulation.

polypectomy, and ERCP [27,29–31]. A wide range of techniques can be demonstrated, including basic biliary cannulation, plastic stent insertion, choledochoscopy, laser lithotripsy, and placement of bilateral hilar metal stents (Video 1.2). EASIE training has been shown to significantly improve technical skill in endoscopic hemostasis in gastroenterology trainees as compared to clinical endoscopy training alone [32]. As will be discussed in detail in other chapters in this book, further adaptations of the *ex vivo* simulator have extended the use of this modality for training in colonoscopy, balloon-assisted small bowel endoscopy, improved simulation of bile duct and pancreatic duct manipulation, EUS with FNA, and even NOTES® [33–36].

Just as in the Lucero et al. experience described above, training sessions using the Erlanger or EASIE models are labor-intensive, with high faculty-to-trainee ratios. Moreover, the advance work to organize and staff workshops using this technology is extensive. Since the compact EASIE is relatively portable, its use may allow easier access to animal simulator training at local sites, but this is counterbalanced by the need to have the required expertise to prepare the animal tissues and "load" the models. For this training technique to be applied widely, many expert teachers will still need to be trained; the feasibility of 1 day "train-the trainer" courses has now been demonstrated [37].

On the other hand, like the static models before it, the EASIE model allows trainees to perform multiple repetitions of the same technique. The use of real tissue and the capability of performing advanced therapeutic procedures make this an attractive simulator for practitioners hoping to learn new techniques and for advanced fellows to practice and improve their skills, as well as to acquire new abilities [38].

By devising a way to allow realistic simulation of diagnostic and therapeutic techniques using a model that is portable, Hochberger set in motion a rapid expansion in the use of hands-on training for GI fellows in the United States and Europe. Workshops at courses such as the annual NYSGE course and at national and regional endoscopy meetings proliferated. Around 2000, under the leadership of Christopher Gostout, the ASGE launched a major initiative to create opportunities for *ex vivo* model training in a central freestanding location. This effort culminated in the creation of the Integrated Technology and Training (ITT) center of the ASGE in Oak Brook, Illinois, and the development of standardized first year fellows' course curriculum, integrating a day of intensive hands-on work in the *ex vivo* laboratory with interactive didactic lectures. The ongoing ASGE and industry support for these courses has led to over 300 fellows each year since 2005 attending the ITT workshop in the summer of their first year of fellowship. Through this effort, *ex vivo* hands-on training to some degree has become part of the standard endoscopy training for US GI fellows. Efforts to extend such opportunities for advanced endoscopy trainees and to individuals in practice have begun, but so far to a more limited extent. Creative solutions to expanding such opportunities are addressed in detail in a later chapter in this book.

Just as important as his role in the development and popularization of the *ex vivo* model, Hochberger made several other key contributions to the evolution of endoscopy training. Expanding

on the course concept of Lucero, he embedded the simulator work into rigorous training programs, which deconstructed instruction according to specific targeted skill sets. Regardless of the endoscopic procedure being taught, each learning station was assigned separate specific learning objectives. Manual hand–eye skills were taught using specially designed coordination exercises. Communication skills between endoscopist and assistant were emphasized. Assessment of skills was broken down by specific procedure steps to ensure that all details received specific attention and instruction. The structure of the workshops he designed in collaboration with his German colleagues and his colleagues from the NYSGE incorporated expert demonstration of proper technique, repetitive practice with sufficient endoscope time per trainee per skill station to do so, self-assessment, and instructor feedback. These components have remained the essential backbone of all subsequent *ex vivo* model-based training. In addition, Hochberger first promoted the concept of "team training", focusing on the importance of coordinating training among the endoscopist and his staff.

Live animal courses

Both research and training courses have employed endoscopy performed on live anesthetized pigs and dogs [38–41]. Using live animals provides the best possible tactile "feel" of real tissue and endoscope movements with conditions most closely resembling those that occur during human endoscopy. Specifically, this includes the presence of luminal fluid, motility, and the ability to cause real bleeding and perforation (Video 1.3). Such courses have been conducted to teach therapeutic techniques, most notably ERCP and EUS [40]. At present, live animal courses are the only means of nonhuman simulation of sphincter of Oddi manometry [41].

Although clearly advantageous for the above reasons, live animal courses also present some substantial drawbacks. Among these are that animals are very expensive to maintain and there are significant ethical considerations in using animals for training. These ethical considerations are magnified by the fact that *ex vivo* alternatives now exist for teaching most techniques and do not require sacrificing any animals solely for this purpose. In contrast to the multiple uses possible on other simulator types, once certain procedures, such as sphincterotomy, are performed, it is difficult or impossible for others to practice the same techniques on the same animal.

For these and other reasons, training on live animals, while potentially more realistic than on inanimate simulators, appears now to be on the wane in the evolution of endoscopic training techniques. It appears likely that live animal courses will be limited to advanced procedures such as sphincter of Oddi manometry, for which no comparable inanimate model exists, and advanced training in ESD and NOTES®. For the latter techniques, many of the skill sets would still be best taught in inanimate tissue models, saving the live animal work for later training in which real physiological conditions and the potential for complication management is required. Live animal endoscopy laboratories remain well suited for clinical investigation. Finally, testing of new accessories and development of new techniques on live animals will likely continue, but much of the groundwork for these tests will have been already completed on inanimate simulators.

Computer simulation

Parallel to the introduction and adoption of *ex vivo* animal tissue models has been the development of increasingly sophisticated computer simulators. The technology has evolved to incorporate two main features, the ability to vary the pathology encountered and refinements of forced feedback or "haptics" to improve the realism of the earlier static models.

A number of investigators have pioneered efforts to produce computer models, which can allow realistic experience handling the endoscope, and are also able to incorporate broad exposure to pathologic images [20,42–52]. Because so many diverse images can be stored, computer simulation offers the best opportunity to expose trainees to a wide range of pathology. Computer-based learning can take place either independently or as part of larger training courses, and progressive tutorials of increasing difficulty can be constructed. Unlimited repetition and drilling in specific infrequently encountered procedures is possible. Moreover, progress during training can be recorded and opportunities for feedback exist.

Computer simulators typically utilize a "real" endoscope passed into a dummy mannequin. Tactile feedback capability, generated by sensors on the endoscope tip, is a key feature. The experience is enhanced by incorporation of real video images. Moreover, insufflation, suction, and bowel wall motility can be reproduced. An ASGE technology assessment statement on simulators describes in detail the innovative technological developments in this field [42]. The images on the display can be derived from interactive video stored on the computer or external storage devices, computer-generated images, or a combination of both.

Two commercially available computer simulators exist for EGD, colonoscopy, bronchoscopy, EUS and ERCP, and a colonoscopy-specific simulator is also in development (Video 1.4).

The AccuTouch® endoscopy simulator (Immersion Medical) system (Figure 1.11) (http://www.immersion.com/products/medical/endoscopy.html) allows training in a number of procedures, including flexible sigmoidoscopy and colonoscopy, as well as bronchoscopy. It is possible to practice mucosal biopsy on this model. The simulator provides direct performance feedback to the trainee. A number of validation studies have been conducted using this simulator [52–55], which will be covered in detail in subsequent chapters in this book.

The GI Mentor II (Simbionix) (Figure 1.12) (http://www.simbionix.com/GI_Mentor.html) offers several diagnostic and therapeutic modules [48]. Upper and lower endoscopy and ERCP are all performed on the same mannequin using a special endoscope for each procedure type. An accessory channel allows the endoscopist to perform a variety of therapeutic techniques, including biopsy, polypectomy, sclerotherapy, and electrocoagulation to control active bleeding, ERCP cannulation, and sphincterotomy. This simulator also includes some manual dexterity training exercises ideal for beginners to develop skills controlling the endoscope dials and using torque. The logical descendent of the Lucero model and progressive training program, the simulator incorpo-

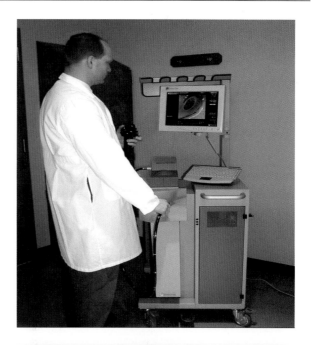

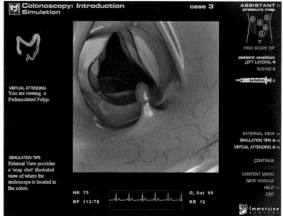

Figure 1.11 Immersion AccuTouch® colonoscopy simulator.

rates a series of cases of varying pathology and technical difficulty. Instructors may delineate specific training programs. Trainees can get immediate feedback during and after completing each simulated procedure. In fact, the computer will even generate an expression of pain for overinsufflation or excessive looping of the instrument. Performance is recorded, including numbers and types of errors made. The instructor can review the progress of each trainee and the written procedure reports to determine whether abnormalities were correctly detected and identified; feedback messages may be sent back to the trainee.

The GI Mentor II computer simulator has been incorporated into a number of European endoscopy courses, most notably in Scandinavia [56–58]. Respondents to questionnaires have expressed great satisfaction with the limited experience on the GI Mentor II simulator. As with the AccuTouch® simulator, a number of objective validation studies have been carried out for

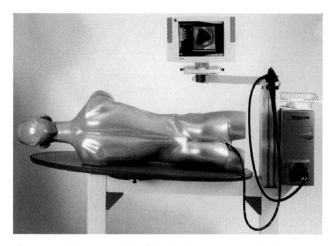

Figure 1.12 GI Mentor II (Simbionix) colonoscopy virtual reality simulator.

the GI Mentor II, and these data are presented in detail elsewhere in this book.

The Olympus colonoscopy simulator is a colonoscopy-specific simulator based on advanced mathematical models and is presently completing development and undergoing rigorous validation evaluation [59,60]. Among its features, this model attempts to better simulate more difficult colonoscope passage and perhaps allows for an accurate enough skills assessment on the model to predict performance on actual procedures. To date, none of the computer simulators have been able to achieve this degree of realism.

If computer simulators are to have a role in credentialing in addition to training, they must be able to distinguish between a novice and an accomplished endoscopist. A study from the Mayo Clinic demonstrated that performance parameters on the simulator vary according to real colonoscopy experience [55]. To date, however, no investigator has shown that a particular performance level measured on a computer or any other simulator is predictive of competent performance on subsequent real endoscopy.

At present, computer simulators appear to have much to offer trainees in terms of showing diverse pathology and teaching beginners hand–eye coordination and endoscope handling. Unique aspects of this type of training are simulation of contractions, feedback on comfort, opportunity for self-instruction without constant expert supervision, quantification of skills, and offsite skills assessment by instructors. Current available models appear less useful for more experienced endoscopists, although capabilities are expanding rapidly. At present, the therapeutic modules for the GI Mentor II simulator are best suited for introductory orientation only to polypectomy, hemostasis, and ERCP.

Computerized technology offers the potential to incorporate didactic lessons, specific questions for the endoscopist concerning accessory setup and generator settings, and opportunities for self-assessment quizzes to complement the hands-on technical experience. However, to date, such potential advances have not yet been incorporated into the existing simulators.

The major obstacle to expanded use of these simulators remains the cost and logistics of making them accessible to trainees. At costs ranging from $50,000 to $70,000, most individual departments cannot afford to purchase computer simulators.

The future of simulators in endoscopy training

Ongoing evolution of endoscopic training

The past two decades have been characterized by rapid expansion of the training modalities at our disposal and the general acceptance of their use. Much work remains to clarify the optimal way to integrate these tools into standard training, training in advanced procedures, and in the uncharted waters of maintaining skills. What will be the next steps in the evolution of endoscopy simulators? A number of scenarios can be envisioned. Some potential developments are described in Table 1.1. Regardless of exactly how this field evolves in the coming years, it is fairly certain that simulators will play an increasing role in teaching and training in gastrointestinal endoscopy.

Several challenges exist as endoscopic training continues to evolve. To date, the vast capacity to incorporate the trove of stored video and photographic content covering endoscopically encountered pathology and how to manage it has been greatly underutilized. The DAVE project [61] has been a significant advance in allowing for free and easy access to view much of this kind of material (Video 1.5). However, there is still very limited incorporation of this material into Web-based interactive learning opportunities. By taking advantage of broadband transmission and Web-based learning, cognitive training might undergo as great a transformation in the coming years as *ex vivo* models have provided for technical skills development.

A second major area for progress is in the area of creation and validation of simulator-based skills assessments that predict performance level and competency on actual procedures. Simulator investigators have long realized that a key milestone would be the development of reliable simulator-based assessments of competency.

A third area that will need to be addressed in coming years is the further integration of some of these new teaching modalities into local programs. For example, the ideal follow-up of the national first year's fellows hands-on training experience at the ITT would be a follow-up hands-on workshop at various intervals run and funded locally with support of local physicians and industry. Funding and logistic issues need to be addressed, but adoption will first require increased acknowledgment by local program directors of the importance of such activities. Expansion of hands-on *ex vivo* simulator training at the local level will also require a considerable effort to train a broader group of trainers on how best to utilize these simulators to teach endoscopy [62].

One other area of real promise is the growing role of simulators and specific training program development in the process of the introduction of new endoscopic technology and techniques. On the part of industry, this begins with the use of models to test early devices and procedures prior to more costly animal studies. Next is the growing recognition that innovative techniques require

Table 1.1 Potential next generation applications of endoscopy simulators.

1. Computer simulators may be used to test innate hand–eye coordination skills of fellowship applicants.
2. More training programs may offer static mannequins to allow novices to practice rudimentary maneuvers with controls on endoscopes and for manual dexterity training prior to handling endoscopes on real patients.
3. GI training programs with sufficient resources may provide access to hospital-based virtual reality simulators, designed to offer training in many GI and non-GI procedures. Hospitals can purchase these for training and credentialing of practitioners in many fields and training of technical assistants for these procedures. Multiuse simulators could justify the cost.
4. The large capital outlay for these simulators could be obviated by regional Web-based virtual reality servers. These might allow hospitals and training programs to subscribe and then "perform" specific procedures on "dummy" terminals at remote sites via cloud computing without purchasing the entire computer and software packages.
5. Interactive quizzes of pathology recognition and correct management decisions based on findings may be integrated into future simulator training along with the hands-on practice of technical skills. Alternatively, an Internet-based tutorial could serve as an introduction to pathology.
6. Simulators and simulator-based workshops might allow skill assessments, which would indicate when trainees were ready to proceed to perform supervised real cases and ultimately independent endoscopic procedures.
7. With validated simulator-based skills assessment, it is conceivable that no procedures would be allowed on human subjects until simulated training has occurred and satisfactory performance measured.
8. Therapeutic workshops using *ex vivo* animal models will proliferate further and become increasingly available at multiple regional locations for trainees and practicing gastroenterologists hoping to learn new skills or polish old ones.
9. GI trainees will be required to attend one such workshop during the first year of fellowship and recommended to attend another early in the third year.
10. A cadre of endoscopy instructors could be trained to run such workshops, including individuals from every region of the country.
11. Possibly, practicing endoscopists will be required in the future to attend such workshops at defined intervals, possibly every 5 years, to maintain privileges for therapeutic endoscopy.

specific training programs to ensure both proper execution of the new procedures and acceptance of the innovation by practitioners. Busy clinicians will not adopt new skills unless an efficient and preferably validated training program is available to ensure that they can develop the proficiency to safely and effectively do the procedure. In contrast to the past when efforts to determine the best ways to train for techniques often came long after the procedure was adopted, in the future, there will be increasing pressure to address training upfront. One hopes that with this additional attention to training in parallel with technology development will come increasing avenues of support for simulator-based training in general. This may be of particular importance as a partial solution to the problem of creating more opportunities for practicing endoscopists who desire to and will need to learn new techniques. The innovators will need to support those they hope will adopt the innovation; simulators are likely to facilitate this growing interdependence.

Conclusion

Training in endoscopy began with a pioneering spirit of self-taught innovators and quickly transitioned to a traditional apprenticeship model of learning during one-on-one proctored clinical experiences. Over the last 10 years, the advent of simulator-based teaching tools and a heightened scrutiny of the optimal methods, components, and endpoints of training have sparked a transformation in the way endoscopy is taught.

On the technology of training, there are now an array of realistic simulators that in sum allow for an excellent training experience in most of the therapeutic procedures comprising current endoscopic practice. There is growing evidence that training using these models is of benefit. These hands-on complementary methods are certainly popular, and thanks to the vision of the leadership of endoscopic societies and the support of the industry, opportunities to use them are increasingly available. The area of simulator-based skills assessment remains a relatively undeveloped field, awaiting increased realism, and the development and validation of proper tests. Still, the combination of static models, *ex vivo* artificial models, *ex vivo* animal models, and computer simulators, collectively represent a substantial and powerful tool for education and training in gastrointestinal endoscopy. It is easy to see the day when there will be ready availability of hands-on training via simulators beyond the gastroenterology fellowship setting. Paralleling the progression of technology and the continuous introduction of new devices and procedures will be a compelling need for hands-on experience on simulators for all such new tools and techniques.

Parallel to this transformation in the methods of training have been key new concepts about how this process ought to occur. Realizing that simulator work is generally costly and labor intensive, attention is being paid to learn how to best time simulator experience during training; for example, work with static models might be more cost-effective for novices than hands-on *ex vivo* workshops. The benefit from such workshops is intuitively greater for trainees who already have attained some basic skills. The growing experience with simulator-based training has taught the value of concepts such as team training of assistants along with the endoscopists, deconstructing complex procedures into their component skills, and increasing emphasis on self-assessment and feedback within the training process.

At the same time, the growing emphasis on maximizing quality in endoscopy has also affected guidelines and attitudes about endoscopic training. From the early days of endoscopy, thought leaders have aimed to train new endoscopists who were competent to perform procedures independently. But recently, the question they have asked has changed from "How many procedures are required for a trainee to become competent?" to "What are the objective measures of competency for a particular procedure and has a trainee reached that level of skill?" There is increasing recognition of the importance of objective measurement of success both during training and beyond. The process of keeping track of outcomes during training has the potential not only to ensure that benchmark end points of training are attained before endoscopists perform procedures independently on patients but also to facilitate that training process itself, by virtue of the feedback this information provides.

Videos

Video 1.1 The EASIE hemostasis *ex vivo* training workshop
Video 1.2 Tips for teaching using *ex vivo* models
Video 1.3 Use of simulator to teach what not to do: improper submucosal lift in EMR leads to perforation on purpose
Video 1.4 Virtual reality colonoscopy simulator training
Video 1.5 A tour of the DAVE project: a free versatile multimedia resource for endoscopy education

References

1 Borland JL: Retraining in endoscopy. *Gastrointest Endosc Clin N Am* 1995;**5**:363–372.

2 American Society for Gastrointestinal Endoscopy: Guidelines for clinical application. Statement on role of short courses in endoscopic training. *Gastrointest Endosc* 1999;**50**:913–914.

3 Modlin IM (ed): *A Brief History of Endoscopy.* Milan, Italy: MultiMed, 2000.

4 American Society for Gastrointestinal Endoscopy: Principles of training in gastrointestinal endoscopy. *Gastrointest Endosc* 1999;**49**:845–850.

5 Friedman LS, Brandt LJ, Elta GH, et al.: Report of the Multisociety Task Force on GI Training. *Gastrointest Endosc* 2009;**70**:823–827.

6 Freeman ML: Training and competence in gastrointestinal endoscopy. *Rev Gastroenterol Disord* 2001;**1**:73–86.

7 Sivak MV: The art of endoscopic instruction. *Gastrointest Endosc Clin N Am* 1995;**5**:299–310.

8 Church JN: Learning colonoscopy: the need for patience (patients). *Am J Gastroenterol* 1993;**88**:1569.

9 Katz PO: Providing feedback. *Gastrointest Endosc Clin N Am* 1995;**5**:347–355.

10 Hawes R, Lehman GA, Hast J, et al.: Training resident physicians in fiberoptic sigmoidoscopy. How many supervised examinations are required to achieve competence? *Am J Med* 1986;**80**:465–470.

11 Marshall JB: Technical proficiency of trainees performing colonoscopy: a learning curve. *Gastrointest Endosc* 1995;**42**:287–291.

12 American Society for Gastrointestinal Endoscopy: Guidelines for advanced endoscopic training. *Gastrointest Endosc* 2001;**53**:846–848.

13 Cass OW, Freeman ML, Cohen J, et al.: Acquisition of competency in endoscopic skills (ACES) during training: a multicenter study [Abstract]. *Gastrointest Endosc* 1996;**43**:308.

14 Cass OW, Freeman ML, Peine CJ, et al.: Objective evaluation of endoscopy skills during training. *Ann Intern Med* 1993;**118**:40–44.

15 American Society for Gastrointestinal Endoscopy: Guidelines for credentialing and granting privileges for gastrointestinal endoscopy. *Gastrointest Endosc* 2002;**55**:780–783.

16 Cohen J: Training and credentialing in gastrointestinal endoscopy. In: Cotton PB, Sung J (eds), *Advanced Endoscopy: Endoscopy Practice and Safety.* Oxford, UK: Blackwell Publishing, 2008.

17 Schindler R: *Gastroscopy: The Endoscopic Study of Gastric Pathology.* Chicago: University of Chicago Press, 1937:74–75.

18 Heinkel VK, Kimmig JM: Megenphantome zur ausbiling in der gastrokamera-magenuntersuchung. *Z Gastroenterol* 1971;**9**:331.

19 Classen M, Ruppin H: Practical training using a new gastrointestinal phantom. *Endoscopy* 1974;**6**:127–131.

20 Williams CB, Saunders BP, Bladen JS: Development of colonoscopy teaching simulation. *Endoscopy* 2000;**32**:901–905.

21 Leung JW, Chung RS: Training in ERCP [Letter]. *Gastrointest Endosc* 1992;**38**:517.

22 Lucero RS, Zarate JO, Espinella F, et al.: Introducing digestive endoscopy with the "SimPrac-EDF y VEE" simulator, other organ models and mannequins: teaching experience in 21 courses attended by 422 physicians. *Endoscopy* 1995;**27**:93–100.

23 Grund KE, Bräutigam D, Zindel C, et al.: Interventionsfähiges Tübinger Simulationsmodell INTERPHANT für die flexible Endoskopie. *Endoskopie heute* 1998;**11**:134.

24 Hochberger J, Neumann M, Hohenberger W, Hahn EG: Neues Bio-Trainingsmodell für die operative flexible Endoskopie. *Endoskopie heute* 1997;**1**:117–118.

25 Hochberger J, Neumann M, Hohenberger W, Hahn EG: Neuer Endoskopie-Trainer für die therapeutische flexible Endoskopie. *Z Gastroenterol* 1997;**35**:722–723.

26 Hochberger J, Maiss J, Hahn EG: The Erlangen EASIE model for a close-to-reality team-training of doctors and nurses in interventional endoscopy. In: Bhutani MS, Tandon RK (eds), *Advances in Gastrointestinal Endoscopy.* New Delhi: Jaypee Brothers Medical Publishers (P) Ltd, 2001.

27 Hochberger J, Maiss J, Magdeburg B, Cohen J, Hahn EG: Training simulators and education in gastrointestinal endoscopy: current status and perspectives in 2001. *Endoscopy* 2001;**33**:541–549.

28 Neumann M, Mayer G, Ell C, et al.: The Erlangen Endo-Trainer: life-like simulation for diagnostic and interventional endoscopic retrograde cholangiography. *Endoscopy* 2000;**32**(11):906–910.

29 Hochberger J, Maiss J, Nägel A, Tex S, Hahn EG: Polypectomy/vital endoscopic staining/mucosectomy—a new structured team-training in a close-to-reality endoscopy simulator (EASIE). *Endoscopy* 2000;**32**(Suppl 1):E23.

30 Hochberger J, Maiss J, Neumann M, Hildebrand V, Bayer J, Hahn EG: EASIE-team-training in endoscopic hemostasis—acceptance of a systematic training in interventional endoscopy by 134 trainees [Abstract]. *Gastrointest Endosc* 1999;**49**:AB143.

31 Hochberger J, Neumann M, Maiss J, Hohenberger W, Hahn EG: EASIE (Erlangen active simulator for interventional endoscopy)–a new bio-simulation model: first experiences gained in training workshops [Abstract]. *Gastrointest Endosc* 1998;**47**:AB116.

32 Hochberger J, Matthes K, Maiss J, Koebnick C, Hahn EG, Cohen J: Training with the compact EASIE biologic endoscopy simulator

significantly improves hemostatic technical skill of gastroenterology fellows: a randomised controlled comparison with clinical endoscopy training alone. *Gastrointest Endosc* 2005;**61**:204–215.

33 Maiss J, Matthes K, Naegel A, et al.: Der coloEASIE-Simulatoro: ein neues Trainingsmodell für die interventionelle Kolo-und REktoskopie [German]. The colo EASIE-Simulator—a new training model for interventional colonoscopy and rectoscopy. *Endoskopie Heute* 2005;**18**:190–193.

34 Sedlack RE, Baron TH, Downing SM, Schwartz AJ: Validation of a colonoscopy simulation model for skills assessment. *Am J Gastroenterol* 2007;**102**:64–74.

35 Matthes K, Cohen J: The Neo-Papilla: a new modification of porcine *ex vivo* simulators for ERCP training (with videos). *Gastrointest Endosc* 2006;**64**:570–576.

36 Raizner A, Matthes K, Goodman AJ: Evaluation of a new endoscopic ultrasound (EUS) simulator (EASIE-R simulator) for teaching basic and advanced EUS. *Gastrointest Endosc* 2010;**71**:AB296.

37 Matthes K, Cohen J, Kochman ML: Efficacy and costs of a one-day hands-on EASIE endoscopy simulator train-the-trainer workshop. *Gastrointest Endosc* 2005;**62**:921–927.

38 Gholson CF, Provenza JM, Silver RC, Bacon BR: Endoscopic retrograde cholaniography in the swine: a new model for endoscopic training and hepatobiliary research. *Gastrointest Endosc* 1990;**36**:600–603.

39 Falkenstein DB, Abrams RM, Kessler RE, Jones B, Johnson G, Zimmon DS: Endoscopic retrograde cholangiopancreatography in the dog: a model for training and research. *Gastrointest Endosc* 1974;**21**:25–26.

40 Noar MD: An established porcine model for animate training in diagnostic and therapeutic ERCP. *Endoscopy* 1995;**27**:77–80.

41 Pasricha PJ, Tietjen TG, Kalloo AN: Biliary manometry in swine: a unique endoscopic model. *Endoscopy* 1995;**27**:70–72.

42 American Society for Gastrointestinal Endoscopy: Technology status evaluation report. Endoscopy simulators. *Gastrointest Endosc* 1999;**50**:935–937.

43 Williams CB, Baillie J, Gillies DF, Borislow D, Cotton PB. Teaching gastrointestinal endoscopy by computer simulation: a prototype for colonoscopy and ERCP. *Gastrointest Endosc* 1990;**36**:49–54.

44 Noar MD: Robotics interactive endoscopy simulation of ERCP/sphincterotomy and EGD. *Endoscopy* 1992;**24**(Suppl 2):539–541.

45 Noar MD: The next generation of endoscopy simulation: minimally invasive surgical skills simulation *Endoscopy* 1995;**27**:81–85.

46 Noar MD, Soehendra N: Endoscopy simulation training devices. *Endoscopy* 1992;**24**:159–166.

47 Beer-Gabel M, Delmontte S, Muntlak L: Computer-assisted training in endoscopy (CATE): from a simulator to a learning station. *Endoscopy* 1992;**24**(Suppl 2):534–538.

48 Bar-Meir S: A new endoscopic simulator. *Endoscopy* 2000;**32**(11):898–900.

49 Baillie J, Jowell P: ERCP training in the 1990s. Time for new ideas. *Gastrointest Endosc Clin N Am* 1994;**4**(2):409–421.

50 Gessner CE, Jowell PS, Baillie J: Novel methods for endoscopic training. *Gastrointest Endosc Clin N Am* 1995;**5**:323–336.

51 Bar-Meir S: Endoscopy simulators: the state of the art, 2000. *Gastrointest Endosc* 2000;**52**:201–203.

52 Gerson LB, Van Dam J: The future of simulators in GI endoscopy: an unlikely possibility or a virtual reality? [Editorial]. *Gastrointest Endosc* 2002;**55**:608–611.

53 Gerson LB, Van Dam J: A randomized controlled trial comparing an endoscopic simulator to traditional bedside teaching for training in flexible sigmoidoscopy [Abstract]. *Gastrointest Endosc* 2002;**55**:AB78.

54 Tuggy ML: Virtual reality flexible sigmoidoscopy simulator training: impact on resident performance. *J Am Board Fam Pract* 1998;**11**:426–433.

55 Sedlack RE, Kolars JC: Validation of computer-based endoscopy simulators in training [Abstract]. *Gastrointest Endosc* 2002;**55**:AB77.

56 Aabakken L, Adamsen S, Kruse A: Performance of a colonoscopy simulator: experience from a hands-on endoscopy course. *Endoscopy* 2000;**32**(11):911–913.

57 Adamsen S: Simulators and gastrointestinal endoscopy training. *Endoscopy* 2000;**32**:895–897.

58 Ferlitsch A, Glauninger P, Gupper A, et al.: Virtual endoscopy simulation for training of gastrointestinal endoscopy [Abstract]. *Gastrointest Endosc* 2001;**53**:AB78.

59 Haycock A, Koch AD, Familiari P, et al.: Training and transfer of colonoscopy skills: a multinational, randomized, blinded, controlled trial of simulator versus bedside training. *Gastrointest Endosc* 2010;**71**(2):298–307.

60 Williams CB, Thomson-Gibson S: Rational colonoscopy, realistic simulation, and accelerated teaching. *Gastrointest Endosc Clin N Am* 2006;**16**:457–470.

61 DAVE project Web site. Available: www.daveproject.org (accessed January 7, 2010).

62 Matthes K, Cohen J, Kochman ML, Cerulli MA, Vora KC, Hochberger J.: Efficacy and costs of a one-day hands-on EASIE endoscopy simulator train-the-trainer workshop. *Gastrointest Endosc* 2005;**62**:921–927.

2

How Endoscopy is Learned: Deconstructing Skill Sets

Gerald M. Fried[1,2,3] & Kevin A. Waschke[1,2]

[1] McGill University, Montreal, QC, Canada
[2] McGill University Health Centre, Montreal, QC, Canada
[3] Montreal General Hospital, Montreal, QC, Canada

Introduction

Proficient performance of flexible gastrointestinal endoscopy requires a combination of technical and cognitive skills. Understandably, comprehensive training in endoscopy requires attention to each of these components. Unfortunately, the medical literature is lacking in evidence supporting the differential effects of specific training modalities. Educational theories, however, suggest that each of these components is best learned using different approaches. With respect to the technical component, literature from a variety of areas has demonstrated that "deconstructing" a procedural skill into smaller, easy-to-master tasks can facilitate teaching and learning. This chapter will focus on providing a general framework for the specific skills required to train individuals in flexible endoscopy. By deconstructing the common gastrointestinal endoscopic procedures in this manner, both trainer and trainee can approach the acquisition, practice, and evaluation of endoscopic skill in a structured manner. Effective training in endoscopy requires more than a simple "how-to" of procedures, as will be illustrated in the remainder of this volume. For this reason, we will also not only discuss the deconstruction of an endoscopic skill set, but at the same time illustrate several key components of a second skill set, that of endoscopic training, which we consider to be distinct and different from endoscopic skill.

Using an approach that involves deconstructing the skills required to perform endoscopy has several advantages for both the trainer and the trainee. The first advantage is that the deconstruction of a task makes both the trainer and the trainee consciously aware of both the specific steps to be learned and their relationship to the overall framework. The importance of this step should not be underestimated, as training in endoscopy requires expertise in training, not only in performance of the procedure. A common observation in both medicine as well as other areas is that expertise in an area does not automatically convey expertise in the teaching of that area. Anyone who has attempted to learn a sport such as golf can attest to the importance of good teaching and good teachers in the learning of complex motor skills.

Sports, music, and avionics are good examples of fields in which training has progressed to include coaching, feedback, training aids, the use of simulators, and other approaches to ensure that efficient and effective learning occurs. There is no doubt that readers of this text can recall excellent endoscopists who simply cannot describe how they performed specific complex acts in a manner that permitted the learner to learn from them. As such, we cannot assume that expert endoscopists are all automatically expert trainers simply by virtue of their endoscopic skill set. The explanation for this apparent paradox can be illustrated by Peyton's stages of learning [1]. A learner is conceptualized as passing through a variety of stages during their development of procedural skill (unconscious incompetence, conscious incompetence, unconscious competence, conscious competence). By the time the endoscopist reaches the unconsciously competent stage, he or she may be highly proficient at endoscopy but, by virtue of the process of skills acquisition, be unable to describe the components of their skill. The very same cognitive process that permits rapid, fluid movement, termed automaticity [2], also prevents the individual from consciously accessing and describing the steps required to perform the task. A sign of unconscious competence is the teacher who, when teaching endoscopy, is required to take the scope from the trainee rather than being able to verbalize what needs to be done. Words fail the instructor because the description of the endoscopic skill is not consciously accessible. Again, a sports analogy is useful here, as a skilled golfer is unlikely to be able to describe or think about all of the steps in a golf swing while they are performing it without it impairing the fluidity of their motion. Explicit explanation of what is to occur and why it is important is a crucial element in skills acquisition, but it does not naturally occur. It is, however, a crucial component in the effective teaching of procedural skills.

This brings us to a second important advantage of deconstructing skill sets, facilitating the generation of specific learning objectives. Learning objectives are a central component in the development of a deliberate approach to training. Ideally, each learning activity involves some element of planning by the endoscopy trainer, even for elements such as practicing a

Successful Training in Gastrointestinal Endoscopy, First Edition. Edited by Jonathan Cohen.
© 2011 Blackwell Publishing Ltd. Published 2011 by Blackwell Publishing Ltd.

previously learned skill. The use of objectives enables a more efficient use of time for teaching, learning, or practice. Even short periods of time can be used to best advantage to attend to a specific learning objective if learning activities are planned appropriately. When feedback is closely tied to performance and aligned with learning objectives, the learning of procedural skills can be markedly enhanced. It is also important to consider motivational aspects, such as encouragement, at this stage. The use of objectives with constructive feedback followed by the correction and optimization of performance forms the basis for deliberate practice with the goal of achieving mastery. This "deliberate practice" is felt to be a determining component of the attainment of expert levels of performance [3] across many areas.

Objectives, along with appropriately timed feedback, also facilitate the learner's reflection upon the learning process. Critical self-reflection [4] is considered in the educational literature to be an important skill for future self-directed learning. Although not reserved exclusively for trainees who are having difficulties, there is no doubt that you have encountered many "difficult" trainees that are unaware of their shortcomings. Providing trainees with a basis upon which to judge their own progress can be a useful tool in such situations, particularly for future occasions when they will no longer be supervised.

Depending on the level of experience of the trainee and the complexity of the endoscopy, having an awareness of the overall breadth of learning objectives can be very useful. In our opinion, it is useful to consider a hierarchy of objectives in teaching that begins with patient safety, progresses to basics of endoscopy, more advanced techniques, and subsequently to cognitive and behavioral aspects. Having a wide variety of teaching scenarios and relevant objectives in mind is particularly useful in situations where unplanned learning opportunities may arise, such as rare occurrences or unusual aspects of endoscopic practice. In some situations, these instructional objectives may be highly specific and involve evaluation using specific criteria, such as withdrawal time, or percentage of mucosa visualized, termed metrics. Metrics can be employed to assess these technical skills, particularly when using simulators, training tasks, or when comparing trainees to a specific standard.

Identification of fundamental endoscopy skills

The terminology used in this chapter is meant to facilitate the reader's deconstruction of endoscopic skill sets and hence the specific terms are less important than the underlying principles they are meant to illustrate. It is hoped that individual trainers will consider the various advantages afforded by deconstructing skill sets in such a manner when designing or adapting their own training programs. Subsequent chapters will cover training in the major endoscopic procedures and in specific techniques using a variety of different perspectives. The reader is encouraged to approach these chapters with their own framework in mind.

In this section, we will discuss the following skills, which we consider to be constant requisites in the technical performance of any form of gastrointestinal endoscopy. It is assumed that prior

to introducing a trainee to the technical components of performing endoscopy that they have already become familiar with the various components of the endoscope, including the function of the air/water and suction buttons, as well as proper holding and handling of the endoscope and other practical aspects such as troubleshooting malfunctioning equipment. Ideally, these basic skills have been introduced to the trainee and practiced in an environment away from the patient until a minimum level of proficiency has been reached.

1 *Introduction of the endoscope:* Comfortable and safe introduction of the scope into the GI tract through an orifice (oropharynx, anus, stoma).

2 *Navigation:* Navigation of a flexible instrument through a tubular conduit until a goal or end-point is reached.

3 *Overcome obstacles:* Strategies to navigate across sphincters, around sharp curves, and through areas of resistance.

4 *Inspection:* Careful and thorough inspection of the mucosal surface

5 *Instrumentation:* Advancing an instrument through an accessory channel to a specific point, while maintaining a stable view of the target and then subsequently performing the desired task.

These skills will be discussed in some detail, including the nuances that affect their learning.

Introduction of the scope

To begin any gastrointestinal procedure, the endoscope must first be inserted into the lumen of the GI tract. Introduction of the endoscope requires a clear understanding of the relevant regional anatomy.

For upper GI endoscopy, this involves direction of the endoscope down the oropharynx into the esophagus. To avoid gagging, retching, and possible laryngospasm, the oropharynx should be appropriately anesthetized with a local anesthetic agent and the endoscope directed away from the vocal cords and into the esophagus. In some cases, intravenous sedation is useful to supplement the topical anesthesia. Appropriate patient positioning and education to avoid efforts at swallowing further add to the smoothness of this phase of the endoscopy. Patients with large anterior osteophytes of the cervical spine may pose particular risks for perforation, as might Zenker's diverticula. Attention to these possibilities is mandatory for safe upper endoscopy.

For lower GI endoscopy, the endoscope needs to be introduced into the lumen, most often through the anus, but under some circumstances, through a stoma. Preceding the introduction of the endoscope with a properly performed digital examination is an essential adjunct to safe and comfortable intubation. This provides the opportunity to lubricate the entry, slowly relax the sphincter, and to evaluate the individual anatomy for direction and for any unexpected pathology or sites of potential obstruction.

Endoscopy through a stoma requires some understanding of stomal varieties. A loop stoma is oriented at right angles to the long axis of the bowel. Imprudent introduction of the scope through the stoma can easily cause perforation through the antimesenteric side of the bowel. This is particularly prone to occur in patients whose bowel has been excluded, resulting in atrophy. End stomas are oriented in line with the long axis of the bowel. Digital examination may disclose angulation or kinks in the intra-abdominal segment of intestine that must be negotiated when introducing the scope.

Methods to evaluate the phase of introduction of the endoscope include rating of patient comfort, time to intubate, the number of attempts to intubate, and any complications related to the endoscope intubation, anesthesia, and sedation.

Navigation

Once the endoscope is successfully introduced, the next goal is advancement of the scope to a specific extent, as indicated by the clinical reason for the endoscopy. For upper GI endoscopy, this is usually down to the 3rd stage of the duodenum; for colonoscopy, it would be to the cecum, terminal ileum, or to an anastomosis, for example. Scope navigation is accomplished by a series of maneuvers that include tip deflection, scope rotation/application of torque, external compression of the abdomen, adjusting the patient position, insufflation and suction of air or fluids, and insertion and withdrawal of the scope.

Control of the tip of the endoscope is necessary when navigating to maintain an adequate luminal view, as well as to assist in advancement of the endoscope. Depending on the type of endoscopy being performed, tip control may be done in different ways by nature of the physical characteristics of the endoscopes. Standard esophagogastroduodenoscopy (hereafter referred to as EGD, or gastroscopy) requires very different maneuvers than ERCP or colonoscopy, for example. In the case of ERCP, the increased endoscope stiffness and oblique viewing angle mandates very different technical skills. Intubation, manipulation of the endoscope tip through the stomach, traversing the pylorus, and positioning in front of the papilla require very different maneuvers and changes in body position than are required for other procedures. It is our preference to train endoscopists to use the left hand to grip the handle of the endoscope and to manipulate the wheels using the thumb of the left hand for all procedures, particularly during colonoscopy. The main advantage of this approach is to reserve the right hand for advancement and withdrawal of the endoscope, and application of torque when necessary. This allows us to focus our trainees' attention upon the sensation of resistance or torque in their right hand. If additional tip deflection is required, small movements of the wheels using the left thumb is typically sufficient. This awareness of changing resistance, possible impending scope movement/stability or response to torque is particularly important when attempting to perform maneuvers such as shortening the endoscope in ERCP, resolving a loop in colonoscopy, or when performing controlled small repositioning maneuvers in endoscopic ultrasound, for example. It is useful to also train in the use of imaging techniques such as fluoroscopy or scope imaging devices [5] for those situations when the endoscopic image does not provide sufficient information to guide scope navigation. Although some endoscopists prefer to use alternative navigation methods such as controlling tip deflection via two hands on both endoscopy wheels while an assistant advances,

rotates, and applies torque to the scope, we feel that this is less than optimal for training purposes for a variety of reasons, particularly for more advanced or difficult endoscopic procedures and maneuvers and techniques.

With appropriate insufflation (of air, water, or carbon dioxide), the lumen of the GI tract can be identified and the scope advanced to the desired limit of examination. Too much insufflation adds to patient discomfort, may precipitate cardiovascular instability, and can increase the risk of perforation or aspiration. Insufflation is required only to achieve sufficient distension of the bowel for adequate imaging of the circumference of the bowel wall, to assist in identifying the lumen or differentiating the lumen from a diverticular opening, and to provide adequate focal distance between the lens of the scope and the object being viewed. The endoscopist should also be trained in the use of pharmacological agents that can assist in maintaining stability of position (e.g., in ERCP) or inspection (e.g., screening for early gastric cancer) by decreasing bowel contractions.

The endoscopist should be familiar with the unique endoscopic characteristics of the portion of the GI tract being examined. For example, the sigmoid, descending colon, colonic flexures, transverse colon, and ileocecal region all have specific endoscopic appearances. In most cases, knowledge of these appearances is useful feedback for the endoscopist in knowing where he is within the colon and what strategies need to be used if advancement of the scope is not successful. This is particularly relevant during colonoscopy in which different strategies may be employed in the right versus the left colon. Furthermore, it is important to understand the concept of paradoxical movement. In this situation, the endoscope is being advanced, but its distal tip is retracting as a loop is forming within the bowel. Similarly, the endoscopist should recognize both in the endoscopic image and in the sensation perceived by the right hand when advancement of the endoscope is not producing an associated advancement of the tip of the scope. This can lead to patient discomfort and increase the risk for perforation. At this point, consideration should be given to strategies for dealing with such difficulties. Depending on the type of endoscopy and patient factors (tortuous anatomy, altered anatomy, presence of surgical adhesions, etc.), strategies may vary.

Attention to landmarks within the upper GI tract such as the Z-line marking the squamocolumnar junction, the location of the hiatus, the various regions of the stomach (cardia vs. fundus, body vs. antrum, lesser curve vs. greater curvature, incisura angularis) should also be considered during upper endoscopic training. In EUS training, knowledge of vascular anatomy forms the linch pin for orientation and imaging of many intrathoracic and intra-abdominal structures. Without this understanding, it is impossible for the endoscopist to accurately communicate the location of observed pathology.

Some knowledge of surgical anatomy is also essential. The endoscopist should know the implications of an end-to-end versus end-to-side versus side-to-side anastomosis. Without this understanding, it is possible to perforate the bowel while attempting to navigate the scope through a dead-end or blind segment.

Evaluation of scope navigation requires the consideration of efficiency, patient comfort, and success at reaching the desired end point. Further evaluation of navigation skills will be incorporated in the section on mucosal evaluation. Clearly, excellent control of the scope is required to thoroughly evaluate the entire mucosal surface.

Coordinating all of these maneuvers may seem overwhelming to a novice endoscopist, particularly if they occur during a particularly challenging point in an endoscopy. This raises several key points for the training of endoscopy. As these points are outlined, consider your own experience with trainees who are attempting to learn how to traverse the pylorus in upper endoscopy or to resolve a loop in lower endoscopy for example. The first training point is the need for using a common terminology during endoscopy. This is particularly important when several trainers are involved in training the same individual over time or when there is a potential for misinterpretation or misunderstanding. It is important to be as specific as possible in instruction so that the trainee understands what is to be accomplished, how it is to be accomplished, and how to evaluate the level of success. As an example, providing a specific instruction, such as giving a directional reference of "12 o'clock," is more useful than "tip up." Whenever possible, orienting the learner to the video image is preferable to providing instruction describing movements [6].

A second important consideration when giving feedback on performance during endoscopy is the influence of cognitive overload or dual task interference [7]. If a specific situation is particularly challenging to an individual, then they may not be able to pay attention to other "distractions" such as the voice of an instructor because all of their concentration is directed to the task at hand. This implies that feedback on performance should not be constant or ongoing, but rather be intermittent. In particular, in situations where decision making may be involved, it may be more useful to have the trainee pause during the endoscopy, stabilize their position, and direct their attention to the trainer. This requires a significant level of trust and rapport between the trainer and trainee, and again illustrates the importance of attending to all aspects of training, including the training environment.

The concept of cognitive overload during endoscopy also illustrates the importance of using specific learning objectives at an appropriate level of difficulty for the learner. Learning activities should be focused on simple, well-defined, and achievable points. Using a stepwise educational program can be useful since as each new skill is acquired, gradual introduction of progressively more difficult components of each task becomes easier as they build on prior successes. Ideally, these steps are acquired along with conscious understanding of the steps and how they were taught, allowing the trainee to become a future trainer.

Overcoming obstacles

This section refers to difficulties that can be encountered in a variety of aspects of endoscopic procedures. Strategies to navigate across sphincters, around sharp curves, and through areas of resistance typically require achievement of a basic level of competence in navigation prior to attempting to master these challenges. Novice endoscopists typically struggle with traversing the

pylorus if they have not mastered when to use small amounts of tip deflection rather than large movements via torque application in order to generate rotation of the scope upon its long axis for example. Another area of uncertainty for trainees is how much resistance is normal, such as when encountering paradoxical scope movement. This becomes particularly important when traversing strictures or altered anatomy (e.g., advanced diverticular disease in colonoscopy, Billroth II anastomosis in ERCP, etc.). Again, this requires both attention to a cognitive component and a technical component of training. Although it may technically be possible to traverse a malignant stricture, clearly consideration must first be given in training to the potential advantages and disadvantages of other modalities or approaches before this is attempted. A similar analogy applies to the difficult cannulation during ERCP. A trainee can too easily become consumed with technical efforts to overcome the obstacle and must not lose sight of the relative indications for persistence as the procedure proceeds. What may seem obvious and commonplace to an experienced endoscopist may not be known or understood by trainees. This also highlights the importance of checking understanding with trainees during endoscopic training, particularly if the trainee is new to the trainer.

Recognition and prevention of difficulties are a major component of ensuring patient safety and comfort. This may require using a lower setting of air insufflation for instance or defining the amount of the procedure that should be performed by trainees (e.g., limiting polypectomy, sphincterotomy, or other therapeutic steps until the preliminary diagnostic skills have been mastered). This emphasizes the importance of establishing clear limits on what the trainee is expected to do during a procedure and when the trainer will take over the procedure. By doing this, the teacher will manage the emotional aspects of learning better and avoid the negative connotation of taking over a procedure. The other important components of training (covered in the next chapter) include the medicolegal aspects, appropriate informed consent, and so on.

Inspection

Once the scope has been advanced to the desired limit, and that location has been confirmed in some way, the next step is to carefully withdraw the scope while thoroughly examining the entire mucosal surface. This requires essentially the same skills as in scope navigation. Again, although this can be viewed as a technical component, there is no doubt that cognition plays an important role. Detection of specific lesions, such as the findings of celiac disease, eosinophilic esophagitis, and so on, are more related to an awareness of what is being looked for rather than being solely based upon technique. This is particularly relevant to endoscopic reporting, in which a thorough description of tumor characteristics and relation to landmarks may have great implications for the surgical approach for instance, and a repeat endoscopy will be required if communication between endoscopist and the surgeon is not sufficiently specific and detailed. Training in the cognitive aspects of image interpretation and assessment can be developed by didactic resources such as review of atlases and by direct mentored experience. The development of such cognitive skills should occur at the same time that the trainee learns to carefully inspect the entire mucosa, as these skills are complementary and dependent on one another.

The technical requirements of inspection differ somewhat depending on the nature of the procedure. In upper endoscopy, for example, the papilla and medial wall of the duodenum are common blind spots without careful and deliberate inspection, and may not always be easily obtained during EGD. In EUS or ERCP, the oblique viewing nature of the endoscope provides particular limitations and careful attention must be paid. In EUS imaging, the ultrasound view has very specific requirements to ensure that adequate imaging of specific structures has occurred. Depending on the indication for the procedure, repositioning of the patient, addition of fluid in the lumen, removing mucous, using chromoendoscopy, or narrow band imaging may be particularly useful. For enteroscopy or colonoscopy, inspection is a crucial aspect that has been highlighted by recent trials of adenoma detection. Slow withdrawal of the endoscope must be achieved, while at the same time using frequent movement of the tip of the endoscope to ensure that the entire circumference of the mucosa is inspected. Proper insufflation is helpful in effacing the mucosa, making polyps more easily identified. In several areas, repositioning of the patient may also be useful. Care must be taken to avoid rapid expulsion of the scope as this may occur when the tip of the endoscope is not anchored in place. To avoid unintended sudden changes in endoscope position, careful attention to both the endoscopic image and sensation in the right hand is necessary. Scope readvancement may be required if a region of the wall is not seen on first pass. Flexures and folds in the colon may create potential blind spots in colonoscopy for instance, or in the case of EUS, there are known blind spots in the stomach or regions that are outside of the limit of the ultrasound image. The endoscopist must always be aware of these locations and ensure that they are properly evaluated. Complete examination of specific areas within the GI tract, such as the distal rectum and anorectal junction, or the gastric fundus, requires the endoscopist to be able to retroflex the endoscope in the rectum. This may also be required for complex polypectomy or other therapeutic maneuvers elsewhere in the GI tract. In the upper GI tract, complete inspection of the stomach requires the endoscopist to be able to retroflex the scope to provide a complete view of the cardia and fundus. Retroflexion requires the endoscopist to understand the concept of paradoxical movement; as the retroflexed scope is withdrawn, the tip gets closer to the esophagogastric junction. Once the scope is retroflexed, the endoscopist can more accurately view the entire lesser curvature with a good view of the incisura angularis and the proximal lesser curvature. The hiatal opening can be viewed from below, and lesions in the cardia and fundus can be accurately evaluated. The combination of retroflexion, withdrawal of the scope, and rotation are required to fully evaluate the stomach.

Evaluation of mucosal inspection can be done in terms of the percent of mucosal surface evaluated. This is best done using virtual reality simulators, where these metrics are readily obtained electronically. A skilled endoscopist can achieve this more effi-

ciently than a novice, but it must be emphasized that quick endoscopy that does not provide complete mucosal inspection is a poor trade-off. At the present time, documentation of imaging quality in lower GI procedures typically involves photo or video documentation of specific landmarks such as the terminal ileum, ileocecal valve, and appendiceal orifice. In addition, aspects such as bowel preparation and residual bodily fluids may impair visualization of subtle lesions, and trainees should be encouraged to evaluate and document their presence. In endoscopic ultrasound, training should give consideration to the evaluation and documentation of the adequacy of examination on an intent-to-image basis.

Instrumentation

A fundamental skill that should be in the skill set of any GI endoscopist is to be able to use instrumentation placed through the accessory channel to accomplish biopsy, snare a polyp, perform an injection, or apply energy for tissue destruction or hemostasis. Virtually, all GI endoscopes have a working channel through which instruments can be introduced. Although side-viewing endoscopes are used in ERCP, or linear EUS have an elevator that can be used to deflect the angle of accessories that exit the scope tip, most upper and lower endoscopes do not have a separate deflector for the instrument channel, hence control of the instrument must be achieved by orienting the working channel properly using the combination of tip deflection and torque of the scope to provide the best working angle between the instrument and the target. The endoscopist must be able to maintain a stable endoscopic position and clear view at all times when performing therapeutic procedures. At times, it may be helpful to have an assistant hold the endoscope in place while advancing the instrument, particularly if a stable position is hard to maintain.

Accurate targeting is a learned skill that can be practiced and evaluated. Metrics to evaluate targeting include time required to instrument the "lesion" once the target mucosa has been visualized, accuracy of placement of the instrument relative to the target, and number of attempts to direct the instrument to the target. This is relevant to a number of procedures such as biopsy in EGD, fine-needle aspiration in EUS, cannulation in ERCP, and polypectomy in colonoscopy. Again, mastery of these tasks requires sufficient skill in scope handling and navigation, as well as an understanding of the cognitive aspects, such as indications for the intervention, potential complications, alternatives, and so on. This final stage of training is typically only reserved for advanced trainees who have successfully demonstrated proficiency in the fundamental earlier stages and will be discussed in later chapters of this volume.

Summary

The training of endoscopic skill is an important component of residency training that has not been the focus of extensive study. In this chapter, we have attempted to illustrate that although performing endoscopy involves highly complex psychomotor skills, a structured approach to training using deconstruction of relevant skill sets can be a useful starting point to designing training. Although current training programs are no doubt producing competent endoscopists, and many have learned endoscopy on their own in the past, observations from a variety of perspectives have demonstrated that there is room for improvement. A careful examination of current training methods using a framework for both endoscopy and training, such as that described in this chapter as a starting point, can assist endoscopy trainers in providing efficient, timely, and comprehensive training to future endoscopists.

Video

Video 2.1 Acquisition of technical and procedural skills: lessons learned from teaching laparoscopic surgery

References

1 Peyton JWR: The learning cycle. In: Peyton JWR (ed), *Teaching and Learning in Medical Practice*. Rickmansworth, UK: Manticore Europe Limited, 1998:13–19.

2 Logan GD: Toward an instance theory of automatization. *Psychological Review* 1988;**95**:492–527.

3 Ericsson KA, Krampe RT, Tesch-Romer C: The role of deliberate practice in the acquisition of expert performance. *Psychological Review* 1993;**100**:363–406.

4 Schön DA: *Educating the Reflective Practitioner: Toward a New Design for Teaching and Learning in the Professions*. San Francisco, CA: Jossey-Bass, 1987.

5 Shah SG, Brooker JC, Williams CB, et al.: Effect of magnetic endoscope imaging on colonoscopy performance: a randomised controlled trial. *Lancet* 2000;**356**:1718–1722.

6 Wulf G, Prinz W: Directing attention to movement effects enhances learning: a review. *Psychon Bull Rev* 2001;**8**:648–660.

7 Pashler H: Dual-task interference in simple tasks: data and theory. *Psychol Bull* 1994;**116**:220–244.

3

Training to Become a High-Quality Endoscopist: Mastering the Nonprocedural Aspects

Sahar Ghassemi[1] & Douglas O. Faigel[2]

[1]Santa Rosa Community Hospital, Santa Rosa, CA, USA
[2]Mayo Clinic, Scottsdale, AZ, USA

Quality is not an act, it is a habit

—Aristotle

It is quality rather than quantity that matters

—Seneca

In training programs across the country, there is a growing pressure to perform a higher volume of procedures in a patient population that is often new to the institution and referred through open access without prior clinic visitation. With these increased demands on quantity, the urgency to provide the highest quality of care requires deliberate effort and defined standards. The practice of medicine is fraught with the same limitations as the human health it serves to restore. Medical procedures are imperfect even in the most competent of hands, and unrealistic patient expectation and overzealous legal litigation are real factors in the climate within which we practice medicine. With the advent of more involved therapeutic procedures comes a growing responsibility toward the patient prior to the initiation of sedation and long after the completion of the therapeutic task. Apart from gaining competence in procedural skills, a trainee must exhibit a mastery of the quality measures by which his/her procedure will be assessed.

The American College of Gastroenterology (ACG) and the American Society for Gastrointestinal Endoscopy (ASGE) have used published data and expert consensus to define the major determinants for high-quality endoscopy and have published these guidelines [1]. These measures are increasingly utilized by third parties (hospitals, insurers, and regulatory agencies, lawyers) to assess if proper and careful consideration was performed by a physician. The trainee must understand these standards and learn to make them an integral part of his/her practice. These measures can be broken down into three categories: preprocedure, intraprocedure, and postprocedure quality measures. Each is equally relevant and must be considered separately. Although each type of endoscopic procedure will have specific quality indicators, the common principles are reviewed in the following chapter.

Preprocedure

The preprocedure period encompasses all contact between the care provider(s) and the patient before administration of sedation and commencement of endoscopy. Important quality measures include proper indication for the procedure, informed consent, a focused history and physical exam, appropriate use of prophylactic antibiotics, a management plan for anticoagulants, the sedation plan, and a team pause (Table 3.1).

Studies have shown that when endoscopic procedures are performed for established indications, the yield of these procedures is highest [2]. An important quality measure in the preprocedure period is limiting the number of inappropriate procedures [2,3]. When a procedure is performed outside of standard indications, care should be taken to document the justification for the procedure. Patients with marginal indications, particularly with higher risk procedures such as ERCP, are more likely to incur complications. Importantly, patients referred through open access endoscopy programs know little more than an abnormality was found on imaging or labwork. In this setting, it is imperative to define a patient–doctor relationship that empowers and educates the patient to understand the indication for the procedure and reviews the necessary elements of informed consent. Finally, a focused history and physical exam provides the physician important preoperative risk assessment and reassures the patient that the physician has properly considered their individual health prior to the procedure.

Informed consent

Obtaining an informed consent is a process that requires more than the attainment of a patient's signature. It involves mutual communication, disclosure of procedural limitations, and setting realistic expectations. When done effectively, it is an important risk management tool, transferring the responsibility of risk for an imperfect procedure to a competent patient who acknowledges and accepts that well performed endoscopies can have adverse or

Successful Training in Gastrointestinal Endoscopy, First Edition. Edited by Jonathan Cohen.
© 2011 Blackwell Publishing Ltd. Published 2011 by Blackwell Publishing Ltd.

Table 3.1 Preprocedure quality indicators.

Indication for procedure	The indication is specified, and if a nonstandard indication, the reason is documented
Informed consent	Proper informed consent documenting "PARQ" is documented
Focused history and physical exam	Document any cardiovascular disease, medications, allergies, vital signs, heart and lung exam, airway assessment
Preprocedure risk assessment	Document ASA or Mallampati score
Appropriate use of prophylactic antibiotics	As per published guidelines
Management of anticoagulants and antiplatelet agents	Plan as to whether and when to stop them and when to resume is documented
Sedation plan	Specify depth of sedation planned: minimal, moderate, deep, general anesthesia
Team pause	Ensure that the proper patient is undergoing the proper procedure

limited outcomes [4,5]. Much of our approach to informed consent has been shaped by the culture we live in and the judicial system. In a landmark 1914 ruling "Every human being of adult years and sound mind has a right to determine what is done with his body," the focus of informed consent shifted to a patient-centered approach of self-determination [6]. It is the physician's responsibility to disclose as much information as a *reasonable* patient would wish to know when making a decision [7]. Determining "reasonable" is not a precise science and the physician must simultaneously balance the need to avoid overwhelming the patient with providing pertinent risk information [8]. Certain states, such as Louisiana, have assisted the physician by providing a list of material risks for common medical procedures [9]. It is important to know the legal requirements where you practice [10]. Many physicians use brochures or website-guided tutorials as tools for informed consent. While these instruments can augment informing a patient of a procedure, they should not substitute for the individual conversation between the patient and provider. Although state law varies on who can legally obtain informed consent, most experts recommend that the physician do so personally [1,4].

The process of informed consent requires a thoughtful exchange of seven essential elements between physician and patient. The consent form should be timed and dated and, if possible, witnessed by a third party.

There are seven elements that require discussion in nontechnical terms and should be appropriately documented. These include the following:
1 Nature of procedure
2 Benefits
3 Material risks and complications of the procedure, including their likely incidences and severity
4 Alternatives (including nontreatment)
5 Limitations of procedure
6 Conflict of interest/research evaluation: A physician who has either financial or research gain in enrolling a patient into a specific study or medication must be direct about these affiliations.
7 Opportunity given for patient to ask questions.

Exceptions to informed consent
In a few specific circumstances, a physician can bypass the need to acquire informed consent. Several important exemptions to informed consent include the following [3,4]:

1 *Emergency waiver:* The patient's critical condition incapacitates them from providing informed consent, and delay in performing the procedure can result in unnecessary harm to the patient
2 *Waiver of self-determination:* A patient waives his/her right of informed disclosure and assigns his/her physician the right for decision making
3 *Legal mandate:* A judge or court orders a necessary medical therapy for a patient without their consent
4 *Incompetence:* A patient cannot make a decision and thus this responsibility is given an assigned third party (legal guardian)
5 *Therapeutic privilege:* A physician can withhold information regarding the procedure because of perceived harm to the patient. This is difficult exception and one that can be perceived as an excuse for not informing the patient. Unless there is a clear and compelling evidence of psychological vulnerability, it is best to avoid use of this exception.

Informed refusal
Patients who refuse a procedure must do so in a well-informed way. The physician should document that she/he has explained the purpose of the examination and the consequences of deferring procedure.

Lack of informed consent
If there is no consent or the procedure goes beyond the scope of obtained consent, a charge of battery could be brought upon the physician. Unlike medical malpractice suits, which are a civil offense retributed monetarily, a charge of battery is a criminal allegation. Therefore, when obtaining consent, it may be reasonable to expand the extent of the consent to include foreseeable complications (i.e., surgery in the setting of perforation or blood transfusion in the setting of bleeding). Most malpractice insurances do not cover battery and a physician can be held personally liable. Additionally, a charge of battery can result in restriction of hospital privileges [10].

Documentation
"If you didn't write it, you didn't do it." This often quoted phrase holds true in litigation. A simple note confirming that discussions occurred regarding the nature of the procedure, alternatives, risks (highlighting the major ones), sedation, and an opportunity

was given for patient to ask questions (aka "PARQ"—procedure, alternatives, risks, questions) can confirm a discussion took place with the patient and holds up as an important legal record of the exchange.

Preoperative clinical assessment: focused history and physical exam

Understanding the preoperative health and medical limitations of the patient undergoing a therapeutic procedure is a necessary prerequisite to the successful undertaking of the procedure. The risks of sedation can be assessed using the American Society of Anesthesiologists (ASA) score (Table 3.2) [11]. The ASA score correlates with sedation-related complications during endoscopy and is helpful in determining the need for anesthesiology support. The cardiopulmonary risks of sedation correlate with the depth of sedation, and for that reason, the sedation plan (minimal, moderate, deep, or general anesthesia) should be specified before the procedure begins [12,13]. In minimal sedation, previously referred to "anxiolysis," the patient is fully awake and cardiorespiratory functions are unaffected. In moderate sedation, previously referred to as "conscious sedation," the patient has purposeful response to verbal or tactile stimuli, there is spontaneous ventilation, and cardiovascular function is maintained. In deep sedation, there is only purposeful response to painful stimuli, the airway may require support, but cardiovascular function is preserved. In general anesthesia, there is no response to painful stimuli, the airway frequently requires support, and cardiovascular function may be impaired [14].

A careful review of patient's medical history, pertinent medications/drug allergies, and preoperative physical exam should be undertaken and documented. Certain medications (narcotics, benzodiazepines, anticoagulants, antiplatelet agents, alcohol, and illicit drugs) may impact the choice of sedatives and therapeutic maneuvers. Any medication allergies as well as any adverse events with sedation or anesthesia in the past should be noted. The timing of the last oral intake should be noted. The patient should undergo a focused physical exam measuring vital signs, auscultation of the heart and lungs, and performing an airway assessment.

Prophylactic antibiotics should be used when indicated. PEG placement and endoscopy for gastrointestinal bleeding in a cir-rhotic patient call for prophylactic antibiotics as these have been shown to decrease infectious complications and, in cirrhosis, decrease mortality. In most cases, antibiotics will not be indicated for prophylaxis against endocarditis or infection of implanted devices [15]. The management plan regarding anticoagulants and antiplatelet medications should be specified, including if and when they are to be discontinued, for how long, and if stopped, when they should be resumed.

Lastly, there is an increasing mandate among institutions for a team pause in which the patient and named procedure is identified prior to the start of sedation. The purpose is to ensure that the proper patient is receiving the proper procedure and that all necessary equipment is available. Although there are no data supporting the benefit of the team pause in improving quality of endoscopic procedures, the ASGE/AGE guidelines recommend it as a best clinical practice and a preprocedure quality measure [1].

Intra-procedure

This period begins with the administration of sedation and extends to the end of the procedure when the scope is withdrawn (Table 3.3). An important consideration during this period is the appropriate documentation of care provided to the patient in the form of written intraprocedure record (sedation records) and photo documentation. During the procedure, important vital sign documentation should occur at intervals no greater than 5 minutes for pulse, oxygenation, and blood pressure. Photos should be taken to establish important landmarks were met for completion of exam. For example, photo of cecal base or of the duodenum confirms the maximal depth of scope insertion was achieved. In addition to photos of important landmarks, care should be taken to photograph abnormalities found or therapies performed [1,11,14]. To improve the safety and efficacy of sedation, the use of reversal agents (flumazenil, naloxone) or discontinuation of propofol due to excessive sedation should be recorded. While data on reversal agents may be used for staff education and quality improvement, it should not be used to penalize physicians as this may cause reluctance to use these life-saving medications.

As previously stated, specific endoscopic procedures have specific quality indicators associated with their technical aspects.

Table 3.2 ASA classification.

ASA 1: Healthy patient
ASA 2: Patient with well-controlled mild systemic disease (HTN, DM) with minimal functional impairment
ASA 3: Patient with severe systemic disease with moderate functional impairment
ASA 4: Patient with severe systemic disease that is constant threat to life
ASA 5: A severely ill patient who is not expected to survive without an operation
ASA 6: A brain-dead patient whose organs are being removed for donor allocation

Table 3.3 Intra-procedure quality indicators.

Patient monitoring	Vital signs (BP, pulse, oxygenation) recorded at least Q5 minutes
Medications	Dose, route, and timing of all medications used is recorded
Photodocumentation	Major landmarks and findings are photodocumented
Sedation reversal	Need to reverse sedation with naloxone, romazicon, or cessation of propofol due to oversedation is recorded

Table 3.4 Post-procedure quality indicators.

Discharge criteria	Documentation that the patient has achieved predetermined criteria prior to discharge
Patient instructions	Written instructions including resumption of diet, activities (driving), and medications
Pathology follow-up	The plan for follow-up of any pathology results is specified
Procedure report	A complete procedure report is prepared (see text for required elements)
Complications	The unit has a policy for monitoring complications
Patient satisfaction	Patients are periodically surveyed as to their level of satisfaction with their endoscopic experience
Communication	Documentation of communication with referring provider(s)

Training in endoscopy should also include a thorough familiarity with these indicators.

Post-procedure

This period extends from scope removal through patient discharge, referring provider communication and pathology follow-up (Table 3.4). Each endoscopy unit should have an established policy regarding the criteria required before unit discharge. Detailed instructions should be provided to the patient which address diet, activity, and medication restrictions. Patients should be provided a means of contacting the provider should questions or concerns arise. Finally, feedback to the patient regarding findings and therapies performed should be undertaken [1].

Documentation of procedure

Individual style practices aside, important documentation of the following should be included within each procedure report:

- Time, date of procedure
- Patient name and identifier
- Endoscopists and assistants
- Indication and informed consent
- Documentation of relevant history and physical findings
- Type of instrument
- Medication used
- Anatomic extent of procedure
- Findings
- Limitations or complications of procedure and interventions
- Tissue acquisition, use of instruments
- Diagnostic impression
- Results of therapeutic intervention
- Disposition
- Recommendations for subsequent care and follow-up.

Feedback to referring provider

It is the responsibility of the endoscopist to inform the referring provider of the results of the procedure. If pathology is sent or further imaging is ordered, a clear plan outlining responsibility to follow these results must be provided in correspondence to the patient and referring provider.

Recognition of complications

Complications may be recognized immediately during the procedure or after the procedure has been completed. Some complications may be delayed in onset by several hours (e.g., post-ERCP pancreatitis) or may not occur until weeks later (e.g., post-polypectomy hemorrhage). It is the responsibility of the endoscopist and endoscopy unit to identify complications and institute proper therapy in a timely manner. Complications should be recorded and each unit should have a procedure for doing so. For some procedures, the expected frequency of complications is high enough that this may be used as a quality endpoint in and of itself (e.g., post-ERCP pancreatitis). However, most procedures' complications are rare and therefore their occurrence, or lack of occurrence, is an unreliable marker of an individual's competency. Instead, complications should be used as a tool towards quality improvement. Complications should be regularly reviewed, such as quarterly, in a nonconfrontational forum that focuses on the educational aspects with the goal of improving the quality of care.

Patient satisfaction

All endoscopy units should periodically consider surveying their patients for feedback regarding preprocedure (prep instructions, day of instructions), intraprocedure (endoscopy unit), and postprocedure (follow-up calls and reporting) experiences. The benefit of this interval review is that it provides information specific to the individual practice as seen from their client base. In these modern times, patient reviews on the internet are common practice and capturing this feedback for internal improvement may be helpful in improving the quality of care as seen from the patient's perspective.

Medicolegal issues

Gastroenterologists have an ethical and legal obligation to provide the highest quality of care to their patients. Use of quality markers during the pre-, intra-, and post-procedural period are important to optimizing patient outcome, minimizing patient dissatisfaction, and may be useful for avoiding malpractice litigation. There are limited data on malpractice trends in gastroenterology. One physician insurance carrier, the Physician Insurers Association of America (PIAA) showed that gastroenterology ranked 21st among 28 medical subspecialties in terms of frequency sued and accounted for 2% of claims. Interestingly, in the majority of the suits (60%), the basis of claims involved cognitive decision making rather than therapeutic misadventures [16,17]. In a separate ASGE survey, 42% of gastroenterologist that had been sued reported that informed consent was an issue [18]. Thus medical malpractice actions can be brought on because of failure to obtain informed consent (regardless of outcome) as well as civil wrong or harm brought on by medical negligence.

Elements of malpractice

In the setting of medical negligence or "civil wrong," four basic legal elements must be proven in a malpractice suit [4,10]:

1 The physician had a duty to the patient (patient–physician relationship).

2 The physician breached the duty by violating the standard of care.

3 The breach resulted in injury.

4 The injury is compensable.

The standard of care is often determined through expert testimony, published data, and accepted practice guidelines, with the most important of these being expert testimony. It is important to note that this standard of care is what is customary among the majority of competent gastroenterologists and not what a few noted experts in the field would do in specific circumstances [10].

The best defense against malpractice suits is good medical practice. Perform procedures that are within the accepted indications and avoid risky cases when possible. Use the process of informed consent to educate the patient on the inherent risks and limitations of the procedure, thus transferring some of the responsibility to a well-informed patient. Employ good documentation of adverse events, decision-making, and patient communication. In the setting of complications, be vigilant in communicating honestly with the patient and their family and provide timely and appropriate management.

Training in quality assurance and improvement

It is important that trainers teach their trainees both the importance of quality and also methods of quality assurance and improvement. The apprenticeship model of postgraduate medical training means that the mentors must have the proper mindset and the institutions the proper support. Faculty must be good role models for their trainees in their adherence to best clinical practice. The institutions should establish QA and QI programs that include trainee participation. These are skills that trainees can then take with them into their own practices.

Specific curricula in quality assurance and improvement for trainees are unusual. Most institutions have lectures on obtaining informed consent and medicolegal responsibilities. It is also common to have morbidity and mortality conferences where complications and adverse events may be discussed with the goal of improving quality and patient outcomes. Most other aspects are learned through the apprenticeship of the training program: preprocedure patient assessment, proper indication, proper procedure performance, procedure reports, communication with referring providers, etc.

Specific curricula in QA and QI would include didactic lectures on quality assurance and improvement topics, drawing from the rapidly expanding literature. They should focus on the quality improvement cycle: measuring quality indicators to identify areas of underperformance, instituting an improvement plan, and then remeasurement to document improvement. Trainees could immediately begin to incorporate relevant quality indicators into their own training (e.g., cecal intubation). Measuring these indicators during training could be used to track performance improvement and ultimately to document attainment of procedural competency.

Conclusion

Quality measures are important in optimizing patient care and minimizing error, patient harm, and legal recourse. Trainees should familiarize themselves with the key quality measures required in the preprocedural, intraprocedural, and postprocedural time periods. Proper documentation, communication, and follow through are critical in maintaining the highest standards of care. These quality measures represent best clinical practice and may be used for continuous quality improvement.

References

1 Faigel DO, Pike IM, Baron TH, et al.: Quality indicators for gastrointestinal endoscopic procedures: an introduction. *Gastrointest Endosc* 2006;**63**(4):S3–S9.

2 Froehlich F, Respond C, Mullhaupt B, et al.: Is the diagnostic yield of upper GI endoscopy improved by use of explicit panel based appropriateness criteria? *Gastrointest Endosc* 2000;**52**(3):333–341.

3 Balaguer F, Llach J, Castells A, et al.: The European panel on the appropriateness of gastrointestinal endoscopy guidelines colonoscopy in an open access endoscopy unit: a prospective study. *Ailment Pharmacol Ther* 2005;**21**:609–613.

4 Feld AD: Informed consent: not just for procedures anymore. *Am J Gastroenterol* 2004;**99**(2):977–980.

5 Zuckerman MJ, Shen B, Harrison ME, et al.: Guideline: informed consent for GI endoscopy. *Gastrointestinal Endosc* 2007;**66**(2):213–217.

6 Schloendorff vs. Society of New York Hospital, 1914:211 NY 123.

7 Feld AD: Malpractice, tort reform, and you, an introduction to risk management. *Am J Gastroenterol* 2004;**99**(2):977–980.

8 Berg JW: *Informed Consent: Legal Theory and Clinical Practice.* New York: Oxford University Press, 2001.

9 *Louisiana Rev Stat Ann* 1997;9:2794.

10 Frakes JT: Medicolegal issues. In: *ERCP.* Philadelphia, PA: Saunders Publishing, 2008:3–11.

11 American Society of Anesthesiologists Task Force on Sedation and Analgesia by Non-Anesthesiologists: Practice guidelines for sedation. Anesthesiology 2002;**96**:1004–1017.

12 Sharma V, Nguyen C, Crowell M, et al.: A national study of cardiopulmonary unplanned events after GI endoscopy. *Gastrointest Endosc* 2007;**66**(1):27–34.

13 Vargo JJ, Holub JL, Faigel DO, et al.: Risk factors for cardiopulmonary events during propofol-mediated upper endoscopy and colonoscopy. *Alim Pharm Therap* 2006;**24**:955–963.

14 Waring J, Baron T, Hirota W, et al.: Guidelines for conscious sedation and monitoring during gastrointestinal endoscopy. *Gastrointest Endosc* 2003;**58**(3):317–322.

15 Banerjee S, Shen B, Baron, T et al.: Antibiotic prophylaxis in GI endoscopy. *Gastrointest Endosc* 2008;**67**:791–798.

16 *PIAA Risk Management Review: Gastroenterology.* Rockville, MD: Physician Insurers Association of America, 2005.

17 *A Risk Management Review of Malpractice Claims: Gastroenterology Summary Report.* Rockville, MD: Physician Insurers Association of America, 2005.

18 Levine EG: Informed consent: a survey of physician outcomes and practices. *Gastrointest Endosc* 1995;**41**:448–452.

Training in the Major Endoscopic Procedures

4 Esophagogastroduodenoscopy (EGD)

Lauren B. Gerson & Shai Friedland

Stanford University School of Medicine, Stanford, CA, USA

Introduction to EGD training

Need for training

Upper endoscopy is often the first procedure performed by gastroenterology fellows during the training period. Compared to other procedures performed by gastroenterologists, diagnostic upper endoscopy has the most straightforward learning curve and lowest complication rates. Esophageal intubation can be mastered earlier by trainees compared to intubation of the cecum during a colonoscopy [1]. Indications for upper endoscopy include evaluation of symptoms including heartburn, dyspepsia, dysphagia, chest or abdominal pain, nausea and/or vomiting, and chronic diarrhea. Diagnostic EGD is also indicated in patients with iron-deficiency anemia, acute or chronic GI blood loss, and/or weight loss. Training in therapeutic endoscopy can include acquisition of skills in endoscopic hemostasis, variceal ligation, foreign body extraction, stricture dilation, percutaneous endoscopic gastrostomy (PEG), and stent placement. Currently, guidelines recommend up to 100 upper endoscopic procedures before credentialing should be considered in upper endoscopy [2].

Format of training

Training in upper endoscopy typically commences on the first day of an ACGME (Accreditation Council for Graduate Medical Education) certified fellowship in gastroenterology. Most gastroenterology fellows learn endoscopy during inpatient and night or weekend on-call rotations during the first year of training. While this format gives fellows exposure to more challenging endoscopic procedures, including gastrointestinal hemorrhage, foreign body extraction, and management of varices, these cases often require intervention by the attending physician while the first year fellow is in the steepest learning curve for EGD. During the second and third years of training, most of the EGDs performed are elective cases on outpatients. However, exposure to inpatient EGDs continues while the trainee is on call.

Bedside training, involving a trainer and a trainee, remains the cornerstone of endoscopic training. Alternative methods to training using simulators will be discussed below, but have not yet replaced bedside training due to cost of the available simulators and lack of evidence that they can replace bedside teaching.

Requirements for EGD training

Trainee

There do not appear to be any formal guidelines for trainee prerequisites other than the fact that the trainee must be enrolled in an ACGME-approved training program in gastroenterology or general surgery. The ACGME has mandated that programs in surgery and gastroenterology must provide experience to each resident in the performance of EGD and colonoscopy during their training programs.

Trainer

The trainer should be an experienced endoscopist who possesses the ability to teach endoscopic skills. Particularly, this requires an ability to verbalize endoscopic maneuvers, demonstrate working of the dials and channels, and be able to participate in the evaluation process. It is important that the trainer enjoy teaching and possess patience so that he/she can allow the trainee adequate time to perform a thorough examination while receiving verbal coaching. A trainer who takes away the endoscope from the trainee consistently during the procedure or who is unable to teach with a hands-off approach will be less effective.

Setting

EGDs should be performed in the outpatient as well as inpatient setting. The ASGE has recommended 100 EGDs as the threshold for the assessment of competence. However, a study by Cass and colleagues in 1995 demonstrated that the esophageal intubation rate was about 75% after 100 cases, suggesting that more than 100 EGDs were needed for the acquisition of technical skills [1]. The trainee should be encouraged to keep a procedural log so that the number of cases can be documented by the fellowship program at the end of the training period. The procedural log should contain the number of diagnostic and therapeutic procedures performed, including ligation or sclerotherapy of varices, endoscopic hemostasis of ulcer disease or other vascular lesions, stricture dilation, foreign body removal, and PEG tube placements.

EGD training

Cognitive aspects

Indication for the EGD

It is important to perform EGD for an appropriate indication. Published data, for example, has demonstrated that many patients undergo repeat EGDs for dyspepsia, where the yield of a second EGD is very low, particularly in patients without alarm symptoms. In series assessing appropriate indications for EGD, approximately 15–20% of cases have been determined to be nonindicated examinations [3]. Similarly in patients with chronic GERD who have an initial normal EGD, the yield of repeated endoscopic examinations remains low and performance of an esophageal motility study or measurement of esophageal pH may yield more diagnostic information in patients who are failing to respond to PPI therapy [4]. However, in patients with repeated hematemesis or ongoing melena, studies have demonstrated a miss rate of 15–20% for lesions in the upper GI tract, including PUD, vascular lesions, GAVE, AVMs, and other pathology, demonstrating the importance of a second-look endoscopy in patients with ongoing acute or chronic GI hemorrhage [5].

Administration of conscious sedation

In addition to understanding the appropriate indications for the procedure, other important cognitive aspects of EGD training include the administration of conscious sedation. Studies have demonstrated that the administration of conscious sedation increases the probability of a successful examination, patient satisfaction, and willingness to repeat the examination [6]. It is important to train fellows that some patients may be able to undergo an EGD with topical anesthesia and without the administration of conscious sedation. Patients who request to undergo endoscopy without sedation should be advised regarding symptoms that they might experience during the procedure. They should be provided with the opportunity to undergo a sedated procedure if they are unable to tolerate esophageal intubation without sedation. Prior studies have demonstrated, however, that only a minority of patients in the United States are willing to undergo an EGD without sedation [7]. However, transnasal endoscopy without sedation has been shown to be acceptable to many patients who are offered this examination and equally effective for screening and surveillance of Barrett's esophagus [8].

In some patients, routine administration of conscious sedation may not be effective. This includes patients who consume moderate to large amounts of alcohol and patients using concomitant benzodiazepines and/or narcotics. These patients should be advised that the administration of conscious sedation may not produce significant sedation. In some of these patients, utilization of propofol or general anesthesia may be required and has been shown in some studies to be associated with a higher probability for a complete examination [9]. In addition, in alcoholics requiring upper endoscopy for gastrointestinal hemorrhage, general anesthesia may be required for sedation during active alcohol withdrawal. These examinations are best performed in the intensive care unit for any patients with active gastrointestinal hemor-rhage. Intubation should be strongly considered for patients with massive hematemesis because of the risk of aspiration during the procedure.

Landmark and pathology recognition

It is important for the trainee to recognize and document important landmarks during the EGD. The location of the esophagogastric junction (EGJ) in centimeters from the endoscope insertion point should be noted. In order to characterize this landmark, trainees must be able to discern the top of the gastric folds by identification of longitudinal palisade vessels seen in either normal esophageal mucosa or the folds themselves, which are accentuated by the gentle application of suction. The location of the Z line is often required, for example, for placement of subsequent wireless pH monitoring to evaluate for the presence of pathologic reflux. The appearance of the EGJ should be described as regular, irregular, and with or without erosions or tongues of salmon-colored mucosa. A standard classification system (such as the Los Angeles Classification System, Figure 4.1) should be used for all examinations where erosive esophagitis is present [10]. If Barrett's esophagus is suspected or present (Figure 4.2), the Prague grading system should be used to document the length and circumferential involvement of the intestinal metaplasia [11]. If a hiatal hernia is present, the endoscopist should mark the proximal and distal end of the hernia sac and whether erosions are present.

Other important landmarks to note include the appearance of the gastric body and antrum (Figure 4.3), views of the gastric fundus and cardia during the retroflexed view (Figure 4.4), pyloric intubation (see Figure 4.13), appearance of the duodenal bulb (Figure 4.5) and first and second portions of the duodenum (Figure 4.6).

During the course of training in EGD, the fellow must learn to recognize a number of other key commonly encountered pathological findings. These would include inlet patch, esophageal candidiasis, features suggestive of eosinophilic esophagitis, rings, diverticula, achalasia, fundic gland gastric polyps, early superficial cancers of the oropharynx, esophagus, stomach, gastric antral vascular ectasia (GAVE), features suggestive of *H. pylori* and NSAID-associated gastritis, Bruenner's gland hyperplasia, duodenal and ampullary adenomas, celiac disease, lymphangiectasias, angioectasias, hemobillia, graft versus host disease, and other abnormalities that can occur in the upper digestive tract (Figure 4.7).

Technical aspects

The most important technical aspects for the trainee to master include successful esophageal intubation, pyloric intubation, ability to perform retroflexion in the stomach, proper inspection of the proximal duodenum, and the ability to perform biopsy and other therapeutic maneuvers required for endoscopic hemostasis.

Equipment

The standard current video-endoscope consists of a control head with dials and air and water suction buttons, the instrument shaft, and a deflectable tip (Figure 4.8). A CCD (charge couple device)

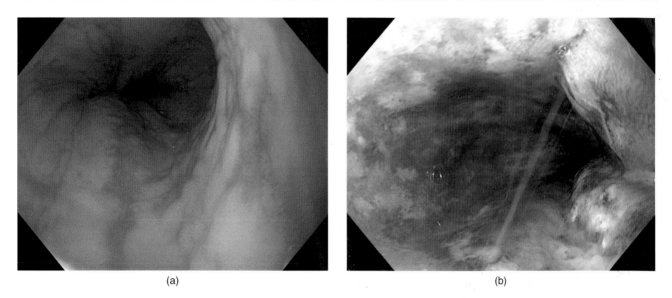

(a)   (b)

Figure 4.1 (a) High-resolution white light image demonstrates the furrows of mucosal erosion found in early erosive esophagitis (Mayo Clinic, Jacksonville, USA). (b) Los Angeles Grade 4 gastroesophageal reflux-induced esophagitis (University of Utah Health Sciences Center). (Contributed with permission from *Advanced Digestive Endoscopy: Comprehensive Atlas of High-Resolution Endoscopy and Narrowband Imaging*. Edited by J. Cohen. Blackwell Publishing. 2007: p. 177.)

chip allows for transmission of the image to a television monitor. The operating channel ranges in size from 2.0 mm for transnasal endoscopes to close to 4 mm for therapeutic endoscopes. The endoscope diameter ranges from approximately 5 mm for ultra-slim or transnasal endoscopes to 9–10 mm for diagnostic endoscopes and up to 10–13 mm for therapeutic EGDs. The larger channels for the therapeutic endoscopes allow for more effective suctioning of blood and gastric contents and passage of larger accessories.

Diagnostic accessories include guide wires for subsequent placement of motility catheters or stents, a variety of biopsy forceps, and brushes to obtain specimens for microbiology or cytology. Therapeutic accessories include sclerotherapy needles, polypectomy snares, rat tooth and other types of forceps, baskets, endoscopic banding devices, probes for thermal coagulation or argon plasma coagulation, through the channel balloon dilators, and stents.

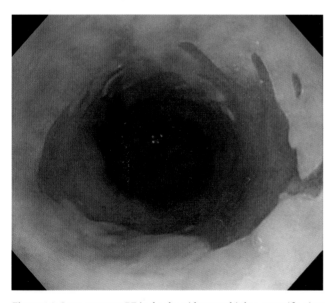

Figure 4.2 Long-segment BE is clearly evident on this low-magnification white light HRE view (University of Amsterdam). (Contributed with permission from *Advanced Digestive Endoscopy: Comprehensive Atlas of High-Resolution Endoscopy and Narrowband Imaging*. Edited by J. Cohen. Blackwell Publishing. 2007: p. 182.)

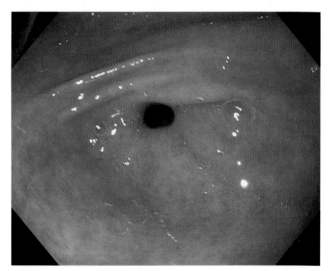

Figure 4.3 White light view of a normal gastric antrum (University of Utah Health Sciences Center). (Contributed with permission from *Advanced Digestive Endoscopy: Comprehensive Atlas of High-Resolution Endoscopy and Narrowband Imaging*. Edited by J. Cohen. Blackwell Publishing. 2007: p. 215.)

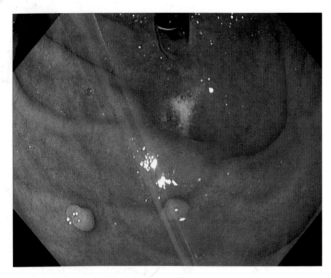

Figure 4.4 HRE white light low magnification image of normal fundus with two small fundic gland polyps and hiatal hernia seen in turnaround view (Mayo Clinic, Jacksonville, USA). (Contributed with permission from *Advanced Digestive Endoscopy: Comprehensive Atlas of High-Resolution Endoscopy and Narrowband Imaging*. Edited by J. Cohen. Blackwell Publishing. 2007: p. 214.)

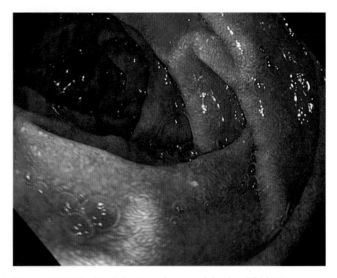

Figure 4.6 HRE white light view of a normal duodenal fold. The villiform architecture is readily discernable (Medical University of South Carolina). (Contributed with permission from *Advanced Digestive Endoscopy: Comprehensive Atlas of High-Resolution Endoscopy and Narrowband Imaging*. Edited by J. Cohen. Blackwell Publishing. 2007: p. 246.)

Diagnostic endoscopy

Patient positioning

Patient positioning is important to a successful examination. The patient should lie on the left side, which may reduce aspiration by allowing gastric contents to pool in the fundus. The head can be supported by a small pillow. One exception to this position would be during placement of a PEG tube, where the patient would be placed in the supine position to facilitate transillumination and placement of the PEG. Vital signs should be obtained prior to

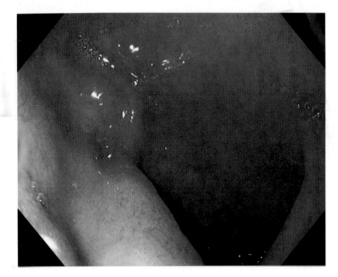

Figure 4.5 White light image of a normal duodenal bulb. The villiform architecture is indistinct (University of Utah Health Sciences Center). (Contributed with permission from *Advanced Digestive Endoscopy: Comprehensive Atlas of High-Resolution Endoscopy and Narrowband Imaging*. Edited by J. Cohen. Blackwell Publishing. 2007: p. 245.)

initiation of conscious sedation, and nasal oxygen administered. A bite block, either with or without a neck strap, should be placed prior to the administration of conscious sedation. The patient should be instructed not to talk to the physician or staff after administration of conscious sedation so that appropriate response to sedation can be monitored and in an attempt to create a quiet environment to help with the effects of sedation.

Handling of the endoscope

The trainee should be instructed not to handle the endoscope until the patient has been adequately sedated, as the light from the endoscope tip may distract the patient and result in need for further conscious sedation. Some physicians place a washcloth over the patients' eyes in order to prevent the distraction from visualization of the endoscopy equipment. Once sedation has been achieved, the endoscopist should stand facing the patient with the endoscope held in a curve towards the patient's mouth. The patient's head should be flexed with the chin towards the chest, to facilitate esophageal intubation.

The trainee should be instructed to hold the control head of the endoscope in his/her left hand, using the thumb to control the up/down control dials with the rest of the fingers resting on the shaft (Figure 4.9). The first finger can be applied on the water and air suction buttons. The trainee should be encouraged to learn to use the thumb to control the up/down buttons, rather than taking the right hand away from the endoscope to control the dials, as this technique may lead to increased loop formation, particularly during colonoscopy.

Esophageal intubation (Video 4.1)

It is preferable and safer to teach insertion of the endoscope using the direct visual technique, rather than under finger guidance. The latter technique may be needed, however, if the patient is unable to swallow the endoscope upon command. Under the direct technique, the trainee should first align the scope so that the tongue will be at the top of the screen as the scope is inserted into the mouth. The tip of the endoscope should be gently advanced over the midline of the tongue, past the uvula and the epiglottis as the tip is dialed up. If the teeth are visualized, the endoscope should be withdrawn, and re-introduced. Once the base of the vocal cords is visualized, the tip of the endoscope should be placed

under the cricoaryenoid cartilage on either side with temporary nonvisualization of the mucosa (Figure 4.10). The trainee should ask the patient to swallow and maintain gentle pressure so that the instrument will be directed into the proximal esophagus. Trainees should be alerted to the relatively rare possibility of entering a Zenker's diverticulum; in this case, the endoscope should be slowly withdrawn while searching for the entrance to the esophagus. If esophageal intubation is not easily achieved, more sedation may

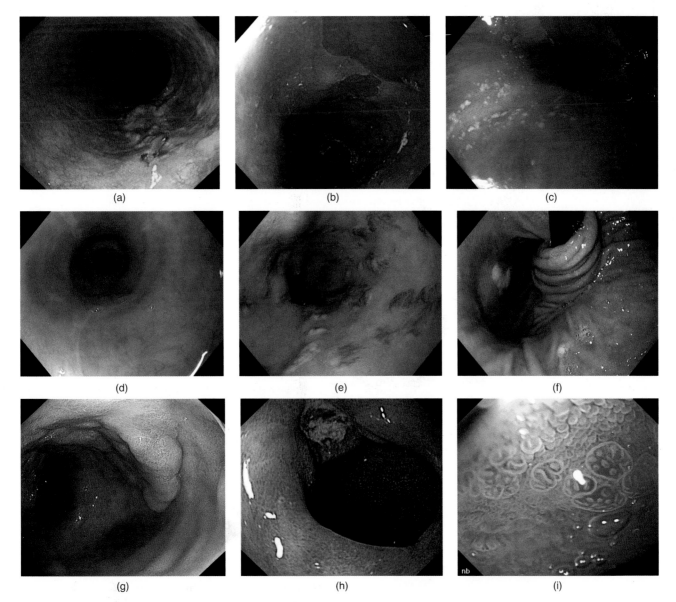

Figure 4.7 (a) White light magnified view of squamous cell esophageal carcinoma. Histology revealed an invasive well-differentiated SCC (University of Amsterdam). (b) White light low-magnification endoscopy reveals a gastric inlet patch upon slow withdrawal of the endoscope from the esophagus (Mount Sinai School of Medicine). (c) Multiple tiny white plaques suggesting Candidiasis actually represent eosinophilic esophageal microabscesses. White light nonmagnified view (NYU School of Medicine). (d) Normal magnification white light provides a good assessment of this smooth benign esophageal stricture (Mayo Clinic, Jacksonville, USA). (e) High-resolution image demonstrating the white, curd-like exudate of Candidal esophagitis. White light view is sufficient to make this diagnosis (Mayo Clinic, Jacksonville, USA). (f) Nissen-type fundoplication, with wrap well intact in this HRE white light view (Mayo Clinic, Jacksonville, USA). (g) White light HRE view of an early gastric carcinoma in a background of intestinal metaplasia and atrophy (University of Amsterdam). (h) Nonmagnified white light view of benign appearing gastric ulcer with smooth regular borders (Institut Arnault Tzanck). (i) Bruener's gland hyperplasia of the duodenal bulb seen in white light HRE magnification view (Institut Arnault Tzanck). (*continued*)

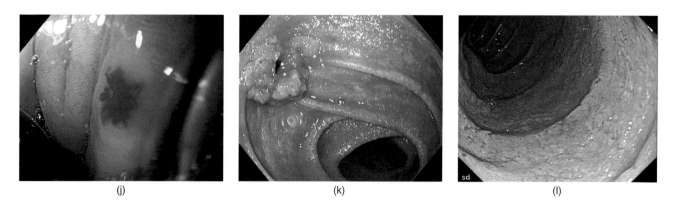

(j)   (k)   (l)

Figure 4.7 (*Cont.*) (j) Arterio-vascular malformation viewed with high-resolution white light (Mayo Clinic, Jacksonville, USA). (k) Bile duct adenoma with high-grade dysplasia seen here with high-resolution white light (note yellow colored bile) (Mayo Clinic, Jacksonville, USA). (l) Complete villous atrophy, HRE white light low-magnification view (Institut Arnault Tzanck). (Contributed with permission from *Advanced Digestive Endoscopy: Comprehensive Atlas of High-Resolution Endoscopy and Narrowband Imaging*. Edited by J. Cohen. Blackwell Publishing. 2007: pp 170, 208, 207, 206, 178, 239, 229, 223, 246, 260, 256, 259.)

be required for patients who still have a strong gag reflex or a more experienced endoscopist should attempt intubation.

Examination of the esophagus and stomach

Once entered, the esophagus should be examined for any structural abnormalities, including ulcerations, varices, strictures, rings, webs, or other findings. While routine endoscopy does not replace the information obtained during esophageal motility, a global assessment of motility can often be ascertained. In particular, patients with achalasia will be noted to have an absence of esophageal peristalsis, in addition to a dilated esophagus and tight-appearing EGJ that does not easily open with air insufflation. In patients with esophageal varices, air insufflation should occur in order to accurately stage varices, determine the number of columns present, the extent in centimeters, and the presence of any stigmata. The location of the EGJ should be noted in centimeters along with its appearance and whether salmon-colored

mucosa is present in the tubular esophagus. The proximal extent of the gastric folds should be identified. The diaphragmatic hiatus can be identified by asking the patient to take a deep breath. If a hiatal hernia is present, the size of the hernia should be measured and a patulous hiatus documented on retroflexed view of the cardia.

Any fluid present upon entrance to the stomach should be suctioned if possible to avoid subsequent aspiration or reflux. Adequate examination of the stomach requires extensive air insufflations and up-close inspection of each segment. Retroflexion is necessary for complete visualization of the fundus and cardia (Video 4.2). Commonly missed lesions in the stomach include varices in the fundus and Dieulafoy's lesions near the cardia when endoscopy is performed after bleeding has ceased. Subtle mucosal abnormalities in early gastric cancer and the erythematous lesions of GAVE are also commonly missed.

Retroflexion in the stomach is important to further examine pathology in the gastric cardia and fundus that can be missed,

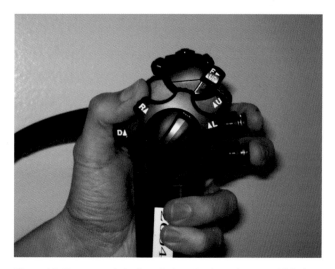

Figure 4.8 Recommended grip technique for the endoscope with index and middle fingers free to activate air/water and suction buttons and thumb to control up/down dials.

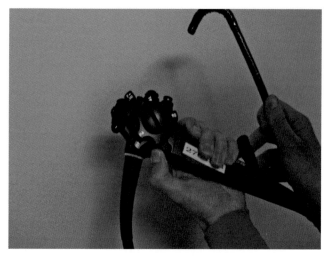

Figure 4.9 Upwards tip deflection demonstrated with the thumb pushing the up/down dial counter-clockwise.

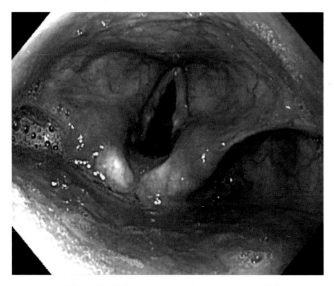

Figure 4.10 This white light HRE clearly shows erythema of the aryepligottic folds in this patient with endoscopically confirmed active GERD and throat clearing (NYU School of Medicine).

including ulcerations, varices, and malignancies. In order to perform retroflexion, the tip of the endoscope should be in the antrum and the stomach insufflated with air. By angulating the tip 180° and gently advancing the endoscope, views of the fundus and cardia can be obtained. In this position, the shaft should then be rotated 180° in both directions. With the instrument retroflexed, the endoscope should be withdrawn to obtain close-up views of the fundus and cardia (Video 4.2).

Examination of the duodenum (Video 4.3)

After retroflexion is performed, the endoscope should be straightened out and advanced to the antrum. Once the pyloric channel is visualized, attempts should be made to place the endoscope tip into the pyloric channel so that duodenal intubation can occur. The duodenal bulb should be carefully examined more than once as pathology can be missed particularly in the superior bulb and posterior wall. The scope is advanced past the duodenal bulb while dialing up and right to enter the second portion. The scope is typically advanced deep into the second portion of the duodenum during a reduction maneuver: with the tip dialed up and right, the shaft is pulled back and torqued clockwise to straighten the scope and remove the loop of scope that inevitably forms in the stomach during insertion.

In a patient with acute upper gastrointestinal hemorrhage, the bulb, first, and second portions should be examined multiple times to assure that no pathology was left undetected, particularly in the blind portion of the first duodenum. Sometimes, a duodenoscope is useful in examining the duodenal bulb, as for example, when looking for a bleeding site when the examination with the standard endoscope fails to identify a source. With modern high-resolution scopes, duodenal villi are easily visualized and trainees should be taught to routinely evaluate the villi and search for evidence of blunted villi from celiac sprue. The ampulla should be identified if possible (a side-viewing duodenoscope is usually required for a detailed examination of the ampulla; see Chapter 7) and inspected for any abnormalities that may require tissue sampling. In order to obtain optimal visualization of the duodenum, it is recommended that the endoscopist angle the tip of the endoscope down and withdraw in a hooked position to see the bulb, then angle up again to advance over the superior duodenal angle, and rotate 90° clockwise while angling the endoscope up and right to enter and view the descending duodenum (Figure 4.11).

Routine tissue biopsy (Video 4.4)

Biopsies in the esophagus can be useful to determine the presence or absence of Barrett's esophagus, the presence of histologic changes consistent with gastroesophageal reflux, and the presence of eosinophilic esophagitis. It is recommended that at least five biopsies be obtained from the distal, mid and proximal esophagus in order to accurately diagnose eosinophilic esophagitis. In the stomach, biopsies are most useful to distinguish benign fundic gland polyps associated with PPI usage from adenomatous lesions and to determine if *H. pylori* infection or any premalignant changes are present. Duodenal biopsies should occur if celiac sprue is suspected in a patient presenting with a variety of symptoms, including abdominal pain, diarrhea, iron-deficiency anemia, or

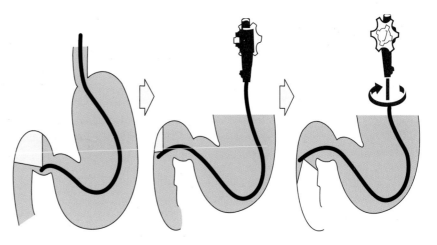

Figure 4.11 Angulation and hooking of the endoscope tip to aid with duodenal intubation and visualization.

weight loss. In order to obtain tissue biopsies, the biopsy forceps should be introduced through the endoscope working channel. The forceps should be opened and placed on to tissue for sampling. The forceps should close in order to grasp the tissue and then collect it for the laboratory analysis.

In the esophagus, routine biopsy may be more challenging, given the tubular nature of the esophagus. Particular care should be exercised while pushing the forceps out into the narrow lumen. The scope shaft may need to be rotated to bring the forceps close to the target area of mucosa. It is sometimes helpful to apply suction in order to bring the esophageal wall into close proximity to the biopsy forceps so that tissue can be obtained.

Therapeutic endoscopy

Hemostasis

In the setting of GE bleeding due to ulcer disease, it is important for the trainee to note the appearance of the ulceration in order to guide the need for endoscopic therapy and a further hospital stay. When the EGD demonstrates an ulceration with a clean base, the subsequent rate of rebleeding has been estimated to be under 5%, while ulcerations with active bleeding and/or visible vessels have rebleeding rates over 50% [12]. The trainee should record the associated Forrest classification in the endoscopy report [13]. Injection of epinephrine in a 1:10,000 dilution using a sclerotherapy needle around the base of the ulceration is not effective as solo therapy to decrease rebleeding rates, but can be used for initial hemostasis, to improve visualization in the setting of active bleeding and in combination with either thermal coagulation therapy or hemoclips [14]. When using thermal therapy, the trainee should be taught to apply direct probe pressure on the vessel until coagulation is achieved. Hemoclips should be applied directly on or around the vessel and can be repeatedly applied until bleeding has stopped. The utilization of hemoclips may be more challenging in angulated areas such as the first portion of the duodenum.

Variceal ligation

In patients with acute or chronic blood loss due to esophageal varices, hemostasis can be applied using sclerotherapy or banding. Sclerotherapy can be accomplished using sodium morrhuate (5%) or sodium tetradecylsulphate (1%) injected in 1–2 cc aliquots, directly into the varix, until a total of 20–30 mL are injected. However, sclerotherapy has been largely replaced in many centers by variceal ligation due to the associated complications of esophageal ulcers and strictures. Variceal banding is performed using a banding device that is placed on the tip of the endoscope; a wire that runs through the endoscope channel is connected to an inner cylinder that is loaded into the top of the channel. After suctioning a varix into the sleeve of the banding device, the cylinder is turned, releasing a band around the varix. Several varices are commonly treated in one session.

Gastric varices can be particularly challenging to treat. In Europe and Asia, cyanoacrylate glue injection is commonly utilized. However, the glue is not approved for this use in the United States, and there is a small probability of fatal pulmonary embolism [15].

Stricture dilation

Options available for stricture dilation include mercury-weighted dilators that do not require endoscopy or sedation, wire-guided bougie dilation, or through the scope (TTS) balloon dilators, which allow for dilation under direct endoscopic visualization. The TTS balloon dilators are 3–8 cm in length and range from 6–20 mm in diameter. The soft tip of the balloon dilator is passed gently through the stricture under direct vision and the balloon is inflated under direct vision. For complex strictures, fluoroscopy is useful to confirm that the tip of the balloon is in the lumen beyond the stricture and to delineate the anatomy. Dilation carries a significant perforation risk of approximately 1–2%, and it is common to dilate strictures gradually over a period of days to weeks [16].

PEG placement

Placement of PEG tubes are important means of providing enteral nutrition to patients with chronic feeding problems from neurologic conditions, malignancies, or other associated medical disorders. The trainee should learn that there are contraindications to placement of PEGs, including the presence of bowel distension or obstruction, ascites, obstructing esophageal or gastric carcinoma, or the presence of portal hypertension or other hypercoagulable states. The pull technique is illustrated in Chapter 29 of this book (Figure 29.1) and remains the most popular method of placement. With the patient in the supine position, the endoscope is advanced into the stomach. A point of maximum transillumination should be identified, and at that point, indentation of the abdominal wall by an assistant or second physician should be seen by the endoscopist. If this is unable to be achieved, there may be overlying bowel loops or fluid, and PEG placement should not occur via endoscopic means.

Once the insertion site is identified, the second physician should make a small skin incision at the site incision on the anterior abdominal wall after local anesthesia has been applied with 1% lidocaine. The trocar with the introducer needle should then be advanced through the incision, maintaining the trocar at a 30° angle. The needle should then be removed, and a guide wire is placed through the trocar. The endoscopist should then grasp the guide wire with a snare and remove the endoscope and guide wire through the mouth. The suture loop attached to the PEG tubing and bumper should then be tied to the snare, and the guide wire gently pulled so that the PEG can be pulled into the stomach until the bumper is attached. It is recommended to re-introduce the endoscope to confirm proper placement of the PEG bumper. Once confirmed, the PEG external bumper can be fastened, the tubing cut to the desirable length and the PEG can be used within 12 hours if the site is intact, and abdominal exam is benign.

Stenting

Placement of endoscopic stents can be considered for palliative treatment of malignant strictures, for refractory benign esophageal strictures and for treatment of esophageal perforations and fistulas. Uncoated self-expanding metal stents (SEMS) are associated with extensive hyperplastic tissue ingrowth that can prevent removal and can eventually result in obstruction [17]. Coated SEMS and self-expanding plastic stents (SEPS) can generally be

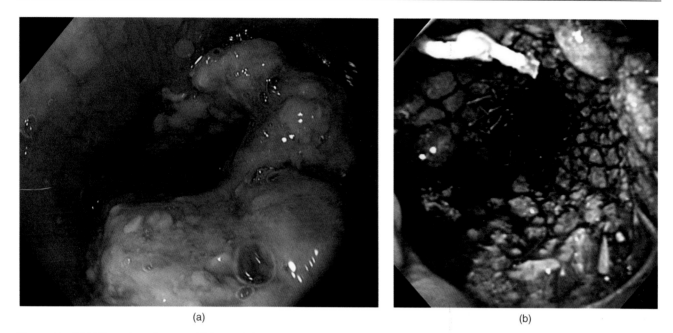

Figure 4.12 (a) Mid-esophageal cancer with luminal obstruction. (b) Subsequent stent placement over the area occupied by the neoplasm.

removed (Figure 4.12) and have therefore been used for strictures that do not respond to standard dilation. However, stents have significant risks of migration and perforation, so for benign strictures, it is reasonable to initially attempt at least three standard endoscopic dilations and consider the addition of four quadrant steroid injection of the stricture prior to stenting. Stent placement is usually performed over a guide wire with fluoroscopy to confirm positioning. Small bowel and colonic stents are placed TTS, while the bulkier esophageal stents do not fit TTS and are instead delivered over a wire after first removing the endoscope (in some cases, the scope is inserted alongside the stent delivery system to observe the deployment).

Alternatives for EGD training—Simulator-based training

Simulator-based training in upper endoscopy includes computer simulators and animal models. Advantages associated with usage of computer simulation models include didactic videos, tactile force feedback system, a series of cases with varying degrees of difficulty and pathologic findings, and the ability to receive feedback from the virtual patient. Advantages associated with *ex vivo* porcine models have been the ability to perform endoscopic hemostasis and other therapeutic maneuvers.

Computer simulators

The two major computer simulators available for training in upper endoscopy include the Immersion Medical simulator (Immersion Medical Inc., San Jose, CA. Figure 4.13) and the Simbionix Simulator (Simbionix USA Corporation, Cleveland, OH, USA). Both

simulators feature mannequins and endoscopes, which allow for endoscope steering, torque, air insufflation, diagnostic, and therapeutic maneuvers. Both simulators feature libraries of simulated cases that escalate in terms of procedural difficulty. The Simbionix GI Mentor II system also features eye–hand coordination modules containing virtual games that are recommended prior to the endoscopic training. Both systems feature a virtual attending that can provide feedback, and the virtual patients are able to voice discomfort. The Immersion Medical system uses a proxy endoscope based on the Olympus endoscope, while the Simbionix simulator uses a Pentax endoscope. Disadvantages currently for both systems include inability to customize training modules and high cost ($75,000–$100,000).

In two initial validation studies using computer simulators in novices and experts, both simulators were able to distinguish between novices and experts [17,18]. In a subsequent prospective Italian study, 22 novice fellows were randomly assigned to 10 hours of preclinical training on the Simbionix simulator while the other group did not undergo such training. Each trainee then performed EGD in 20 subjects. The trainees who received simulator training demonstrated more complete procedure rates and less instructor assistance [19]. Another study using the Simbionix simulator in 20 medical residents randomized one half to 5 hours of simulator-based training in EGD and demonstrated that this group demonstrated higher skills for performance parameters measured during subsequent live EGD cases [20] (Figure 4.13).

Animal models

The primary animal model used has been the Erlangen Endo-Trainer (ECE Ltd., Erlangen, Germany) or the compact Erlanger Active Simulator for Interventional Endoscopy (EASIE)

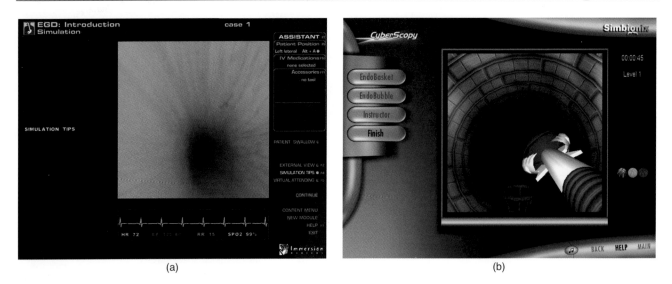

Figure 4.13 (a) Illustration of the pyloric channel with the Immersion Medical simulator upper endoscopy module. (b) Hand-eye coordination game illustrated on the GI Mentor II simulator.

simulator. Both models feature a rotatable plastic torso in which organ packages can be placed for training. In the compactEASIE model, a roller pump has been used to drive an artificial blood circulation through major organ arteries and simulate spurting arterial bleeding. Initial comparison of both models used during endoscopic courses showed no difference in trainee preferences between the two models [21]. Subsequent analyses of data generated from training courses showed that trainees all improved in endoscopic skills [22] and that the usage of the EASIE simulator improved skills over bedside training alone [23]. In a multicenter study enrolling novices in endoscopy, a one-week course with the Erlangen Endo-trainer was associated with significant improvements in the tested endoscopic parameters, but no control group was used [24]. In a subsequent 2006 study where fellows were randomized to education only versus simulator training in EGD with the Erlangen Endo-Trainer, the learning curve for the simulator-trained group after 9 months of fellowship significantly improved compared to the group receiving education alone [25].

Assessment of performance

Assessment of performance in EGD should include the following aspects:
• Recognition of landmarks including EGJ, gastric body, antrum and pylorus, duodenal bulb, and second duodenum.
• Recognition of pathology including esophagitis and/or varices with appropriate grading, gastritis, ulcerations, and other mucosal abnormalities such as villous blunting in the second duodenum.
• Ability to perform retroflexion.
• Ability to take adequate tissue samples.
• Performance of tissue sampling for appropriate indications, such as in suspected Barrett's esophagus.

• Performance of EGD for an appropriate indication.
• Comprehensive documentation of the procedure, findings, and recommendations.
• Plan for communication of results to the patient and adequate follow-up to incorporate the procedural findings into the plan of care.
• Physicians obtaining credentialing in therapeutic endoscopy should be skilled in endoscopic hemostasis, variceal ligation, stricture dilation, PEG placement, foreign body retrieval, and stent placement, if applicable.

In addition to the 100 EGDs set forward by the ASGE as the minimal threshold for competency [26], the ACGME has defined procedural competence to include the following features [2]:
• Completion of an ACGME-approved fellowship program with structured experience in endoscopy
• Demonstration of proficiency in endoscopic procedures and adequate clinical judgment as determined by faculty proctors
• Documentation of the number of cases performed during the training period
• Ability to correctly interpret endoscopic findings and integrate them into medical or endoscopic therapy
• Ability to recognize limitations of endoscopic procedures and personal skills and acknowledge when help is required

Conclusions

Proper training in upper endoscopy remains a vital skill and backbone for trainees in endoscopic training programs. Fellows should be trained not only in landmark recognition and procedural ability, but also in the determination of when the procedure is indicated and the recognition of important clinical findings. Skills in therapeutic endoscopy, particularly in the management of endoscopic hemostasis, are important, and thresholds exist for the determination of competence for each therapeutic modality. Simulation in EGD is available through computer and animal models; both models have shown that trainees improve endoscopic skill sets with simulation compared to no simulation, but further studies are needed to determine if simulation alone can reduce or even ultimately replace bedside training.

Videos

Video 4.1 Esophageal intubation
Video 4.2 Retroflexion in the stomach
Video 4.3 Advancing into the duodenum
Video 4.4 Endoscopic biopsy

References

1 Cass OW: Objective evaluation of competence: Technical skills in gastrointestinal endoscopy. *Endoscopy* 1995;**27**:86–89.

2 American Society for Gastrointestinal Endoscopy: Principles of training in gastrointestinal endoscopy. *Gastrointest Endosc* 1999;**49**:845–853.

3 Rossi A, Bersani G, Ricci G, et al.: ASGE guidelines for the appropriate use of upper endoscopy: Association with endoscopic findings. *Gastrointest Endosc* 2002;**56**:714–719.

4 Stoltey J, Reeba H, Ullah N, Sabhaie P, Gerson L. Does Barrett's oesophagus develop over time in patients with chronic gastro-oesophageal reflux disease? *Aliment Pharmacol Ther* 2007;**25**:83–91.

5 Fry LC, Bellutti M, Neumann H, Malfertheiner P, Monkemuller K: Incidence of bleeding lesions within reach of conventional upper and lower endoscopes in patients undergoing double-balloon enteroscopy for obscure gastrointestinal bleeding. *Aliment Pharmacol Ther* 2009;**29**:342–349.

6 Abraham NS, Fallone CA, Mayrand S, Huang J, Wieczorek P, Barkun AN: Sedation versus no sedation in the performance of diagnostic upper gastrointestinal endoscopy: A Canadian randomized controlled cost-outcome study. *Am J Gastroenterol* 2004;**99**:1692–1699.

7 Madan A, Minocha A: Who is willing to undergo endoscopy without sedation: Patients, nurses, or the physicians? *South Med J* 2004;**97**:800–805.

8 Jobe BA, Hunter JG, Chang EY, et al.: Office-based unsedated small-caliber endoscopy is equivalent to conventional sedated endoscopy in screening and surveillance for Barrett's esophagus: A randomized and blinded comparison. *Am J Gastroenterol* 2006;**101**:2693–2703.

9 Meining A, Semmler V, Kassem AM, et al.: The effect of sedation on the quality of upper gastrointestinal endoscopy: An investigator-blinded, randomized study comparing propofol with midazolam. *Endoscopy* 2007;**39**:345–349.

10 Armstrong D, Bennett JR, Blum AL, et al.: The endoscopic assessment of esophagitis: A progress report on observer agreement. *Gastroenterology* 1996;**111**:85–92.

11 Sharma P, Dent J, Armstrong D, et al.: The development and validation of an endoscopic grading system for Barrett's esophagus: The Prague C & M criteria. *Gastroenterology* 2006;**131**:1392–1399.

12 Lau JY, Chung SC, Leung JW, Lo KK, Yung MY, Li AK: The evolution of stigmata of hemorrhage in bleeding peptic ulcers: A sequential endoscopic study. *Endoscopy* 1998;**30**:513–518.

13 Zaragoza AM, Tenias JM, Llorente MJ, Alborch A: Prognostic factors in gastrointestinal bleeding due to peptic ulcer: Construction of a predictive model. *J Clin Gastroenterol* 2008;**42**:786–790.

14 Yuan Y, Wang C, Hunt RH: Endoscopic clipping for acute nonvariceal upper-GI bleeding: A meta-analysis and critical appraisal of randomized controlled trials. *Gastrointest Endosc* 2008;**68**:339–351.

15 Marion-Audibert AM, Schoeffler M, Wallet F, et al.: Acute fatal pulmonary embolism during cyanoacrylate injection in gastric varices. *Gastroenterol Clin Biol* 2008;**32**:926–930.

16 Ukleja A, Afonso BB, Pimentel R, Szomstein S, Rosenthal R: Outcome of endoscopic balloon dilation of strictures after laparoscopic gastric bypass. *Surg Endosc* 2008;**22**:1746–1750.

17 Ferlitsch A, Glauninger P, Gupper A, et al.: Evaluation of a virtual endoscopy simulator for training in gastrointestinal endoscopy. *Endoscopy* 2002;**34**:698–702.

18 Moorthy K, Munz Y, Jiwanji M, Bann S, Chang A, Darzi A: Validity and reliability of a virtual reality upper gastrointestinal simulator and cross validation using structured assessment of individual performance with video playback. *Surg Endosc* 2004;**18**:328–333.

19 Di Giulio E, Fregonese D, Casetti T, et al.: Training with a computer-based simulator achieves basic manual skills required for upper endoscopy: A randomized controlled trial. *Gastrointest Endosc* 2004;**60**:196–200.

20 Shirai Y, Yoshida T, Shiraishi R, et al.: Prospective randomized study on the use of a computer-based endoscopic simulator for training in esophagogastroduodenoscopy. *J Gastroenterol Hepatol* 2008;**23**:1046–1050.

21 Hochberger J, Euler K, Naegel A, Hahn EG, Maiss J: The compact Erlangen Active Simulator for Interventional Endoscopy: A prospective comparison in structured team-training courses on "endoscopic hemostasis" for doctors and nurses to the "Endo-Trainer" model. *Scand J Gastroenterol* 2004;**39**:895–902.

22 Maiss J, Wiesnet J, Proeschel A, et al.: Objective benefit of a 1-day training course in endoscopic hemostasis using the "compactEASIE" endoscopy simulator. *Endoscopy* 2005;**37**:552–558.

23 Hochberger J, Matthes K, Maiss J, Koebnick C, Hahn EG, Cohen J. Training with the compactEASIE biologic endoscopy simulator significantly improves hemostatic technical skill of gastroenterology fellows: A randomized controlled comparison with clinical endoscopy training alone. *Gastrointest Endosc* 2005;**61**:204–215.

24 Neumann M, Hahn C, Horbach T, et al.: Score card endoscopy: A multicenter study to evaluate learning curves in 1-week courses using the Erlangen Endo-Trainer. *Endoscopy* 2003;**35**:515–520.

25 Maiss J, Prat F, Wiesnet J, et al.: The complementary Erlangen active simulator for interventional endoscopy training is superior to solely clinical education in endoscopic hemostasis—The French training project: A prospective trial. *Eur J Gastroenterol Hepatol* 2006;**18**:1217–1225.

26 Eisen GM, Baron TH, Dominitz JA, et al.: Methods of granting hospital privileges to perform gastrointestinal endoscopy. *Gastrointest Endosc* 2002;**55**:780–783.

5 Colonoscopy

Robert E. Sedlack

Mayo Clinic, Rochester, MN, USA

Introduction

All trainees in gastroenterology must acquire competence in the basic endoscopic procedures of esophagogastroduodenoscopy (EGD) and colonoscopy. Though some skills learned in EGD may translate to colonoscopy, overall the skills required for colonoscopy are more technically demanding and require more time to achieve competence. This chapter focuses on the specific skills required in colonoscopy. For each skill, we will also examine available data on how best to teach/learn these skills and finally methods to assess competence in each of these skills.

Specific skills

The skills required in colonoscopy can be broken down into two main groups: motor and cognitive skills. Traditionally, the focus of many previous colonoscopy-training chapters published has been almost exclusively on the motor skills. However, the cognitive skills are just as, if not more, important. In this chapter, we will try to address both skill sets.

These two skill groups can be broken down further into "early" and "intermediate" skills as shown in Table 5.1. It is well established in the surgical literature that the most effective method for teaching any technical procedure is to break the overall procedure down into individual skills [1]. These skills can then be taught in a stepwise fashion, from the most basic towards the more complex, building on one another. Colonoscopy is no different. These beginning and intermediate skills are simply the skills required to complete routine screening colonoscopy safely and reliably. More advanced endoscopic skills such as complex polypectomy and hemostasis techniques will be covered in other chapters in this text. Depending on how a training program is structured, many trainees will have performed a fair number of EGDs prior to attempting colonoscopy and may have some basic mastery of a few of the early skills such as how to hold a scope correctly and use of the scope controls. Many of the other early skills, however, are specific to lower endoscopy, hence even with some EGD experience, these specific skills will be quite new.

These skills should not be confused with the metrics used to assess competency. Though these skills are an integral part of those metrics, the latter includes additional parameters such as cecal intubation times and success rates, withdrawal times, and polyp detection rates, as well as many others that will be discussed later.

Early skills

Early cognitive skills

Before a fellow attempts a colonoscopy for the first time, there needs to be a fundamental understanding of the colonic anatomy, basic elements of the colonoscopy exam, indications/contraindications for performing such an exam, the risks and benefits of the exam, and finally preparation and sedation. This section will focus on each these issues.

Anatomy

The colonic anatomy can be broken down into various segments, each with some defining characteristics that can help the endoscopist keep track of the scope's location in the colon (Figure 5.1) (Video 5.1). The anal canal is lined with squamous mucosa. Inside the internal sphincter and puborectalis muscles, the anus transitions to the rectum at the dentate line. This line represents the transition between the anal squamous mucosa and the columnar epithelium found throughout the intestines and stomach (Figure 5.2). The rectum progresses posteriorly in the retroperitoneum. Within the rectum, there are three semicircular folds called the valves of Houston (Figures 5.2 and 5.3). These folds differ from the rest of the colon in that they are not circumferential but rather span roughly 50% of the circumference of the lumen. At the peritoneal reflection the colon leaves the retroperitoneal space and moves into the peritoneum. At this reflection, the sigmoid colon begins and deflects anteriorly, inferiorly, and to the left in the peritoneal space. This portion of the colon varies in length and configuration from one individual to the next and accounts for a majority of the looping and difficulty with scope advancement encountered during colonoscopy, due to its mobile and circuitous nature. As one moves more proximally, the sigmoid continues towards the left flank and posteriorly to its junction with the descending colon. The descending colon rises up the left posterior abdomen in a fairly straight manner. This segment of the colon, along with the ascending colon, is partially fused to the posterior

Successful Training in Gastrointestinal Endoscopy, First Edition. Edited by Jonathan Cohen.
© 2011 Blackwell Publishing Ltd. Published 2011 by Blackwell Publishing Ltd.

Table 5.1 Listed are the core motor and cognitive skills trainees must acquire to be minimally competent in colonoscopy. These are broken down into early and intermediate skills to ensure the foundation of basic skills are established before building upon this with more complex abilities.

	Motor	Cognitive

Early	• Correct holding of the scope
	• Use of the scope controls
	• Scope insertion
	• Scope advancement
	    – Tip control
	    – Torque
	• Lumen identification
	• Withdrawal/mucosal inspection
		• Anatomy
		• Preparation
		• Scope selection
		• Sedation management
		• Assessment of indication and risks

Intermediate	• Loop reduction • Angulated turns • TI intubation	• Pathology identification • Therapeutic devices • Complication management

peritoneum along the colonic gutters and as a result is relatively nonmobile. In some instances, however, these segments may be freely mobile, making endoscopic advancement quite difficult. At the splenic flexure, the colon acutely deflects anteriorly and to the right, marking the transition between the descending colon and the transverse colon. Like the sigmoid, the transverse colon is mobile in the peritoneal space attached only by the mesentery. It too can be quite variable in length and redundant, leading to difficult scope advancement. The lumen of the transverse colon also differs from the other segments of the colon in that the three tinea coli running the length of the colon produce a triangular appearance as opposed to the circular appearing folds elsewhere

in the colon (Figure 5.4). As the transverse colon sweeps to the right side, it again moves posteriorly, and at the hepatic flexure, the colon deflects posteriorly and downward, becoming the ascending colon. This segment is normally fixed to the right posterior gutter of the peritoneal cavity. At the hepatic and splenic flexures, external organs such as the liver or spleen can often be seen through the wall of the colon as bluish-gray discoloration (Figure 5.5). The ascending colon proceeds down along the right posterior flank to the cecum. The cecum marks the most proximal portion of the colon and is the location where the three tinea coli come together along the external surface of the colon and meet at the appendix. From the luminal view, this appears in the cecal base as three

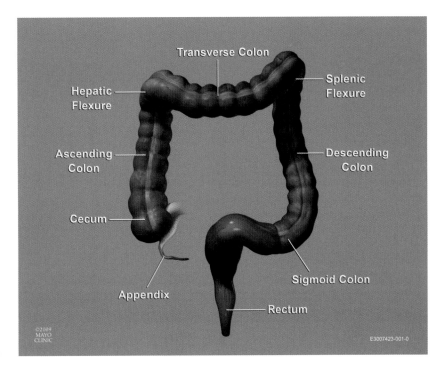

Figure 5.1 Colon anatomy. This illustration demonstrates the anatomy of the colon. (Copyrighted and used with permission of Mayo Foundation for Medical Education and Research.)

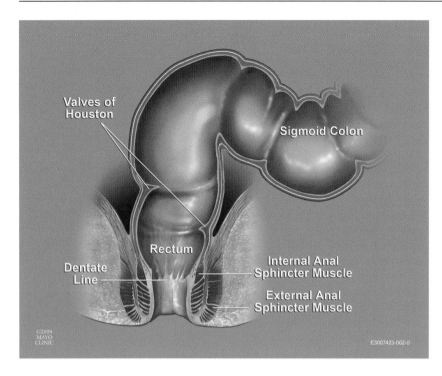

Figure 5.2 Rectal anatomy. Just inside the anal sphincter muscles, the dentate line marks the transition from the squamous mucosa lining the anal canal to the columnar epithelium of the rectum. The rectum is notable for its semilunar (half-circle) folds called the Valves of Houston. (Copyrighted and used with permission of Mayo Foundation for Medical Education and Research.)

longitudinal folds coming together adjacent to the appendiceal orifice (Figure 5.6). These folds are often referred to as the "crow's foot" or "Mercedes sign" as it resembles the clawed foot of a crow or the emblem of the well-known automaker. The cecum transitions to the ascending colon at the level of the ileocecal valve that rests on the first major haustral fold above the appendiceal orifice. The valve can be identified by the asymmetric prominence of this first fold and with careful inspection, torque, and dial control, the valve os can be directly visualized and intubated.

Basics of endoscopic anatomy

Endoscopists use anatomical landmarks to help them identify where their scope is at any given point of the procedure to ensure pathology is correctly located for the purposes of documenting disease extent, for future re-examination, or for locating pathology for possible surgical intervention. Another method to identify location is by checking the scope length markings at the anal verge. These markings will inform the endoscopist how many centimeters of scope are inside the patient. However, relying on the scope

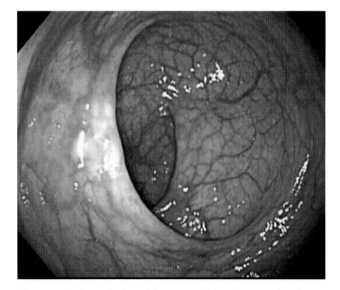

Figure 5.3 Endoscopic view of the rectum. This endoscopic view shows the semilunar folds of the rectum (Valves of Houston).

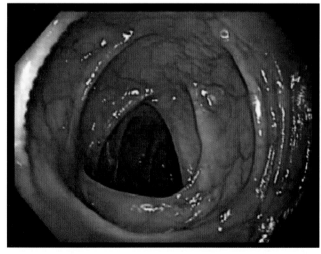

Figure 5.4 Endoscopic view of the transverse colon. The transverse colon is easily identified by the triangular appearance of the lumen. Externally, the tinea coli are located at the apexes of the triangular folds.

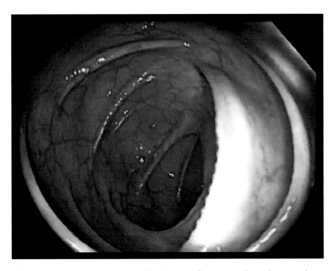

Figure 5.5 Endoscopic view of the hepatic flexure. At the splenic and hepatic flexure, the purplish hue of the spleen or liver can often be seen through the wall of the colon.

length from the anal verge is unreliable especially in the right colon where variances in the anatomic length of an individual's colon segments can lead to marked variability. Also, using the scope markings during the insertion phase of the exam is also prone to error as looping can greatly increase the length of scope inserted and greatly alter the reliability of these numbers as they correlate to location. As a rule, these numbers are only used as a crude estimate of location, typically only in the left half of the colon and only during the withdrawal phase of the exam. Instead, the

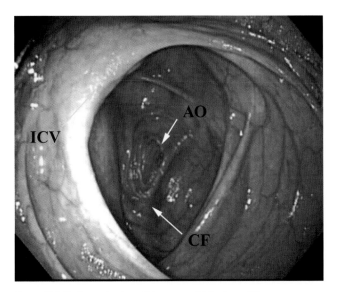

Figure 5.6 Endoscopic view of the cecum. This view of the cecum demonstrates the small semilunar os of the appendiceal orifice (AO) as well as the indentations of the tinea coli coming together externally to make up the "Crow's foot (CF)". The ileal–cecal valve (ICV) can be seen at the thickening of the first major fold above cecal base.

anatomical landmarks of the colon are in general more reliable markers of location than scope depth.

The major landmarks during withdrawal start with the appendiceal orifice, crow's foot, and ileocecal valve of the cecum. The next major landmark is the acute angulation in the colon with the purplish hue of the liver representing the hepatic flexure. The triangular folds of the transverse colon make it readily identifiable. At the distal end of the triangular lumen is a second acute angulation with a purplish hue of the spleen, which signifies the splenic flexure, and is located at roughly 50 cm from the anal verge. Just past this acute turn, one often encounters a collection of retained liquid stool that collects at this point as the proximal segment of the descending colon is the most gravity-dependent portion of the colon with the patient in the left lateral decubitus position. The descending colon is marked by a long straightaway from roughly 50 to 30–35 cm from the anal verge, followed by a number of acute turns and the more muscular haustra of the sigmoid colon. The rectosigmoid junction is located at roughly 15 cm from the anal verge. Distal to the junction, the rectum is identified by the increase in lumen caliber and the three prominent semi-lunar folds called the valves of Houston (Figure 5.3). The dentate line is seen on retroflexion in the rectum.

Preparation

One of the most important steps in successfully achieving the goals of colonoscopy is adequate cleaning of the colon. Without this, polyp detection or pathology identification may be hindered and adequate visualization to enable safe scope advancement may not be possible.

There are a number of different methods that have been used to prepare the colon. These fall under two main groups: osmotic and nonosmotic agents. Ingestion of highly osmotic agents, such as sodium phosphate, magnesium citrate, or mannitol, function by creating a large osmotic gradient between the bowel lumen and interstitial tissue, resulting in a large influx of fluid from the bowel lining into the lumen. This fluid is then passed, cleansing the colon in the process. These agents have been used successfully; however, they do have significant drawbacks that have lead to limitations or even the discontinuation of their use in some instances. As a group, the osmotic agents result in large intravascular and intracellular fluid shifts. In healthy individuals, symptoms of dehydration are not uncommon, however, in patients with significant heart or renal disease, these fluid shifts can lead to significant heart failure or worsening of renal function. Additionally, magnesium citrate and sodium phosphate result in some absorption of their elements and can lead to dangerous elevations of magnesium or phosphate in patients. This is especially true in the elderly or patients with renal insufficiency. Mannitol, on the other hand, is a nondigested carbohydrate and does not get absorbed, which would limit the problem of electrolyte disturbances; however, colonic bacteria can metabolize this carbohydrate, leading to the production of methane and hydrogen gases within the colon. Not only do these gases lead to distention and greater patient discomfort, but they are also extremely flammable and can lead to combustion with the use of electrocautery during polyp removal.

Lavage of the colon using nonosmotic agents has become the most common method of preparation. These agents use various preparations of polyethylene glycol (PEG) in electrolyte solutions. Like mannitol, PEG is nondigestible and nonabsorbable molecule. In addition, it cannot be fermented by colonic bacteria. PEG preparations are formulated so that concentrations of electrolytes and PEG are isoosmotic to patients' interstitial fluids. This results in no significant fluid shifts in either direction, leaving the patient's fluid status largely unaffected by the preparation with no dangerous electrolyte imbalances. This makes PEG a safer alternative to cleanse the colon, especially in patients with cardiac or renal disease. The strengths of these PEG preparations, however, are also their weaknesses. Since there is no fluid recruitment from the patient's interstitial fluid as seen with the osmotic agents, the entire volume of cleansing fluid must be ingested. This requires drinking large volumes (traditionally 4 liters) of solution to achieve the preparation goals. These solutions are generally not very palatable, also limiting the tolerability of these. Some variations have tried to ameliorate this by concentrating the solution into a smaller volume followed by drinking a predetermined amount of free water. Another formulation places PEG in capsules, so the patient does not have to taste the medication. This pill preparation, however, requires ingesting >30 capsules over a short period of time and still requires ingesting large amounts of water or clear soda to provide the fluid volume needed to clean the colon and ensure an isoosmotic concentration in the intestines. Despite these drawbacks, PEG preparations still remain the safest, most effective, and most commonly used preparations.

Scope selection

One decision that needs to be made prior to initiating endoscopy is what instrument to use. There are a number of different types of endoscopes in the gastroenterologist's armamentarium that can be selected to perform lower endoscopy. These include the standard adult colonoscope, pediatric colonoscope, flexible sigmoidoscope, or even a gastroscope that is dedicated to lower procedures (Figure 5.7). Understanding the advantages/disadvantages of each is an important cognitive skill that can improve ones chances of successfully achieving the goals of a lower endoscopy.

In general, the standard adult scope is slightly larger in diameter than the other scopes (measuring roughly 12.8 mm in diameter) and is one of the most commonly used scopes for colonoscopy. Its thickness results in it being somewhat stiffer than the others. As a result of being slightly stiffer, it tends to loop less than other scopes especially in patients with a very mobile sigmoid or redundant transverse colon. By the same token, its larger diameter and decreased flexibility can also make it more difficult to navigate through fixed, sharply angulated colons. Such fixation and angulation can be seen in patients with prior abdominal or pelvic surgeries (hysterectomy, C-sections, etc.), prior radiation, or significant prior peritoneal infection (ruptured appendix or other infection). In these patients, a pediatric scope can sometimes succeed in navigating through a difficult fixed sigmoid where an adult scope could not. This is primarily due to the greater flexibility of this scope resulting from its smaller diameter

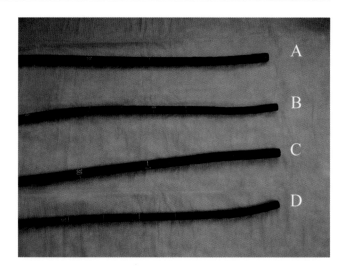

Figure 5.7 Endoscope options. Four different endoscopes can be used for lower endoscopy. Depicted here are: A adult colonoscope (12.8 mm diameter), B pediatric colonoscope (11.3 mm diameter), C sigmoidoscope (12.8 mm diameter), and D gastroscope (8.8 mm diameter). The diameter of the endoscope may vary slightly based on the manufacturer.

(11.3 mm diameter). In a long redundant, highly mobile colon, however, this flexibility can result in excessive proximal looping, requiring greater experience and skill to advance the scope to the cecum.

Gastroscopes are also used in special circumstances for lower endoscopy. Because of their smaller caliber (8.8 mm diameter), gastroscopes are ideal for lower endoscopy of an ileostomy or in a patient with an ileoanal pouch. The smaller diameter is also useful in patients who have left-sided colonic strictures (within reach of the shorter gastroscope) that prevent the passage of either of the larger colonoscopes. For routine colonoscopy, however, these scopes loop quite a bit due to their flexibility and their short length prevents them from reaching the cecum in most cases.

Flexible sigmoidoscopes are useful if only the left colon is to be examined. Traditionally, this was the primary method for routine colon cancer screening when paired with testing such as a barium enema or fecal occult blood testing to screen the remaining colon for malignancies. For this purpose, however, colonoscopy has largely replaced flexible sigmoidoscopy (FS). FS is still useful in evaluating the severity of a flare of known ulcerative colitis, suspected ischemic or infectious colitis, to obtain colon biopsies in suspected microscopic colitis or to evaluate radiographic abnormalities seen in the left colon.

Learning when to use each scope is a skill that comes with guidance and experience and can vary from one individual to another. Just as a golfer learns which club he/she can use most effectively in given circumstances, the endoscopist too must develop an understanding of which scope they can best employ from one case to the next. When a particular type of scope is preferred for a procedure, trainees should get in the habit of including that request at the time of booking, to better ensure that it will be available in the endoscopy unit when it is time to perform the case.

Sedation

From the patient's perspective, sedation and analgesia are two of the most important issues linked to procedure satisfaction. Considering that success of colonoscopy as a screening exam relies on serial evaluations at least every 10 years, a patient's avoidance of pursuing repeat evaluations due to prior bad experiences can lead to potential premalignant lesions or other disease going undetected and advancing to more serious disease. Sedation, analgesia, and patient monitoring in endoscopy are covered in greater detail in another chapter of this text. In general, the use of a benzodiazepine (midazolam or diazepam) in combination with analgesia (meperidine or fentanyl) provides adequate conscious sedation for lower endoscopy. These agents work synergistically in providing sedation while the benzodiazepine provides an added amnestic effect. However, in some instances, deeper sedation may be needed. Diprivan or even general anesthesia can be used for these patients.

Indication/contraindications

All trainees need a solid understanding as to when a colonoscopy should be performed, and perhaps more importantly when it should be avoided. One of the most common indications for a colonoscopy is as a screening exam for colorectal cancer. In the general population, these exams begin at the age of 50 years, and if normal, every 10 years thereafter. If a few small polyps are found, this frequency is increased to every 5 years. Certain other indications, such as more numerous polyps, larger polyps, advanced dysplasia, villous architecture, or hereditary polyposis syndromes, can result in initiating early screening before the age of 50 or increase the frequency of exams to every 3 years. In the case of particularly large or advanced polyps, a follow-up examination within 3 months may be required to ensure complete resection of the lesion. Screening guidelines are frequently updated and every endoscopist must keep current with the most recent recommendations. These guidelines can typically be found online at professional society Web sites such as the American Society for Gastrointestinal Endoscopy (ASGE), American College of Gastroenterology (ACG), or American Gastroenterology Association (AGA) [2,3].

Other indications for colonoscopic exam are primarily symptom driven. Of these, suspicion for GI bleeding (iron deficiency anemia, positive stool occult blood tests, or even frank hematochezia) is likely the most common cause for lower endoscopy [4]. A change in bowel habits (stool caliber, constipation, or chronic diarrhea), suspicion of inflammatory bowel disease, abdominal pain, and abnormal radiographic imaging studies are all common indications to pursue colonoscopy as well. Other less common causes include foreign body removal, volvulus reduction or decompression of colonic pseudo-obstruction.

As stated earlier, there are times when it is not safe to proceed with colonoscopy. These include recent colon surgery, recent myocardial infarction (MI), the presence of severe colitis, supratherapeutic anticoagulation, or the presence of hemodynamic instability [4]. It is advised to delay colonoscopic exam for 3 months following colonic surgery, such as a new stoma or other colonic anastomosis. In the case of a recent MI, there are no specific guidelines regarding this. For elective procedures, one should wait until well after the even and base timing on the patient's clinical status. Emergent colonoscopy for gastrointestinal bleeding following an MI has been studied. Though there is roughly a ninefold increase in complications (9% vs. 1%), these complications are usually minor and generally the patients benefit more from timely intervention [5]. These are relative contraindications and earlier exams can be performed if clinically required. In "severe" colitis (as can be associated with infections, Crohn's, ulcerative colitis, or ischemic colitis), it is generally advised to reduce the colonic inflammation before proceeding with endoscopy; however, limited exams can be indicated if the cause of colitis is unclear or to monitor the response to therapy. Mild to moderate colitis typically do not pose a contraindication to colonoscopy. For patients on anticoagulation therapy (such as Warfarin, Clopidogrel, or ASA), institutions vary with the level of acceptable risk, but in general, low-risk diagnostic exams can likely be safely performed on some level of therapeutic-range anticoagulation [6]. Therapeutic measures (such as biopsy or polypectomy) may require lower anticoagulation thresholds or even discontinuation of therapy prior to colonoscopy for safety reasons. Endoscopy should be delayed if levels of anticoagulation are supratherapeutic. Trainees should read and remain current on published guidelines on the practice of endoscopy for patients taking anticoagulation medications which are available online at www.asge.org.

Early motor skills

How to hold scope

The scope handle is held in the left hand with the umbilical cable that connects to the video processor resting between the thumb and index finger (Figure 5.8). The base of the scope handle is held between the palm and the fourth and fifth digit. The left elbow is bent in a comfortable position to allow the arm to carry the weight of the scope for long periods of time. The right hand holds the shaft of the scope and is kept within 20–30 cm from the anal opening to allow maximum control of the shaft. The height of the bed should be at a level that allows the endoscopist to stand with the hips and back straight to avoid overuse of the back muscles. In this position, the right elbow should also be bent at roughly 90°. Trainees need to be instructed early on how to correctly set the high of the bed, proper posture, and position of the arms. Improper posture or form can lead to muscle fatigue and chronic musculoskeletal problems over an endoscopist's career [7].

Scope dials

On the medial side of the scope, there are two dials with sprockets (Figure 5.9). These dials control the deflection of the flexible scope tip and are used to steer the scope during advancement and to direct the video camera's field of view during mucosal inspection on the withdrawal phase of the exam. The large inner dial deflects the scope tip up (counterclockwise dial rotation) and down (clockwise). The smaller outer dial controls left (clockwise) and right (counterclockwise) tip deflection. Since the orientation of the camera in the scope's tip is fixed in relation to the control mechanisms, the direction of tip deflection is always in relation to the video image on the display monitor, regardless of how the scope is torqued. Ideally, both dials are controlled with the left thumb, but as you will see later, the smaller dial is used less

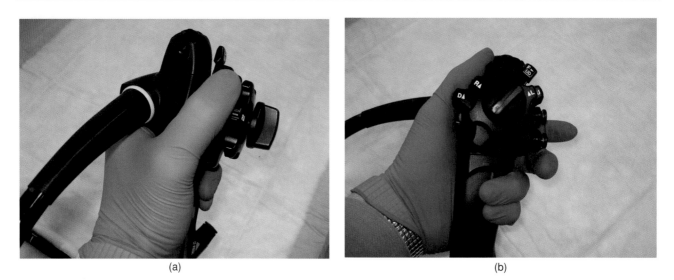

(a)   (b)

Figure 5.8 How to hold the scope? These images demonstrate the proper manner in which to hold a colonoscope. (a) The scope is held in the left hand with the cable exiting posteriorly between the thumb and index finger. (b) The handle is held with the fourth and fifth digits freeing the thumb and remaining fingers to operate the controls.

frequently as most steering directions can be achieved with rotation of the scope and the up/down control alone.

Next to these dials there are two levers that can be used to lock their respective dial in place in order to hold the scope tip in a deflected position and free up the endoscopist's hands during therapeutic maneuvers. In general, however, it is important to remember that during the scope advancement or withdrawal, these dials should be "unlocked" in order to reduce the risk of colonic perforation due to a rigid scope tip.

Scope valves

In the front of the scope handle, there are two valves (Figure 5.10). The upper "red" color-coded valve provides suction through the

working channel of the scope. When pressed all the way in, the suction can be used to remove air from the colon and improve mucosal visualization by suctioning up retained liquid within the colon, or when a trap is employed in the suctioning circuit, it can be used to retrieve removed polyps (Figure 5.11). This valve is typically controlled with the left index finger.

The lower "blue" valve has dual functions of air insufflation and water rinse of the camera lens. This valve can be controlled with either the index finger or middle finger. When the fingertip is lightly placed occluding the hole in the middle of the valve, air is forced down the scope, resulting in inflation of the colon lumen. One common error many trainees make is to "rest" their finger over this opening, resulting in over inflation. Care must be

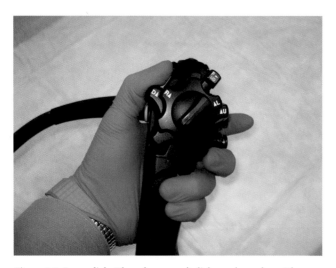

Figure 5.9 Scope dials. The colonoscope's dials are shown here. The large inner dial deflects the scope tip up or down as indicated by the arrows. Similarly, the small outer dial deflects the scope tip left or right.

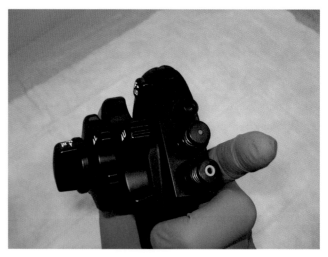

Figure 5.10 Scope valves. The top "red" valve activates the scope's suction when pressed. The "blue" valve controls air insufflation when lightly touched as well as water to rinse off the lens when fully pressed.

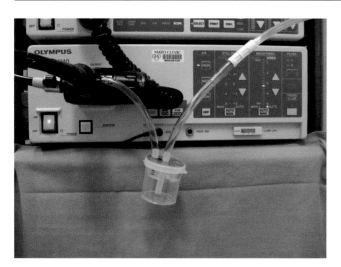

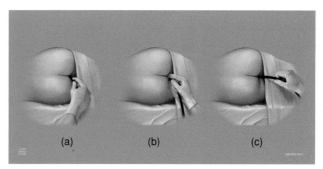

Figure 5.12 Rectal intubation techniques. This illustration demonstrates the three common methods of inserting the scope through the anal canal: (a) tangential approach, (b) along-side finger, and (c) straight insertion. (Copyrighted and used with permission of Mayo Foundation for Medical Education and Research.)

Figure 5.11 Trap in suction circuit. When a polyp is removed with a snare, a trap is needed to collect the tissue. This trap is placed in the circuit of the scope's suction line. This trap allows liquid and air to be suctioned normally but traps larger particles such as polyp tissue in a small chamber. This allows the removed polyp to be collected by suctioning it up through the working channel of the scope by pressing the red valve.

taken to limit the amount of air used during endoscopy as excessive distention of the colon results in greater patient discomfort as well as increasing the risk of colonic perforation (particularly in the thin-walled cecum). The second function of the valve (water rinse of the camera lens) is achieved by pressing the blue valve in completely. This results in a fine jet of high pressured water to be sprayed horizontally across the tip of the scope, rinsing away adherent debris that can reduce or obscure the camera's visualization of the colon. Some colonoscopes also include a special port for irrigation of the colon controlled by a foot pedal. This can be used to clean the colonic mucosal to improve inspection when suboptimal preparations are encountered. An alternative to this is simply injecting water through the biopsy port of the scope using a large syringe. A small amount of simethicone can be added to this water if bubbly or foamy fluid is encountered.

Scope insertion

Prior to insertion of the scope, a digital rectal exam is performed for the dual purpose of lubricating the anal canal as well as examining the canal for pathology and patency. The right hand is ideally double gloved so that following the rectal exam the outer glove can be removed and discarded without the need for regloving. The scope handle is draped over the endoscopists left shoulder or laid on the bed freeing the left hand to lift the upper gluteal fold exposing the anal canal. The anal area is visually inspected for pathology and then the rectal exam performed with the right index finger. Following the exam, the outer glove is discarded. The distal 20 cm of the scope is then liberally lubricated. The scope insertion into the rectum is then performed by one of the following manners (Figure 5.12) (Video 5.2):

1 *Tangential approach:* The scope is held in the right hand at about 10 cm with the index finger down near the tip. The scope tip is then positioned at the anal canal at roughly a 45° angle. The index finger then gently pushes the tip of the scope though the anal canal and the scope is then advanced. This technique gives better control of the tip during insertion. With this technique and the next, the second (outer) glove on the right hand remains on until after scope insertion and can then be removed and discarded.
2 *Along-side finger:* The right index finger is inserted into the anal canal and the scope is inserted along side this as the finger is withdrawn.
3 *Straight insertion:* The scope is held with the right hand at about 20 cm from the tip and is positioned perpendicular to the anal canal. The scope tip is the then inserted straight into the rectum. This is probably the most direct approach and most commonly used method.

Scope advancement

Once in the rectum, the objective is to advance the scope quickly and safely to the cecum. In order to accomplish this, the endoscopist needs to be able to steer the scope tip in the direction desired. This is done with a combination of the scope dials as well as torque of the scope. Being able to locate the colonic lumen when lost is also a mandatory early skill. Barring looping of the scope or tight angulations, the cecum can sometimes be reached with these simple techniques alone. Other skills such as loop reduction, navigation of angulated turns, and TI intubation will be covered later in this chapter.

Tip control

The large (up/down) dial is controlled with the thumb. The scope's camera is fixed in relation to the scope's axis, hence the up or down deflection described earlier is always in relation to the image on the video monitor. "Up deflection" of the camera (or "thumb down" on the dial) will always deflect the scope towards the top of the image displayed on the video screen and "down deflection" (or "thumb up") will always aim the camera towards the bottom of the screen. For the teacher and student alike, it helps for the training center to conform to a single use of terms describing the desired

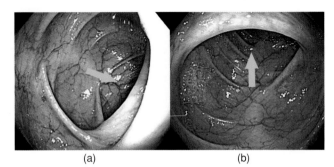

(a)　　　　　　　　(b)

Figure 5.13 Torque to change from horizontal to vertical. The two images depict the same turn but in different orientations. In the first image (a), the turn goes off to the right and would require the use of the small left/right dial to navigate. However, after torque of the scope shaft 90° clockwise, this turn is now oriented vertically (b) and can now be navigated with the large dial alone.

action such as always using the terms "steer up" and "steer down" vs. "thumb down" and "thumb up." Most find that describing which direction you want the camera to steer in relation to the video image as the most intuitive method as opposed to advising which way to turn the wheel with their thumb.

Torque

As trainees will quickly find, reaching the thumb to the smaller right/left dial can be difficult and awkward. Many trainees early in their training will be tempted to remove their right hand from the scope shaft and use this hand to turn the small dial. Fortunately, with correct technique, the use of this dial can be minimized. The most efficient method of steering is combining torque with use of the up/down dial. In general, experienced endoscopists would agree that, rather than using excessive right/left dial control, it is better to teach the use of scope torque in either direction to reorient the right or left turns in the lumen so that they are oriented towards the top or bottom of the screen. This is accomplished with the right hand rotating the shaft of the scope. Firm torque of the scope's shaft in the desired direction can rotate the entire shaft of the scope inside the patient and realign a horizontal turn in the lumen to one that is vertically oriented (Figure 5.13). Once in this position, the large up/down dial can be used to steer in the direction desired.

Scope advancement techniques

There are three techniques used to handle the scope.

The "one-handed" technique is the one most commonly used by experienced colonoscopists as it provides the most uninterrupted control of the scope shaft and is best suited to the predominant use of torque to maneuver the instrument (Figure 5.14). In this method, the dials are controlled with the left hand alone, relying primarily on the up/down dial. The right hand remains on the shaft of the scope providing torque, advancement, and withdrawal of the scope. Occasionally, the right can be brought up to control the smaller right/left dial but only with particularly tight turns, such as the splenic or hepatic flexure, where torque and up/down deflection may not be sufficient.

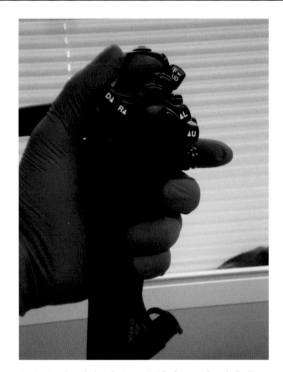

Figure 5.14 One-handed technique. With the one-handed advancement technique, all of the dial control is done by the left hand, primarily using the large dial. The right hand is responsible for providing torque and advancement, and generally does not leave the scope shaft.

The "two-handed" technique is favored by some experts who feel that when the thumb is used to cross over to the small dial, fine control of the large dial is not possible. Additionally, the left thumb cannot maximally deflect the small dial in either direction. Once the right hand has turned the small dial, it can be temporarily locked in this position to hold the intended deflection while the right hand returns to the scope shaft (Figure 5.15). The major drawback to this technique is the intermittent interruption of control of the scope shaft with the right hand. When the hand is off the shaft, the scope frequently can fall back unintentionally or rotate due to loops. Many endoscopists who employ the two-handed technique can compensate for this decreased shaft control by positioning the scope shaft so that it hangs down by the side of the table, pinning the scope shaft between the endoscopist's thigh and the side of the bed and rapidly moving the right hand back and forth between shaft and the outer small dial. Another stabilization method is to loop the left fifth digit around the scope shaft, pinning it against the left palm while the right hand is busy maneuvering the right/left dial [8].

A third method is called the "two-person" technique and is rarely used. It involves the endoscopist using the two hands to control the dials exclusively while an assistant advances the shaft of the scope at their order.

Lumen identification

During endoscopy, experienced endoscopists occasionally find it difficult to identify where the lumen is due to factors such as

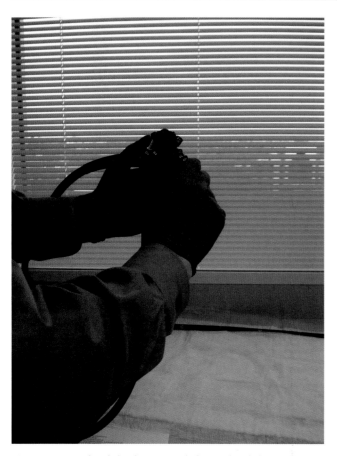

Figure 5.15 Two-handed technique. With the two-handed technique, the right hand is moved back and forth between the shaft of the scope and the small right/left dial, while the left thumb controls the large inner dial.

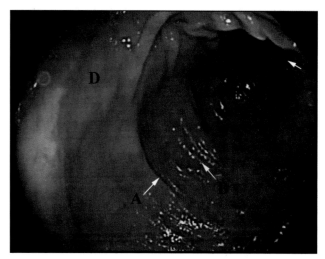

Figure 5.16 Lumen identification. When the lumen cannot be readily identified, clues such as (A) the arcs of the colon folds, small arcs of reflected light off of the ripples of muscular rings (B), or the area of shadow behind a bright fold (C) can help. Following the indentation of the tinea coli (D) can also guide the endoscopist around acute angulations.

acute angulations, numerous large diverticula, or inadequate colon preparation. Novice endoscopists, however, find factors such as red-out (tip of the scope up against the colon wall), or inability to recognize clues to indicate the direction of the lumen, to be far more common. In the case where the lumen cannot be seen, it is always advisable for the trainee to slowly pull back on the scope until they are away from the wall or until the lumen again becomes visible. In order to avoid perforation, a trainee should never continue pushing inward on the scope if the lumen is not visible.

Once away from the wall and red-out corrected, there are a number of clues that can help the endoscopist identify the direction of the lumen. The most common is observing the direction of the haustral folds. The concave portions of the folds point in the direction of the lumen. The second is the use of shadows. When identifying a bright fold close to the scope and a dark shadow behind this, the lumen is often behind this fold. A third method that is often helpful in guiding the endoscopist is following the tinea coli. The length of any of the three tinea coli will point in the direction the lumen is turning.

Similar to following the haustral folds as described above, ripples in the colon wall created by the circular muscle layer of the colon can also be used. When the colonoscope light reflects off

of these arcuate ripples, steering the scope towards the concave portion of the arc should guide the endoscopist in the direction of the lumen.

All of these techniques can be used alone or in combination to help the endoscopist find their way to the cecum (Figure 5.16) (Video 5.3).

Withdrawal/inspection

Once the cecum is reached, the most important portion of the exam begins, that is careful inspection of the colon for pathology. In many instances, pathology such as polyps will be seen during the insertion phase and if desired can be treated at that time. Many endoscopists may also simply note the location of the lesion during insertion and take care of it during the withdrawal phase.

The first key to adequate visibility is adequate insufflation. Instilling air into the colon requires a balance between ensuring the colonic folds are adequately distended yet without creating too much tension on the colon wall and discomfort for the patient. Trainees often make the mistakes of using too little air or conversely leaving their finger on the air valve all of the time. Care must be taken and the endoscopist must always be cognizant of the degree of insufflation of the colon and patient comfort levels.

The second important factor of proper withdrawal technique is to ensure the colonic mucosa and the camera lens is clean enough to allow optimal visualization. The colon preparation often does not completely clear the colon of fecal debris. Suction can be used alone or in combination with water lavage. Some scopes are capable of having automatic water lavage controlled by a foot pedal while others require manual injection of water. With the latter, water can be instilled to lavage the colon using a large (60 cc) syringe injected through the biopsy port just below the scope handle. As one injects, the scope is aimed with the dials and torque at the area in need of cleansing. After cleansing, suctioning is then used by positioning the scope so that the suction port is below the surface of the puddle but the camera lens in not. The location of this port varies modestly based on the model and type of scope used. The suction button is then used and the scope repositioned as needed until the liquid is removed. This process often needs to be repeated multiple times throughout the colon to achieve adequate visualization. Trainees will frequently put the scope tip too deep into a puddle and obscure their view or repeatedly suctioning too close to the colon wall resulting in the mucosa being pulled into the suction port. If this occurs, the suction holding the mucosa in the port can be broken by either pulling the scope tip away from the mucosa or by briefly breaking the seal of the rubber biopsy port cap at the scopes handle base, thereby relieving the vacuum in the biopsy channel of the scope.

The next important skill is the development of a slow, careful inspection pattern. Inspection is carried out by developing a circular inspection pattern as the scope is slowly pulled back. This circular pattern does not necessarily need to be done with the scope tip but more with the eyes and only augmented by minor deflections of the scope tip as needed to see the entire circumference of the lumen. Scope readjustments are an ongoing process involving not only the use of the dial controls but also torque of the scope to keep the tip in the center of the lumen. As the scope passes larger folds, it is often necessary to readvance the scope just above the fold and use greater deflection of the scope tip with the dials to view behind the fold and ensure pathology is not missed. In experienced endoscopists, it is felt that a minimum of 6–7 minutes is needed to examine the entire colon adequately [9,10]. For trainees, this process initially takes much longer due to their developing skills of scope control, inspection behind folds and pathology recognition. As skills advance, this inspection time will gradually decline. Trainees must clearly understand that while average withdrawal time is a surrogate marker for a careful exam, the key objective is complete mucosal inspection; areas poorly seen due to the colonoscope "jumping" past folds or due to puddles must be reexamined, even if it means reinserting the scope as needed to reinspect.

The final maneuver of a colonoscopy is retroflexion within the rectum. This is performed to better inspect the distal rectum for very low-lying polyps, internal hemorrhoids, or other perianal pathology. This is best accomplished by returning the patient to their left side if they have been repositioned during the exam. The scope is then inserted to the first (or most distal) semilunar valve in the rectum at roughly 10–12 cm from the anal verge. The large dial is then deflected maximally upwards while at the same time the shaft of the scope is torqued in either direction roughly 180° and the scope inserted another few centimeters. When these three steps are done simultaneously, it should result in a view of the distal rectum with the scope shaft entering the rectal vault (Figure 5.17). The scope is then torqued in either direction to obtain views of the entire circumference of the distal rectum. On some occasions, maximal deflection of the large dial is not enough and the addition of small dial deflection in one direction or the other is needed in order to successfully retroflex the scope. This maneuver should be done with care as it is often uncomfortable for the patient and can

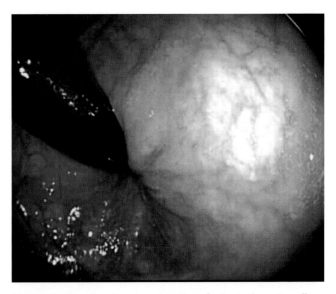

Figure 5.17 Retroflex views in rectum. Retroflexion in the rectum allows for better visualization of the distal rectum where polyps or other pathology such as internal hemorrhoids can often be found.

result in perforation of the rectum if too much force or torque is used against resistance. If difficulty is encountered, maximally bending the knees towards the chest can also aid in retroflexion, though this is usually not necessary.

Intermediate skills

In this section, the focus will be on those cognitive and motor skills required to be proficient at routine colonoscopy. Specifically, this section will address the cognitive skills of pathology recognition, the selection and settings of basic therapeutic devices, and the management of complications. The motor skills addressed here will include the basic management of loops, difficult turns, TI intubation, and the use of the basic biopsy cable and snare. More advanced skills such as those needed in complex or therapeutic endoscopy will be covered in later chapters.

Intermediate cognitive skills

Pathology recognition
Colonoscopy is not simply reaching the cecum and performing a careful inspection during withdrawal; it also involves the ability to identify and manage potential pathologic findings such as polyps or inflammation. Skilled detection of abnormalities requires a careful inspection process and rapid recognition of variances in the mucosa. The method of inspection was discussed earlier in this chapter. Here, the stress will be on the development of recognition of abnormalities. This skill of rapid pathology identification by experienced endoscopists is a result of the cognitive skill of pattern recognition. Pattern recognition is the ability to quickly identify small changes and understand their meaning, much like a master chess player can look at a complex arrangement of chess pieces on a board and quickly understanding the implications,

such as which player will eventually win the game and how it can be done. This pattern recognition is the key factor that allows an experienced endoscopist to quickly scan the mucosa and continue the withdrawal with greater speed than trainees. This skill typically is acquired only with experiencing first-hand the broad spectrum of normal and abnormal findings with considerable repetition (Figure 5.18). Over time and with careful supervision and guidance by instructors, this skill is eventually acquired to a sufficient level to operate independently (competence), but skills will

continue to be honed throughout the lifetime of the endoscopist. Education researchers have suggested that it takes roughly 10,000 hours of experience to become a "master" at whatever it is one wishes to do, be it playing chess, sports, or performing endoscopy [11]. Basic competence, however, occurs much earlier, yet what defines basic competence in this skill is difficult to assess. Later in this chapter, we will discuss how best to teach these skills of pathology recognition as well as how best to assess these skills as the trainee works towards competence.

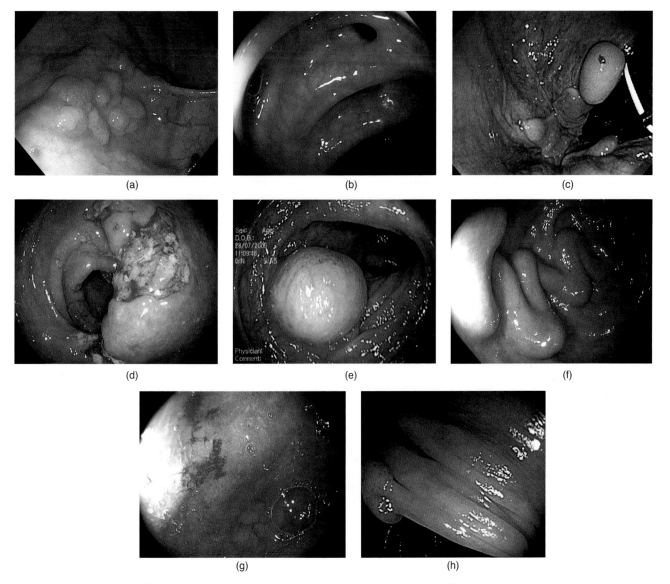

Figure 5.18 Some examples of key colonic abnormalities that trainees should be able to recognize and properly identify: (a) Laterally spreading adenoma in cecum. (Mount Sinai School of Medicine.) (b) HRE white light nonmagnified view of a diverticulum. (NYU School of Medicine.) (c) Retroflexed view in rectum of hypertrophied anal papilla. (Mount Sinai School of Medicine.) (d) Ulcerated cecum in a patient with confirmed celiac disease and ASCA positive Crohn's disease. (NYU School of Medicine.) (e) White light HRE view of colon lipoma.

(Hospital Sao Marcos.) (f) Tortuous rectal varix under white light low-magnification HRE view. (NYU School of Medicine.) (g) Nonmagnified white light HRE view of a cecal angioectasia. (NYU School of Medicine.) (h) Prior India ink tatoo with polyp partially hidden behind a fold. (Mount Sinai School of Medicine.) (Contributed with permission from *Advanced Digestive Endoscopy: Comprehensive Atlas of High-Resolution Endoscopy and Narrowband Imaging.* Edited by J. Cohen. Blackwell Publishing. 2007: pp 269, 271, 295, 304, 306, 307, 311, 312.)

Device selection and settings

As fellows begin to identify pathology such as polyps, the next cognitive skill that must be acquired is how to best manage the abnormality. Part of this management is the hands-on motor skills of applying therapy and will be covered later in this chapter. The cognitive components of this skill include selection of the ideal device, such as a cold/hot biopsy forceps or cold/electrocautery snare. Additionally, if electrocautery is used, one must also understand what settings to use on the current generator to ensure ablation of the pathologic findings yet minimize risks of post-treatment ulcerations, bleeding, or perforation. As with all skills that require coordination with an assistant, trainees must become facile with communication of directions. This section will focus on these basic issues as they pertain to simple polyp removal.

The goal of polyp removal is for both diagnostic purposes (histology) as well as therapeutic to ensure no residual adenomatous tissue remains. Very small polyps (<3 mm) can typically be removed effectively with simple cold biopsy (i.e., no electrocautery). This is performed by grasping the polyp with a biopsy forceps. The open forceps is placed over the polyp and closed to grasp the entire polyp. With a quick tugging maneuver, the polyp is plucked off the mucosal surface and the cable withdrawn. The tissue is saved for diagnostic microscopic examination. This process results in only a small amount of oozing at the biopsy site and rarely results in any immediate or delayed complications.

Slightly larger polyps (3–5 mm) pose a different problem. Simple cold biopsy tends not to completely remove the polyp. Some endoscopists will commonly take multiple cold biopsies until the polyp appears removed. This approach is safe but runs the risk of leaving some small amount of adenoma behind. One alternative is to convert to using "hot" biopsy (i.e., biopsy augmented with electrocautery.) This uses a special biopsy cable that also acts as a monopolar conductor that is connected to a power generator. Monopolar devices require placement of a grounding pad on the patient (typically on the hip or thigh), which is also connected back to the ground outlet on the power source to complete the circuit. The polyp is then grasped by the biopsy cable. The polyp is lifted tenting up its attachment to the colon wall. Care is taken to ensure the cable or gasped tissue is not touching any other part of the colon, such as the wall opposite the polyp. This is to ensure collateral cautery injury does not occur. The endoscopist then pushes a foot pedal that activates the generator sending a current of electricity down the cable, through the polyp and patient to the grounding pad and back to the generator's ground. This current results in heat due to the conductive resistance of the tissue, resulting in destruction of tissue at the polyp site. Typically pure coagulation current is used with a power setting of 15–20 watts [12]. Some would argue lower settings can reduce the risk for post-polypectomy ablation complications [13]. The polyp is then plucked off as with cold biopsy and collected for pathologic examination. The heating effect created by the current is most intense at the cable/tissue interface and as the current runs deeper through the tissue, this effect dissipates based on the distance from the cable/tissue interface. Although this results in good ablation of polypoid tissue, this also results in injury of surrounding tissue. As this injury heals during the ensuring days, the injured tissue sloughs off and an ulcer develops at the site as part of the body's attempt to clear injured tissue. In most cases, this does not result in problems and these ulcerations will heal without symptoms to the patient. In some instances though, as the ulcer develops, it can erode into a vessel, resulting in sudden onset of GI bleeding. This complication typically occurs 4–7 days after the procedure. Deeper tissue injury can also result in serosal inflammation (resulting in post-polypectomy electrocoagulation syndrome of focal peritoneal pain) or even transmural injury with perforation [14,15]. These two complications are of particular concern with the use of cautery in the cecum where the colon wall is the thinnest. These complications are uncommon yet great care must be taken to minimize injury to adjacent tissue. The depth and degree of injury is dependent on the power used (watts) and duration of current (how long the foot peddle is pressed). Fellows not uncommonly use current for too long of a period. For most polyps, using power settings of 15–20 watts is reasonable with the duration limited to just long enough to see a *hint* of desiccation (white halo of tissue ablation) around the polyp base. This is typically accomplished in roughly one second, but this can vary depending on the polyp's size. In the cecum, cold techniques (biopsy or snare as below) are preferable, but if cautery is needed, a lower setting such as 12–14 watts should be used [12].

The use of cold snare polyp removal is becoming an increasingly used alternative to hot biopsy for polyps in the range of 3–8 mm. This is with the idea that it might reduce the risk of post-electrocautery complications as outlined above. This technique is performed by placing an open snare around the polyp with the snare's catheter near the base of the polyp (Figure 5.19). The snare is then slowly closed by an endoscopy assistant until the wire loop is snuggly around the base of the polyp. Care must be taken to ensure as little normal surrounding tissue is caught within the loop of the snare but also that the entire polyp is included. The assistant is then instructed to apply greater force to cause the wire loop to close further and cut through the tissue at the base of the polyp. The snare is then removed and the polyp tissue is then suctioned up through the scope and collected in a trap placed in the suction circuit. Cold snare polyp removal is quite effective for these slightly larger (3–8 mm) polyps and does not result in much immediate bleeding despite their increased size.

If the polyp is too large, the snare will not be able to cut through the thick tissue without the assistance of electrocautery. For polyps greater than roughly 8 mm in size, electrocautery is typically used with the snare. The process is identical to the cold snare technique except once the polyp is grasped snuggly in the snare, a monopolar current is then passed through the snare wire. To allow the wire to cut through the thicker tissue and to prevent bleeding, a blended current (both cutting and coagulation) is often used with the same power settings as in hot biopsy; however, many practitioners often utilize pure coagulation current. As the current flows through the polyp base, the endoscopy assistant applies greater force on the closing loop, allowing the wire to cut through the polyp base. This current also helps ablate any tiny foci of adenomatous tissue around the perimeter of the polypectomy site. The assistant should be advised not to close the snare too quickly as this can reduce the cautery effects on the underlying vessels and result in bleeding

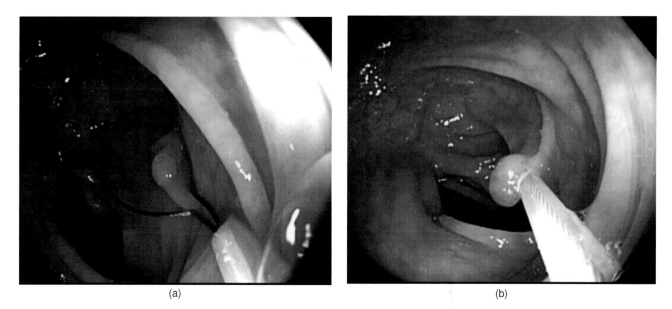
(a)   (b)

Figure 5.19 Snare polypectomy. When a snare is required to remove a polyp, the loop of the snare is opened and placed around the polyp base (a) with the end of the catheter tip near the polyp. The snare is then closed around the polyp base (b) and removed either with or without cautery by fully closing the snare loop.

at the polypectomy site. Like hot biopsy, however, electrocautery snare also runs the risk of post-polypectomy ulceration and complications. To help minimize deeper tissue injury, once the polyp is grasped by forceps or snare, the polyp should be lifted up away from the wall to "tent" up the mucosal away from the deeper layers. Again, great care must be taken to avoid touching the opposite wall or adjacent folds with the cautery device or polypoid tissue to avoid inadvertent thermal injury to these unintended areas. If the wall is too taught to lift it up, suction can be used to reduce the wall tension and "soften-up" the area to allow better lifting. For larger polyps, the mucosal layer can be lifted using an endoscopy needle to inject saline (or other agent) to create a fluid cushion between the mucosa and the deeper layers [16]. This technique will be covered in a later chapter.

The use of any monopolar device (biopsy cable, snare, argon plasma coagulation) all work by sending a current through the patient and need to be used with great care in patients with pacemakers or defibrillators, as the current can cause these devices to malfunction or discharge (defibrillator), resulting in harm to the patient or injury to the endoscopist. If monopolar cautery is to be used, the patient should have cardiac monitoring and the defibrillator should be turned off while cautery is in use. Pacemakers should be interrogated by a specialist following endoscopy to ensure proper functioning. As discussed in the section on preparation, cautery should be avoided in an unprepared or poorly prepared colon due to the risk of igniting the flammable gases present in the colon.

Complication management

As with any procedure, colonoscopy has risks. These range from over-sedation, hypoxia, and other airway or hemodynamic problems to complications more directly related to the scope itself, such as bleeding or perforation. Sedation complications and endoscopic hemostasis will be discussed elsewhere in this book. This section will address the management of colonic perforation.

One of the most feared complications is perforation of the viscera. The risk for this is low with perforation rates of roughly 1 in 1,000 for colonoscopy [17]. Perforation can occur in a number of ways. One cause is from the scope tip exerting too much pressure on the wall of the colon when incorrect technique is used by attempting to advance the scope while in "red-out." This occurs when novices attempt to blindly push the scope around tight turns in the colon or when the endoscopist inadvertently intubates a diverticulum. For this reason, all trainees are warned from day one of training, not to advance the scope if the lumen is not visualized. This is the most avoidable method of perforation. When a trainee cannot find the lumen, it is always advisable to slowly pull the scope back specifically to avoid perforation. The second, and probably one of the more common causes of perforation with more experienced endoscopists, is injury to the sigmoid due to excessive looping in this region even though the scope tip may be well beyond this portion of the colon (Figure 5.20). An excessive loop can exert too much lateral pressure on the colon wall, causing a tear. This can be avoided by using repetitive loop reduction techniques and avoidance of excessive pushing force against significant resistance. Severe patient discomfort can also be a warning of excessive loop force against the colon wall. Excess air insufflating the colon can also lead to perforation. This leads to ballooning of the colon and subsequent perforation of the cecum (thinnest wall of the colon). Finally, retroflexion in the rectum also can lead to perforation due to incorrect technique or simply due to attempting the maneuver in a rectum that is too small to accommodate the maneuver. This maneuver should be avoided in patients with significant active inflammatory bowel disease

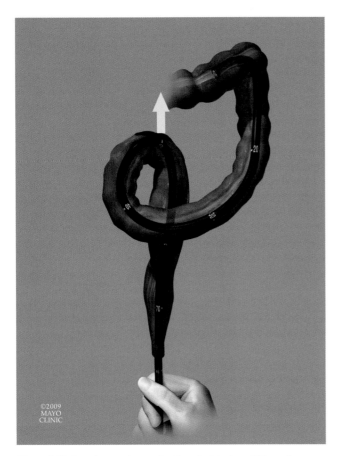

Figure 5.20 Looping causing perforation. In this sigmoid loop, the scope is pushing against the wall of the sigmoid colon in the direction of the arrow. One cause of perforation is due to excessive lateral pressure against the colon wall from a loop in the colon and scope. (Copyrighted and used with permission of Mayo Foundation for Medical Education and Research.)

involving the rectum. In the hands of more experienced endoscopists, perforations still occur but typically with therapeutic maneuvers, such as complex polypectomy.

The key to managing colonic perforation is early recognition. Often if the perforation is caused by the scope's tip, the peritoneal cavity, organs, or serosa will be readily visible to the camera lens. When perforation occurs as a result of looping, the defect and fresh blood will commonly be identified during withdrawal. Commonly with perforations, the patient will develop increased distention of the abdomen due to free air or worsening abdominal pain either during the procedure or in recovery. If perforation is at all suspected, immediate evaluation with a flat and upright abdominal X-ray is indicated to evaluate for free peritoneal air. If identified, immediate evaluation and likely intervention by a surgeon is required. Delay in intervention can lead to sepsis and even death. Attempts at endoscopic closure of perforations using hemoclips or other closure devises will be discussed in another chapter; however, surgical intervention is still the gold standard. Endoscopic closure of defects should only be attempted by skilled endoscopists. Less commonly, perforations may be retroperitoneal

(as can occur in the distal rectum) and walled off. In these cases, free air will not be identified on abdominal X-ray. In these cases CT scanning would be needed to identify and locate the problem. These can often be managed more conservatively with fasting and IV antibiotics with close inpatient monitoring. Occasionally, incidental radiographic findings of free air in the peritoneal cavity occur following endoscopy, yet in the absence of any clinical symptoms of perforation. The clinical significance, if any, of these findings is unclear, yet conservative management and close observation also is recommended.

Training fellows to manage perforations is difficult, as these do not occur often. The main teaching point is to never underappreciate or deny to oneself the possibility of a perforation. If there is any suspicion that a perforation has occurred, this needs to be aggressively pursued with diagnostic and therapeutic intervention as needed. In the event of a perforation, it is also paramount that the endoscopist personally stays in direct communication with the patient and family and not to simply ship the patient off to the emergency room and distance oneself from the case.

Intermediate motor skills

Loop reduction

One of the hardest skills for trainees to master is the prevention and adequate reduction of loops that develop during scope advancement. This section will address the common types and locations of loops that form and how to manage these effectively. One key concept to understand with loop formation is that of "force vectors." Force vectors are where and in what direction the majority of the pushing force is being delivered in the colon. If a scope is perfectly straight, all of the force is being translated directly into tip advancement. If there is a 90° or greater turn, much of this force is directed at the wall of the colon on the outside part of the turn (Figure 5.21). As the wall pushes back, some of this opposing force gets delivered forward to the scope tip, resulting in advancement, some back to the operator as resistance and some absorbed by the elastic nature of the colon wall as a loop. Reducing and straightening these loops not only removes the force against the colon wall but with correct technique can result in prevention of recurrent loop formation and better delivery of the pushing force to the scope tip.

The sigmoid colon is the location where most loops occur. This is due to the serpentine nature of this section of colon accompanied by the fact that it is freely mobile within the abdominal cavity. The most common natural course of the sigmoid is a clockwise spiral between the rectum and descending colon. As the tip of the scope makes the first acute turn from the rectum into the sigmoid and the scope is advanced, the shaft of the scope behind the flexible scope tip tends to be pushed upwards in the abdomen as the force vector of the scope is still relatively straight-in from the anus and rectum (Figure 5.22). This results in loss of "one-to-one" motion; a term meaning the scope is not advancing as much (or not at all) as the shaft of the scope is being pushed in. This extra inserted scope that is not resulting into tip advancement is instead contributing to the development of a loop. Looping can also result in "paradoxical

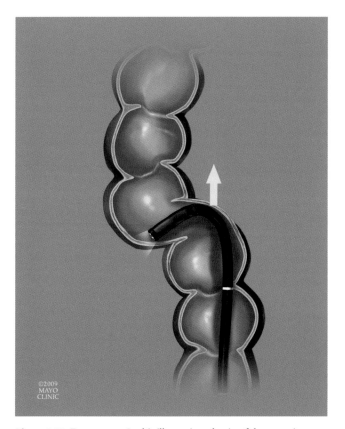

Figure 5.21 Force vector. In this illustration, the tip of the scope is deflected greater than 90° around an acute turn in the colon. In this configuration, the force vector (FV) of any attempts to advance the colon will be directed against the wall of the colon on the outside turn. This will be felt by the endoscopist as resistance to advancement or will result in looping of the scope shaft here or elsewhere in the colon. (Copyrighted and used with permission of Mayo Foundation for Medical Education and Research.)

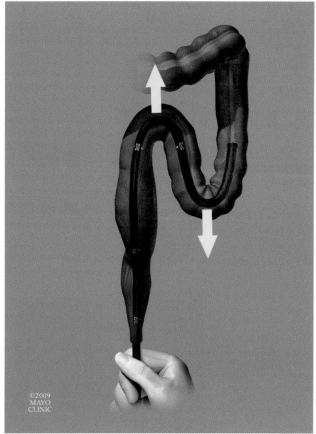

Figure 5.22 Sigmoid loop. As the scope makes multiple turns in the sigmoid colon, advancing the scope frequently results in the force being transmitted laterally against the sigmoid walls (arrows) resulting in loop formation. (Copyrighted and used with permission of Mayo Foundation for Medical Education and Research.)

movement" of the scope, which is when the scope tip actually moves in the opposite direction as the shaft is pushed or pulled.

There are three main types of loops that develop in the sigmoid colon. The "alpha-loop" is one of the most common and is termed this because the sigmoid is looped in a counterclockwise spiral in the shape of the Greek letter of its name (Figure 5.23) (Video 5.4). The second most common loop is the "N-loop" called this because it too is shaped like the letter of its name (Figure 5.24) (Video 5.5). This loop follows and exaggerates the normal S-shaped spiral of the sigmoid colon. Less common than these two is the "reverse alpha-loop" that follows a similar spiral to the alpha-loop but the more proximal sigmoid passes behind the more distal sigmoid (Figure 5.25) (Video 5.6). Which type of loop forms is likely due to variances in sigmoid anatomy? The method best suited for reduction of these sigmoid loops varies depending on the type of loop. In each of the loops, it is generally advisable to attempt to advance the scope beyond the splenic flexure, or other acute turn, if possible before attempting reduction. This allows the flexible portion of the scope tip to hook around this flexure and act as an anchor. This allows for greater direct force on the loop itself

during reduction and torques maneuvers. Once anchored, the dials are held with the left thumb to prevent the scope tip from straightening out and slipping back into the descending colon. The two most common types of loops (alpha- and N-loop) respond to slow scope withdrawal augmented by clockwise scope torque (Figures 5.23 and 5.24). During this maneuver, the tip of the scope may advance or simply remain motionless as the scope shaft is withdrawn. Clockwise torque and withdrawal of the shaft is continued until the scope tip begins to respond by starting to move backwards in a one-to-one manner. This is evidence that the loop has been reduced. Torque is key to the maneuver as this will untwist the spiral nature of the sigmoid and create a straighter lumen if done correctly. The most common cause for failure of this technique is either failure to withdraw enough scope to re-establish one-to-one motion or inadequate clockwise torque of the scope shaft during withdrawal. It is not uncommon to require 360° of torque or more during sigmoid reduction to adequately remove the spiral nature of this segment of the colon. Another cause of failure is the presence of a reverse alpha-loop. Suspicion of this should arise if the usual clockwise maneuver repeatedly fails.

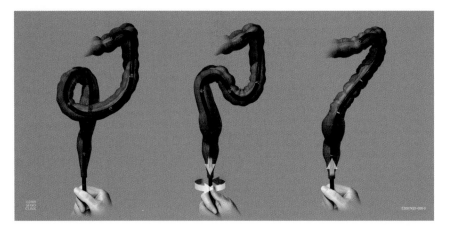

Figure 5.23 Alpha-loop. One of the most common types of sigmoid loop formation is the alpha-loop. This can be reduced with clockwise torque of the scope shaft as it is slowly pulled back. Once the loop is reduced, the scope shaft is again straight and can be readily advanced again. (Copyrighted and used with permission of Mayo Foundation for Medical Education and Research.)

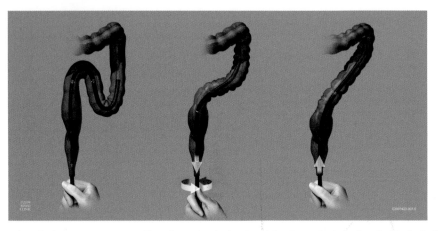

Figure 5.24 N-loop. The N-loop is also a common type of loop formation in the sigmoid and can also be reduced with clockwise torque and slow withdrawal like the alpha-loop. (Copyrighted and used with permission of Mayo Foundation for Medical Education and Research.)

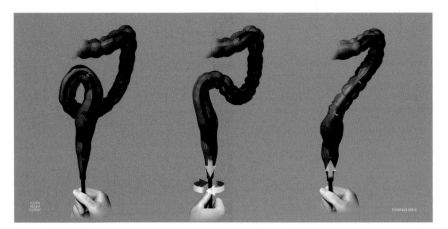

Figure 5.25 Reverse alpha-loop. A reverse alpha-loop follows a similar configuration as an alpha-loop; however, the loop passes posteriorly to the scope shaft. Attempts at clockwise torque of the scope shaft will typically result in tightening of this loop and a sensation of increasing resistance to torque attempts by the endoscopists. Instead, counterclockwise torque and withdrawal is needed to reduce this type of loop. (Copyrighted and used with permission of Mayo Foundation for Medical Education and Research.)

In cases such as this, attempts at counterclockwise torque during scope withdrawal may result in successful loop reduction. Other clues that the direction of required torque should be reversed are if one experiences increasing resistance to scope shaft rotation during torque attempts, or if the tip of the scope moves backwards with the torque maneuver. In general, the correct direction of torque should result in a sensation of decreasing resistance to shaft rotation and modest scope tip advancement. Once a loop is reduced and the scope is straight, the torque that was used in the reduction can be undone. If the scope is straight, this should not result in any reproduction of the spiral but rather simply rotate the entire shaft of the scope back to a comfortable position. Some scopes are equipped with a variable stiffness feature that is controlled by a dial at the base of the handle. If this feature is available, increasing the stiffness of the scope, now that the loops are removed, can help prevent the reformation of these loops as the scope is advanced. This increased stiffness should be removed during subsequent attempts at loop reduction and reengaged when pushing forward. External pressure can also help prevent the reformation of loops and will be discussed below.

The other mobile section of the colon, the transverse colon, also frequently requires loop reduction. Looping here is mainly caused by redundancy of this section of the colon looping down, resulting in multiple changes in the force vector of the scope. The reduction technique is similar to loop reduction in the sigmoid. If possible, the flexible tip of the scope should be advanced around the hepatic flexure and hooked around this turn by holding the scope dials in place. With appropriate torque and withdrawal, the transverse colon will be straightened out. The scope tip may advance considerably down the right colon during this maneuver (Figure 5.26) (Video 5.7). The direction of torque here can vary, however, like the sigmoid; the correct direction of torque should result in a sensation of decreasing resistance and modest scope tip advancement.

Angulated turns

Acute turns can be encountered predominately in the sigmoid colon and flexures but can occur in any colon segment. These pose a significant problem to early trainees because they often cause the fellow to develop significant loops of the scope shaft as well as over-inflation of the colon as they struggle to round the turn. This over-inflation can lead to increasing the acuity of the angulation. The difficulty by trainees is predominantly due to incorrect technique of overusing the dials to accomplish these turns. Attempting to use the dials to steer around turns results in acute angulation of the scope shaft at the junction between the steerable tip and the less flexible scope shaft. With this acute bend in the scope, the force vector with advancement will be directed along the scope shaft at the outside wall of the turn rather than where the scope tip is pointing (Figure 5.27a). This resistance to scope advancement will be transmitted back along the scope shaft to the endoscopist's hand or to an area of mobile colon where a loop will develop. In acute turns such as these, the one-handed technique of using torque as the primary means of opening up the fold of a turn often results in less acute angulation of the scope tip and avoidance of this problem. This is accomplished by advancing the scope tip just beyond the fold on the inside portion of the acute turn. Up or down deflection is used just enough to begin hooking the turn. The scope is then gently pulled back just keeping the scope tip off of the wall of the outside turn while just enough deflection or torque is used to keep the scope hooked around the fold on the inside of the turn (Figure 5.27b) (Video 5.8). This hooking and slight withdrawal maneuver pulls this first (inside turn) fold out of the way until the lumen beyond the turn can be visualized (Figure 5.27c). Now with scope shaft still relatively straight, the force vector from pushing will translate directly into scope tip advancement.

With less acute turns, torque alone, without hooking and pulling, can often push the inside fold out of the way. Again the scope tip is advanced beyond the first fold and the scope is then

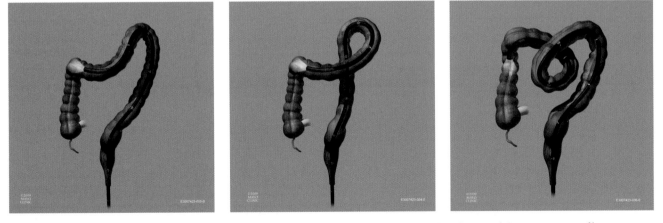

Figure 5.26 Transverse colon loop. Like the sigmoid, the transverse colon is also typically very mobile and can result in an assortment of loops. Reduction techniques vary but often require a combination of torque with slow shaft withdrawal. The direction of torque required will depend on the nature of the loop. (Copyrighted and used with permission of Mayo Foundation for Medical Education and Research.)

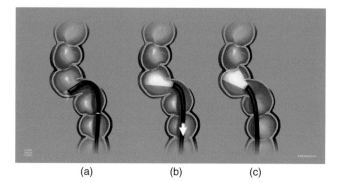

(a)   (b)   (c)

Figure 5.27 Acute turn. When attempting to navigate and acute turn novices will often rely on excessive use of the dials, resulting in the scope tip flexing greater than 90° around the turn and in poor position to be advanced (a). Correct technique involves passing the fold on the inside of the turn and gently flexing the scope tip just enough to hook the fold (b). The scope shaft is then slowly pulled back, pulling the inside fold back until the lumen can be seen past the next fold (c). This leaves the scope in better position to be advanced once the turn is opened. (Copyrighted and used with permission of Mayo Foundation for Medical Education and Research.)

torqued into the turn while keeping the scope tip straight. This torque pushes the fold aside until lumen beyond it is seen and the straight scope can then be readily advanced (Figure 5.28). Often these techniques are done over and over in opposite directions in the sigmoid colon until the descending colon is reached. An adult colonoscope is preferable with this technique as the added stiffness allows greater ability to push folds aside with torque. This technique is difficult when the sigmoid or area of acute turn is fixed in position due to adhesions. In instances like this, a pediatric scope and two-handed dial technique may be a more effective method to pass a turn. Endoscopists tend to favor one technique or scope type over another, but experienced endoscopists must master all techniques and equipment to accommodate any type of colonic anatomy.

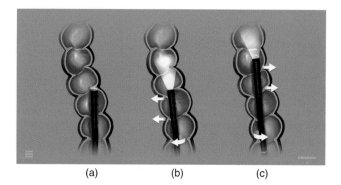

(a)   (b)   (c)

Figure 5.28 Torque to open folds. When less acute turns are encountered, the folds can often be pushed aside by advancing the scope tip just past the fold and torquing the scope shaft into them (a). This allows a straight shaft to allow easy advancement (b). This technique is often used repeatedly in opposite directions, especially through the sigmoid colon (c). (Copyrighted and used with permission of Mayo Foundation for Medical Education and Research.)

Another area where acute turns result in a disruption of the force vector is commonly encountered in the right colon. Once the tip has made it around the hepatic flexure, it is not uncommon to lose the one-to-one motion of the scope even after loop reduction. This is due to a significant change in the force vector caused by this turn or the accumulation of multiple turns distal to this. In cases like this, attempts at scope advancement often simply results in recurrent loop formation. When this occurs, there are multiple techniques that can be employed. The first is simply to use suction to deflate the colon in order to reach the next turn in the colon. Often once around this next turn, better reduction of the scope can be achieved. Another is the use of abdominal pressure. Experienced endoscopy assistants can palpate the abdomen and feel the location of scope looping. External abdominal pressure can then be applied over that area in an attempt to keep the scope from looping again. This simply translates the force of scope advancement further along the shaft rather than being used up in loop development. If there is a question as to where the best sight for external pressure might be, viewing the video display while palpating various spots in the abdomen might give a clue. While palpating, a site that results in slight scope tip advancement may be an ideal location for application of external pressure [18]. Conversely, a site that results in slight scope retreat might hinder scope advancement and increase the likelihood of loop formation. Another method used to prevent recurrent looping is to reposition the patient to a supine position (and in rare instances to a prone position) [19]. This tends to be of benefit by changing the orientation of how the colon is laying in the abdominal cavity and often can result in an orientation more favorable to reaching the cecum. This repositioning is most effective while navigating through the right colon but can also be used to relax acute angulations encountered elsewhere in the colon.

Ileocecal valve

Intubation of the ileocecal valve is really no different than navigating an angulated turn as described above. The location of the valve is readily identifiable by the asymmetric thickened fold just above the cecum. The valve lies within the thickened fold. In difficult-to-identify valves, the appendiceal orifice can serve as a clue to its location. Following the concave portion of the appendiceal orifice as if it were a bow shooting an arrow, the valve should be located in the direction this "bow" would shoot the arrow.

Occasionally, the os can be seen without special maneuvering and entered directly. More often, however, navigating through the valve requires the use of the torque or dial technique to open up the folds just as described in the angulated turn section above. One should advance the scope just past the valve so it is just off the screen. Slight torque or dial deflection is used in the direction of the valve as the scope is very slowly withdrawn. The stress on this is to only use "slight" torque or dial deflection as too great of deflection will simply hook the tip of the scope behind the valve. The tip should just lightly brush across the folds of the valve as the shaft is pulled back (Figure 5.29) (Video 5.9). Once the first fold (cecal side) is seen, the withdrawal is stopped and gradually increasing torque or deflection is used to steer the scope tip between the two folds making up the valve. Puffs of air, by tapping on the air valve,

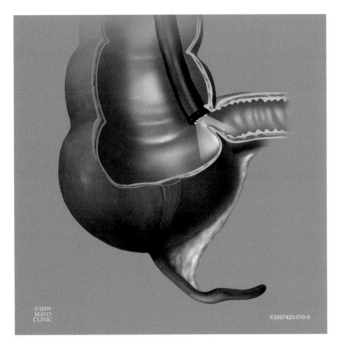

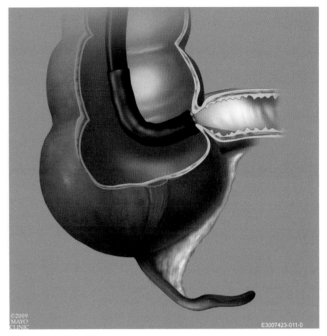

Figure 5.29 Terminal ileum intubation. To intubate the ileocecal valve, the scope tip should be brought alongside the valve and gentle deflection of the tip towards the valve used as the scope is slowly drawn back. Too much deflection will often result with the scope tip simply hooking behind the valve in the cecum. Once past the first fold of the valve, the endoscopist stops withdrawing and uses a combination of torque and slightly more tip deflection to open the valve. This leaves the scope in better position to be advanced once the os is intubated. (Copyrighted and used with permission of Mayo Foundation for Medical Education and Research.)

Figure 5.30 Incorrect TI maneuver. Like the acute turns, novice endoscopists will often rely on excessive dial controls to attempt to intubate the Ileocecal valve. This makes the scope difficult to advance, typically resulting in the scope loop advancing into the cecum and the tip falling out of the valve. (Copyrighted and used with permission of Mayo Foundation for Medical Education and Research.)

can keep the mucosa off of the lens, allowing better identification of the os. Once the os is identified, the scope shaft can be advanced, pushing the scope tip into the terminal ileum. One further pearl for advanced students to consider is to gently pull back the scope when the valve is visualized en face in the retroflexed position in the cecum if this maneuver is carefully performed to view behind the cecal folds and valve.

A common mistake of trainees is simply coming alongside the valve and trying to use all dials in hopes that the scope tip will fall into the terminal ileum. Occasionally, this does work, but as described in the previous section, this results in a very angulated scope tip and loss of the force vector (Figure 5.30). Pushing the scope in this scope configuration will simply advance the scope shaft into the base of the cecum, which often leads to paradoxical regression of the scope tip, causing it to fall out of the valve. In instances where the ileocecal valve is inverted towards the base of the cecum, advanced endoscopists will utilize a maneuver of retroflexing the scope tip in the cecum to view the valve en face. In this scope configuration, the inverted valve can then intubated by slowing pulling back on the scope. This maneuver can create significant pressure along the cecal wall however, thus should be used cautiously and only by experienced endoscopists when cecal intubation is necessary.

How to teach and assess colonoscopy skills

Identifying methods best suited to teach colonoscopy can be quite difficult. Traditionally, these skills have been taught at the bedside during patient-based endoscopy. However, with the recent advent of computer simulation models, as well as live and *ex vivo* animal models, evidence would suggest that these alternatives to patient-based endoscopy can impart some of these motor and cognitive skills [20,21]. In the case of early motor skills, this can also be done more safely, economically, and with better patient outcomes [22].

A second problem with the current state of colonoscopy education is that skills are primarily taught all together from the first day without differentiation between beginning or intermediate skills. In traditional training, a trainee attempts to learn intermediate skills such as loop reduction and navigation of fixed angulated turns at the same time he/she is learning simply how to use the dials and steer the scope. This produces a great deal of stress for the trainee not to mention some element of discomfort or even increased risk for the patient. Breaking the procedure down into individual skills, greater utilization of alternate teaching tools such as texts, multimedia, and simulation, training can proceed in a more stepwise fashion, starting with focused instruction of the most basic skills first and then on to more advanced skills when ready. Education literature has well established that building skills in a stepwise fashion is the most effective learning model [23]. This is not to suggest that these teaching aids will replace patient-based training, but rather these training tools can be used to effectively augment patient-based training and improve on the traditional training model. In this final section, we will examine the methods by which each of these skill groups previously outlined can best be taught.

The focus of this chapter will also be on methods to assess the mastery of these required skills by trainees. Accrediting bodies have placed a growing emphasis on assessment and documentation of competency, yet few programs do any type of formal evaluation other than a global subjective assessment of skills towards the end of training. This type of informal global assessment is fraught with biases inherent to subjective assessments. It also fails to identify struggling trainees early enough to provide timely remediation. Instead, assessment must be an ongoing process from the first scope performed during fellowship to the last. In general, there are four different types of assessment: written tests, performance tests, clinical observation methods, and a group of miscellaneous tests made up of oral examinations, portfolios, and the like [24]. Each can be used in a formative (testing primarily for the purposes of feedback or learning) or summative (testing for grading purposes) manner, yet as we will discuss, a specific testing method may be better suited for assessment of a particular skill. This chapter will address the best methods to provide continuous assessment of trainees' cognitive and motor skills (Table 5.2).

Early cognitive skills

Before hands-on endoscopy training begins, trainees need to undergo a curriculum that ensures the early cognitive skills (anatomy, preparation, scope selection, sedation, and indications/contraindications) have been acquired. Like many other aspects of endoscopy, training has been traditionally accomplished at the bedside under direct supervision. Cognitive skills however need not be learned entirely "on-the-job." In fact, it is likely of great benefit to us and our patients to have the bulk of these cognitive skills learned prior to introduction to the endoscopy suite. This will save valuable teaching time and make the teaching experience more meaningful for the trainee and teacher alike. For all of the specific early cognitive skills outlined, each can be generally be achieved through multiple instructional media, including anatomy atlases, textbooks, and pertinent journal articles such as professional society practice guidelines. Common to all is that these methods are primarily "self-directed" learning tools. The trainee only needs ready access and guidance as to what materials are most pertinent to ensure all cognitive skills are covered and that the materials are of appropriate quality. This is best accomplished by assigning trainees a set of required readings that cover intended topics and learning goals. The rest is done as self-study. Didactic lectures can also be included to augment these learning materials. At the Mayo Clinic, new fellows undergo a series of "Core

Table 5.2 How skills can be taught and assessed?

	Teaching methods	Assessment methods
Early skills (first 50 procedures)		
Cognitive	1. Self-directed learning – Texts – Articles – Multimedia aids 2. Lectures	1. Written exams – Board-type questions 2. Formative assessment during didactics 3. Simulation – Sedation/airway/complication management
Motor	1. Patient-based training 2. Simulation training – Computer simulator – *Ex vivo* course	1. Early formative assessment 2. Objective structured clinical examinations (OSCE)
Intermediate skills (50–250 procedures)		
Cognitive A. Pathology recognition	1. Self-directed learning – Text – Atlases – Multimedia (DAVE project)	1. Written exams – Pathology recognition
B. Decision-making	2. Patient-based training – Socratic method 3. Self-directed learning – Multimedia (GESAP)	2. Patient-based training – Socratic method 3. Written exams – Board-type questions 4. Ongoing assessment – Standardized assessment tool
Motor	1. Patient-based training 2. Simulation – Ex vivo models 3. Scope locating device – ScopeGuide	1. Continuous assessment tool 2. OSCE – Bovine model

Endoscopy Lectures" during the first two months of fellowship in addition to their required readings. Each lecture focuses on one of the core cognitive competencies. Lectures or discussion groups can ensure that students have the opportunity to ask questions and clarify misunderstandings that may arise from their self-directed learning. When trainees participate in interactive sessions, these didactic discussions can also allow for formative assessments of the trainees' fund of knowledge.

Assessment is the other important half of any educational endeavor but is the one often neglected. For cognitive skills in general, the use of brief written exams can be an easy means to reliably and objectively measure the acquisition of these skills. As with any assessment, these can be used as self-assessment exams for feedback (formative assessment) or as higher-stakes exams that must be passed prior to advancing to patient-based practice (summative assessment). Regardless how an institution uses the assessment, it should be carried out to ensure the learning goals of a curriculum are being met. Both education and assessment goals can be met through the use of computer multimedia tools where self-assessment quizzes can be linked directly to the learning material and provide real-time feedback on areas where the trainee may have answered incorrectly.

Sedation skills are unique in that simulation training can also be effectively employed to augment the other self-directed learning tools. Much of sedation training involves airway management taught to all medical students in basic and advanced life support courses. Even as fellows, these skills should be renewed periodically based on American Heart Association recommendations and endoscopy training programs should ensure that these skills or equivalent training is up to date. The use of airway and anesthesia mannequins can help teach the skills of basic airway management, monitoring, titration of medications, and management of sedation complications such as the appropriate use of reversal agents. These simulation tools can also be used for skills assessment where trainees must be able to demonstrate adequate ability in the management of these various sedation skills. Which specific modalities an institution uses for early cognitive training will depend largely on the resources available. Whichever are used, however, a concerted effort should be made to ensure these basic skills are taught prior to initiating patient-based training, and some form of assessment (even if informal formative feedback) is used and documented as part of the fellows training folder.

Early motor skills

The basic skills of holding the scope correctly and orientation to the various dials and buttons are simple first steps. This initial orientation to the scopes mechanics is brief and takes only 10–15 minutes. Frequently, this is done just prior to the first patient-based colonoscopy but can be accomplished outside the endoscopy suite, with a basic scope. A computer simulator, static mechanical model or an *ex vivo* animal model set-up can also provide the same basic exposure but can quickly be followed by the next step of learning how to insert and advance the scope through a lumen. Either one of these simulator environments affords the trainee the liberty to experiment with the early motor skills (controls, insufflation, scope advancement, mucosal inspection) in a safe

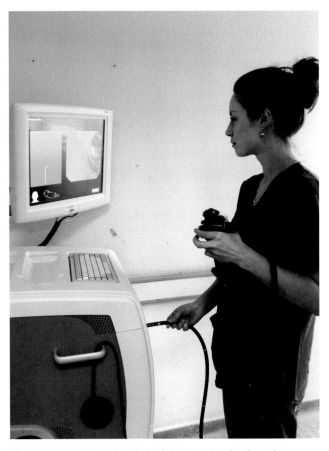

Figure 5.31 A trainee using the Endo TS-1, a virtual reality colonoscopy simulator made by Olympus KeyMed.

environment away from patients and in a low stress environment without concerns for patient pain, procedure completion issues, or the usual time constraints. Research has shown that the use of computer simulators during initial training of novice endoscopists can indeed teach basic scope steering, lumen identification, and scope advancement as well, if not better than traditional patient-based training [22,25,26] (Figure 5.31). In this research, GI fellows who had received computer simulation training over a 6-hour curriculum (20–25 simulated cases) outperformed traditionally trained fellows over the first 20–30 patient-based cases. These fellows were nearly twice as likely to reach the cecum independently and did so with greater speed, better lumen visualization, and most importantly with greater patient comfort than traditionally trained fellows. This performance advantage was observed for roughly 30 patient-based procedures, after which the skills for the traditionally trained group statistically caught up. On the basis of these positive results and others like it, some institutions, such as the Mayo Clinic, have adopted early training curricula around computer simulation, requiring all GI fellows to perform roughly 20–30 simulated colonoscopies prior to being allowed to begin patient-based training. Could longer simulation training provide an even greater performance advantage seen in the simulator-trained group? This is possible, as similar research to the study above has shown 10 hours of simulator training, imparting a measurable benefit in skills in up to 80 live cases [20]. However, other data examining the learning curves of performance metrics during simulation training have found that a trainee's performance on the simulator tends to plateau after roughly 20–25 cases, suggesting that a computer simulator has taught a trainee all it can during this length of training [27,28]. This is likely due to the modest level of difficulty of the cases currently available on computer simulators [29,30]. As the realism of looping, haptic feedback, and case complexity improves on these models, the benefits computer simulation training could conceivably extend well beyond the initial training of novices. Currently, however, it is recommended that computer simulation be used primarily for teaching early motor skills [31]. Simulators are also still prohibitively expensive ($75K–$100K), and as a result are found primarily at larger academic teaching institutions. One solution that would allow for smaller training programs to reap the benefits of these teaching tools would be the development of regional training centers. This initial simulation training of 20–25 cases could easily be completed over a weekend course and sponsoring such courses could provide a return on an investment for institutions that have already purchased such devices. Regional training centers could also serve as testing centers. As computer simulators become more advanced, it is inevitable that they will become part of board certification in gastroenterology, where testing of competence in endoscopy skills will be eventually be required. Before this type of high stakes assessment could happen though, the complexity and measured performance metrics of current endoscopy simulators would need to be greatly enhanced and separately validated for such testing purposes.

Static mechanical models such as the Erlangen active simulator for interventional endoscopy colonoscopy model (coloEASIE) consists of a tube of spiraled wired mounted to a platform that allows for practice in navigation and loop management (Figure 5.32) [32,33].

Ex vivo colonoscopy models have also been developed and can be used for teaching early motor skills [33,34] (Figures 5.33a,b). These models utilize harvested bovine or porcine colons that are

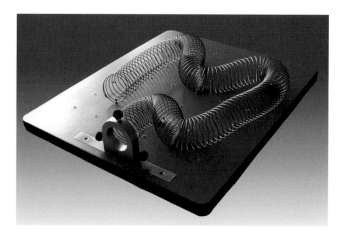

Figure 5.32 ColoEASIE. A static mechanical model, the colonoscopy Erlangen active simulator for interventional endoscopy (coloEASIE) model, is shown here.

laid out on a special platform in a human anatomical configuration. The use of these models are typically limited to more advanced training in skills such as therapeutic hemostasis devices or advanced endoscopy procedures such as ERCP. The ASGE, however, does offer annual training courses to first year fellows, teaching early endoscopy skills with the aid of *ex vivo* models, but requires trainees to travel to their central endoscopy training center, the Interactive Training and Technology [ITT] Center in Oak Brook, IL, for a few days. Another option is to utilize one of a number of commercial entities that offers the delivery and set up a temporary *ex vivo* training laboratory wherever it is needed. As the use of *ex vivo* simulation training for basic skills becomes more common, participation by first year fellows in standardized courses for colonoscopy could become commonplace as a precursor to starting patient-based training.

In addition to the teaching above, the assessment of early motor skills is an important part of training. This ideally should be done

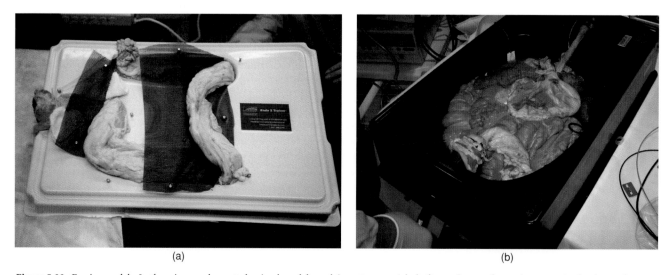

(a)   (b)

Figure 5.33 *Ex vivo* models. In these images, harvested animal models are lain out on special platforms that configure the organs in the shape of a human colon. The Endo-X trainer (a) is designed specifically to accommodate a harvested bovine colon while the Erlangen active simulator for interventional endoscopy model (EASIE-R) (b) platform is shown here with a porcine digestive tract.

in a formative manner to help identify early bad habits such as overuse of the two-handed scoping technique or to extinguish unsafe practices such as pushing while in red-out. This should be done during the simulation phase of training (if used), otherwise very early in the patient-based training experience to prevent bad habits from becoming ingrained.

In summary, the use of computer or *ex vivo* animal models can be used effectively to teach basic endoscopy skills when used prior to beginning patient-based training. Regardless of the type of simulation training used, it should be noted that it is not intended as a replacement to bedside teaching but simply a means to augment traditional training and possibly accelerate the acquisition of skills. There is no training that will ultimately better prepare one to perform colonoscopy on patients than actually performing patient-based exams. If simulation models are not available, seeking out special courses such as those offered by the ASGE would be recommended. If these options are not possible, patient-based training alone is still the standard and completely acceptable means to train these early skills.

Intermediate cognitive skills

The intermediate cognitive skills in colonoscopy hinge on a trainee's ability to recognize abnormalities and the decision-making abilities of what to do about them. As discussed earlier in this chapter, the skill of recognizing patterns of pathology simply requires numerous encounters with various abnormal findings. As the trainee develops the ability to recognize patterns of pathology and their sometimes subtle differences, management decisions will become more refined as well. Instruction in this cognitive skill predominately rests on ensuring that fellows experience a wide variety of findings during patient-based endoscopy. However, if patient exposure is the only means of education, a trainee's ability to recognize certain abnormalities could be limited due to patient selection biases or inadequate volume of certain abnormal findings (i.e., many polyps in a given practice but limited exposure to various presentations of inflammatory bowel disease). Instead, patient-based training should be augmented with self-directed study of photo atlases and multimedia resources that have been identified by instructors to ensure a wide variety (and more importantly, greater repetition) of pathology is experienced by the learner. One such media resource is the Digital Atlas of Video Education (DAVE) project. This free online site (www.daveproject.org) provides many examples of endoscopic images and videos along with case reports and explanations to accompany them. Contributions to the site are peer reviewed by its editorial board and review panel made up of nationally recognized names in gastroenterology. The site also has a curriculum specifically designed for fellows to ensure that a broad spectrum of endoscopic findings is experienced.

Assessment of pathology recognition skills is relatively simple. The most common method is from instructors getting a sense of the fellow's ability to identify pathology during live cases, yet the results of such assessment is rarely recorded in any manner. Formal objective assessments (written tests) can also be developed where images or videos can be presented to trainees at various stages of their training. The trainees can then be graded based on how quickly or accurately they can identify what is depicted. Results of such testing can be used to document the progression towards

cognitive competence and could also lead to earlier identification of deficiencies and timely remediation in some cases [35].

In addition to pathology recognition, the intermediate cognitive skills include the ability to make appropriate management decisions during endoscopy (such as what requires therapy, what devices to use, and what settings to use). This requires a broad fund of knowledge gained from bedside teaching, self-directed learning by reading texts, and supplementary study aids. One such supplement is the GI endoscopy self-assessment program (GESAP) developed by the ASGE. This resource is a computer-based program that provides board-exam type questions with endoscopic images focusing on both diagnostic and therapeutic decision skills. Software such as this can not only provide more repetition with seeing endoscopic pathology but also challenges a trainee's decision-making abilities. More importantly, the program provides instant feedback with explanations of the correct answers that can be used for self-assessment and study purposes. At the bedside, these skills will be honed as a trainee's experience with different pathology grows.

The assessment of decision-making skills is also relatively straightforward. The most common method is again an informal assessment during patient-based training as instructors talk a trainee through the thought process regarding management of specific findings. This "Socratic" teaching method with an actual case is not only one of the most effective teaching methods but is also a very effective form of formative assessment that imparts to the instructor a sense of what the fellow knows and how they come to their management decisions. As a result, feedback on errors in reasoning can be corrected on the spot. Assessment of this requires follow-up to ensure that the same errors in reasoning have been corrected. To accomplish this, a more formal and reproducible means of assessment is needed. Assessment must be an ongoing process that requires a means to record and evaluate progress in a trainee's skills. A standardized skill assessment form can be used. An assessment tool of this type should ideally be completed by staff during each case and measures a broad spectrum of both cognitive and motor skills, including the knowledgeable selection of device and settings based on pathology encountered. More will be discussed about how to employ this type of ongoing assessment later in this chapter.

Intermediate motor skills

Most trainees should be secure with the basic motor skills relatively quickly (roughly the first 30–50 colonoscopies). After that, the long process of mastering the intermediate skills becomes the next hurdle towards competence. These skills of navigating acute turns and managing loops are the most difficult skills for trainees to acquire. The nuances of these skills require a heightened awareness and understanding between what the eyes are seeing and what the right hand is feeling in respect to the degree of resistance, effectiveness of torquing, and fixation of the colon. It is also often difficult for staff to know how to manage a specific difficult turn or loop without taking the scope personally to get a sense of how things "feel." This makes teaching these skills difficult. More often than not, staff will simply take over the scope and advance the scope past the area of difficulty and then return the scope to the trainee with little explanation of exactly how this was accomplished. In order for fellows to grasp these nuances, a keen understanding of what is going on 3-dimensionally with the scope and loops of colon are key. Multimedia video can be of utility so that conceptually trainees can understand in general how loops develop, how different maneuvers can be used to open up turns, and how force vectors can be affected by these different techniques. Simulation can also help trainees practice some of these techniques and begin to get a sense of how these situations "feel." *Ex vivo* models comes close to mimicking the elasticity and feel of live tissue, however, nothing thus far can completely replace actual practice during live endoscopy [36]. For advanced endoscopic motor skills such as hemostasis techniques, training with *ex vivo* models have been shown to translate to improved patient-based hemostasis skills and improved outcomes [37]. More will be discussed on this elsewhere in this text.

A less common but much more effective teaching device is the use of an external scope locating device such as ScopeGuide® (Olympus, Center Valley, PA) [38]. This device can create real-time visual image of how the scope is looped or positioned in an actual human colon during live cases. It does so by using a magnetic field to passively detect special markers along the length of a scope (or along a special cable in a regular scope's biopsy channel). The real-time images allow the fellow to correlate what is being felt and seen with what is actually happening inside the patient. It can also show the effectiveness of reduction maneuvers. Despite the usefulness of such a device, these are rarely used due to cost, availability in the United States, and limited awareness of such tools. Instead most trainees gain a sense of what is occurring inside the patient simply with greater and greater volumes of experience during patient training.

Assessment of these motor skills can be achieved by a number of means. Spot checks of these skills can be accomplished using *ex vivo* simulation models where a set of set tasks need to be performed satisfactorily and are graded in a standardized method. These types of exams are referred to as Objective Structured Clinical Examinations (OSCE) and are frequently used in surgical training [39–41]. The ideal model for this would be a bovine *ex vivo* colon model (Figure 5.34) (Videos 5.10 and 5.11). This model has been validated as a tool for assessment of competence in intermediate colonoscopy skills [34]. It has some distinct advantages over computer simulation in that the anatomy can be made as easy or difficult as desired based on the skill level of the user. Additionally real endoscopes and therapeutic devices are used as opposed to the simulated tools used with computer simulators. This advantage can also be a major disadvantage, as the need for endoscopy equipment and laboratory space dedicated to animal training are not available at most institutions. Two alternative options to setting up a dedicated laboratory would be to utilize regional training centers such as the ASGE's animal laboratories or to bring in a group that will set up a temporary *ex vivo* training laboratory. Regardless of the method used, OSCE exams in general are costly from the respect of time to set up and personnel to precept exams. As such, OSCEs are best used as a summative type of exam (for a grade or for some form of certifying exam). For most centers, however, the assessment of these intermediate motor skills will still simply take place in the endoscopy suites during clinical cases. It should be stressed that

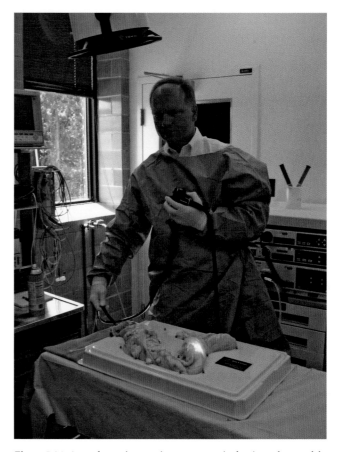

Figure 5.34 An endoscopist practices on an *ex vivo* bovine colon model.

this bedside assessment should incorporate objective measures that are recorded using a form such as the standardized assessment tool as discussed below. This assessment method is cheap, efficient, and can provide continuous monitoring of both cognitive and motor skills during fellows' progress through training. This can be performed with every procedure, which provides the most accurate assessment of a trainee's progress or on a periodic basis such as monthly or alternatively during every 25th or 50th colonoscopy.

For terminal ileum intubation skills, there really is no substitute for patient-based experience. Computer and *ex vivo* animal models do not recreate the valve adequately to be effective either for learning or for assessing this skill. Instead practice of valve intubation with every colonoscopy should be encouraged during training. This allows the required repetition needed both to gain this skill as well as to allow programs to accurately assess and monitor ileal intubation rates in an ongoing manner.

Ongoing assessment

Suggestions as to the ideal method for training and assessment have been made for each of the cognitive and motor skills addressed in this chapter (Table 5.2). In each section, reference to the need for ongoing assessment was made. This is to allow the ability to document when a fellow has reached the threshold of competence and more importantly to help define what factors equate to competence. This continuous monitoring is something rarely done at most institutions. For greater than 15 years, experts in endoscopy education have been calling for continuous measurements of fellows' skills as they progress towards competency [42,43]. In recent years, greater emphasis has been placed on the documentation of competence by professional organizations such as ASGE and training regulatory bodies such as the Residency Review Committee (RRC) of the American College of Graduate Medical Education (ACGME). This section will focus on the development and use of one such method of ongoing skills assessment from the beginning of training until graduation.

Many institutions utilize a global evaluation system, where, towards the end of training, supervising staff make subjective recommendations as to the preparedness of the trainee to operate alone. Though commonly used, this type of assessment is profoundly subjective in nature and is prone to significant biases. It also does not allow for early identification of learners below the average learning curve nor provide ample time as graduation draws close to remediate these fellows. Instead, professional societies have tried to develop recommendations in order standardize training. Unfortunately, these recommendations are based on a few publications of learning curve data that have very small numbers of subjects, are predominantly retrospective data, and focus on a very narrow definitions of competency based primarily on cecal intubation rates [42–45]. As a result of these data, it has been suggested that a minimum of 140 colonoscopies should be performed by a trainee before competency can be assessed [46]. However, these competency guidelines make only one suggestion as to what benchmarks define competence (Cecal intubation rate). The ASGE suggests that an "80–90% technical success" at reaching the cecum is needed to be deemed minimally competent [47]. Though better defined, this is still only one parameter of performance and does not take into account all of the other motor or cognitive skills. The RRC guidelines state, "Assessment of procedural competence should not be based solely on a minimum number of procedures performed, but on a formal evaluation process." What is needed is the development of an ongoing, formalized assessment that assesses a broad range of both motor and cognitive skills (Table 5.3).

One such evaluation process is called the Direct Observation of Procedural Skill (DOPS) form. This form focuses on six broad motor skill parameters and was developed by researchers as a means of assessing these skills following an intensive hands-on training course [26,48]. Another standardized skill evaluation form has been developed at the Mayo Clinic (Rochester, MN), which grades a spectrum of both cognitive and motor skills of trainees during colonoscopy. These component skills of colonoscopy were identified by a panel of expert endoscopists and educators and are based on the general training and competency recommendations outlined by professional societies [49]. From this, a blueprint for the evaluation tool was created, and based on this blueprint, the Mayo colonoscopy skills assessment tool (MCSAT) was developed (Table 5.4). This survey has been in use for over 4 years and is completed on every colonoscopy from the first day of a fellows training until graduation. The supervising staff enters this data directly into the institution's endoscopy database during the procedure so that the performance data is connected to other procedural data such as cecal intubation time

Table 5.3 Competency metrics for continuous assessment

Cognitive skills
Appropriate use of initial sedation

Continuous monitoring and management of patient comfort and depth of sedation

Identification of landmarks/awareness of scope location

Accuracy and sophistication of pathology recognition

Selection of appropriate tools and settings for therapy

Motor skills
Safe scope advancement

Loop reduction techniques

Depth of independent scope advancement

Cecal intubation time

Success/failure at TI intubation

Mucosal inspection during withdrawal

Application of tools for therapy

and withdrawal times as well as special therapies applied, polyp detection, and complications. Linking this evaluation to the procedural database has allowed the avoidance of having staff duplicate much of the data already generated automatically as part of the procedure. Admittedly, the goal of fellow skills assessment with every procedure is labor-intensive and daunting but can certainly be accomplished. Alternatively, the use of assessment forms such as the DOPS or MCSAT could be performed on a periodic basis, giving instructors a "snap-shot" in time of how a trainee compares to the expected learning curve.

The data collected from such an ongoing evaluation system allows reporting of a fellow's performance at any given point in their training as well as the comparison of the individual's scores to the average learning curve of his/her peers at the same points in training (Figure 5.35). In the examples shown, progress reports can graphically depict the learning curves of any of the various competency parameters. In this example, the progress of three different first year fellows – A, B, and C (above, at, and below average, respectively) is shown. This allows program directors to spot early those trainees who are falling off the learning curve and provide intervention earlier in training. Additionally, these metrics and average learning curves are valuable data for establishing criteria to define what performance equates to "competence" in a reliable, reproducible, and generizable manner. The concept of "competence" at present is rather limited in scope and defined as roughly a minimum of 140 procedures and cecal intubation rates of about 80%. A method that can formally define and assess competence such as Mayo's Colonoscopy Skills Assessment Tool or DOPS can be powerful tools. Each teaching institution should be encouraged to adopt some form of continuous assessment process whether using a comprehensive form such as the one described here or an ongoing skills assessment in a more limited form. Eventually, professional organizations and regulating organizations will require some type of direct measures of competence for all training

Table 5.4 Mayo colonoscopy skills assessment tool (MCSAT). This survey is completed by staff during each colonoscopy and grades a fellow's various cognitive and motor skills. This form is meant to augment the data already collected by the procedural database (such as medications administered, cecal intubation, and withdrawal times). Such a form allows for continuous assessment of a fellow's individual skills as they progress towards competence. (Copyrighted and used with permission of Mayo Foundation for Medical Education and Research.)

Mayo Colonoscopy Skills Assessment Tool

Date:
Fellow Pager
Staff Pager:
Pt MC#

> **Instructions to Staff:**
> – Check the appropriate box for each question.
> – A separate form should be completed for each procedure in which a fellow participated.

Pre-Procedure

1. Fellow's knowledge of the Indication & Pertinent Medical Issues (INR, Vitals, Allergies, PMH etc.)

   ☐ 0- NA- fellow observed;
   ☐ 1- Novice (Poor knowledge of patient's issue, or started sedating without knowing the indication);
   ☐ 2- Intermediate (Missed an Important element, i.e. Allergies, GI Surgical History or INR in pt on Coumadin);
   ☐ 3- Advanced (Missed minor elements);
   ☐ 4- Superior(Appropriate knowledge <u>and</u> integration of patient information).

2. Use of Initial Sedation during this procedure:

   ☐ 0- N/A- Fellow Observed,
   ☐ 1- Novice (Sedated without attention to titration or no assessment of level of sedation before intubating).
   ☐ 2- Intermediate (Initial titration was somewhat too rapid or slow, or too light/heavy).
   ☐ 3- Advanced (Initial sedation was appropriate.)
   ☐ 4- Superior (Fellow independently monitors vitals, and level of sedation to achieve ideal sedation before intubating.)

Procedure Skills:

3. Fellows participation in this procedure

   ☐ 0- N/A - Observed only,
   ☐ 1- Novice – (Performed with significant hands-on assistance)
   ☐ 2- Intermediate – (Performed with significant coaching or limited hands-on assistance)
   ☐ 3- Advanced (Performed Independently with limited coaching),
   ☐ 4- Superior (Performed Independently without coaching).

4. What is the farthest landmark the fellow reached **without** any hands-on **assistance**:

   ☐ 0- N/A - fellow observed only **or** Procedure terminated before completion.
   ☐ 1- Rectum,
   ☐ 2- Sigmoid,
   ☐ 3- Splenic flexure,
   ☐ 4- hepatic flexure,
   ☐ 5- Cecum, **No TI attempt** (completed cecal intubation without hands-on assistance and **no attempt at TI**)
   ☐ 6- Cecum, **Failed TI attempt** (completed cecal intubation without hands-on assistance and **Failed attempt at TI**)
   ☐ 7- Terminal Ileum (Successful intubation of TI)
   ☐ 9- Other-Post surgical anatomy encountered, fellow reached maximal intubation.

5. Safe Endoscope Advancement techniques:

   ☐ 0- N/A, Fellow observed;
   ☐ 1- Novice (Pushes blindly or Against fixed resistance/requires significant hands-on assistance);
   ☐ 2- Intermediate (Slow advancement/Repeated red-out/needs considerable coaching);
   ☐ 3- Advanced (Able to keep lumen in center and advance at a reasonable pace, limited coaching);
   ☐ 4- Superior (Safe technique, expedient independent advancement without the need for coaching)

6. Loop Reduction Techniques (Pull-back, External pressure, Patient Position Change)

   ☐ 0- N/A, Fellow observed;
   ☐ 1- Novice (Unable to reduce/avoid loops without **hands-on assistance**);
   ☐ 2- Intermediate (Needs **considerable coaching** on when or how to perform loop reduction maneuvers);
   ☐ 3- Advanced (Able to reduce/avoid loops with **limited coaching**);
   ☐ 4- Superior. (**without prompting**, uses appropriate ext. pressure/position changes/loop reduction techniques, Peds Scope)

Table 5.4 (*Cont.*)

7. Monitoring and management of patient Discomfort during this procedure:

  ☐ *0- N/A Fellow observed;*

  ☐ *1- Novice (Does not quickly recognize patient discomfort or requires repeated staff prompting to act);*

  ☐ *2- Intermediate (Recognizes pain but does not address loop or sedation problems in a timely manner);*

  ☐ *3- Advanced (Adequate recognition and correction measures);*

  ☐ *4- Superior (Proactive assessment and management. i.e. intermittently talks to patient to assess sedation and comfort).*

8. Landmark Recognition/Localization of Instrument

  ☐ *0- NA/Not Assessed*

  ☐ *1- Novice (Generally unable to recognize most landmarks);*

  ☐ *2- Intermediate (Recognizes cecum & some landmarks but generally poor perception of Instrument/pathology location)*

  ☐ *3- Advanced (Recognizes major landmarks; has a general idea of location of instrument/pathology based on landmarks);*

  ☐ *4- Superior. (Ability to recognize all landmarks and clear idea of instrument/pathology location in relation to landmarks)*

9. Adequately visualized mucosa during withdrawal:

  ☐ *0- NA/Fellow Observed Withdrawal;*

  ☐ *1- Novice (red out much of the time, does not visualize significant portions of the mucosa or requires assistance);*

  ☐ *2- Intermediate (Able to Visualize much of the mucosa but requires direction to re-inspect missed areas)*

  ☐ *3- Advanced (Able to adequately visualize most of the mucosa without coaching);*

  ☐ *4- Superior (Good visualization around difficult corners and folds and good use of suction/cleaning techniques.)*

10. Pathology identification/interpretation:

  ☐ *0- N/A, Study was normal;*

  ☐ *1- Novice - Poor recognition of abnormalities (Misses or cannot ID significant pathology);*

  ☐ *2- Intermediate - Recognize abnormal findings but **cannot** interpret ("erythema").*

  ☐ *3- Advanced - Recognizes abnormalities and correctly interprets ("colitis");*

  ☐ *4- Superior - competent Identification and assessment ("Mild chronic appearing colitis in a pattern suggestive of UC").*

11. Interventions Performed by fellow:

CHECK ALL THAT APPLY

  ☐ *N/A – Fellow did not perform any interventions (go to question 12)*

  ☐ *Biopsy*

  ☐ *Snare polypectomy*

  ☐ *Complex Polypectomy*

  ☐ *Other* _____

  11b. Therapeutic tool/cautery setting selection

    ☐ *1- Unsure of the possible tool(s) indicated for pathology.*

    ☐ *2- Able to identify possible appropriate tool choices but not sure which would be ideal*

    ☐ *3- Independently selects the correct tool yet needs coaching on settings*

    ☐ *4- Independently identifies correct tool and settings as applicable.*

  11c. What was the **fellows participation** in the therapeutic maneuver

    ☐ *1- Performed with significant hands-on assistance,*

    ☐ *2- Performed with minor hands-on assistance or significant coaching,*

    ☐ *3- Performed Independently with minor coaching,*

    ☐ *4- Performed Independently without coaching.*

Overall Assessment:

12. The fellows Hands-on **skills** are equivalent to those of a:

  ☐ *1- Novice (Learning basic scope advancement; requires significant assistance and coaching);*

  ☐ *2- Intermediate*

  ☐ *3- Advanced*

  ☐ *4- Competent to perform routine colonoscopy independently.*

13. The fellow's Cognitive Skills (Situational Awareness (SA)/Abnormality interpretation/decision making skills) are:

  ☐ *1- Novice (Needs significant prompting, correction or basic instruction by staff)*

  ☐ *2- Intermediate (Needs intermittent coaching or correction by staff)*

  ☐ *3- Advanced (Fellow has good SA, and interpretation/decision making skills)*

  ☐ *4- Competent to make decisions and interpretations independently.*

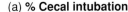
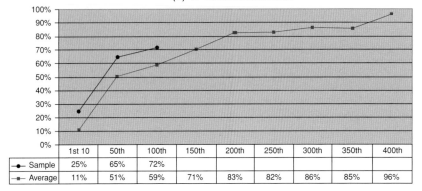

(a) % Cecal intubation

	1st 10	50th	100th	150th	200th	250th	300th	350th	400th
Sample	25%	65%	72%						
Average	11%	51%	59%	71%	83%	82%	86%	85%	96%

(b) % Cecal intubation

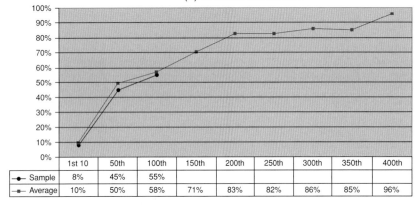

	1st 10	50th	100th	150th	200th	250th	300th	350th	400th
Sample	8%	45%	55%						
Average	10%	50%	58%	71%	83%	82%	86%	85%	96%

(c) % Cecal intubation

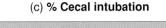
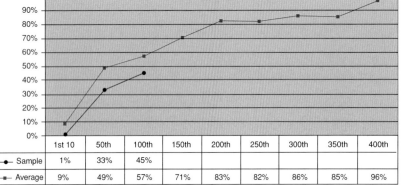

	1st 10	50th	100th	150th	200th	250th	300th	350th	400th
Sample	1%	33%	45%						
Average	9%	49%	57%	71%	83%	82%	86%	85%	96%

Figure 5.35 Learning curves. Mayo's colonoscopy skills assessment tool (MCSAT) allows ongoing monitoring of various metrics of an individual trainee's performance throughout training. These three images demonstrate how the learning curves of three different fellows (blue lines) might appear for the parameter of cecal intubation rates as compared to the average learning curves of their peers (Magenta). Fellow A is above the learning curve (a), B is following the curve closely (b), and C is repeatedly below the curve and might be identified for early remediation (c). (Copyrighted and used with permission of Mayo Foundation for Medical Education and Research.)

portfolios as the parameters of cognitive and motor competence are increasingly better defined [50].

Videos

Video 5.1 Endoscopic anatomy of the colon
Video 5.2 Rectal intubation techniques
Video 5.3 Locating the lumen
Video 5.4 Alpha-loop
Video 5.5 N-loop
Video 5.6 Reverse alpha-loop
Video 5.7 Transverse colon loop
Video 5.8 Acute turn
Video 5.9 Intubation of the ileal–caecal valve
Video 5.10 *Ex vivo* colonoscopy model overview
Video 5.11 *Ex vivo* colonoscopy model set-up
Video 5.12 Subtle lesions of colon
Video 1.4 Virtual reality colonoscopy simulator training
Video 1.5 A tour of the DAVE project: a free versatile multimedia resource for endoscopy education

References

1 Reznick RK, MacRae H: Teaching surgical skills—Changes in the wind. *N Engl J Med* 2006;**355**:2664–2669.

2 Levin B, Lieberman DA, McFarland B, et al.: Screening and surveillance for the early detection of colorectal cancer and adenomatous polyps, 2008: A joint guideline from the American Cancer Society, the US multi-society task force on colorectal cancer, and the American College of Radiology. *CA Cancer J Clin* 2008;**58**:130–160.

3 Winawer SJ, Zauber AG, Fletcher RH, et al.: Guidelines for colonoscopy surveillance after polypectomy: A consensus update by the US multi-society task force on colorectal cancer and the American Cancer Society. *Gastroenterology* 2006;**130**:1872–1885.

4 ASGE Consensus Statement: Appropriate use of gastrointestinal endoscopy. *Gastrointest Endosc* 2000;**52**:831–837.

5 Cappell MS: Safety and efficacy of colonoscopy after myocardial infarction: An analysis of 100 study patients and 100 control patients at two tertiary cardiac referral hospitals. *Gastrointest Endosc* 2004;**60**:901–909.

6 ASGE: Management of antithrombotic agents for endoscopic procedures. *Gastrointest Endosc* 2009;**70**:1061–1070.

7 Buschbacher R: Overuse syndromes among endoscopists. *Endoscopy* 1994;**26**:539–544.

8 Guelrud M: Improving control of the colonoscope: The "pinkie maneuver." *Gastrointest Endosc* 2008;**67**:388–389.

9 Barclay RL, Vicari JJ, Doughty AS, et al.: Colonoscopic withdrawal times and adenoma detection during screening colonoscopy. *New Engl J Med* 2006;**355**:2533.

10 Sawhney MS, Cury MS, Neeman N, et al.: Effect of institution-wide policy of colonoscopy withdrawal time > or = 7 minutes on polyp detection. *Gastroenterology* 2008;**135**:1892–18.

11 Norman G: Expertise in medicine and surgery. In: Ericsson KA, Charness N, Feltovich PJ, Hoffman RR (eds), *The Cambridge Handbook of Expertise and Expert Performance.* New York: Cambridge University Press, 2006.

12 Williams CB: The use of hot biopsy. *Endosc Rev* 1985;**6**:12–17.

13 Kadakia SC, Goldner FH: Is hot biopsy appropriate for treatment of diminutive colon polyps? In: Barkin J, O'Phelan CA (eds), *Advanced Therapeutic Endoscopy,* Second edn. New York: Raven Press, 1994.

14 Waye JD, Kahn O, Auerbach ME: Complications of colonoscopy and flexible sigmoidoscopy. *Gastrointest Endosc Clin N Am* 1996;**6**:343–377.

15 Nivatvongs S: Complications in colonoscopic polypectomy: An experience with 1555 polypectomies. *Dis Colon Rectum* 1986;**28**:825–830.

16 Norton ID, Wang L, Levine SA, et al.: Efficacy of colonic submucosal saline solution injection for the reduction of iatrogenic thermal injury. *Gastrointest Endosc* 2002;**56**:95–99.

17 ASGE Standards of Practice Committee: Complications of colonoscopy. *Gastrointest Endosc* 2003;**57**:441–445.

18 Prechel JA, Young CJ, Hucke R, et al.: The importance of abdominal pressure during colonoscopy techniques to assist the physician and to minimize injury to the patient and assistant. *Gastroenterol Nurs* 2005;**28**:232–236.

19 East JE, Suzuki N, Arebi N, Bassett P, Saunders BP: Position changes improve visibility during colonoscope withdrawal: A randomized, blinded, crossover trial. *Gastrointest Endosc* 2007;**65**:263–269.

20 Cohen J, Cohen SA, Vora KC, et al.: Multicenter, randomized, controlled trial of virtual-reality simulator training in acquisition of competency in colonoscopy. *Gastrointest Endosc* 2006;**64**:361–368.

21 Sedlack RE: Simulators in training: Defining the optimal role for various simulation models in the training environment. *Gastrointest Endosc Clin N Am* 2006;**16**:553–563.

22 Sedlack RE, Kolars JC: Computer simulator training enhances the competency of gastroenterology fellows at colonoscopy: Results of a pilot study. *Am J Gastroenterol* 2004;**99**:33–37.

23 Ericsson KA: Deliberate practice and the acquisition and maintenance of expert performance in medicine and related domains. *Acad Med* 2004;**79**:S70–S81.

24 Downing SM, Yudkowsky R: *Assessment in Health Professions Education.* New York: Routledge, 2009.

25 Gerson LB: Can colonoscopy simulators enhance the learning curve for trainees? [Review]. *Gastrointest Endosc* 2006;**64**:369–374.

26 Haycock AV, Koch AD, Familiari P, et al.: Training and transfer of colonoscopy skills: A multinational randomized blinded controlled trial of simulator versus bedside training. *Gastrointest Endosc* 2010;**71**(2):298–307.

27 Sedlack RE, Kolars JC: Colonoscopy curriculum development and performance-based assessment criteria on a computer-based endoscopy simulator. *Acad Med* 2002;**77**:750–751.

28 Eversbusch A, Grantcharov TP: Learning curves and impact of psychomotor training on performance in simulated colonoscopy: A randomized trial using a virtual reality endoscopy trainer. *Surg Endosc* 2004;**18**:1514–1518.

29 Aabakken L, Adamsen S, Kruse A: Performance of a colonoscopy simulator: Experience from a hands on course. *Endoscopy* 2000;**32**:911–913.

30 Sedlack RE, Kolars JC: Validation of a computer-based colonoscopy simulator. *Gastrointest Endosc* 2003;**57**:214-8.

31 Sedlack RE: Simulators in training: defining the optimal role for various simulation models in the training environment. *Gastrointest Endosc Clin N Am* 2006;**16**(3):553–563.

32 Maiss J, Matthes K, Naegel A, et al. The ColoEASIE simulator: A new training model for interventional colonoscopy and rectoscopy. *Endosk heute* 2005;**18**:190–193.

33 Hochberger J, Maiss J: Currently available simulators: Ex vivo models. *Gastrointest Endosc Clin N Am* 2006;**16**:435–449.

34 Sedlack RE, Baron TH, Downing SM, et al.: Validation of a colonoscopy simulation model for skills assessment. *Am J Gastro* 2007;**102**:64–74.

35 Thomas-Gibson S, Saunders BP: Development and validation of a multiple-choice question paper in basic colonoscopy. *Endoscopy* 2005;**37**:821–826.

36 Sedlack RE, Petersen BT, Kolars JC: The impact of a hands-on ERCP work shop on clinical practice. *Gastrointest Endosc* 2005: **61**; 67–71.

37 Hochberger J, Matthes K, Maiss J, et al.: Training with the compactEASIE biologic endoscopy simulator significantly improves hemostatic technical skill of gastroenterology fellows: a randomized controlled comparison with clinical endoscopy training alone. *Gastrointest Endosc* 2005;**61**:204–215.

38 Williams CB, Thomas-Gibson S: Rational colonoscopy, realistic simulation, and accelerated teaching. *Gastrointest Endosc Clin N Am* 2006;**16**:457–470.

39 Patil NG, Saing H, Wong J: Role of OSCE in evaluation of practical skills. *Med Teach* 2003;**25**:271–272.

40 Cerilli GJ, Merrick HW, Staren ED: Objective structured clinical examination technical skill stations correlate more closely with postgraduate

year level than do clinical skill stations. *Am Surgeon* 2001;**67**:323–326.

41 Tang B, Hanna GB, Carter F, et al.: Competence assessment of laparoscopic operative and cognitive skills: Objective structured clinical examination (OSCE) or observational clinical human reliability assessment (OCHRA). *World J Surg* 2006;**30**:527–534.

42 Cass OW: Training to competence in gastrointestinal endoscopy: A plea for continuous measuring of objective end points. *Endoscopy* 1999;**31**:751–754.

43 Tassios PS, Ladas SD, Grammenos I, et al.: Acquisition of competence in colonoscopy: The learning curve of trainees. *Endoscopy* 1999;**31**:702–706.

44 Marshal JB: Technical proficiency of trainees performing colonoscopy: A learning curve. *Gastrointest Endosc* 1995;**42**:287–291.

45 Chak A, Cooper GS, Blades EW, et al.: Prospective assessment of colonoscopic skills in trainees. *Gastrointest Endosc* 1996;**44**:54–57.

46 ASGE/ACG Taskforce on Quality in Endoscopy: Ensuring Competence in Endoscopy. Available: http://www.asge.org/WorkArea/showcontent.aspx?id=3384 (accessed June 3, 2009).

47 ASGE Standards of Training Committee: Principles of training in gastrointestinal endoscopy. *Gastrointest Endosc* 1999;**49**:845–853.

48 Thomas-Gibson S, Bassett P, Suzuki N, Brown GJ, Williams CB, Saunders BP: Intensive training over 5 days improves colonoscopy skills long-term. *Endoscopy* 2007;**39**:818–824.

49 Rex DK, Bond JH, Winawer S, et al.: Quality in the technical performance of colonoscopy and the continuous quality improvement process for colonoscopy: Recommendations of the U.S. multisociety task force on colorectal cancer. *Am J Gastro* 2002;**97**:1296–1308.

50 Sedlack RE: The Mayo Colonoscopy Skills Assessment Tool: Validation of a unique instrument to assess colonoscopy skills in trainees. *Gastrointest Endosc* 2010;**72**:1125–1133.

6 Endoscopic Ultrasound

Thomas J. Savides[1] & Frank G. Gress[2]

[1] University of California, San Diego, CA, USA
[2] State University of New York (SUNY), Downstate Medical Center, New York, NY, USA

EUS requires different skill sets than standard endoscopy

EUS is difficult to learn for several reasons. There are new cognitive skills regarding anatomy and disease states, there are endoscopic technical skills to master, and there are ultrasound concepts to learn.

Most importantly from a cognitive viewpoint, gastroenterologists usually are not trained to understand extraintestinal three-dimensional anatomy. This needs to be mastered before attempting to understand the EUS imaging of these areas. Additionally, much of EUS is related to the diagnosis, staging, and treatment of cancer, which is not taught in depth during fellowship [1–9]. Endosonographers must understand the diagnosis and management of gastrointestinal, pancreaticobiliary, and thoracic malignancy at a level where they can communicate effectively with medical and surgical oncologists. They must also have sufficient knowledge of cytology and pathology to maximize diagnostic yield with their pathologists.

From an endoscopic technical point of view, endoscopic ultrasound equipment is quite different than standard endoscopes, with extra buttons, balloons, and ultrasound processors to master. The scopes are often larger, with greater outer diameters and longer bending sections at the tip, and with oblique viewing, which makes scope passage and manipulation more difficult than standard endoscopes. These larger, stiffer scopes also may increase the risk of complications, such as perforation, if not used carefully. After learning how to handle the instruments and maneuver them, trainees must acquire dexterity with the fine adjustments in scope position necessary to bring the ultrasound image into focus.

Another major challenge is that endoscopists now need to learn the fundamentals of ultrasound imaging. This is not taught during GI fellowship. Specifically, trainees need to understand ultrasound physics, impact of imaging frequency on resolution, and depth of penetration, characteristics of various tissue structures (i.e., air, fluid, blood, soft tissue, bone), as well as imaging artifacts [10,11].

Learning resources for EUS

A number of skill sets will be described, which are needed to learn EUS (Table 6.1). To master these skill sets, one needs a variety of learning tools. These tools include textbooks, instructional videos, attending national, regional, and local courses, internet web sites, observing experts, or performing formal training at a center of excellence in advanced endoscopy. Table 6.2 lists a number of these resources for self-study, and Table 6.3 lists some of the programs offering advanced endoscopy training or "fourth year" EUS training fellowships. Note that these training resources constantly change over time, but provide a good base from which to start training. In addition, some GI societies such as the American Society of Gastrointestinal Endoscopy (ASGE) post and update a comprehensive list of advanced endoscopy training programs on their websites.

The skill sets needed to learn EUS

While there is no single way to learn anything, EUS learners need to focus on the core skill sets required for successful performance of EUS. The trainee should generally learn this in a sequential order, although simultaneous learning often occurs. These skills can be learned using a variety of sources such as textbooks, training videos, short courses, and mentored training [10,11].

Anatomy

This must be reviewed in detail prior to learning the EUS imaging of anatomy. This is best done by reviewing anatomy textbooks. Special attention is given toward the structures immediately adjacent to the luminal gastrointestinal tract, as this is what will be visualized with EUS. More recently, there have been anatomy textbooks and training software created based on digitalized human sections, such as from the Center for Human Simulation at the University of Colorado (www.uchsc.edu). Most importantly, the anatomy must be learned in such a way that the relationship of one structure to another is appreciated, both in cross-sectional

Successful Training in Gastrointestinal Endoscopy, First Edition. Edited by Jonathan Cohen.
© 2011 Blackwell Publishing Ltd. Published 2011 by Blackwell Publishing Ltd.

Table 6.1 Key skill sets for learning EUS.

1. Anatomy
   a. Peri-intestinal organs and structures
   b. Cross-sectional and oblique viewing structural relationships
2. Diseases and conditions assessed with EUS
   a. Malignancy (esophageal, gastric, pancreatic, rectal, lung)
   b. Benign pancreatico–biliary disease (stones, obstruction, cysts, pancreatitis)
   c. Luminal and extraluminal masses (subepithelial masses, cysts)
   d. Muscle disorders (anal sphincters, lower esophageal sphincter)
3. Ultrasound principles
   a. Physics
   b. Variables affecting ultrasound imaging (frequency, resolution, penetration, flow)
   c. Common artifacts
4. EUS image interpretation
   a. Understand common appearances
   b. Various appearances of same condition (i.e., different depths of tumor invasion)
   c. Impact or prior surgery or patient body weight on imaging
   d. Common artifacts
5. How to operate EUS equipment
   a. Scope buttons and balloon tip
   b. EUS console
   c. Troubleshooting common problems
6. Use of EUS scope
   a. Passage through upper esophageal sphincter, lower esophageal sphincter, pylorus
   b. Inflation/deflation of balloon to help with positioning
7. Diagnostic EUS imaging
   a. Improving acoustic coupling of transducer (water in balloon/lumen, avoid air)
   b. Placement of EUS transducer in proper position of given indications
   c. Positioning of patient for various indications (i.e., left lateral, supine, prone)
   d. Obtaining appropriate views required for disease specific indications
   e. Using both the radial and linear scope
8. EUS FNA
   a. Which lesions to FNA and when
   b. Risks of FNA
   c. When to use various needles
   d. How to prepare needle (i.e., heparin flush)
   e. How to use FNA scope (i.e., use elevator)
   f. How to pass needle through the scope channel
   g. FNA puncture
   h. FNA aspiration (suction)
   i. Movement of needle during pass through highest yield areas of the lesion
9. EUS FNA cytologic evaluation
   a. Expressing material from needle onto slides or fixative
   b. Special stains used to evaluate material
   c. Fixative solutions for cellblocks, flow cytometery, immunostains
   d. Estimate if adequate material for analysis
   e. Identify different cytopathologies
   f. Understand advantages and disadvantages of immediate cytologic evaluation

Table 6.1 (*Cont.*)

10. Interventional EUS
    a. Fine-needle insertion/injection (drugs, wires, stents, fiducicals)
    b. Understand risks, benefits, and when investigational
11. Report generation and communication with referring physicians
    a. Include pertinent positive and negative findings related to disease
    b. Express differential diagnose to explain imaging
    c. Suggest next management options
    d. Contact referring physician with results

Table 6.2 Resources for learning EUS.

Textbooks

Anatomy

Ultrasound

Oncology

Cytology

Endoscopic ultrasound textbooks:

   Gress and Savides. *Endoscopic Ultrasonography*, Wiley & Co, 2009.

   Hawes and Fockens. *Endosonography*, Elsevier Saunders, 2006.

   Bhutani and Deutsch. *Digital Human Anatomy and Endoscopic Ultrasonography*, Peoples' Medical Publishing House, 2004.

   Dietrich. *Endoscopic Ultrasound*, Thieme, 2006.

Training EUS Videos

American Society for Gastrointestinal Endoscopy Learning Library DVDs

Industry sponsored meetings (i.e., EUS 2010)

Local Hospital Conferences

Tumor Board

Medical–Surgical Conference

GI Pathology Conference

Radiology Conference

National Courses

Mayo Clinic EUS Course

Harvard EUS Course

NYSGE Annual Course EUS Hands-on Workshop

Web Sites

Visible Human dissector program to learn anatomy www.uchsc.edu/sm/chs/gallery/dissector/movies/flip.html

Digital Atlas of Video Endoscopy (DAVE Project) to see videos examples of various EUS exams www.daveproject.org

Table 6.3 EUS fourth year fellowship programs.

Institution	EUS training director	Email
University of Alabama, Birmingham	Mohamad Eloubeidi, M.D.	meloubeidi@uabmc.edu
University of California, Irvine	Kenneth Chang, M.D.	kchang@uci.edu
University of California, San Diego	Thomas Savides, M.D.	tsavides@ucsd.edu
Stanford University	Jacques Van Dam, M.D.	jvandam@stanford.edu
University of Colorado, Denver	Raj Shah, MD	raj.shah@ucdenver.edu
Yale University	Harry Aslanian, M.D.	Harry.aslanian@yale.edu
Moffit Cancer Center, Tampa, Florida	James Barthel, M.D.	barthejs@moffit.usf.edu
Mayo Clinic, Jacksonville, Florida	Michael Wallace, M.D.	Michael@mayo.edu
University of Chicago	Irving Waxman, M.D.	iwaxman@medicine.bsd.uchicago.edu
Indiana University, Indianpolis, IN	John DeWitt, M.D.	Jodewitt@iupui.edu
Indiana Medical Associates, Fort Wayne, IN	Maurits Wiersema, M.D.	wiersema.mauritsgi@gmail.com
Massachusetts General Hospital, Boston, MA	William Brugge, M.D.	wbrugge@partners.org
Brigham & Women's Hospital, Boston, MA	David Carr-Locke, M.D.	cthompson@partners.org
Johns Hopkins Hospital, Baltimore, MD	Marcia Canto, M.D.	mimicanto@jhmi.edu
University of Michigan, Ann Arbor, MI	James Scheiman, M.D.	jscheima@med.umich.edu
Mayo Clinic, Rochester, MN	Michael Levy, M.D.	Levy.michael@mayo.edu
University of Minnesota, Minneapolis, MN	Shawn Mallery, M.D.	Shawn.mallery@co.hennepin.mn.us
Washington University, St. Louis, MO	Steven Edmundowicz, M.D.	sedmundo@im.wustl.edu
Duke University, Durham, NC	Paul Jowell, M.D.	Jowell001@mc.duke.edu
State University of New York, Brooklyn	Frank Gress, M.D.	Frank.gress@downstate.edu
Columbia University, New York, NY	Peter Stevens, M.D.	pds5@columbia.edu
University Hospitals, Cleveland, OH	Amitabh Chak, M.D.	Amitabh.Chak@UHhospitals.org
Oregon Health Sciences, Portland, OR	Douglas Faigel, M.D.	faigeld@ohsu.edu
University of Pennsylvania, Philadelphia, PA	Michael Kochman, M.D.	michael.kochman@uphs.upenn.edu
Thomas Jefferson University, Philadelphia, PA	Thomas Kowalski, M.D.	Thomas.Kowalski@jefferson.edu
MD Anderson, Houston, TX	Manooh Bhutani, M.D.	Manoop.Bhutani@mdanderson.org
Scott and White Clinic, Temple, TX	Richard Erickson, M.D.	rerickson@swmail.sw.org
GI Consultants, Milwaukee, WI	Marc Catalano, M.D.	mfcatalano@aol.com
Cedars-Sinai, Los Angeles, CA	Simon Lo, M.D.	Simon.Lo@cshs.org
Cleveland Clinic, Cleveland, OH	John Vargo, M.D.	vargoj@ccf.org
Northwestern University, Chicago, IL	John Martin, M.D.	j-martin3@northwestern.edu
University Florida	Chris Forsmark, M.D.	forsmce@medicine.ufl.edu

Source: American Society for Gastrointestinal Endoscopy Website: www.asge.org.

as well as oblique viewing (as would occur with varying imaging planes in EUS) [10].

Understand diseases and conditions assessed with EUS

Trainees should learn about the indications for EUS and specifically the different disease states for which EUS is applied, and how EUS impacts not only the diagnosis, but also treatment and follow-up. These include the broad areas of malignancy (e.g., esophageal, gastric, pancreatic, rectal, anal, lung), benign pancreatico–biliary diseases (i.e., stones, obstruction, cysts, pancreatitis), luminal and extraluminal masses (subepithelial masses, peri-intestinal cysts), and disorders of the intestinal musculature (anal sphincters, lower esophageal sphincter, pylorus, fistulas and abscesses, etc.). This learning is usually done with textbooks of gastroenterology, oncology, surgery, endosonography, as well as Web-based resources. In addition, attending hospi-

tal Tumor Boards and GI/Surgery conferences is a very valuable learning resource for clinical correlation and to understand how different disease states are managed by referring physicians.

Ultrasound principles

Ultrasound principles can be learned using a textbook of ultrasonography, as well as video instruction. This is usually addressed in dedicated EUS textbooks [10,12–14]. Initial focus is on understanding ultrasound principles and artifacts. There are courses on ultrasound for nonradiologists, and they can also be very useful (such as for imaging the liver) for learning the basics. Finally, spending some time with an ultrasound technician or radiologist as they perform and interpret ultrasound images can be very helpful to understand basic principles and to start applying this to learning the EUS anatomy from the transabdominal percutaneous approach [9].

EUS image interpretation

Learning EUS image interpretation is the most important and lengthy part of learning. This is a cognitive skill of pattern recognition and not a technical endoscopic skill. Initially, this should be done by reading EUS textbooks and studying EUS training videos (such as from the American Society for Gastrointestinal Endoscopy) [9]. EUS computer simulators have been created to assist in this training step, but these are still investigational and very few exist [11]. EUS interpretation is best learned by watching an experienced endosonographer, either one-on-one as the endosonographer does cases or via video or live-demonstration courses. The goal here is to see large numbers of cases since images vary based on pathology, normal variants, and patient issues such as prior surgery and body habitus. Learning EUS is a two-step process: interpreting images and endoscopic manipulation.

When learning at this stage, the trainee should always be trying to identify different structures seen on the screen and ask the mentor to confirm if correct. It is critical at this point to start understanding relational anatomy, for example, if you see the confluence of the portal vein and superior mesenteric vein, you should also expect to see the superior mesenteric artery. The instructor can help in teaching here by quizzing the trainee on different anatomical structures and by highlighting the importance of having a routine in terms of visualizing structures. Different instructors use different concepts (i.e., "stations," "pull-back method," "push method"), but the general concept is that one wants to have a standardized approach to visualize all the anatomy.

How to operate EUS equipment

Learning how to operate the EUS equipment is the next stage. This first involves learning to understand the scope and processor anatomy. Understanding the scope requires learning the air and water buttons differ from standard endoscopes, and how to place a balloon on the tip and how to fill the balloon with water. It is also important to understand how to utilize the ultrasound processor to obtain optimal images, by using different presets, imaging frequencies, gain, magnification, Doppler flow, and labeling. This should also include troubleshooting common problems such as no image on the screen, poor image quality, or settings/buttons unintentionally changed during wiping down of ultrasound processor surface during room turn over. These skills can be taught by endosonography mentors, GI nurses/technicians, and equipment company representatives.

Initially, the equipment inservicing should be taught outside the patient's body. The trainee can be shown the parts of the scope and asked to try using various buttons (i.e., inflate and deflate scope tip balloon). The scope can then be placed into a water-filled container that contains gauze to show how the image can be identified, how to troubleshoot, and to show how to manipulate the ultrasound processor settings to enhance imaging. This can also be done in a plastic or porcine model.

Use of EUS scope

Learning to pass the EUS scope through a patient's mouth, intubate the esophagus, and position it properly for EUS imaging ideally requires one-on-one training with a mentor. Because the scopes are larger and stiffer, care must be used in passing the scope through the mouth, the lower esophageal sphincter, and the pylorus/duodenal sweep in order to avoid trauma. Sometimes, these skills can be learned outside the body by manipulating the scope in a training model such as an *ex vivo* simulator or pig stomach [15]. We will discuss simulator models later on in the chapter.

Initially, this skill should be taught in a well-sedated patient. It is important to emphasize to the trainee not to push with force if resistance is met. If there is resistance, then the trainer should take the scope to feel why there is resistance and instruct how to resolve the problem. Often, this is just a matter of repositioning the scope or inflating the balloon slightly.

Diagnostic EUS imaging

Diagnostic imaging is learned once the scope is in place and can be easily manipulated. Skills to be learned at this point also include how and when to inflate water into the transducer balloon, as well as removal of air and placement of water within the lumen to optimize ultrasound imaging. Instruction must also include where and how to place the transducer for imaging and includes patient positioning (i.e., lateral, prone, supine, head of bed elevated, etc.). This should include learning the appropriate maneuvers for obtaining the necessary images for disease-specific indications; for example, if evaluating for a pancreatic mass, one needs to visualize the pancreas parenchyma, pancreatic duct, common bile duct, liver, and peripancreatic blood vessels and lymph nodes. Considerable time is required to master this skill set, as one needs to get comfortable in a variety of disease-specific conditions, patient body habitus states, and sedation levels. Additional time is also needed to become familiar with and ultimately learn to use all available EUS equipment including both radial and linear EUS echoendoscopes and catheter-based ultrasound probes. There is no consensus on whether both linear and radial should be introduced at the onset together or should the trainee master one before starting with the other.

When the trainee initially is learning at this point, emphasis should just be on examining limited areas with EUS. For example, starting with the easiest things such as finding the aorta or gallbladder, then progressing to identifying the pancreas, and finally to visualizing the common bile duct. A balance must be found between expediting the patient's exam and trainee learning time. Usually, the fellow should have short amounts of time to find structures so as not to significantly prolong the sedation for the patient. It is important for the fellow to realize that during this learning phase, not every structure needs to be visualized. As the fellow progresses in ability, emphasis should focus on identifying the pertinent anatomy related to the disease state (such as examining the left adrenal gland in a patient with mediastinal adenopathy and suspected lung cancer).

EUS-guided fine-needle aspiration (FNA)

Once the trainee can reliably identify pertinent normal structures as well as pathology (diagnostic EUS), then, and only then, EUS-guided FNA can be learned. It is critical to have a good understanding of normal and abnormal EUS findings, because one needs to understand which lesions should and should not undergo EUS FNA. Additionally, the trainee needs to understand the risks associated with FNA and when to administer prophylactic antibiotics, such as with pancreatic cysts and possibly during EUS-guided celiac plexus block procedures. One must also learn the differences between EUS FNA needle systems including the different-sized and designed needles (19, 22, and 25 gauge needles, the celiac plexus needle, etc.) and when to use one versus the other. Needle preparation must be learned. One must also learn how to safely advance the needle through the EUS scope's working channel without puncturing the channel, how to adjust the sheath length, how to use the elevator, and what to do if the needle does not come out the scope tip (deflect the scope tip down). Once these skills are mastered, one can learn to puncture a lesion under EUS guidance, remove the stylet, utilize suction if indicated, and move the needle in and out through the lesion in parts, which have the highest yield for diagnostic material. Perhaps, most important is learning and understanding not only when to do FNA, but when not to do FNA, such as for obvious mediastinal cysts (which can get infected) or for peritumoral lymph nodes that can only be reached by passing the needle through intervening tumor (risk of seeding a benign lymph and getting a false positive cytology). Learning how to do EUS FNA can be done with EUS textbooks and videos, as well as using phantom models, simulators, porcine models, or under direct mentorship during live patient cases.

When trainees first learn EUS FNA, it is best to start with the easiest lesions to FNA, those in which the scope tip does not need much deflection. This will usually be a transesophageal or transgastric EUS FNA, or a mediastinal or celiac lymph node, or a pancreatic body lesion. Initially, the trainee may do best by holding the scope tip in order to get comfortable with identifying the lesion and keeping the needle visualized as the needle is moving within the lesion. Once this is mastered, then the trainee can operate the needle while the mentor holds the scope. The mentor should demonstrate to the trainee different techniques (elevator, tip deflection, and scope withdrawal) to change the needle position with a lesion, as well as when to use suction. Finally, once the trainee has mastered transesophageal and transgastric FNA, then one can move to the more difficult transduodenal FNA (i.e., pancreatic head mass lesions) in which the scope tip is torqued and keeping the transducer on the lesion can be more difficult.

EUS FNA cytologic evaluation

The next step is learning how to get the material from the needle, onto the slides and into fixatives, staining and processing the material, and then interpreting the prepared material. These steps are generally performed by the endoscopy technician and cytology technician, but it is critical that the endoscopist understand these steps thoroughly as they can impact the diagnostic yield of FNA. The endosonographer needs to understand how to get material from the needle onto the slides and into the fixative (usually using the stylet to push material forward slowly), the different stains used for interpretation and how they differ (i.e., hematoxylin and eosin stain vs. Papanicolaou stain), and how to determine if adequate cellular material for evaluation (vs. just blood), and ideally the

ability to identify different types of pathologic cytology (i.e., adenocarcinoma). The endosonographer must also understand the advantages and disadvantages of immediate cytologic evaluation of the material by a cytotechnician or cytopathologist. Cytology skills for EUS can be learned by reading EUS textbooks and by observing and working with your cytotechnician and cytopathologist as they prepare and examine these specimens. This is much easier if immediate cytologic evaluation is performed during the case.

Interventional EUS

Once diagnostic EUS and EUS FNA have been mastered, one can consider learning interventional techniques. These procedures generally involve placing a needle into an area of the body using EUS guidance and then inserting something (wire, drug, marker) into that area. These therapeutic EUS procedures include pseudocyst drainage, celiac plexus block, injection of chemotherapy agents into tumors, insertion of metal fiducials to help stereotactic radiosurgery, puncture into obstructed biliary or pancreatic systems to assist ERCP techniques, and the transluminal placement of stents to drain obstructed fluid or abscess collections. These techniques are often extensions of existing skill sets from EUS and ERCP, and so are often learned by reading published articles on the techniques as well as observing videos or live demonstrations. Having prior ERCP training (or another physician assisting who is trained in ERCP) is required for those procedures that are really combined EUS/ERCP, for example, EUS-guided pseudocyst drainage or EUS-guided rendezvous. It is important to note that this is a rapidly evolving field and that one needs to constantly keep up with the literature on these procedures as some are investigational and best performed in a research setting or by tertiary centers of excellence.

Report generation and communication with referring physicians

This is actually one of the most important, and yet least emphasized, parts of the EUS procedure. The exact wording used in reports is important, in that for different indications, there will be different required/expected parts of the exam to be described. For example, for a pancreatic mass EUS FNA, it is important to describe the mass appearance, size, location, relation to other structures, remainder of pancreatic parenchyma, bile duct size, pancreatic duct size, peripancreatic lymph nodes, peripancreatic blood vessels, liver, number of EUS FNA passes, and preliminary cytologic diagnosis (if available). The endosonographer needs to record subtle areas of uncertainty as well, because this can be important in decision-making by oncologists and surgeons. For example, in staging a rectal cancer, it is better to say that a tumor involves the muscularis propria and may barely invade into the superficial perirectal fat and call it a EUS stage T2 versus superficial T3, rather than definitely proclaim a certain stage only to be found wrong at surgical resection. A few incorrect EUS stagings by a beginning endosonographer can result in a lack of confidence from the referring surgeons and oncologists in that endosonographer's abilities. Depending on one's referring physicians, the report impression or recommendations sections can also anticipate the clinical decision-making and provide suggested recommendations, such as suggesting preoperative chemoradiation for an esophageal cancer that extends into the periesophageal fat (T3) and has periesophageal malignant-appearing lymph nodes (N1). Finally, it is important that for time-sensitive cases (such as suspected cancer waiting staging prior to initiating therapy), the endosonographer immediately communicate the findings with the referring physicians.

Trainees should write the first draft of the EUS reports, but this should be modified by the instructor together with the trainee in order to explain why subtle changes are made to the report. Additionally, the trainee should initially listen as the mentor discusses with the referring physicians the findings, as well as the patient and patient's family and eventually the trainee should be able to gradually do this independently (i.e., directly contact the referring providers, etc.).

Pathways for EUS training

There are two main pathways to learning EUS: either as part of a mentored fellowship program (either part of traditional 3-year fellowship training or fourth year advanced endoscopy fellowship) or self-learning for practicing gastroenterologists. Because the skill sets of understanding extraluminal anatomy and ultrasound are not taught in standard 3-year fellowship, learning EUS requires significant focused training to perform competent diagnostic and therapeutic studies. Several of the core skill sets can initially be learned by reading textbooks, watching training videos, attending short courses, and watching an experienced endosonographer. The main difference in learning in a fourth year fellowship versus self-training for a practicing gastroenterologist is in the volume of patient material encountered and the immediate feedback during learning.

EUS fellowship training
Most fellowship training in EUS in the United States is conducted as part of fourth year advanced endoscopy training, which may be dedicated to only EUS, or to all advanced endoscopy techniques (i.e., EUS, ERCP, endoscopic mucosal resection, deep enteroscopy, etc.). With the advent of increasing numbers of interventional EUS procedures, it seems that combined training in all aspects of advanced endoscopy allows the endosonographer to apply therapeutic techniques most effectively. A few fellowships teach EUS during the second and third years of standard fellowship, and it is possible that this may become more common in the future.

There are no guidelines for who is competent to be a EUS trainer during fellowship, but the general assumption is that the trainer is highly skilled and experienced in performing EUS exams. It is often useful that a new faculty member just out of fellowship not be the trainer initially, because that endosonographer is still learning to do EUS exams independently without the mentor. After 12 months of independent EUS exam performance, a recently trained endosonographer will be in a much better position to train others. Also, different endosonographers have learned different

"tricks of the trade" from their mentors, so it is often advantageous to learn EUS from several different instructors for exposure to a variety of techniques.

If one is interested in applying for an advanced endoscopy or EUS fourth year fellowship, the best place to start is the American Society for Gastrointestinal Endoscopy website (www.asge.org). The website has a section on "EUS Training Programs." This will list nearly all of the training programs available and is updated periodically for accuracy. This list increases in number every year, and there may be excellent training programs besides those on the ASGE list. This list provides the names of the institutions, training directors (with email address), and what types of training are provided. Most of these fellowships are for a 1-year period, although some are for 2-year periods. As of 2010, the ASGE has tried to work with the training directors to establish some common application dates, with the current expectation that programs start interviewing no sooner than January during the GI fellow's second year (18 months before starting the EUS fellowship) and that positions are not offered until April 15 (approx. 15 months prior to starting EUS fellowship). This informal agreement among EUS and advanced endoscopy training directors will likely be modified to improve upon the system each year, and so one should go to the ASGE website for current status. Note that a number of programs will give preference to their own internal second year GI fellow and only offer positions to outside fellows if they do not have interest from their internal fellows.

EUS training for established practitioners
Established practitioners start learning EUS on their own by reading books, watching videos, and attending courses. There are very limited opportunities for practicing endosonographers in the United States to get short-term (i.e., few weeks) hands-on training in EUS because of a variety of regulatory issues. Some practitioners will seek short hands-on training at facilities outside of the United States. This can help in the early learning curve of how to use the equipment and get mentored training in moving the scope, visualization, and perhaps FNA. Some practitioners will start doing EUS on their own patients in their hospital, but start with the least complicated lesions such as subepithelial masses and at the same time look at other structures to improve their skills. Over time, they develop their experience and supplement this with ongoing reading of published work on EUS, as well as attending EUS courses and/or observing established endosonographers. After a period of time, they may feel comfortable imaging lesions such as mediastinal nodes or pancreatic masses and want to perform FNA. Often the training for FNA will begin with hands-on courses using nonpatient models (i.e., gelatin phantom or porcine models) to understand the technique, and then they will perform these on their own patients. This path requires ongoing dedication to continued medical education in this area. In one study, the author used his own experience by retrospectively analyzing the first 57 EUS-guided FNAs of pancreatic masses performed. The study showed that the sensitivity for the diagnosis of pancreatic cancer was greater than 80% for the last 20 of the 57 cases, a level that was maintained for cases 51 through 80 [16].

Barriers to EUS training

There are several barriers to training in EUS, which may vary depending on whether for someone in fellowship or an established practitioner. For GI fellows, the greatest barrier is the limited number of competent mentors to train physicians, although in the past few years there has been a great expansion of fourth year EUS fellowship programs as formally trained individuals have gone on to start their own training programs. It must be appreciated that there is a wide range of learning experiences within these "Fourth Year EUS Fellowships" depending on the mentors' training, the number of years the mentors have been doing EUS, the equipment available, the number of cases, the duration of training, and the variety of cases. Therefore, not all fourth year EUS training experiences will be the same, and there is probably significant variability among programs.

For gastroenterologists who are in established practices, the barrier is how to competently learn EUS without doing a prolonged period of EUS fellowship training. Practitioners in the pathway may find alternative training in terms of study materials, short courses, observation of expert endosonographers, EUS in animal models or simulators, and rarely limited hands-on 7–14 day hands-on human training.

Regardless of the training pathway, learning continues beyond the training period and follows the endosonographer as he/she begins practicing on his/her own. A common problem is that after completing a training experience, the advanced endoscopist then goes to a new practice or hospital and frequently either does not own equipment or has old equipment. This can often lead to loss of skill sets. Given the expense of EUS equipment, even well-trained endoscopists sometimes find that because of lack of equipment, they end up not doing EUS in their practices.

Complementary training options

Simulators

The specific modality of EUS that would serve as the best training tool has yet to be determined. Furthermore, the question arises of whether it is better to teach manual skills outside the clinical setting [9]. Some have looked to simulators as a training tool to reduce medical errors by trainees and enhance teaching, as the financial pressures of the current economic crisis take a toll on the time that academic faculty used to have available for teaching. Endoscopic simulators, both vital and nonvital models, have the potential to play a unique role in EUS training based on the ability to simulate visual and tactile experiences that one would encounter during EUS procedures [11]. For example, one study showed that teaching EUS with live pig models significantly increased competence in diagnostic procedures; participants improved in abilities to visualize various anatomical structures, perform FNA, and carry out EUS-guided celiac neurolysis as assessed on the model itself [15,17].

Since EUS involves a steep learning curve, simulators have recently been used to explore other options for improving EUS training. Proponents of simulation learning believe that learning systems that involve artificial intelligence and other forms of simulation might be better than patient-based learning. In addition, simulators may be more beneficial to patients particularly by its avoidance of medical errors. Simulators for procedural training currently include animal models and computer simulation models [11].

Several studies have been conducted that have demonstrated the value of various training courses for improving knowledge and competence in various skills [18–20]. Furthermore, studies have previously reported that simulators can provide a certain degree of visual realism primarily because of new tissue materials that offer more pliability that closely correlates with human anatomy. These devices are utilized as teaching modalities to allow trainees to improve various skills. One such modality is the EUS Mentor (Simbionix Corp, Cleveland, OH, USA), which is a computer-based simulator that provides the experience of virtual endoscopy with more realism when compared to videotapes, CD-ROM, and DVD-ROM learning materials (see Figures 6.1a,b) [6]. Another modality is the EUS-FNA phantom wherein images are produced that replicate the echotexture of human structures, including, for example, hypoechoic structures that simulate suspicious masses and normal structures like lymph nodes (see Figure 6.2) [10]. The phantom modality also allows for the practice of EUS-guided FNA; however, a limitation is that it does not allow for simultaneous real-time video imaging of FNA [10]. In effect, this modality does not simulate or teach actual manipulation but rather offers experience with setting up and advancing the FNA needle and tracking the needle as it is advanced under real-time EUS into the "target" lesion [21].

The live swine model had been used frequently as a teaching modality, given the similarity in anatomy to humans. One study utilized a swine model with real-time EUS guidance to create a submucosal and a focal mediastinal lesion, to perform FNA, and to confirm the site of a sham (using saline solution) celiac block [15]. Another study by same author showed that the swine model is of value in teaching trainees normal EUS anatomy and may serve as a helpful tool in teaching EUS-guided intervention [17]. A recent study in France looked at 17 trainees who had hands-on experience with EUS to investigate whether there would be an improvement in competence in diagnostic procedures in specific anatomical areas, including splenic mesenteric vein, vena cava, splenic mesenteric artery, celiac tree, pancreatic gland, and bile duct after teaching EUS with a live pig model [18]. The study showed there was a significant increase in competence in actual diagnostic procedures with regard to visualizing anatomical structures, performance of FNA, and, to a lesser extent, EUS-guided celiac neurolysis.

Recently, a variation of the EASIE training model, previously used for teaching hemostasis and new endoscopic techniques such as endoscopic mucosal resection (EMR), has been developed for EUS [22]. This simulator, known as EASIE-R (Endosim, LLC (Berlin, MA), has been developed for EUS (Figures 6.3a,b). Several studies, reported in abstract form only, have described the potential role of this modality for teaching EUS. In one study, expert endosonographers attended a hands-on session and spent an hour working on the model. Afterwards, they completed a survey evaluation form regarding the device and its potential as a teaching tool for EUS. On the basis of the evaluations, it appears that this

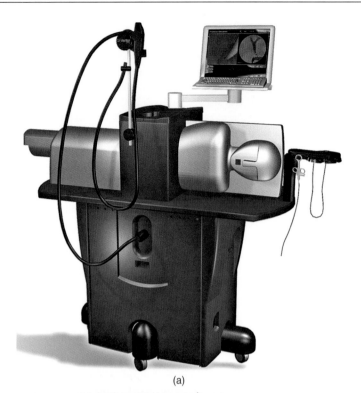

(a)

(b)

Figure 6.1 (a) Computerized EUS simulator (GI Mentor II, Simbionix Inc, Cleveland, OH). (b) Image obtained from GI Mentor EUS simulator (GI Mentor II, Simbionix Inc, Cleveland, OH).

simulator may serve as a useful teaching tool for basic and advanced EUS skills. There is some data regarding the benefit of EASIE as a teaching modality based on a pilot study where the aim was to determine whether hands-on training with the EASIE-R simulator can improve the acquisition of gastroenterology fellows' EUS skills in intubation, recognition of basic anatomical structures and abnormal pathology, as well as acquisition of advanced skills utilization such as performance of FNA. In this study, first, second, and third year gastroenterology fellows with minimal to no exposure to EUS procedures underwent a 1-day training session, which consisted of a morning session of didactics, a pretraining session on EUS simulator, followed by a 2-hour hands-on training session

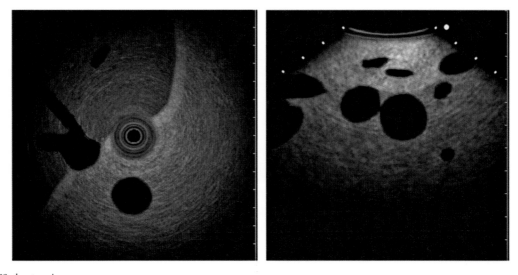

Figure 6.2 EUS phantom images.

with an expert endosonographer trainers. The fellows were asked to perform a series of tasks on the model during the pretraining session and again after the 2-hour hands-on training session. The fellows were evaluated both times, and their surveys were graded by an experienced endosonographer trainer. Scores were recorded and statistical analysis performed. The results concluded that GI fellows undergoing a 1-day training session including didactics followed by a hands-on simulation training session with the EUS EASIE-R simulator performed significantly better on the postsimulation training evaluation. Skills of EUS significantly improved with regard to ability to recognize basic and advanced anatomical structures, utilize the different modalities of EUS, and perform FNA after training on the simulator [23].

However, there has to date been no validation of the benefits of simulators in clinical applications with EUS as performed on actual patients. Furthermore, the length of time needed to practice with simulators to reach a level of competence is also unknown. However, there are such data looking at therapeutic upper endoscopy and colonoscopy training. One randomized, controlled trial was performed to compare the effects of a 7-month period of hands-on training in hemostatic techniques via the use of a compact EASIE model (a modified light weight version) and clinical endoscopic training with only clinical training in endoscopic hemostasis [20]. In this study, the investigators found that the compact EASIE simulator training in 3 full-day sessions over 7 months combined with clinical endoscopic training resulted in an improvement in endoscopic hemostatic techniques as tested on the model, and participants undergoing such training had a significantly higher success rate in clinical practice.

Virtual endoscopy simulators are computer-based devices that offer an alternative option to animal models, and based on data from the EASIE training model and other animal model, data should offer the same benefits, including reduced time to reach competency in endoscopy without the need for using animal models, associated costs for anesthesia, vet care, etc. or to purchase animal GI tract kits required for EASIE [11]. Virtual simulators

work by using three-dimensional pictures, generated in real time by a computer while the endoscope is moved through the GI-torso. Data about the location and movements of the scope are transmitted via sensors located at the tip and shaft of the endoscope. A force feedback module simulates resistance whenever the virtual GI-tract walls are touched, to provide a realistic "feel" during the procedure. One recent study, investigated whether the GI-Mentor (Simbionix, Tel Hashomer, Israel), a personal computer-based simulator with tactile feedback, can distinguish between beginners and experts in gastrointestinal endoscopy [24]. This virtual endoscopy simulator was able to identify differences between beginners and experts in gastrointestinal endoscopy and a 3-week training program appeared to improve the performance of beginners significantly.

To date, a variety of EUS training models/simulators have been developed, from live animal to the EASIE system to computer-based virtual endoscopy models, to assist in EUS training. Although no randomized trials have yet to be performed, prospective data demonstrates that the use of endoscopy simulators is likely to improve training and to shorten the learning curve in patients [11]. Simulators provide visual realism by having anatomical structures correlate to humans and some have a certain degree of tissue pliability allowing for a tactile experience to correlate as closely as possible to human tissue. In addition, these training models offer the opportunity to improve dexterity and fine motor skills required for performing EUS FNA and other therapeutic techniques.

Assessing EUS quality performance

Regardless of the training path followed, once an endoscopist is performing EUS, the expectation is that they are performing high-quality procedures. While difficult to define, this generally means having a diagnostic accuracy and complication rate similar to published results. Data is available from the literature in terms of

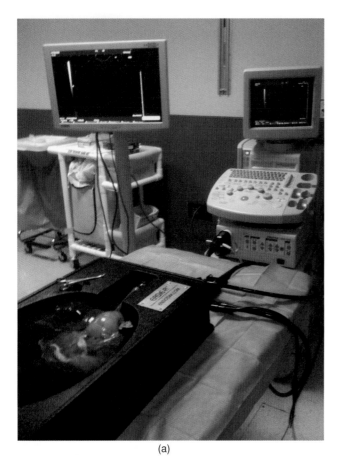

(a)

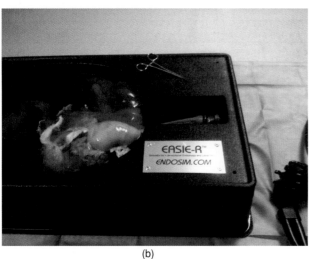

(b)

Figure 6.3 (a) EASIE-R EUS simulator. (b) Depicts a close up of the Easie-R EUS simulator.

expected complication rates (i.e., perforations, infections, pancreatitis) as well as diagnostic yield from FNA of pancreatic masses (see Table 6.4). In addition, one recent study reported on the EUS-guided FNA diagnostic yield of malignancy in solid pancreatic masses as a potential benchmark for quality performance measurement [25]. The aim of the study was to determine the

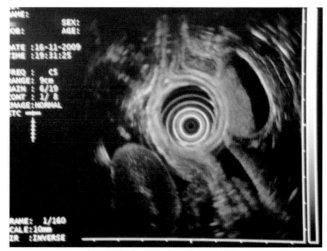

Figure 6.4 Depicts an EUS image produced from the EASIE-R simulator.

cytologic diagnostic rate of malignancy in EUS-FNA of solid pancreatic masses and to determine if variability exists among endoscopists and centers. The median diagnostic rate per center was 78% (range, 39–93%; 1st quartile, 61%) and per endoscopist was 75% (range, 0–100%; 1st quartile, 52%). This study concluded that EUS-FNA was diagnostic of malignancy in 71% of solid pancreatic masses and that endoscopists with a final cytologic diagnosis rate of malignancy for EUS-FNA of solid masses that was less than 52% were in the lowest quartile and should evaluate reasons for their low yield.

It is also clear that there are endosonographers who perform high-quality EUS exams and who were self-trained, and that there are endosonographers who perform low-quality EUS exams and who had fourth year EUS fellowship training. In an attempt to better define quality, the American College of Gastroenterology (ACG) and the American Society for Gastrointestinal Endoscopy (ASGE) created a joint task force to review and establish quality indicators to aid in the recognition of high-quality EUS examinations. The levels of evidence supporting these quality indicators were graded according to evidence-based criteria. Such indicators will hopefully permit the development of quality assurance programs and enable endosonographers to share their personal quality measures with their patients and GI departments [26].

There are few studies available that examine the learning curve for EUS [27–30]. However, there have been several well-done studies assessing learning curves for standard endoscopic procedures (upper endoscopy and colonoscopy) and for endoscopic retrograde cholangiopancreatography [31–33]. Guidelines exist for standard of practice for endoscopy as well [34]. More recently, guidelines for EUS training and recommendations on the minimum threshold number of EUS procedures required for competency have been developed by the American Society of Gastrointestinal Endoscopy (ASGE) based on available data [35]. According to the ASGE guidelines, the minimum number of EUS procedures recommended to reach competency is 150, including 75 mucosal tumors, 75 pancreaticobiliary cases, and 40 submucosal abnormalities. The guideline also recommends a

Table 6.4 Benchmark data for the yield of EUS FNA for diagnosing pancreatic mass lesions.

		Diagnostic Characteristics of EUS FNA for Pancreatic Mass Lesions		
	n	Sensitivity (%)	Specificity (%)	Accuracy (%)
Giovannini [Endoscopy 1995;27(2)]	43	75	100	79
Cahn [AJS 1996;172(5)]	50	88	100	87
Bhutani [Endoscopy 1997;28(9)]	47	64	100	72
Chang [GIE 1997;45(5)]	44	92	100	95
Erickson [AFP 1997;55(6)]	28	–	–	96
Faigel [JClinOnc 1997;15(4)]	45	72	100	75
Gress [GIE 1997;45(3)]	121	80	100	85
Wiersema [Gastro 1997;112(4)]	124	87	100	88
Binmoeller [GIE 1998;47(2)]	58	76	100	92
	560	81%	100%	86%

minimum of 50 FNA cases, 25 of which should be pancreatic FNA [35].

Achieving a level of competence to utilize EUS efficiently as a diagnostic and therapeutic modality requires practice. One particular study conducted in a prospective trial by a single endosonographer showed that the learning curve for EUS-FNA of solid pancreatic masses, a technically challenging procedure, does in fact continue beyond fellowship [27]. Yet, despite this data, a recent survey of training programs revealed that most GI fellows are unable to attain the minimum number of procedures recommended before completing their fellowship and entering practice [36].

Conclusion

EUS training is significantly different than standard GI endoscopy training, but can be achieved by mastering a series of skill sets. Learning EUS requires significant self-study that incorporates textbooks, atlases, and training videos, as well as instruction from experienced endosonographers. Because of the significant amount of material to learn, most EUS training is now being done as part of an additional year of advanced endoscopy/EUS training, but it is possible for practicing gastroenterologists to learn as well using a training plan tailored to individual needs. Simulators (computer or animal based) will increasingly be utilized to avoid early patient exposure with its inherent risks. Ultimately, the goal is to provide excellent patient care with high-quality examinations. Good initial training, followed by ongoing practice and continued medical education in EUS, should result in increasing availability of high-quality EUS procedures.

Video

Video 6.1 Training in endoscopic ultrasound

References

1 Rice TW, Boyce GA, Sivak MV Jr: Esophageal ultrasound and the preoperative staging of carcinoma of the esophagus. *Surgery* 1991;**101**:536–544.

2 Takemoto T, Itoh T, Fukumoto Y, Aibe T, Okita K: Endoscopic ultrasonography in preoperative staging of esophageal cancer. In: Dancygier H, Classen M (eds), *5th International Symposium on Endoscopic Ultrasonography*. Munich: Demeter Verlag (Z. Gastroenterol Suppl), 1989:34–38.

3 Caletti GC, Brochhi E, Gibilaro M, Ferrari A, Carfagna L, Barbara L: Sensitivity, specificity and predictive value of endoscopic ultrasonography in the diagnosis and assessment of gastric cancer [Abstract]. *Gastrointest Endosc* 1990;**36**:194–195.

4 Tio TL, Schouwink MH, Cikot RJLM, Tygat GNJ: Preoperative TNM classification of gastric carcinoma by endosonography in comparison with the pathological TNM system: A prospective study of 72 cases. *Hepato-Gastroenterology* 1989;**36**:51–56.

5 Rösch T, Braig C, Gain T, et al.: Staging of pancreatic and ampullary carcinoma by endoscopic ultrasonography. *Gastroenterology* 1992;**102**:188–199.

6 Mitake M, Nakasawa S, Tsukamoto Y, Kimoto E, Hayashi Y: Endoscopic ultrasonography in the diagnosis of depth invasion and lymph node metastasis of carcinoma of the papilla of Vater. *J Ultrasound Med* 1990;**9**:645–650.

7 Yasuda K, Mukai H, Fujimoto S, Nakajima M, Kawai K: The diagnosis of pancreatic cancer by endoscopic ultrasonography. *Gastrointest Endosc* 1988;**34**:1–8.

8 Pappalardo G, Reggio D, Frattaroli FM, et al.: The value of endoluminal ultrasonography and computed tomography in the staging of rectal cancer: A preliminary study. *J Surg Oncol* 1990;**43**:219–222.

9 Rösch T: State of the art lecture: Endoscopic ultrasonography: Training and competence. *Endoscopy* 2006;**38**(S1):S69–S72.

10 Kefalides P, Gress F: Training in endoscopic ultrasonography. In: Savides TJ, Gress FG (eds), *Endoscopic Ultrasonography*, 2nd ed. London: John Wiley Co., 2009.

11 Kefalides PT, Gress F: Simulator training for endoscopic ultrasound. *Gastrointest Endosc Clin N Am* 2006;**16**:543–552.

12 Hawes R, Fockens P: *Endosonography*. Philadelphia, PA: Saunders, 2006.

13 Bhutani MS, Deutsch JC: *Digital Human Anatomy and Endoscopic Ultrasonography*. Hamilton, ON: BC Decker, 2005.

14 Dietrich CF: *Endoscopic Ultrasound: An Introductory Manual and Atlas*. Munich: Thieme Georg Verlag Inc., 2006.

15 Bhutani M, Stills HF, Aveyard MA: Further development in the swine model for teaching diagnostic and interventional endoscopic ultrasound. *Gastrointest Endosc* 1998;**47**(4):AB44.

16 Mertz H, Gautam S: The learning curve for EUS-guided FNA of pancreatic cancer. *Gastrointest Endosc* 2004;**59**(1):33–37.

17 Bhutani M, Aveyard M, Stills H: Improved model for teaching interventional EUS. *Gastrointest Endosc* 2000;**52**(3):400–403.

18 Barthet M, Gasmi M, Boustiere C, Giovannini M, Grimaud JC, Berdah S: EUS training in a live pig model: Does it improve echo endoscope hands-on and trainee competence? *Endoscopy* 2007;**39**:535–539.

19 Harewood G, Yusuf T, Clain J, Levy M, Topazian M, Rajan E: Assessment of the impact of an educational course on knowledge of appropriate EUS indications. *Gastrointest Endosc* 2005;**61**(4):554–559.

20 Hochberger J, Mathes K, Koebnick C, Hahn E, Cohen J: Training with compactEASIE biologic endoscopy simulator significantly improves hemostatic technical skills of gastroenterology fellows: A randomized controlled comparison with clinical endoscopy training alone. *Gastrointest Endosc* 2005;**61**(2):204–215.

21 Matsuda K, Tajiri H, Hawes R: How shall we experience EUS and EUS-FNA before the first procedure? The development of learning tools. *Dig Endosc* 2004;**16**:S236–S239.

22 Raisner A, Gromsky M, Goodman A, et al.: Evaluation of a new endoscopic ultrasound (EUS) simulator (the EASIE simulator) for teaching basic and advanced EUS. *AJG* 2010;**105**(10):214A.

23 Raisner A, Goodman A, Ho S, et al.: Evaluation of a new endoscopic ultrasound (EUS) training simulator (the EASIE-R simulator) for teaching basic and advanced EUS: A prospective assessment of basic and advanced EUS skills using objective performance criteria. *Gastrointest Endosc Gastrointest Endosc* 2010;**71**(6):451A.

24 Ferlitsch A, Glauninger P, Gupper A, et al.: Evaluation of a virtual endoscopy simulator. *Endoscopy* 2002;**34**:698–702.

25 Savides TJ, Donohue M, Hunt G, et al.: EUS-guided FNA diagnostic yield of malignancy in solid pancreatic masses: A benchmark for quality performance measurement. *Gastrointest Endosc* 2007;**66**(2):277–282.

26 Jacobson BC, Chak A, Hoffman B, et al.: Quality indicators for endoscopic ultrasonography—ASGE/ACG taskforce on quality in endoscopy. *Am J Gastroenterol* 2006;**101**:898–901.

27 Eoubeidi MA, Ashutosh T: EUS-guided FNA of solid pancreatic masses: A learning curve with 300 consecutive procedures. *Gastrointest Endosc* 2005;**61**(6):700–708.

28 Fockens P, Van den Brande, Van Dullemen H, et al.: Endosonographic T-staging of esophageal carcinoma: a learning curve. *Gastrointest Endosc* 1996;**44**:58–62.

29 Bhutani MS, Gress FG, Giovannini M, et al.: The No Endosonographic Detection of Tumor (NEST) Study: a case series of pancreatic cancers missed on endoscopic ultrasonography. *Endoscopy* 2004;**36**(5):385–389.

30 Gress FG, Hawes RH, Savides TJ, et al.: Role of EUS in the preoperative staging of pancreatic cancer: a large single-center experience. *Gastrointest Endosc* 1999;**50**(6):786–791.

31 Cass OW, Freeman ML, Peine CJ, Zera RT, Onstad GR: Objective evaluation of endoscopy skills during training. *Ann Int Med* 1993;**118**:40–44.

32 Marshall JB: Technical proficiency of trainees performing colonoscopy: a learning curve. *Gastrointest Endosc* 1995;**42**:287–291.

33 Jowell PS, Baillie J, Branch S, Affronti J, Browning C, Bute B: Quantitative assessment of procedural competence: a prospective study of training in endoscopic retrograde cholangiopancreatography. *Ann Intern Med* 1996;**125**:983–989.

34 American Society for Gastrointestinal Endoscopy: *Principles of Training in Gastrointestinal Endoscopy*. Manchester, MA: ASGE, 1998.

35 Eisen GM, Dominitz JA, Faigel DO, et al.: Guidelines for credentialing and granting privileges for endoscopic ultrasound. *Gastrointest Endosc* 2001;**54**:811–814.

36 Azad JS, Verma D, Kapadia AS, Adler DG: Can U.S. GI fellowship programs meet American Society for Gastrointestinal Endoscopy recommendations for training in EUS? A survey of U.S. GI fellowship program directors.

7 ERCP

Joseph Leung[1,2] & Brian S. Lim[3]

[1]University of California, Davis School of Medicine, Sacramento, CA, USA
[2]VA Northern California Health Care System, Mather, CA, USA
[3]Kaiser Permanente, Riverside Medical Center, Riverside, CA, USA

Introduction to ERCP training

The need for training

Endoscopic retrograde cholangiopancreatography (ERCP) is an established diagnostic and therapeutic modality for patients with pancreaticobiliary diseases. Although its role as a diagnostic test has been partially replaced by magnetic resonance cholangiopancreatography (MRCP), ERCP remains the gold standard for the diagnosis of suspected biliary pathologies, including ductal stones and strictures. Therapeutic ERCP offers an alternative to surgical treatment and indeed is the preferred method for the management of bile duct stones and for the palliation of malignant obstructive jaundice. More recently, prolonged biliary stenting with multiple plastic stents has offered significant benefits in patients with benign bile duct strictures [1].

ERCP is the one of the most challenging endoscopic procedure performed by gastroenterologists. Optimal performance requires broad knowledge of pancreaticobiliary pathologies, considerable manual dexterity, proper understanding of the equipment being used, and familiarity with alternative diagnostic and therapeutic approaches [2]. It also carries substantial risks, even in the hands of experts. For these reasons among others, it has become very clear that one should be properly trained in order to be competent with ERCP and minimize risks to the patients.

The format of training

Traditional ERCP training takes the form of the teacher–apprentice system with supervised hands-on practice on patients. The trainees learn the basic and advanced skills under the tutelage of the local ERCP trainer and perform the procedure with the help of a trained GI assistant. Sometimes, the trainee or trainer would serve the role of an assistant. For many trainees, they receive their ERCP training as part of a 3-year GI fellowship program, usually in their senior year of training after mastering the techniques of upper and lower GI endoscopy. Because of the lack of sufficient number of patients, many programs cannot offer ERCP training to all of the trainees enrolled in fellowship training. Instead, ERCP training is now being offered to a selected few and in the form of an advanced fellowship where trainees spend an additional (fourth) year in special ERCP training.

The types of training—from clinical to simulation

Clinical experience results from performance of the procedure on patients using real scope and accessories. This is the traditional way by which many endoscopists learn and master the ERCP skills. Supervised hands-on practice offers learning opportunities but the limited number of patients has restricted the trainees' access to patients and thus practice opportunities. Because of the high risks and complications involved with therapeutic ERCP procedures, many trainers do not feel comfortable with allowing trainees to perform these procedures independently. Although many trainees have admitted to not completing the required number [as recommended by the American Society for Gastrointestinal Endoscopy (ASGE) or Accreditation Council on Graduate Medical Education (ACGME)] before graduation, majority of them want to practice ERCP, hoping that they will improve their imperfect skill with practice on patients in the daily unsupervised practice. This poses increased risks to patients as failure and complications tend to increase with inexperienced endoscopists.

Trainers have resorted to alternative methods for hands-on experience to provide trainees with more practice and learning opportunities. Such practice settings include the use of the live anesthetized animal model, the *ex vivo* porcine stomach model, mechanical simulators, and computer simulators. The details of these simulators are discussed later in the chapter.

Prerequisite for training

Trainee—level of skill and expertise

Following are the trainee prerequisites set forth by the latest ASGE guidelines for advanced endoscopic training [3]:

1 Trainees who are seeking to acquire skills in advanced endoscopic training must have completed standard endoscopy training during an approved GI fellowship (or equivalent training) and have documented competence in general routine (i.e., not advanced) endoscopic procedures.

2 Trainees must have good understanding of the normal anatomy/physiology of the pancreatobiliary system and epidemiology, pathophysiology, diagnosis, and treatment involving this system.

3 The trainee must understand the cognitive as well as technical component of the procedures, including appropriate indications for and the contraindications to performing these procedures. They should have knowledge of pre- and postprocedure evaluations as well as managing procedure-related complications that may occur. The trainee should have the ability to explain the procedure to the patient, including obtaining informed consent. Furthermore, trainees must know that the usage of a side viewing scope changes the orientation of the endoscopic image, although the basic controls are similar. Trainees should receive orientation for the basics of ERCP, including didactic talks on organization of the ERCP room and radiological interpretation of cholangiogram and pancreatogram in order to help them understand the clinical procedure. Although technical skill is gained through practice, trainees should have a good grasp on the cognitive aspect of different ERCP procedures in order to understand the technical component as well as clinical application even prior to getting hands-on training.

Setting—case load

The experience gained by the trainee is affected by the clinical case load (and complexity) in individual training centers. The ASGE stated that trainees should perform a minimum of 180 cases with at least 50% of procedures containing a therapeutic component in order to achieve competency [4]. The Australians have set an even higher standard requiring trainees to have performed 200 unassisted procedures. In order to provide adequate training, the training institution should have cases or referrals more than the minimum number required by fellowship training as there may be difficult cases that the trainees cannot handle, especially at the start of their training. Except for large academic centers, many training programs do not have the sufficient number of patients for training and many trainees have graduated without meeting the minimum standard. Yet in a previous survey of 69 graduates from US fellowship programs, 91% were planning to perform ERCP in their practice despite one-third of them stating that their training was inadequate [5].

Trainer—a skilled technician may not be a good teacher

There are certain prerequisites for a trainer, namely clinical and teaching experience. ERCP trainers have different teaching styles; no two trainers agree on everything and there is no standard of reference. However, a skilled technician may not necessarily be a good teacher if he/she cannot communicate effectively with the trainees. Allowing the trainee to struggle by trial and error may not be in the best interest for the patient. The ability to recognize the errors made by the trainees and to correct their mistakes, giving them specific instructions to complete a procedure without taking away the endoscope would be ideal. Yet, this may be difficult to accomplish. Often times, the trainer may have to take over the instrument and demonstrate to the trainee how to complete a particular step of the procedure and then allow the trainee to con-

tinue. Patience in coaching and allowing the trainees to practice without taking the scope away from them is an important quality for the trainer who must balance trainee learning with the safety of the patient.

ERCP training

Cognitive and technical aspects

ERCP skill can broadly be divided into two components: the cognitive and the technical aspects. Technical skills can be learned with understanding the function and operation of the endoscope and different accessories, and practicing coordination between the endoscopist and the assistant. In principle, many accessories have similar basic design, i.e., exchange over a guide wire, so good coordination as a team is necessary to facilitate the ERCP procedure.

Clinical experience comes with hands-on practice and is acquired with repeat performance on patients with different clinical problems. The number of procedures performed has traditionally been used as a surrogate for the trainees' experience. However, it is important to realize that an inexperienced endoscopist could "waste" much of the clinical time if they have to struggle in handling the different ERCP accessories, thus missing the opportunity to learn the clinical application of the procedure in the management of the patient.

In addition to the technical skills, trainees must have the ability to recognize the different endoscopic pathologies and understand the choice of different accessories. Furthermore, ERCP involves monitoring the position of accessories and manipulating them under fluoroscopic control. Basic education on radiological interpretation of ERCP images is therefore necessary to enable the trainee to recognize the different pathologies, for example, how to differentiate between a stone and an air bubble in the bile duct and diagnosing a benign stricture versus a malignant one. This is of crucial importance since many clinical decisions are made at the time of ERCP using the fluoroscopic information to guide subsequent therapy. This is in contrast to traditional radiological imaging because the decision to go ahead with therapy cannot wait until one receives the radiology report. Thus, the trainee needs to be trained to make such clinical decisions (independently) based on proper interpretation of fluoroscopic images.

Equipment—scope, accessories, diathermy

ERCP utilizes the side viewing duodenoscope to provide proper orientation and alignment with the papilla. Although the channel size of different ERCP scopes can vary, it is preferable to use the large channel therapeutic duodenoscope as it can accommodate larger 10 or 11.5 Fr size accessories and allow more options for endoscopic intervention. Further scope modification includes a newly designed system with a small V-notch on the elevator (Olympus Medical System, Tokyo) for holding the guide wire to facilitate the exchange of accessories over a special short guide wire. Further adaptation with the use of wire lock mechanisms such as the Rapid Exchange (Boston Scientific, Natick, MA, USA) or Fusion System (Cook Endoscopy, Winston Salem, NC, USA) allow anchoring of the short (or long) guide wire to facilitate the exchange of accessories over a stable guide wire. If possible, trainees should become familiar with both long and short wire exchanges and manipulation.

Accessories can be separated into diagnostic and therapeutic categories

A simple catheter or papillotome is used for injection of contrast medium and to achieve diagnostic cannulation of the bile or pancreatic duct. Traction on the papillotome cutting wire helps to deflect the tip of the papillotome and facilitates selective cannulation of the bile duct. Curving the tip of the catheter can also facilitate biliary cannulation. Instead of injecting contrast, a flexible hydrophilic tip guide wire can be used for selective cannulation, avoiding the risk of overfilling the pancreas in repeat attempts at CBD cannulation.

Therapeutic accessories include the papillotome, stone extraction balloon or baskets, dilation catheter or balloon, brush cytology catheter, and plastic or self-expandable metal stents. For large stones, one can consider using the mechanical lithotripter or intraductal lithotripsy methods such as electrohydraulic lithotripsy (EHL) and laser lithotripsy.

Diathermy is generally achieved using monopolar electrocautery via electrosurgical generators such as the ValleyLab (Boulder, Colorado, USA) and Olympus (Olympus Co, Tokyo, Japan) diathermy units. The energy levels (cutting and coagulation) can be preset or adjusted on the machine as well as the wave form (pure cutting, coagulation, or a blended mode). Cutting is controlled by activating the foot pedal. The ERBE unit has a microcomputer control that automatically allows a stepwise cutting (alternating coagulation and cut) of the papilla. Trainees need to be well versed in the setup and desired electrocautery settings of the generator in their unit.

Performance —key steps to technique and trick of trade

Scope handling

Unlike performing upper and lower GI endoscopy where there may be considerable hand and body movement, ERCP requires a steady position of the tip of the duodenoscope to facilitate the procedure. In this setting, the endoscope resembles a launching platform where different accessories are used to achieve cannulation and therapy within the pancreas or the biliary system. It is important to minimize body movement that may be transmitted to the tip of the endoscope (Figure 7.1). In addition, the scope shaft should be held with third, fourth, and fifth digits using only the index finger for both the air and suction button (as opposed to using the index finger for suction and third finger for air while holding the shaft with two fingers as many endoscopists prefer during colonoscopy). This puts less strain on the base of the thumb when moving the elevator (Figure 7.2). This three-finger technique also allows the fifth digit to be used for gripping and stabilizing the guide wire during exchange when using the long-wire method.

In terms of scope manipulation, basically, there is a combination of 12 different maneuvers—up/down, left/right tip deflection (angulations), left/right scope tip rotation by the left wrist, pulling/pushing of the scope, up/down control of the elevator, and finally air insufflation and suction—to change the position of the

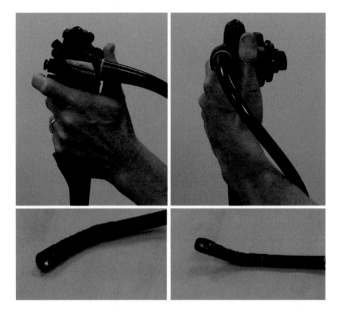

Figure 7.1 Using one finger to control the air and suction button allows easy control of the elevator. Left wrist rotation can alter the scope tip position and change the orientation with the papilla in the duodenum.

scope tip in relation to the papilla in order to achieve and maintain a good orientation and alignment for diagnostic and therapeutic manipulations (Figure 7.3). The wheels should be freed when performing insertion and positioning of the endoscope and locked subsequently to allow a more stable position for manipulation of accessories. A combination of the different maneuvers will serve to position the papilla in the middle of the endoscopy field. In some cases, it may be necessary to reverse some of these manipulations or repeat them in order to regain a proper position.

Cannulation—selective

Selective cannulation of the bile duct and pancreatic duct is achieved using a diagnostic catheter or a wire-guided papillotome. For CBD cannulation, the tip of the scope is inserted further into the duodenum with the catheter approaching the papilla

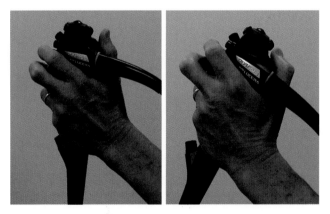

Figure 7.2 Holding the ERCP scope with two fingers on the air and suction buttons (as in a colonoscopy procedure) will limit the left thumb movement and use of the elevator. This will also put unnecessary strain on the base of the thumb when using the elevator.

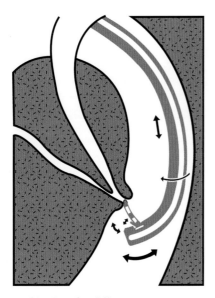

Figure 7.3 A combination of 12 different scope maneuvers to position the catheter for selective cannulation (air insufflation and suction are not shown).

from below and directing towards the 11–12 o'clock position. It is important to avoid impacting the catheter and forceful injection of contrast to prevent submucosal injection, which may traumatize the papilla. Cannulation of the pancreatic duct is achieved by directing the catheter in the 1–2 o'clock position and going slightly more horizontal, i.e., perpendicular to the duodenal wall.

The use of a papillotome allows tip deflection with traction on the cutting wire to align with the biliary axis. If multiple pancreatic injections occur in attempted CBD cannulation, it may be easier to change to the use of a guide wire for selective CBD cannulation. Gentle probing is performed with 5 mm of the tip of the guide wire protruding from the papillotome to aid selective cannulation (see Videos 7.1, 7.2). It is important to note that even though most guide wires have atraumatic flexible tips, they are quite stiff when restrained by the catheter, and forceful manipulation can still lead to trauma and edema of the papilla. Gentle probing in the respective axis of the bile or pancreatic duct while altering slightly the direction of approach if attempts fail will facilitate cannulation. As most papillotomes tend to deviate to the right when traction is applied, it may be necessary to shape the tip of the papillotome to change the orientation of the tip and thus alignment of the guide wire. The use of a rotatable papillotome may achieve similar results (see Video 7.3).

Successful deep cannulation of the bile or pancreatic duct depends on proper alignment of the accessory with the axis of the distal ductal anatomy. It is not uncommon to see that the tip of the catheter or guide wire is abutting against the wall of the ampullary portion of the distal bile duct and further advancement of the accessory is not possible. It is helpful to perform further manipulation under fluoroscopic control to change the alignment of the distal tip of the accessory. Sometimes, dropping the elevator, pulling back the tip of the scope, and gentle rotation to the left will change the accessory orientation and bring back the alignment with the axis of the distal bile duct to facilitate fur-

ther advancement (see Video 7.4). Similarly, manipulation of the scope tip can facilitate deep cannulation of the pancreas, which is more easily achieved using a flexible tip guide wire. There is suggestion (in abstract form) that the use of a loop tip guide wire (Cook Endoscopy, Winston Salem, NC, USA) (which is less traumatic than a pointed tip guide wire) may facilitate cannulation [6]. Other techniques utilized for difficult selective biliary cannulations include wire guided cannulation following wire placement into the pancreatic duct, and after placement of a small diameter pancreatic duct stent. (see Videos 7.5 and 7.6).

Papillotomy—standard

Before performing papillotomy, one has to understand the indication and contraindications for doing the procedure. Different diathermy units are available and each has different design in terms of power (energy) setting and performance (cutting or blended modes), and it is safer to use a unit that one is familiar with.

Papillotomes are designed in a very similar way with a cutting wire that is controlled by varying the traction on the handle and thus the tension applied to the wire while cutting when electrical circuit is completed using the foot pedal. The length of the exposed wire also affects control of the papillotome.

Prior to performing the cut, it is important to have a good assessment of the anatomy of the papilla and adjacent structures such as periampullary diverticulum. The "perfect" axis for a biliary papillotomy is along the axis of the distal bile duct and the intraduodenal portion of the papilla and this is usually considered the 11–12 o'clock orientation, not simply the 11–12 o'clock direction as seen on the endoscopy monitor [7]. Similarly, the pancreatic axis is along the 1–2 o'clock direction. It is important to remember that the alignment of the scope tip with the papilla can change because of scope manipulation but the "perfect" axis will not since this is an anatomical landmark.

Many endoscopists perform papillotomy by putting a lot of tension (traction) on the cutting wire to ensure contact with the papillary structure. However, too much traction tends to cause the cutting wire to deviate to the right and excess pressure on the tissue may result in an uncontrolled cut. The best approach is to maintain minimal traction on the cutting wire (to avoid unnecessary deviation) and using the elevator and up angulation of the scope tip to control the position of the cutting wire and maintain sufficient contact with the tissue. Current is applied in a controlled manner to allow a stepwise cut along the "perfect" axis. A good controlled papillotomy depends on a balance between traction (tension) on the wire and adequate tissue contact. Too little contact will result in only coagulation with a lot of smoke generated but ineffective cutting; too much tension runs a risk of uncontrolled cut and bleeding (see Video 7.7). Occasionally, a long scope position is required to achieve the desirable cutting axis for biliary sphincterotomy (see Video 7.8)

The size of the papillotomy depends on the indication (stent insertion or stone removal) as well as the anatomy of the distal bile duct and intraduodenal portion of the papilla. A long and slender distal bile duct will still give a small cross-sectional diameter even if a relatively long papillotomy cut is performed, whereas a dilated bile duct down to the level of the papilla will give a large opening after a medium-sized cut because of the ductal dilation. It is difficult to predetermine the absolute length of the papillotomy since a lot will depend on the anatomy and prominence of the papilla. We consider it a small cut if the length is less than half of the cuttable papilla (defined as the separation between the papillary orifice and the reflection of the distal bile duct on the duodenal wall beyond which perforation is very likely), a medium cut if half of the papilla and a large cut if it is greater than two-third of the length. Additional methods including balloon sphincteroplasty or the use of lithotripsy may be required for the removal of large bile duct stones.

Stone extraction—balloon and basket

Small- to medium-sized stones (≤ 1 cm diameter) can be removed easily using a retrieval (occlusion) balloon. Stone removal with a retrieval balloon is usually done over a guide wire that allows repeat cannulation of the bile duct and also prevents the risk of subsequent failed cannulation in case of stone impaction that can occur without the guide wire. One should be able to use the two-way stopcock to adjust the amount of air injected into the balloon and thus the balloon size to match the diameter of the bile duct. Excess air will result in a large balloon and stretching or over distension of the bile duct, causing pain to the patient. This can also create an artificial resistance to the pulling or withdrawal of the balloon due to the excess size and friction. On the other hand, if the balloon is too small, particularly when it is in a large bile duct, the stone(s) can move around the balloon, making removal more difficult. Also, the papillotomy must be adequate to allow easy stone passage. If the papillotomy is too small, there is a potential risk that the balloon can deform and slip out alongside the stone but at the same time, impacting the stone at the papillotomy site. If one is uncertain about the ease of stone extraction, an occlusion balloon can be used to gauge the size of the exit passage, i.e., distal bile duct and papillotomy. If the inflated balloon can be removed easily, stones similar to the size of the inflated balloon can be removed easily as well. If, however, there is deformity of the balloon as it comes through, or undue resistance is encountered, stone removal may be difficult.

After an adequate papillotomy, stone(s) can also be removed using stone extraction baskets. For proper engagement of the stone(s), the basket should be manipulated in a closed manner to pass the stones. The basket is then opened above the stone in the common bile duct or common hepatic duct and pulled back in an open manner, shaking gently as the basket is being retracted to engage the stone. Care should be taken to avoid opening the basket below the stone in order to avoid the risk of pushing the stone into the intrahepatic ducts. The ease of engaging the stone also depends on the design of the basket, for example large gaps between the wires may not be good for small stones. The flower baskets (Olympus Medical System, Tokyo, Japan) have a special design that changes the four wires on top into eight wires which close down to a much smaller mesh size and is therefore better for engaging small stones. Ideally, one should control the basket and start removing the bottommost stone first and avoid engaging too many stones in the basket, which will make the extraction more difficult as this resembles removal of a large stone.

When difficulty is encountered in the process of stone extraction with a basket, it is important to apply traction continuously and slowly and allow time for the stone to be removed, especially if the papillotomy is barely adequate. It is important to avoid putting a lot of traction and closing the basket too tightly around the stone as the wires will cut into the stone, running a risk of stone and basket impaction if the stone cannot be removed. Before committing oneself to the risk of stone and basket impaction, it is useful to determine if the stone can be freed from the basket or to look for alternative methods for stone fragmentation, i.e., use of lithotripsy, extending the papillotomy, or using additional balloon sphincteroplasty to avoid this complication.

In removing relatively large CBD stones, it is useful to start with a mechanical lithotripter or with a basket that allows the handle to be connected to a cranking device that allows stone fragmentation to avoid the risk of stone and basket impaction. Usually, we recommend shaking the basket (jiggling up and down) to engage small- to medium-sized common duct stones. With large CBD stone(s), the wires are being compressed and it may be difficult to jiggle the wires. In such cases, it is useful to rotate the scope and basket so that the basket wires can be moved around the stone for proper stone engagement. It may be necessary to advance the metal sheath of the lithotripter to allow better transmission of the rotational force and to allow the basket wires to capture the stone.

Stenting—plastic and metal

Traditional stenting is done using a three layers coaxial system, including a separate inner catheter and pusher over a guide wire. The recently improved OASIS system (Cook Endoscopy, Winston Salem, NC, USA) has combined the catheter and pusher into a single unit and minimizes the exchanges required for stenting. However, this setup requires a stent of a suitable length to be chosen before being loaded onto the stenting system. This delivery system design is shared with many of the different stenting units from other manufacturers.

Stent measurement

The length of the stent usually represents the separation between the proximal and distal flap for a straight stent design or between the pigtails for a double pigtail stent. In an ideal setting, the stent should be placed with the distal flap at the papilla and the proximal flap about 1 cm above the upper level of the obstructing stricture. The length of the stent can be estimated from the plain radiograph by measuring the separation between the papilla (with the tip of the scope against the papilla) and upper level of the stricture using the scope width as a guide for measurement. Alternatively, the guide wire can be pulled back (upon deep cannulation) from the level of the stricture to the level of the papilla (as seen through the transparent accessory), and the distance traveled outward by the guide wire from the accessory port will give the actual measurement of the separation; this distance plus 1 cm equals the length of the stent. Another method is to pull back the accessory over the guide wire, but this time, measuring the distance traveled outward from the biopsy valve. If the separation is measured directly from the fluoroscopic image or a radiograph, it will be necessary to correct for possible magnification, otherwise the stent selected may be too long.

Guide wire negotiation of bile duct stricture

Deep cannulation of the bile duct and negotiating the stricture with a guide wire is easier if a prior papillotomy is performed and if the stricture is not too tight. However, sometimes the stricture takes off at an angle to the distal CBD as seen under fluoroscopy. In this case, it may be necessary to change the scope tip position (as previously discussed) so as to change the orientation (alignment) of the tip of the guide wire and allows it to move in the direction of the stricture to achieve deep cannulation. An alternative is to shape and create a curve at the tip of the guide wire to allow the guide wire tip to loop, and this may facilitate passage of the wire through an angulated stricture. We find that sometimes putting a double curve (S shape) to the tip of the guide wire helps in deflecting and looping of the wire tip to facilitate passage of the guide wire through difficult strictures (see Video 7.9). It may sometimes be necessary to use a papillotome to achieve deep CBD cannulation and deflect the tip of the papillotome to bounce the guide wire tip off the bile duct wall to change the angle and to facilitate passage through the stricture. It may be possible to use an inflated balloon inside the bile duct as a pivot to deflect the tip of the guide wire across a hilar stricture (Figures 7.4 and 7.5).

Dilation of stricture

Standard stricture dilation involves the use of graded dilating catheters or pneumatic balloon dilators. The most important step is to ensure the passage of a guide wire through the stricture. Positioning of the dilator is done using the radiopaque markers placed at the end of the catheter or over the two ends of the dilation balloon. Effective dilation is achieved if the single marker (which represents the widest part of a dilating catheter) is advanced above

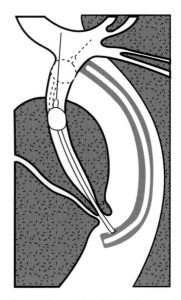

Figure 7.5 An inflated balloon inside the bile duct can be used as a pivot to deflect the tip of the guide wire into the right and left hepatic system.

the level of the obstruction or, in the case of a balloon dilator, the obliteration of the initial waist on the balloon caused by the stricture. Usually, we recommend inflating the dilation balloon according to the pressure recommended by the manufacturer and keeping the balloon inflated for an additional 15–30 seconds after full insufflation or obliteration of the waist. A persistent waist formation on the balloon denotes a very tight bile duct stricture. Choice of the size of the dilation balloon should take into consideration of the diameter of the normal duct, usually the segment below the obstruction in order to avoid damage to the normal portion of the bile duct from excessive dilation.

Brush cytology

Exchange of the brush cytology catheter over the guide wire is done in the usual coordinated fashion. Once the catheter is advanced above the stricture, the brush is pushed out and locked and the whole apparatus is pulled back until the bare brush is positioned through the area of the stricture. A radiograph is taken for documentation. The brush is jiggled in the area of the stricture or dragged through the stricture by left wrist rotation on the scope and subsequently pulled back into the catheter. The catheter is then exchanged over the guide wire.

Stent placement

Most of the current plastic stenting systems have combined the inner catheter and pusher in a single unit using a luer lock mechanism. A stent of suitable length is chosen and loaded onto the stenting system, which is then inserted over the guide wire and positioned across the stricture. Once the stent is in the predetermined position, the inner catheter and pusher are separated and the pusher is used to hold the stent in place while the inner catheter and guide wire are pulled back to deploy the stent. Traditionally, the radiopaque markers were used to help determine the length of the stent, but now with the combined system, a suitable

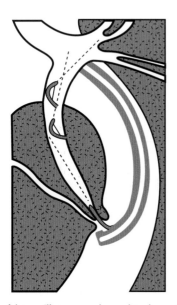

Figure 7.4 Tip of the papillotome can be used to change the orientation of the guide wire tip inside the bile duct to facilitate wire passage into intrahepatic ducts.

length stent is preselected (see section "Stent measurement") and the radiopaque markers are used mainly to determine the position of the catheter and to avoid unnecessary movements during stent deployment. They are especially helpful when it comes to placement of a stent across a hilar stricture into the intrahepatic duct.

With adequate dilation of the stricture, it is easy to advance a stent across a stricture. However, for tight or angulated stricture, the stenting system may not be stiff enough (especially when a 0.025 instead of a 0.035 guide wire is used) to facilitate stent passage. If difficulty is encountered during stent placement, we recommend exchanging the regular guide wire to a stiff guide wire, for example, the Teflon-coated THSF wire (Cook Endoscopy, Winston Salem, NC, USA) or the Amplatz Super Stiff Guide Wire (Boston Scientific, Natick, MA, USA), in order to provide more rigidity to the inner catheter and stenting unit. In addition, pushing the stent against the stricture and then jiggling the inner catheter/guide wire (without actually pulling the unit back) may ease the tip of the stent across the stricture.

In patients with hilar obstruction, where both the right and left systems are obstructed, it is advisable to initially place two guide wires, one into each side of the obstructed liver and to perform balloon dilation prior to stent placement. We prefer to stent the left side first (as described above) because of the angulation and change in axis of the left system followed by placement of the stent into the right hepatic system. It may sometimes be necessary to shape the stent so that it conforms to the anatomy of the left hepatic duct stricture in order to avoid subsequent stent migration (see Video 7.10).

Short wire stenting system for multiple stent insertion

Intraductal exchange (IDE) or intraductal release (IDR) of the guide wire to facilitate stenting using the short wire Fusion system (Cook Endoscopy, Winston Salem, NC, USA) involves the use of a special inner catheter with a side port placed at 2.5 cm from the tip of the catheter. Thus, only a small segment of the inner catheter goes over the guide wire. The stenting system is loaded onto the guide wire and pushed into position using the pusher. In order to release of the stent, the guide wire has to be pulled back to free the tip of the inner catheter, and then the inner catheter and pusher are separated by untwisting the luer lock mechanism. The inner catheter can then be pulled back, deploying the stent in its proper position across the stricture. The real advantage of this stent delivery system is that the guide wire remains across the stricture after the stent is deployed. If there is a need for placement of a second stent, it can be performed easily and there is no need for repeat cannulation and negotiation of the stricture (see Video 7.11).

Pancreatic stenting

There is more and more published data to indicate successful pancreatic stenting offers an advantage in the prevention of post-ERCP pancreatitis [8]. Contrary to biliary stenting, pancreatic stents are often placed just over a prepositioned guide wire in the pancreas. We found that using the short guide wire system allows easy exchange of accessories and placement of the stent over a sta-tionary guide wire, thus minimizing exchange and risk of injury of the pancreatic duct caused by tip of the guide wire. Also, most of the pancreatic stents only have an anchoring mechanism to prevent upward stent migration into the pancreas. Technically, it is easier to use a 0.025″ guide wire for pancreatic cannulation, which is also considered less traumatic compared to the standard 0.035″ guide wire. Most endoscopists prefer to place 5 Fr stents for pancreatic drainage, and to only use larger 7 or 10 Fr stents if there is a significant stricture in the pancreatic duct following dilation or after attempted stone removal. For the purpose of splinting, the pancreatic orifice and drainage following pancreatic sphincterotomy or repeated pancreatic cannulation, a short 3 cm 5 Fr stent can be used as these are more prone to migration after the initial edema settles. An alternative is to place a 9 or 12-cm long 3 Fr stent (Skinny stent, Cook Endoscopy, Winston Salem, NC, USA) in the pancreatic duct with a pigtail end in the duodenum. This is often done after pancreatic sphincter manometry. Even though these stents are long, they still migrate spontaneously with time. If more prolonged drainage is necessary as in cases with a leak or stricture, we recommend placing longer 7 or 9 cm stent in order to bypass the genu so that the end of the indwelling stent lies in the long axis of the pancreatic duct without irritation to the wall or side branches of the pancreas. Sometimes, it may be necessary to shape the polyethylene stents (which are more rigid) to conform to the shape of the pancreatic duct in order to minimize local irritation to the main pancreatic duct. The use of stents made of softer material, such as the Soflex stents (Cook Endoscopy, Winston Salem, NC, USA) and Freeman Pancreatic Flexi-Stent (Hobbs Medical Inc., Stafford Springs, CT, USA), which are more flexible and conform better to the shape of the pancreatic duct, may be less irritating to the pancreas. Although pancreatic stent blockage can occur with time, the incidence of infection and pancreatitis remains very uncommon. However, it is generally recommended to repeat a plain X-ray of the abdomen one week after pancreatic stenting to document if spontaneous stent migration has occurred. It is still advisable to schedule a routine stent pull after several weeks if the stent has not migrated (see Video 7.12).

Special accessories—mechanical lithotripter

For patients with large CBD stones, it may be necessary to fragment the stone using a mechanical lithotripter before removal of the stone fragments. The conventional lithotripters are what we often call lifesavers when we encounter stone and basket impaction. In such situations, it may be necessary to cut the handle of the basket and allow a metal sheath to be inserted either after removal of the duodenoscope or through the channel of the scope and advanced up to the level of the stone (Soehendra lithotripter, Cook Endoscopy, Winston Salem, NC, USA). The end of the basket is connected to a crank handle and traction is applied to the basket wires to fragment the stone against the metal sheath.

Purpose-built lithotripsy baskets are also available, for example, the BML basket (Olympus Medical System, Tokyo, Japan). The setup includes a large and strong basket and a movable metal sheath. Initial cannulation (after an adequate papillotomy) is performed using the Telfon sheath, which makes it easier to manipulate the basket. Once the stone is engaged, the metal sheath is advanced over the Teflon sheath up to the level of the stone. The best position for stone fragmentation is in the mid-CBD (straight portion of the bile duct). Traction is applied to the basket wire by turning the crank handle to allow the wires to cut slowly into the stone.

It is important to remember that large stones produce large fragments and it may be necessary to repeat the lithotripsy before attempting stone removal. If the stones are hard, the wire of the lithotripsy basket are likely to get deformed, and it may be necessary to remove the basket to clean and reshape the basket wires before further attempts at lithotripsy.

Traditionally, we shake the basket to engage the stone, but with large stones, they tend to compress the basket wires and it may be difficult to engage the stone with shaking. It is more useful to advance the metal sheath and rotate the left wrist and using the rotational movement to move the wires around the stone to capture the stone.

Other types of purpose-designed lithotripters are made of Nitinol wires (memory baskets) with a more flexible metal sheath and a special handle that can be adapted onto a cranking device (similar to a caulk gun) that allows continuous traction be applied to the basket to fragment the stone. Examples are Trapezoid basket (Boston Scientific, Natick, MA, USA) and Fusion Lithotripsy Basket (Cook Endoscopy, Winston Salem, NC, USA). These are usually used for medium-sized stones rather than giant stones.

Alternatives for ERCP training

Setting and tools—traditional, caseload, simulator training (comparison)

Certain prerequisites are necessary when we consider alternative methods for ERCP training. It is important to understand that part of the performance is based on the trainees' understanding of the operation of the equipment and accessories. Unless the alternative practice offers the opportunity to use real scope and accessories with hands-on experience, trainees may not be able to reap the benefits of additional or supplemental training. The IDEAL simulator/simulation training should provide trainees with the

learning opportunity to **Improve** their basic skills, **Demonstrates** realism to help trainees understand the anatomy and motility, **Ease** of incorporating into a training program (i.e. inexpensive and portable system that allows repeated practices without special setup), **Application** in training including teaching therapeutic procedures, and **Learning** with real scope and accessories including use of simulation fluoroscopy [9].

Different simulators are available to supplement ERCP training although there is limited published data in the literature regarding the role of individual simulators in training. In particular, there is a paucity of published information on the impact of simulator training on the trainees' clinical performance and outcome of their ERCP procedures.

In general, there are three types of simulators—computer simulator, *ex vivo* porcine stomach model, and mechanical simulator. The computer simulator, for example, the GI Mentor II, is useful for understanding the anatomy, duodenal motility, and basic orientation for cannulation. However, there is a lack of reality and tactile sensation when it comes to the use of different accessories that are represented by special probes (not real tools), and this does not offer the trainees a good feel of the procedure.

A more commonly used training model is the *ex vivo* porcine stomach model with attached biliary system that allows trainees to practice with real scope and accessories. However, the anatomical variation between the porcine model and human papilla makes positioning and cannulation more difficult. Besides, there are separate biliary and pancreatic openings, making it suboptimal to practice selective cannulation. To facilitate proper practice of biliary papillotomy, the porcine model is further improved by attaching a chicken heart (Neopapilla model) to a separate opening created in the second part of the duodenum, which corrects for the anatomical difference and allows multiple (up to five) papillotomy practices to be performed on the chicken heart (Figure 7.6) [10] (see Videos 7.13 and 7.14).

Another form of supplemental training involves the use of mechanical simulators—the ERCP mechanical simulator (EMS) (Figure 7.7) or the X-vision ERCP simulator [11,12]. Both of these simulators utilize a rigid model with special papillae adapted to a mechanical duodenum. Selective cannulation can be achieved using injection of a color solution (X-vision) or using a guide

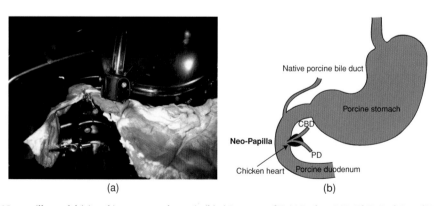

Figure 7.6 Image of the Neopapilla model (a) and its cartoon schematic (b). (Courtesy of Kai Matthes, MD, PhD, Beth Israel Deaconess Medical Center and Harvard Medical School.)

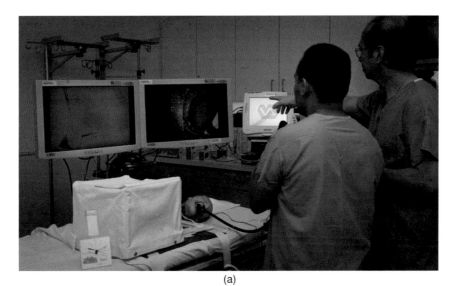

(a)

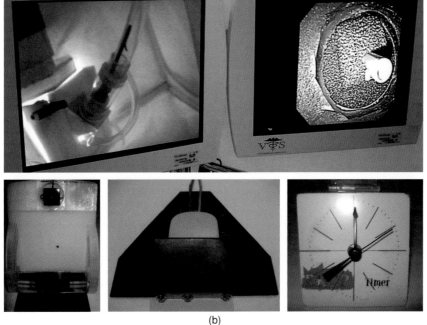

(b)

Figure 7.7 (a) EMS (ERCP mechanical simulator) allows in vitro practices with usage of real scope and accessories; simulated fluoroscopy does not cause radiation exposure. (b) Close-up views of EMS: simulated fluoroscopy showing internal view of the simulator and closer view of endoscopy image (top), small external video camera used for simulated fluoroscopy (bottom left), foot pedal which activates fluoroscopy (bottom middle), and timer for fluoroscopy (bottom right). (Courtesy of Jon-Nolan Paresa, Sacramento VA Medical Center.)

wire with the help of a catheter or papillotome (EMS) [13]. The X-vision model allows practice papillotomy performed on artificial papillae made of a special molded material. The EMS allows practice papillotomy using a foamy papilla soaked with a special conducting gel [14] (see Video 7.15). In addition, the built-in bile duct models for the EMS allow the performance of balloon dilation of stricture, brush cytology, and stenting as well as basket stone extraction and mechanical lithotripsy.

Impact of supplemental simulator training

Despite the different simulators available to supplement clinical training, there is a lack of clinical evidence or published experience to indicate that simulator training improves the clinical outcome. Much of the early studies were limited to commentaries on improving the skill set to perform different techniques or pilot studies to demonstrate that simulators are useful for basic learning. It is generally accepted that basic training using simulator(s) can help trainees to understand the anatomy, issues related to gut motility, as well as being able to practice with real scope and accessories. Currently, there are only two studies, one in an abstract form (Taiwan study) and another recently published (US multi-center study), that report the results of controlled randomized trials to indicate that trainees who received simulator practice (using the EMS) plus usual training achieved a higher clinical biliary cannulation success rate compared to the control group who received usual training only [15,16].

Assessment of performance

Objective assessment of trainee performance is determined by the clinical outcome, i.e., success/failure, complications, and whether the ERCP helped resolve the clinical problem of the patient. This to a great extent depends on ongoing training and practice. Furthermore, the outcome is also affected by the degree of trainer involvement and if the trainee is allowed to perform the procedure in a solo fashion. In a more refined way, assessment can be separated into the clinical knowledge of the procedure and its application. Clinical knowledge reflects on the understanding of the pathologies and interpretation of radiological findings that guide subsequent decision and therapy. The second aspect is technical proficiency and competency in performing the procedure.

ACGME has devised objective endpoints for measuring the different aspects of ERCP training and success of the procedure, but strictly speaking, these end points cannot account for all of the different aspects of this technical procedure [17]. Traditionally, the number of procedures performed is used as a surrogate for the trainee's experience. Jowell et al. reported that a trainee would need 180 ERCPs to achieve an 80% competence, whereas Verma et al. reported that it took 350–400 ERCP procedures for a single endoscopist to achieve 80% success with selective cannulation [18,19]. There is no consensus at present although ASGE recommended that trainees have to perform 180–200 ERCP procedures with at least half being therapeutic [4]. The Australians have a tougher criterion, which requires trainees to perform 200 successful solo procedures without trainer involvement [20].

Conventional assessment involves the local trainer who can assess the trainee performance based on his/her subjective assessment. To some extent, it reflects on their observation of the trainees' performance, both technical competency as well as their knowledge in applying the ERCP procedures in the management of the patient. However, subjective assessment is very arbitrary and no one trainer agrees totally with another on a standard set of guidelines for assessment.

Despite all of the objective assessment criteria, there is no exit examination for technical skills, especially the high-risk ERCP procedures. It can be argued that if one can successfully perform a procedure in front of a panel, one proves his/her ability. However, there are so many variables including the stress of taking a test that can affect the trainee performance and that ultimately might hurt the patient. Setting a limit and monitoring the success and complication rates is another method of ongoing assessment for individual performance. The ability to perform solo procedures successfully without trainer involvement or input reflects on the skill of the trainee. Cumulative data can be collected and analyzed over the whole training period to determine if the trainee shows any improvement. However, true assessment depends on solo performance and this may have to continue into one's practice after graduation since the overall results during training may be attributed to the trainer.

Training and clinical outcome correlation

As discussed, the clinical outcome is affected by the endoscopist skill and degree of difficulty of the ERCP procedure [21]. Despite ACGME and ASGE setting the expectations for fellowship training, many training programs cannot offer the required number of patients for fellows training. The main reason is the lack of sufficient number of patients presenting for ERCP and also the risky nature of the procedure. However, a recent study indicated that over 90% of trainees planned to practice ERCP after their fellowship despite the inadequate training experience. The hope of acquiring more skill in practice with limited training obviously poses certain danger to the patients. Besides, further practice with limited experience and poor technique may not improve the individual's overall skill.

How much volume is needed to maintain skill—retraining and new techniques

Although there is recommendation as to the number of procedures to acquire competence, there is a lack of information as to the optimal number required to maintain the skill. Assuming one acquired the basic ERCP skills, one can probably maintain the skill set if he/she continues to perform the procedure on a regular basis. There is no consensus as to the minimum requirement, and it will probably be up to individual institutions to grant the practicing privilege [22]. However, Freeman et al. reported that centers whose staff physicians each performed an average of more than one sphincterotomy per week had fewer difficult cannulations, lower mean number of pancreatic duct injections, fewer failures of biliary access or drainage after sphincterotomy, fewer hemorrhages, fewer severe complications, and fewer overall complications compared to lower volume centers; there were no significant differences in the rate of pancreatitis [24]. It becomes a more serious concern when one stops doing ERCP for some time and wants to get retraining. Currently, no training programs accept individuals for retraining purposes or to teach them new techniques. Many endoscopists attend ERCP workshops to learn the new advances and then perform the procedures (sometimes with the help of the equipment representatives) if they believe they have the basic skills to handle these new accessories. Hands-on practice under supervision is limited to those undergoing fellowship training. However, it may be possible to use simulators for practice of new procedures or techniques that do not require a patient [23]. Again, credentialing for individuals to perform such procedures lies with the institution.

The role of the assistant

It is important to point out that ERCP is teamwork and an experienced and trained assistant is necessary to accomplish the procedure. Much of the therapeutic ERCP procedure requires a close coordination between the endoscopist and the assistant, even with the short wire systems. Thus, training of the assistant is necessary in the grand scheme of things. In particular, the assistant needs to understand his/her role and is able to observe both monitors during the procedure, helping with stabilizing the guide wire and maintaining the tip of the guide wire position inside the bile duct to facilitate the exchanges. An experienced assistant can also minimize mishaps during exchange of accessories and in coordinating the execution of risky procedures such as papillotomy. Indeed, an experienced assistant can help with the training of inexperienced trainees and in minimizing complications. When available, simulator-training sessions provide an ideal opportunity for combined training of assistants with endoscopists and allow tension-free practice of the all important communication skills necessary for successful ERCP.

Conclusion

ERCP plays an important role in the management of patients with pancreaticobiliary diseases. It is technically challenging and carries substantial risks, even in the hands of experts. Proper training is important for good clinical outcome. The limited availability of patients hampers the training of trainees in many centers. In order to ensure that trainees meet the minimum expectation, many programs offer ERCP training only to a select few, often times in the form of an additional year of advanced fellowship. For a successful ERCP training to occur, certain prerequisites are expected of the trainers and the trainees. During training, the trainee must learn both the cognitive aspect and technical skills of ERCP. To improve the opportunities for hands-on practice, different simulators are used to supplement clinical ERCP training. There is however a paucity of published information on the impact of simulator training on trainees' performance and the clinical outcome. Objective assessment criteria for trainees' performance are equally lacking. More research, including prospective trials, is needed in these areas.

Videos

Video 7.1 Wire-guided cannulation technique

Video 7.2 Wire guided cannulation following pre-cut sphincterotomy

Video 7.3 Maneuvering of the scope for deep biliary cannulation

Video 7.4 Deviated papillotomy and correction

Video 7.5 Shaping of the plastic stent to conform to distorted biliary anatomy

Video 7.6 Multiple stent placement

Video 7.7 Shaping of the guide wire to negotiate difficult turns in pancreatic duct

Video 7.8 Sphincterotome cannulation

Video 7.9 Expert demonstration on the Neopapilla adaptation of the EASIE ex vivo porcine model of pancreatic endotherapy

Video 7.10 Sphincterotomy

Video 7.11 Use of Neopapilla to allow for training in management in post-sphincterotomy bleeding

Video 7.12 Cannulation with pancreatic duct stent

Video 7.13 Pancreatic wire-assisted cannulation

Video 7.14 Sphincterotomy and cholangioscopy

Video 7.15 Papillotomy practice using ERCP mechanical simulator (EMS)

Video 7.16 Billroth II cannulation with rotatable sphincterotome and guidewire

Video 7.17 Billroth II sphincterotomy utilizing a needle-knife over a common bile duct stent

Video 7.18 Impacted stone with a needle knife

References

1 Draganov P, Hoffman B, Marsh W, et al.: Long-term outcome in patients with benign biliary strictures treated endoscopically with multiple stents. *Gastrointest Endosc* 2002;**55**(6):680–686.

2 Cotton P, Leung J: *Advanced Digestive Endoscopy: ERCP*. Oxford: Blackwell Publishing, 2006: 9–16.

3 Eisen GM, Dominitz JA, Faigel DO, et al.: Guidelines for advanced endoscopic training. *Gastrointest Endosc* 2001;**53**(7):846–848.

4 Chutkan RK, Ahmad AS, Cohen J, et al.: ERCP core curriculum. *Gastrointest Endosc* 2006;**63**(3):361–376.

5 Kowalski T, Kanchana T, Pungpapong S: Perceptions of gastroenterology fellows regarding ERCP competency and training. *Gastrointest Endosc* 2003;**58**(3):345–349.

6 Ayala JC, Labbe R, Vera E: The loop tip wire guide: a new device to facilitate better access through the papilla. *Gastrointest Endosc* 2007;**65**(5):AB236.

7 Leung JW, Leung FW: Papillotomy performance scoring scale—a pilot validation study focused on the cut axis. *Aliment Pharmacol Ther* 2006;**24**(2):307–312.

8 Freeman ML: Pancreatic stents for prevention of post-endoscopic retrograde cholangiopancreatography pancreatitis. *Clin Gastroenterol Hepatol* 2007;**5**(11):1354–1365.

9 Leung J, Yen D: ERCP Training - The potential role of simulation practice. *J Interv Gastroenterol* 2011;**1**(1):14–18.

10 Matthes K, Cohen J: The neo-papilla: a new modification of porcine ex vivo simulators for ERCP training (with videos). *Gastrointest Endosc* 2006;**64**(4):570–576.

11 Leung JW, Lee JG, Rojany M, Wilson R, Leung FW. Development of a novel ERCP mechanical simulator. *Gastrointest Endosc* 2007;**65**(7):1056–1062.

12 von Delius S, Thies P, Meining A, et al.: Validation of the X-Vision ERCP training system and technical challenges during early training of sphincterotomy. *Clin Gastroenterol Hepatol* 2009;**7**(4):389–396.

13 Leung J, Lim B, Wilson R, et al.: Mechanical simulator practice speeds up selective cannulation time of novice trainees in "standard" but not "distorted" simulator settings. *Gastrointest Endosc* 2008;**67**: AB231.

14 Leung J, Lim B, Yen D, Wilson R, Leung F: Didactic teaching and practice papillotomy cuts facilitate trainees' understanding of the essence of a "perfect cut." *AJG* 2008;**103**:S86.

15 Leung JW, Liao WC, Wong SP, et al.: A RCT of mechanical simulator practice and usual training vs. usual training on novice trainee clinical ERCP performance. *Gastrointest Endosc* 2009;**69**(5):AB141.

16 Lim BS, Leung JW, Lee J, Yen D, Beckett L, Tancredi D, Leung FW: Effect of ERCP Mechanical Simulator (EMS) Practice on Trainees' ERCP Performance in the Early Learning Period: US Multicenter Randomized Controlled Trial. *Am J Gastroenterol* 2011;**106**(2):300–306.

17 ACGME statement of residency training.

18 Jowell PS, Baillie J, Branch MS, Affronti J, Browning CL, Bute BP: Quantitative assessment of procedural competence. A prospective study of training in endoscopic retrograde cholangio-pancreatography. *Ann Intern Med* 1996;**125**(12):983–989.

19 Verma D, Gostout C, Petersen B, Levy M, Baron T, Adler D: Establishing a true assessment of endoscopic competence in ERCP during training and beyond: a single-operator learning curve for deep biliary cannulation in patients with native papillary anatomy. *Gastrointest Endosc* 2007;**65**:394–400.

20 Conjoint Committee for Recognition of Training in Gastrointestinal Endoscopy: *Information for Supervisors: Change to Endoscopic Training,* Sydney, 1997.

21 Schutz SM, Abbott RM: Grading ERCPs by degree of difficulty: a new concept to produce more meaningful outcome data. *Gastrointest Endosc* 2000;**51**:535–539.

22 American Society for Gastrointestinal Endoscopy: Methods of granting hospital privileges to perform gastrointestinal endoscopy. *Gastrointest Endosc* 2002;**55**:780–783.

23 Freeman ML, Nelson DB, Sherman S, et al.: Complications of endoscopic biliary sphincterotomy. *N Engl J Med* 1996;**335**(13):909–918.

24 Leung J, Lee W, Wilson R, Lim B, Leung F: Comparison of accessory performance using a novel ERCP mechanical simulator. *Endoscopy* 2008;**40**:983–988.

8 Capsule Endoscopy

Felice Schnoll-Sussman[1] & David E. Fleischer[2]

[1]Cornell University, New York, NY, USA
[2]Mayo Clinic, Scottsdale, AZ, USA

Introduction

Capsule endoscopy (CE) has revolutionized many aspects of small bowel imaging and is an important diagnostic procedure in the investigation of obscure gastrointestinal bleeding (OGIB), suspected Crohn's disease, small-bowel tumors, polyposis syndromes, and celiac disease [1]. Despite its widespread use and expanding indications, there remain no currently validated credentialing guidelines or accreditation process for CE. This discussion will focus upon training to read studies with the capsule endoscopes developed by Given Imaging (Yoqneam, Israel) and Olympus America Inc. (Center Valley, Pennsylvania, USA). Recently, other capsule systems that are similar have been developed in Korea (Mirocam) and China (OMOM).

Description of the capsules

Different types of capsules have been developed to investigate the small bowel, esophagus, and colon. Each is made of biocompatible materials sealed with biocompatible adhesive. The small bowel capsule (Figure 8.1) is cylindrical and measures 11 mm in diameter and 26 mm in length. It has one optical dome with a 156° field of view, 1:8 magnification, and minimum size of detection of about 0.1 mm. White light-emitting diodes (LEDs) illuminate the bowel wall through the optical dome. The acquired image is focused by a lens on a complementary metal oxide semiconductor (CMOS) camera or on a charge-coupled device (CCD), depending on the manufacturer. The capsule contains two 8-hour long silver oxide batteries. It captures two images per second and transmits over 50,000 images during a typical exam. An application-specific integrated circuit (ASIC) transmitter sends the radiofrequency signal to an external data recorder worn by the patient. The esophageal capsule (Figure 8.2) (PillCam Eso, Given Imaging) is the same size as the small bowel capsule but has two optical domes that capture seven images per second (for a total of 14 images per second). Its smaller battery allows for a 20-minute examination length. The colon capsule (Figure 8.3) (PillCam Colon 2, Given Imaging) is larger, measures 31 by 11 mm, and has two optical domes, each of which captures two frames per second. In order to facilitate complete imaging of the colon, it shuts down 3 minutes after ingestion and "wakes up" 1 hour and 45 minutes later [2–4].

The capsule endoscopy unit

CE is typically performed in the outpatient setting but may be performed in an endoscopy unit or inpatient setting. There are minimal space requirements to house the equipment, which includes a desktop computer, printer, recording device, interface device between recorder and computer, and data recorder battery charger (Figure 8.4). Once downloaded from the recording device to the workstation, a capsule study may be transferred to a transportable device (DVD, memory key) and read at an off-site location on a personal laptop on which the reader software has been installed. There is no consensus on whether CE studies must be stored, and each practice should develop its own policy and be consistent.

Once the patient demographic information is entered into the workstation, the data recorder can be initialized. The capsule ingestion may then be performed in any location that has a bed or examination table. The patient lies down to have the leads placed on the abdomen. A razor may be necessary to shave any hair that may impair good adhesion of the leads to the skin. It is most efficient to have a trained nurse or other assistant involved in preparation of the equipment and patient. They may enter the demographic information into the workstation, initialize the data recorder, apply the leads, educate the patient on their activities, and then, at the end of the day, collect the equipment and download the study.

Preparing the patient

Informed consent reviewing the risks, benefits, and alternatives of CE should be obtained in writing prior to administration of the capsule. The two most pertinent risks being the possibility of missed lesions and capsule retention, which may require surgery. As with all endoscopic procedures, it is imperative that a thorough history be obtained. There are few absolute contraindications to CE. Patients with known small bowel obstructions, strictures, or fistulas should be avoided. However, a history of previous bowel

Successful Training in Gastrointestinal Endoscopy, First Edition. Edited by Jonathan Cohen.
© 2011 Blackwell Publishing Ltd. Published 2011 by Blackwell Publishing Ltd.

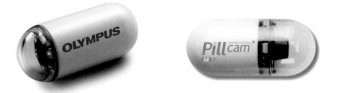

Figure 8.1 Small bowel capsule. Image Courtesy of Olympus America Inc.

obstruction, abdominal surgery, or intestinal resection is not a contraindication to CE. Although the FDA packaging still restricts administration in patients with pacemakers, there are multiple studies proving safety in patients with nondependent cardiac pacemakers (see section "Administering the Capsule"). For standard ingestion, patients should be capable of swallowing a pill. In the pediatric population, an attempt at teaching how to swallow a pill should be entertained. A simple strategy has been devised to assess children's ability to tolerate the swallow by having them practice swallowing with sequentially larger ingestible surrogates. All patients are screened with the "Jelly Bean Test" [5]. Patients start with a mini M&M$^®$, advance to a TicTac$^®$, followed by a regular sized M&M$^®$. If they are able to swallow all of these, the child is then asked to practice swallowing with a Brach's$^®$ jellybean. The 20 mm × 15 mm Brach's$^®$ jellybean is comparable to the PillcamSB$^®$ capsule which is 26 mm × 11 mm (Figure 8.5). Practicing with candies helps alleviate the anxiety patients feel about swallowing the capsule, increasing the likelihood of a successful ingestion. Other specific issues that should be addressed prior to capsule ingestion include swallowing disorders (e.g., achalasia), known Zenker's diverticulum, gastroparesis, and pregnancy.

Although there are few restrictions prior to the examination, several medications require specific instructions. As this is a noninvasive technique, patients requiring anticoagulants and antiplatelet agents may continue on their standard medications. Many patients with iron-deficiency anemia will be on iron supplementation. As iron may darken secretions within the small bowel, it may impair interpretation of images (especially within the distal small bowel), as such it should be stopped 3–5 days prior to the procedure. As with any procedure requiring fasting, dosage adjustments may be required with some medications (e.g., oral hypoglycemics, insulin). Patients are instructed to bring their standard medications with them on the morning of the procedure as they may be taken 2 hours after capsule ingestion. As sedatives are not administered, patients do not require an escort. They should wear comfortable clothing. Women are instructed to wear separates and avoid one piece dresses. Many patients prefer to have a loose shirt or jacket that can make the belt and data recorder inconspicuous. There are minimal restrictions on activities; how-

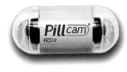

Figure 8.2 Esophageal capsule.

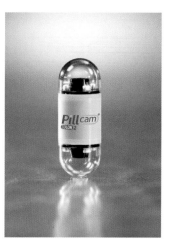

Figure 8.3 Colon capsule.

ever, they should avoid strenuous activities and not undergo an MRI until capsule passage is confirmed.

Unlike standard endoscopic procedures, there is no mechanism of clearing the visual field, which may be impaired by secretions, bubbles, and coating of the capsule by intestinal residue. As such the efficacy of the examination is highly dependent upon the quality of the bowel preparation. A fast of approximately 12 hours before small bowel CE and 4 hours before esophageal CE is necessary. There is an ongoing debate over the need for a bowel purgative or motility agent. In a recent meta-analysis, eight studies comparing sodium phosphate, polyethylene glycol, or simethicone were compared with simple fasting before small bowel CE [6]. Bowel visualization was scored as "good" in 78% of examinations with bowel preparations and 49% without ($P < 0.0001$). There were no significant differences in transit times or cecal intubation. The authors prefer a bowel preparation of a clear liquid diet the day prior to the procedure along with 2 L of PEG solution the evening prior to capsule ingestion. In addition to bowel preparation, another factor that may affect obtaining complete visualization of the entire small bowel mucosa is incomplete passage of the capsule to the cecum, which may happen in up to 20% of CE cases. Interestingly, gum chewing may assist in the transit time of the capsule. In a pilot trial [7], patients were instructed to chew one piece of sugarless gum for approximately 30 minutes every 2 hours following capsule ingestion. The percentage of complete capsule passage into the cecum was higher in the chewing-gum group compared with control (83.0% vs. 71.7% respectively, $p = 0.19$). Both gastric transit time and small bowel transit time were significantly shorter in the chewing gum versus control group. Chewing gum may represent an inexpensive and convenient method to increase the likelihood of complete passage of the capsule to the cecum.

The rate of capsule retention appears to be dependent upon the indication for CE (Table 8.1) [8]. Obtaining a good medical history is essential to avoiding capsule retention. Patients with abdominal pain, distension, and nausea or those with known Crohn's disease, should be suspected of having potential for capsule retention. Only 0.75% of patients require intervention for retention of CE

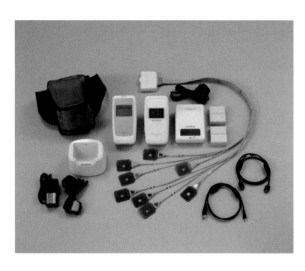

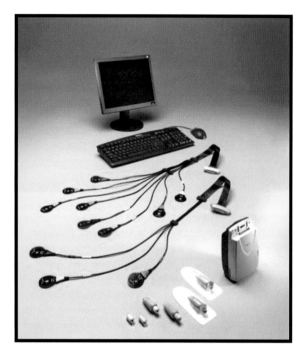

Figure 8.4 Capsule endoscopy equipment (desktop computer, printer, recording device, interface device between recorder and computer and data recorder battery charger).

[9]. Ideally, however, one would know prior to capsule ingestion if there was a stenotic area that would impede safe capsule passage. There are multiple examples within the literature that suggest that neither small bowel follow-through nor CT enterography can rule out the presence of a stenosis [10].

Although there is currently no widely accepted means of accurately predicting capsule retention, the Agile patency system (Given Imaging Ltd, Yoqneam, Israel) has been developed to determine bowel patency in patients who have possible strictures (Figure 8.6). It consists of a dissolvable capsule that contains a small radiofrequency ID (RFID) tag that can be detected by a hand-held scanner and barium, which can be localized by fluo-

roscopy. There are two timer plugs at each end, which come out 30 hours postingestion at which time the gastrointestinal secretions enter the capsule and degrade it. The patient is instructed to ingest the capsule (there is no need for any bowel preparation) and return close to but not after 30 hours to evaluate for the persistent presence of the capsule within the intestinal tract. If the scanner indicates that the capsule is still present, an abdominal plain X-ray is obtained to attempt to isolate the location of the capsule retention (it may merely be still within the colon, indicating safe passage). The Agile patency capsule seems to be a safe and reliable means for detecting asymptomatic stenoses prior to CE [11]. The use of this device, however, has not been widely accepted; this may be in part due to the fact that this procedure is still considered investigational and as such is not widely reimbursed by insurance companies.

Administering the capsule

The usual CE exam begins around 8–9 a.m. with capsule ingestion. During the procedure day, patients may return to home, work, or

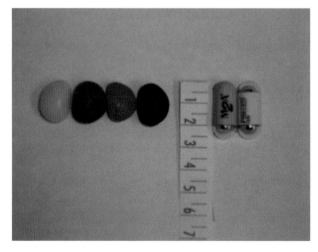

Figure 8.5 Jelly Bean Test.

Table 8.1 Rate of capsule retention based upon indication for CE examination.

Normal volunteers	0%
Suspected Crohn's disease	1.4%
Obscure GI bleeding	1.5%
Known Crohn's disease	5%

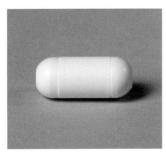

Figure 8.6 Agile patency system.

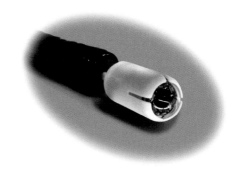

Figure 8.7 AdvanceCE device.

other activities. They should avoid activities such as strenuous exercise, which may cause lead dislodgement. The equipment is removed 8 hours later (correlating with battery length). Some centers allow patients to remove the equipment themselves and return it the following day. If the equipment is to be sent back in the mail, the patient should be instructed to take out insurance covering the full value of the equipment and capsule in case it were to be lost. The patient should be provided a letter, with an emergency contact number, that documents the patient is wearing specialized equipment for a medical examination.

Prior to the ingestion, the patient is outfitted with the procedure-specific sensor equipment (esophageal or small bowel), which is attached to the abdomen. The data recorder is within a pocket attached to a waist belt or harness.

The small bowel capsule endoscope is ingested in the natural way with some water. Very rarely, a patient, despite reporting no previous problems with pill ingestion, may have some initial difficulty swallowing the capsule. It is important to recognize that capsule ingestion should be without coughing or pain. If a patient starts to choke after ingestion, the pill may be within the airway and necessary measures taken (Heimlich maneuver, bronchoscopy). There may be a sensation of pill retention associated with some mild discomfort within the neck or thorax after ingestion. This should be brief and may be mitigated by allowing for additional water ingestion to aid in movement of the pill out of the esophagus. If the symptoms persist, the real-time viewer can be useful in assuring that the capsule has entered the stomach.

In patients with known anatomic or motility disorders, which may impair capsule ingestion, endoscopy-guided capsule delivery may be necessary [9]. The mode of placement is based upon the reason for difficulty with capsule ingestion. For those patients with esophageal pathology such as a Zenker's diverticulum or luminal narrowing, the capsule may be directly delivered with an accessory such as the US Endoscopy (Mentor, Ohio, USA) Roth net or AdvanceCE device. When attempting placement with the Roth net, one must pay careful attention to avoid trauma during intubation of the esophagus and inadvertent release of the capsule from the net within the oropharynx. The AdvanceCE device (which is specifically outfitted for the Given capsule) is a catheter-based system that passes through the endoscope channel. The capsule is placed within a holder that allows for direct placement of the capsule within the small intestine. Releasing the capsule may be difficult if the scope is not in a straight position (Figure 8.7). An overtube

may also be used to enable safe passage of the capsule within the esophagus. This approach is limited by the large size of overtube necessary to accommodate the capsule and accessory device (Roth net, snare). In patients with gastroduodenal pathology impeding capsule passage, patients may be allowed to swallow the capsule normally and then immediately undergo endoscopy, where the capsule is retrieved with an accessory device and then directly placed within the duodenum. Most importantly, if endoscopy is necessary to guide capsule placement, every attempt should be made to deliver the capsule to the duodenum and avoid possible gastric retention and subsequent incomplete small bowel evaluation.

The esophageal capsule has a unique ingestion protocol to help slow the transit time in the esophagus and hence increase the number of images acquired. The Pillcam ESO is an ingestible, disposable capsule that is identical in size to the Pillcam SB (11 × 26 mm). It is able to acquire images from both ends during passage through the esophagus at a rate of 7 frames/second from each end (for a total of 14 fps) of the capsule (Figure 8.2). It also transmits images via radiofrequency communication to an external data recorder. After a 4 hour fast, the patient is instructed to drink 100 mL of water in the standing position, then they are placed in the right decubitus position and asked to ingest the pill with a single sip of water from a cup with straw. After pill ingestion, the patients are instructed to sip 15 mL of water through the straw twice a minute for 7 minutes (Figure 8.8). No head or body movements or talking is allowed. After 7 minutes, the patient sits upright and drinks an additional sip of water and then allowed to walk for the next

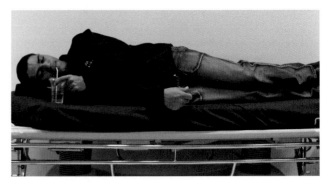

Figure 8.8 Simplified ingestion protocol (SIP).

15 minutes, at which time the equipment is removed and the video is downloaded and read. This simplified ingestion protocol (SIP) improves visualization of the Z-line by increasing the number of images acquired and decreasing the amount of overlying bubbles and saliva. [12]

The colon capsule (Figure 8.3) requires a more aggressive bowel cleanse to prepare the colon mucosa. In the colon capsule clinical trials, patients are kept on a clear liquid diet the day before the examination, administered 3 L of PEG in the evening, and another liter in the early morning of the examination. Additionally, later in the day, they receive two doses of sodium phosphate solution as a "booster" to help propel the capsule through the fluid-filled colon [3]. The lower sensitivity for both polyps and colon cancer in comparison to standard colonoscopy had held back FDA 510K clearance of the original colon capsule. The new PillCam Colon 2 with advanced optics and 172° field of view from each imager has recently received European approval [4] and ongoing trials will help establish the appropriate preparation requirements (in the face of most sodium phosphate products being taken off the market) and its utility in colon polyps and cancer detection.

Although the FDA-approved package insert still lists pacemakers as a contraindication to CE, there have been multiple studies that have proven that small bowel CE can be safely performed in patients with nondependent cardiopacemakers implanted in the chest. Patients that are pacemaker-dependent should continue to be monitored during CE. Small bowel CE can be safely performed in patients with ICDs implanted in the chest. However, until more data is available, it is recommended that these procedures be done in the hospital under continuous monitoring, with support from the patient's cardiologist. No data is available on patients undergoing esophageal CE or in patients with CPs or ICDs implanted in the abdomen. These patients should undergo CE in a monitored environment [13].

Capsule endoscopy reading in clinical settings

CE should be the first imaging modality used for evaluating patients with OGIB after unremarkable upper and lower endoscopy [14]. The positive predictive value of CE in the evaluation of OGIB is in the range of 43–72% [15,16]. The highest diagnostic yield is in patients who have ongoing bleeding or have recently bled [15] (Video 8.1).

In order to assist in the identification of bleeding lesions, a red blood indicator was developed, which automatically marks images with red areas felt to correlate with suspected blood. A multicenter trial, however, concluded that there are many false-negative and false-positive images identified by the software [17].

It is also important to recognize that not every lesion found at CE for the evaluation of OGIB is significant. Saurin et al. stratified patients into those with low- and high-bleeding potential and showed that lesions with a high bleeding potential made up only 50–60% of the total number of CE findings identified [18].

CE has been shown in several clinical situations to be a useful investigation in patients with suspected or known Crohn's disease [19,20]:

- Identification of Crohn's disease involvement in additional areas of the small intestine out of reach of colonoscopy and upper endoscopy
- Patients with high clinical suspicion of Crohn's disease and negative endoscopic work up
- Indeterminate colitis
- Detection of recurrence of Crohn's earlier after ileocecal resection

As with OGIB, not all lesions found at CE in the evaluation of a patient with suspected Crohn's disease necessarily confirm the diagnosis. In order to increase the specificity of the diagnosis, the examination should be performed in an appropriate clinical setting and must provide an accurate description of the type and severity of the lesions identified. Specifically, patients should be prescreened for NSAIDs and aspirin usage, which are known in both short- and long-term administration to lead to small intestinal mucosal injury, which may be misconstrued as Crohn's-type lesions [21,22]. The risk of capsule retention may limit the use of CE in patients with Crohn's disease [23,24]. The Agile patency capsule (discussed above) may help prescreen those patients deemed at high risk for retention.

In the evaluation of diseases of the esophagus, the esophageal capsule has been shown to have a moderately high sensitivity in the screening of patients with chronic reflux disease for Barrett's esophagus (BE) (67%) and in patients with portal hypertension for esophageal varices (86%). Improvements in the ingestion protocol have assisted in better visualization of the esophagogastric junction (see SIP) [12]. It has not been demonstrated in either setting to be more cost effective than EGD [25,26]. The Food and Drug Administration approved CE for use in adults to detect abnormalities in the esophagus and in certain clinical situations serves as a potential alternative to EGD for screening of esophageal varices and BE (Figures 8.9 and 8.10).

Reading capsule endoscopy study

There are two modes in which one is able to view a capsule video: manual and automatic. The manual-viewing mode allows for review of every image captured during pill passage. The automatic-viewing mode combines repetitive images, allowing the reader to focus on images that show change (Figures 8.11 and 8.12) (Videos 8.2 and 8.3).

The video may be viewed in single, dual, or quad view. It is generally felt that quadview affords maximum efficiency in reading because it allows more time per image than DualView or Single view when viewing at the same frame rate. Additionally, in the Given platform, there is a Quick View v5 mode that allows for a fast preview of a small bowel video while highlighting images that may be of interest in the video stream. The trade-off of higher efficiency at reading studies for a higher false-negative rate must be balanced.

When an image of interest is identified, the video stream is stopped and the reader toggles over the abnormality to evaluate its significance and thumbnail it. Clearly, the most challenging part of reading a capsule examination is diagnosing an abnormality that

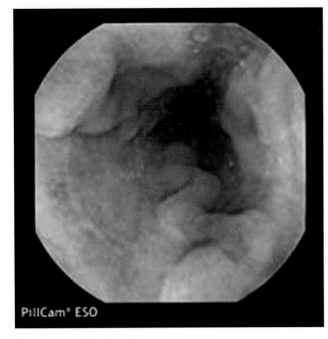

Figure 8.9 Esophageal varices.

is only identifiable on a single frame. How can you reliably make a diagnosis? If possible, it is always best not to make a diagnosis on a single image. Look at the surrounding mucosa for additional clues. View the video flow of images to see the intestinal lining before and after the lesion in question and look for similar abnormalities to the image in question (Video 8.4). It is also important to select an appropriate frame rate by which to read. This is best done by

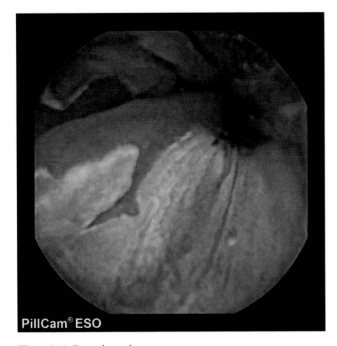

Figure 8.10 Barrett's esophagus.

identifying a single frame abnormality (i.e., red spot) and setting the reading speed at the maximum speed in which the abnormality is able to be clearly identified. For a novice reader, this rate is typically no faster than 15 fps.

While there may be many different styles in which to read a video capsule, the authors advocate the following three stages—preview, review, and report.

- Preview
  - Use QuickView (Given) or a high frame rate to scan video while creating thumbnails of landmark locations (first gastric image, first duodenal image, first cecal image) and images of interest.
  - Review red indicator software images, especially if evaluating a patient with gastrointestinal bleeding.
- Review
  - Review entire video with automatic mode.
  - Thumbnail images of interest.
  - Viewing speed 10–25 fps depending on experience.
- Report
  - Review selected thumbnails and delete unnecessary images. Add comments to significant thumbnail images.
  - Generate formal report with selected annotated thumbnails.

The inability to take biopsies or obtain additional images beyond those acquired by passive migration of the capsule may make establishing a diagnosis very challenging. This is especially true in the case of submucosal lesions that are one of the most difficult to interpret findings in CE. Bulges in the bowel wall may be created by another loop of bowel overlying the loop being observed during CE and be misinterpreted as a submucosal process. When a potential submucosal lesion is encountered, the reader should view the video stream instead of single images. Adjacent loops will move with peristalsis and will not change the appearance of the villi. On the other hand, overlying bowel edema and inflammation may indicate the presence of a submucosal lesion (i.e., carcinoid, GIST, leiomyoma). The following findings attest to a submucosal or infiltrative process and not a bulge of adjacent bowel loops (Video 8.5):

- Immobility with peristalsis
- Surface ulceration (Figure 8.13)
- Central umbilication (Figure 8.14)
- White appearance of stretched and thinned mucosa
- Lobulated mucosa—not a single smooth bulge typical of an adjacent bowel loop (Figure 8.15)
- Bridging folds—folds come up to but not across the bulge (Figure 8.16)

A scoring system has been developed to provide a common language to quantify small bowel inflammatory changes [27]. It may help facilitate communication and standardization for assessing disease states, monitor the progress of treatment, and provide a threshold for a differential diagnosis. The score is based upon three scoring parameters—villous edema (villous width is equal to or greater than villous height), mucosal ulceration, and the presence of stenotic lesions. The score provides a common language to quantify mucosal changes associated with any inflammatory process. The score does not diagnose or measure disease but merely differentiates normal small bowel from disease states.

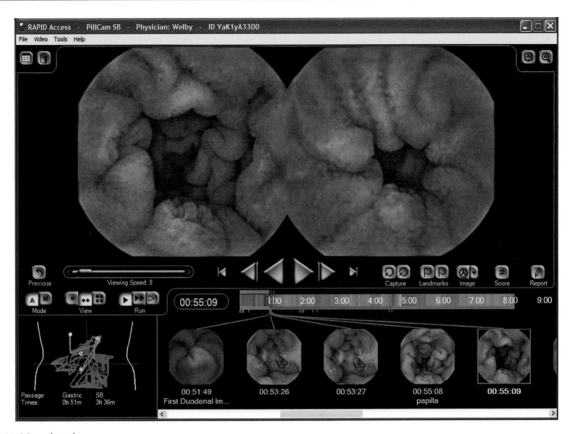

Figure 8.11 Manual mode.

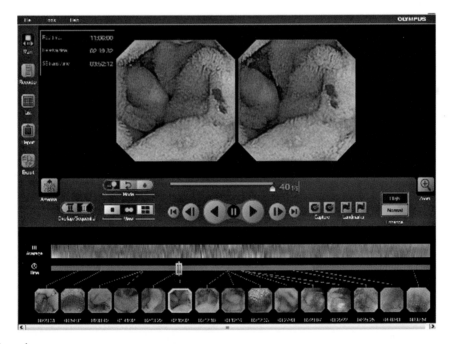

Figure 8.12 Automatic mode.

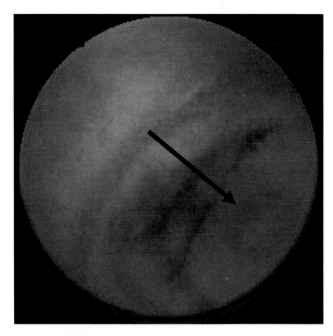

Figure 8.13 Surface ulceration.

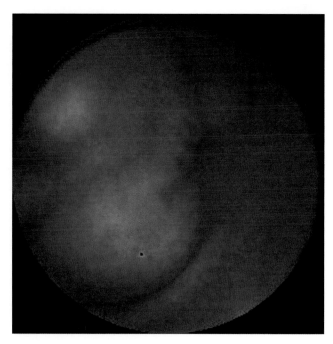

Figure 8.15 Lobulated mucosa.

Credentialing the capsule endoscopist: current guidelines

Unlike nearly all other endoscopic techniques, VCE requires little if any technical competence and is merely based upon *interpretive* competence. Mastery of this technique requires physicians to reliably detect and correctly diagnose abnormalities based on their appearance at VCE. The practitioner is unable to control the location of the capsule as it moves passively (forward, backward, and tumbling) through the small intestine aided only by peristalsis. The reader is reliant upon the images captured. It may at times be frustrating to be unable to get additional images of an area of interest or biopsy confirmation of a visualized abnormality. The images obtained from CE are also slightly different from traditional endoscopy since there is no air distension of the bowel wall and the capsule is at times located within millimeters of

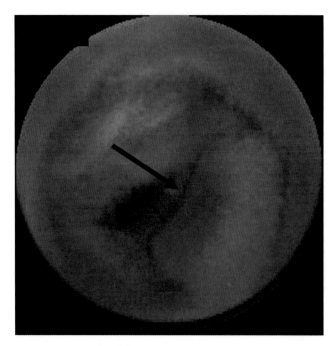

Figure 8.14 Central umbilication.

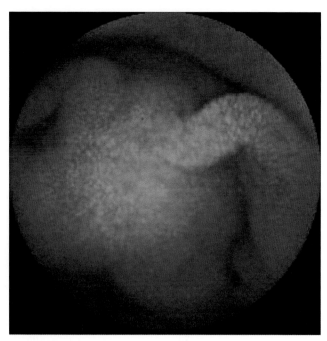

Figure 8.16 Bridging folds.

the mucosa. Recognizing normal anatomy or variations of normal anatomy that do not, in fact, represent diagnostic abnormalities may be difficult especially for the novice reader.

Perhaps as a consequence of the ease of "performing" this technique in comparison to classic endoscopic procedures, there are still no universally agreed upon benchmarks for competence to read VCE studies independently. Although many GI trainees receive direct training in VCE as part of their core GI fellowship, most training programs do not have a structured curriculum for teaching CE [28]. There are few published data regarding the learning curve for VCE. The 2007 GI core curriculum [29] recommends reading a minimum of 25 cases to achieve competency, and it suggests that "most experienced endoscopists who have completed a formal GI fellowship can readily master this technique." However, it goes on to state that the minimum training requirements needed to competently perform WCE have not been evaluated. ASGE guidelines recommend that training within GI fellowship must include didactic tutoring and an adequate case volume so the trainee attains a level of competence similar to that of the mentor [28]. As with other techniques, the necessary case volume may vary among trainees, may be influenced by the length of time the training is spread over and depend upon when during the fellowship the training is undertaken [26].

The ASGE recently published a guideline for credentialing and granting privileges for CE [30] (http://www.asge.org/WorkArea/showcontent.aspx?id=2994). This consensus recommends the following training guidelines before competency can be assessed:

- Completion of a GI fellowship program (or equivalent)
- Competence in performing upper endoscopy, colonoscopy, and push enteroscopy
- Clear understanding of the indications, risks, and potential complications of CE
- Familiarity with CE hardware and software systems
- One of the following two options:
  ○ Formal training in CE in the context of a gastroenterology fellowship
  ○ Completion of a hands-on course with at least 8 hours CME credit, which has been endorsed by a national or international GI or surgical society and review of first 10 capsule studies by a credentialed capsule endoscopist.

Although this seems like a surmountable number of exams to complete, doing so under the tutelage of another endoscopist outside of a training program may not be easily feasible. The authors recommend that those in practice may consider reviewing another endoscopist's previously read examinations. Additionally, at the early stages of independent reading, the practitioner may want to establish a relationship with a seasoned capsule endoscopist to help review indeterminate lesions.

The ASGE holds multiple courses throughout the year tailored to the needs of both the novice and advanced capsule user. These sessions include didactic lectures on capsule equipment and setup, clinical indications and contraindications to the exam, and a review of the clinical outcomes date for specific disease processes. Additionally, attendees have hands-on opportunity to review cases under the tutelage of expert capsule endoscopists.

Although an important benchmarking tool, there has to date been no published data validating the efficacy of such training.

Other regional gastrointestinal societies and the individual capsule companies also host multiple regional and online training seminars that can provide an opportunity to gain additional capsule reading experience.

To date, there are two English language texts on CE—*The Atlas of Video Capsule Endoscopy* [31], which provides an excellent overview of the technology, indications, and images in WCE, and *Capsule Endoscopy* [32], which provides technical information on the procedure with clinically relevant guidance on how CE may be used to facilitate the diagnosis and management of diseases of the small intestine. Still images are contextualized by the accompanying CD that provides videos of many of the images that are in each chapter. The RAPID software has an embedded reference atlas that can aid in the interpretation of images. Saved thumbnails may be used in a side-by-side comparison with hundreds of images stored according to CEST terminology (show image). Additionally, Given Imaging's sponsored Web site (www.capsuleendoscopy.org) and the DAVE project (www.dave1.mgh) are both excellent Web resources that provide case summaries and videos archived with references.

Training the capsule endoscopist: current literature

There are to date no evidence-based training guidelines for physicians to perform and interpret capsule. There are also no universally agreed upon benchmarks of expert practice to establish competence in reading CE studies independently. There are, however, several studies from which we can extrapolate an understanding of the amount of training necessary to reach competency.

Several studies have been performed, which compare experienced CE physicians (gold standard) with gastroenterology fellows, nurses, and medical students (see Table 8.1). In the largest, Sidhu et al. [33] assessed the ability of nine gastroenterology trainees with endoscopic experience (200–3,500 gastroscopies, 20–500 colonoscopies, no CE), one CE-experienced trainee (50 CE studies), five medical students (no endoscopy experience), and one CE expert (>700 CE studies). When comparing the ability to interpret CE abnormalities detected, trainees were more likely to reach a correct diagnosis after identification of the corresponding abnormalities on the videos compared to the students ($p = 0.001$, OR 3.6, CE 1.8–7.4). This finding suggests that prior endoscopy experience is beneficial in CE reporting.

In one study, Adler et al. [34] compared the capsule reading accuracy of a senior therapeutic endoscopist experienced in both CE and push enteroscopy to a fourth year "advanced" endoscopy fellow. The fellow's training experience consisted of a review of 15 previous capsule examinations. In this prospective study of patients with OGIB, there was complete agreement in 18/20 (90%) of capsule studies ($k = 0.69$). In one patient, each reader saw a finding the other did not see, and in one patient, the unblinded reviewer saw a finding the blinded reader did not. None of these findings were felt to represent definitive causes of gastrointestinal bleeding. This study suggested that the learning curve for reading CE among physicians with some degree of endoscopic experience was short.

To further define what type of training would be necessary, Postgate et al. [35] evaluated a structured CE training program with two experienced GI fellows and a senior endoscopy nurse. The physicians had each performed more than 1,000 colonoscopies. Neither the physicians nor the nurse had any CE experience. The trainees were introduced to the CE software to allow for independent reporting of landmarks, thumbnail capture, and report writing. The fellow trainees then read a series of CE videos. Each CE video had been graded in difficulty from 0 (easy) to 12 (hard) based on the number of lesions present, type of difficulty of the lesion identification, and the degree of impairment in view quality. The videos were grouped in blocks of three, which increased in difficulty with the intention that changes in performance over time could be compared against baseline performance as they progressed through the training program. Comprehensive feedback and teaching was given by an expert capsule endoscopist after each block of three studies was completed. The physician trainee each performed 12 complete CE studies (number recommended by current guidelines) in four blocks and the nurse performed 22 capsule studies (assuming their lack of hands-on endoscopy experience would necessitate additional training) in seven blocks. Each report was analyzed against the expert's report, which represented the gold standard. A global score was given for performance of each capsule. "0" = unsatisfactory—significant lesions missed and incorrect diagnosis, "1" = average (nonexpert)—significant lesions missed but correct diagnosis, "2" = good (expert)—no significant lesions missed and correct diagnosis and management. Reading speed was not assessed. Overall, the trainees achieved a correct diagnosis in 75–83% of cases with the majority of incorrect diagnoses occurring early on in training. Physician trainees and the nurses demonstrated consistent improvement in diagnostic accuracy; however, physician trainee 2 showed no improvement over time (correlation coefficient -0.06, $p = 0.81$). Additionally, physician trainee recommended inappropriate management in four of the last six studies even when a correct diagnosis had been made. The overall performance score improved in all trainees but only approached statistical significance in the nurse trainee (correlation coefficient 0.41, $P = 0.06$).

We can surmise from this study that, as in other endoscopic techniques, there is variability in skill acquisition and that management recommendation may not be appropriate even when a correct diagnosis is made. Importantly, even at the end of training, none of the trainees had achieved an overall score equivalent to expert performance and that a longer training program (more than 12 for physicians and 22 for nurses) would be necessary to achieve independent reading competency. It is difficult to draw many conclusions about the gastroenterology trainee learning curve with only two subjects analyzed; still this data does underscore key points universal to all endoscopic training:
• Trainees learn at different rates.
• Cognitive competency includes recognition of whether an image is normal or not, correct identification of those abnormal findings that are recognized, and appropriate interpretation

of the significance of this finding as reflected in management recommendations.
• Experienced endoscopists should have a considerable advantage over nonendoscopists and even trainees, particularly with the management decisions based on findings.

Another recent prospective educational evaluation study by Postgate et al. [36] developed an interactive, computer-based training module for improving lesion recognition skills at CE. The two primary end points were to examine the differences in performance among participants with different levels of experience and then to examine the change in performance on a test module after training. The training module developed included a comprehensive range of CE images, including normal anatomical appearances, common incidental findings, and pathological findings. The images were annotated with relevant background information and detailed diagnostic features. The module provided a menu-driven teaching resource that included a key work index, learning objectives, links to related resource, and an integrated feedback mechanism. The testing module included 60 40-second videos that were played back at five frames per second and presented as multiple-choice questions with one correct answer among five possible options. Four CE experts (median of 300 CE studies) and one experienced CE research nurse (> 300 CE studies) were used to benchmark expert performance on the testing module.

Subsequently, 14 medical students (without CE, EGD, or colonoscopy experience) and 14 gastroenterology trainees (no CE experience, median of 800 EGD, and 325 colonoscopies) were recruited prospectively to test the training and evaluation modules in a pretest–posttest design. Following training, there was a significant improvement (15%) in test performance for both the medical students and the gastroenterology trainees ($p < 0.001$), which confirmed the ability of the training module to improve lesion recognition skills at CE after a relatively short training intervention. Not surprisingly, however, the trainees did not achieve the benchmark "expert" performance. This study helps substantiate the potentially significant role of computer-based training and testing in CE. As we continue to strive to achieve a validated educational tool to teach and assess competence at CE, it seems reasonable that a module such as this is a reasonable expectation to have available as an independent learning tool either through courses or in a Web-based learning forum.

In two other studies available in abstract form only [37,38], 50 CE videos were preread by a specially trained GI nurse who thumbnailed abnormalities detected for interpretation by the gastroenterologist. There was complete agreement between the nurse and gastroenterologist for all 12 normal cases. Complete interobserver agreement was achieved for 93 of the 96 lesions categorized as "significant" by the physician (96%). In the other study, 20 consecutive capsule exams were reviewed by one gastroenterologist, one endoscopy nurse, and resident. The gastroenterologist's sensitivity for "overall lesions" was lower and specificity higher compared with both nurse and resident. The interobserver agreement for "overall lesion" was discrete to moderate and excellent for "significant lesion" (kappa = 1 for all readers). In these two studies, the concept of employing physician extenders as prereaders or even independent readers is suggested. These readers do not have formal training in gastrointestinal endoscopy and were merely trained in reviewing CE images. As such, intensive training in image identification may be suitable to identify the "significant lesions" and these lesions only reviewed by a trained endoscopist with subsequent diagnosis and management.

The speed with which a capsule study is read is easily measured; however, it may have no considerable relationship to skill level. Especially, early on in learning CE, a faster reading rate may be a deterrent to accurate image identification. As previously discussed, the set reading rate should be no faster than that which permits identification of a single frame abnormality. In the novice reader, this is typically in the range of 15 fps. This variable may be useful in the design of future studies on competency after training, during which interpretation of unknown examinations can be scored for both time and accuracy.

Conclusions

CE is a valuable innovation with potentially lifesaving benefits and expanding indications. There is increasing awareness that proficiency should be based upon competence rather than merely numbers performed. There is a paucity of data regarding training and credentialing of CE physicians. Evidence-based training guidelines should be developed to assist in CE education. The ability to take full advantage of interactive computer-based learning using still and video images makes this technique amenable to effective short courses and independent learning opportunities. Better tools to assess competency following training will both improve the quality of CE in the community and expand its use by providing practitioners with more confidence to perform VCE. Despite this representing a "noninvasive" endoscopic technique, the training and credentialing afforded it should be as effective and vigorous as any other "invasive" technique in an endoscopist's armamentarium.

Videos

Video 8.1 Introduction to reading a capsule examination
Video 8.2 How to read a Given Endoscopy video capsule
Video 8.3 How to read an Olympus Endocapsule video
Video 8.4 At what speed should I read a capsule endoscopy video examination?
Video 8.5 How to identify a submucosal lesion at capsule endoscopy?
Video 8.6 Lymphatic structures identified at capsule endoscopy

References

1 Mergener K, Ponchon T, Gralnek I, et al.: Literature review and recommendations for clinical application of small-bowel capsule endoscopy, based on a panel discussion by international experts. Consensus statements for small-bowel capsule endoscopy, 2006/2007. *Endoscopy* 2007;**39**:895–909.

2 Eliakim R, Fireman Z, Gralnek IM, et al.: Evaluation of the Pill-Cam Colon capsule in the detection of colonic pathology: results of the first multicenter, prospective, comparative study. *Endoscopy* 2006;**38**:971–977.

3 Schoofs N, Deviere J, Van Gossum A: PillCam Colon capsule endoscopy compared with colonoscopy for colorectal tumor diagnosis: a prospective pilot study. *Endoscopy* 2006;**38**:971–977.

4 Van Gossum A, Navas MM, Fernandez-Urien I, et al.: Capsule endoscopy versus colonoscopy for the detection of polyps and cancer. *NEJM* 2009;**361**:3.

5 Sockolow R, Solomon A. The Jelly Bean Test: a novel technique to help children swallow medications. In: Andrew Mulberg (ed), *Concepts and Applications of Pediatric Drug Development*. New York: John Wiley & Sons. (In press.)

6 Niv Y: Preparation for capsule endoscopy. *World J Gastroenterol* 2008;**14**(9):1313–1317.

7 Apostolopoulos P, Kalantzis C, Graknek IM: The effectiveness of chewing-gum in accelerating capsule endoscopy transit time: a prospective randomized, controlled pilot study. *Aliment Pharmacol Therapeut* 2008;**15**:405–411.

8 Cave D, Legnani P, deFranchis R: ICCE consensus for capsule retention. *Endoscopy* 2005;**37**(10):1065–1067.

9 Storch I, Barkin JS: Contraindications to capsule endoscopy: do any exist? *Gastrointest Endosc Clin N Am* 2006;**16**:329.

10 Delvaux M, Laurent V, Regent D, et al.: Should an entero-CT scanner necessarily precede capsule endoscopy recording when exploring patients with suspected intestinal disease? *Gastrointest Endosc* 2004;**59**:AB175.

11 Herrerias M, Leighton JA, Costamagna G, et al.: Agile patency system eliminates risk of capsule retention in patients with known intestinal strictures who undergo capsule endoscopy. *Gastointest Endosc* 2008;**67**:902–909.

12 Gralnek IM, Rabinowitz R, Afik D, Eliakim R: A simplified ingestion procedure for esophageal capsule endoscopy initial evaluation in healthy volunteers. *Endoscopy* 2006;**38**:913–918.

13 Leighton JA, Sharma VK, Srivathsan K, et al.: Safety of capsule endoscopy in patients with pacemakers. *Gastrointest Endosc* 2004;**59**(4):567–569.

14 Faigel DO, Cave DR: 6th international conference on capsule endoscopy. *Endoscopy* 2007;**39**:895–909.

15 Hindryckx P, Botelberge T, De Vos M, De Looze D: Clinical impact of capsule endoscopy on further strategy and long-term clinical outcome in patients with obscure bleeding. *Gastrontest Endosc* 2008;**68**:98–104.

16 Pennazio M, Santucci R, Rondonotti E, et al.: Outcome of patients with obscure gastrointestinal bleeding after capsule endoscopy: Report of 100 consecutive cases. *Gastroenterology* 2000;**118**:197–200.

17 D'Halluin Pn, Delvaux M, Lapalus MG, et al.: Does the "suspected blood indicator" improve the detection of bleeding lesions by capsule endoscopy? *Gastrointest Endosc* 2005;**61**:243–249.

18 Saurin JC, Delvaux M, Vahedi K, et al.: Clinical impact of capsule endoscopy compared to push enteroscopy: 1- year follow-up study. *Endoscopy* 2005;**37**:318–323.

19 Bourrelille A, Jarry M, D'Halluin PN, et al.: Wireless capsule endoscopy versus ileocolonoscopy for the diagnosis of postoperative recurrence of Crohn's disease: a prospective study. *Gut* 2006;**55**:978–983.

20 Maunoury V, Savoye G, Bourreille A, et al.: Value of wireless capsule endoscopy in patients with indeterminate colitis. *Inflamm Bowel Dis* 2007;**13**:152–155.

21 Smecuol E, Pinto Sanchez MI, Suarez A, Argonz JE, et al.: Low-dose aspirin affects the small bowel mucosa: results of a pilot

study with a multidimensional assessment. *Clin Gastroenterol Hepatol* 2009;7(5):524–529.

22 Goldstein JL, Eisen G, Lewis B, Gralnek IM, et al.: Video capsule endoscopy to prospectively assess small bowel injury with celecoxib, naproxen plus omeprazole, and placebo. *Clin Gastroenterol Hepatol* 2005;3(2):133–141.

23 Cheifetz AS, Lewis BS: Capsule endoscopy retention: is it a complication? *Tech Gastrointest Endosc* 2006;8:175–181.

24 Li F, Gurudu SR, De Petris G, Sharma VK: Retention of the capsule endoscope: a single-center experience of 1000 capsule endoscopy procedures. *Gastrointest Endosc* 2008;68(1):174–180.

25 Sharma P, Wani S, Rastogi A, et al.: The diagnostic accuracy of esophageal capsule endoscopy in patients with gastroesophageal reflux disease and Barrett's esophagus: a blinded, prospective study. *Am J Gastroenterol* 2008;103:525–532.

26 de Franchis R, Eisen GM, Laine L, et al.: Esophageal capsule endoscopy for screening and surveillance of esophageal varices in patients with portal hypertension. *Hepatology* 2008;47:1595–1603.

27 Gralnek IM, Defranchis R, Seidman E, et al.: Development of a capsule endoscopy scoring index for small bowel mucosal inflammatory change. *Aliment Pharmacol Ther* 2008;27:146–154.

28 Erber JA: Wireless capsule endoscopy: where and how to learn? *Gastrointest Endosc* 2008;68(1):115–117.

29 American Association for the Study of Liver Diseases, American College of Gastroenterology, American Gastroenterological Association, and American Society for Gastrointestinal Endoscopy: *Gastroenterology Core Curriculum*. 3rd ed. 2007. Available: http://www.asge.org/ Training Education Index.aspx?id-502#curriculum (accessed October 14, 2007).

30 Faigel DO, Baron TH, Adler DG, et al. ASGE guideline: Guidelines for credentialing and granting privileges for capsule endoscopy. *Gastrointest Endosc* 2005;61:503–505.

31 Keuchel M, Friedrich H, Fleischer DE: *The Atlas of Video Capsule Endoscopy*. New York: Springer Link Publishing, 2007.

32 Faigel D, Cave D: *Capsule Endoscopy*. Philadelphia, PA: Saunders Elsevier, 2008.

33 Sidhu R, Sakellariou P, McAlindon ME, et al.: Is formal training necessary for capsule endoscopy? The largest gastroenterology trainee study with controls. *Dig Liver Dis* 2008;40:298–302.

34 Adler DG, Knipschield M, Gostout C: A prospective comparison of capsule endoscopy and push enteroscopy in patients with GI bleeding of obscure origin. *Gastrointest Endosc* 2004;59:492–498.

35 Postgate A, Haycock A, Fitzpatrick A: How should we train capsule endoscopy? A pilot study of performance changes during a structured capsule endoscopy training program. *Dig Dis Sci* 2009;54(8):1672–1679.

36 Postgate A, Haycock A, Thomas-Gibson S: Computer-aided learning in capsule endoscopy leads to improvement in lesion recognition ability. *Gastrointest Endosc* 2009;70(2):310–316.

37 Sigmundsson HK, Das A, Isenberg G: Capsule endoscopy (CE): interobserver comparison of intrepretation. *Gastrointest Endosc* 2003;57:AB165.

38 Mergener K, Enns R. Interobserver variability for reading capsule endoscopy examinations. *Gastrontest Endosc* 2003;57:AB85.

9 Deep Enteroscopy

Patrick I. Okolo[1] & Jonathan M. Buscaglia[2]

[1]Johns Hopkins University School of Medicine, Baltimore, MD, USA
[2]State University of New York, Stony Brook, NY, USA

Introduction

Small-bowel endoscopy refers to endoluminal examination of the small bowel using any method, including wireless capsule enteroscopy (CE) and push enteroscopy. Deep enteroscopy excludes push enteroscopy and refers specifically to those procedures that permit endoluminal examination of the small bowel using an assistive device. The term device-assisted enteroscopy may be interchangeably used to encompass all forms of deep enteroscopy. Deep enteroscopy is technically challenging and requires a finely honed confluence of skills derived from other endoscopic procedures. Considerable experience in other forms of endoscopy (especially colonoscopy) coupled with specific and comprehensive training in deep enteroscopy is a prerequisite for performing this procedure.

This chapter considers the prerequisite technical and cognitive skills that prospective trainees should possess before attempting to learn to perform deep enteroscopy and detail the specific components of the procedures that they must master. Guidance for the optimal current pathway to gaining skill in this field will be offered. The procedures to be considered in this chapter include the following:

1 Spiral-tip overtube enteroscopy
2 Balloon-assisted enteroscopy
  i Single-balloon enteroscopy
  ii Double-balloon enteroscopy

The small bowel can be approached in an anterograde manner via the mouth and frequently in a retrograde manner via the colon or an enterostomy. The choice of a primary route often depends on the pathology sought within the small bowel.

Prerequisites for training in deep enteroscopy

Trainee

There are no formal guidelines for trainee prerequisites in deep enteroscopy. However, it is prudent that the trainee must have completed formal training requirements in upper endoscopy and colonoscopy before learning deep enteroscopy. The second international consensus statement suggests enteroscopy training should be contemplated by advanced trainees only, even though a

definition of advanced is not offered [1]. Given the complexity and breath of skills necessary to perform enteroscopy, the trainee must demonstrate skills beyond basic competence at upper endoscopy and colonoscopy.

Deep enteroscopy is often a therapeutic procedure and as such competence in a number of therapeutic maneuvers common to standard endoscopic procedures is a prerequisite for performing deep enteroscopy. These would include sufficient prior training in hemostasis methods such as argon plasma coagulation, injection sclerotherapy and tattooing, endoscopic polypectomy, and hydrostatic dilation of strictures. Endoscopists with a background in interventional endoscopy may also need to perform ERCP or placement of enteral stents using deep enteroscopy to access the biliary tree. ERCP in the setting of altered anatomy is considerably more difficult than standard ERCP, thus mastery of ERCP is requisite when contemplating ERCP in this setting. For this reason, it is advisable for trainees who intend to perform ERCP using these methods either to be enrolled or to have already completed a higher-tier advanced endoscopy fellowship.

In addition to these technical prerequisites, deep enteroscopy requires sufficient cognitive skills related to small-bowel pathology, interpretation and use of CE, and noninvasive imaging. The ability to understand the natural history of small-bowel lesions and in-depth understanding of both endoscopic and nonendoscopic treatment options for small-bowel diseases are necessary for the proper performance of deep enteroscopy.

Trainers

The trainer must be an experienced endoscopist who possesses the ability to teach endoscopic skills. The major attribute is the ability to verbally impart the skills necessary for performing deep enteroscopy. These procedures often require two operators, and the trainer must be able to impart by verbalization and demonstration the necessary maneuvers to operate the enteroscope and the accompanying overtube. A disposition towards teaching in combination with patience and a good working relationship with the trainee enhances the trainer's effectiveness.

Setting

Enteroscopy is performed in both ambulatory and inpatient settings. Operational logistics often dictate that most units will house the equipment in the inpatient units if these are separate. Most future trainees will receive their formal training in this setting. Deep enteroscopy is still relatively early in its evolution and supernumerary training using multistage focused workshops may be appropriate for advanced endoscopists. The training curve for learning enteroscopy using modular nontraditional settings has been described for double-balloon and spiral enteroscopy [2,3].

Cognitive component of deep enteroscopy

Indications for deep enteroscopy

It is important that enteroscopy is performed for the appropriate indications. There are other complementary methods that are in current clinical use, and the role and timing of these technologies are pivotal to proper clinical outcomes. It is useful to describe the specific clinical situations where deep enteroscopy may be considered in the evaluation of patients. Enteroscopy is most often used in the setting of mid-gastrointestinal bleeding. *Mid-gastrointestinal bleeding has been recently defined as bleeding from the ampulla of vater to ileocecal (IC) valve* [4] in contrast to upper gastrointestinal bleeding which is now defined as bleeding from the upper esophageal sphincter to the ampulla of vater.

Obscure GI bleeding is defined as bleeding from the GI tract that persists or recurs without an obvious etiology after esophagogastroduodenoscopy (EGD), colonoscopy, and/or radiologic evaluation of the small bowel, such as small-bowel follow-through or enterocolysis [5–7]. Obscure GI bleeding can be occult or overt based on whether or not there is clinically evident bleeding [8].

The indications for deep enteroscopy include mid-gastrointestinal bleeding, endoluminal interventions within the small bowel, and diagnostic evaluation of inflammatory and mass lesions in the small bowel. Deep enteroscopy may be indicated for the placement of jejunostomy feeding tubes and for the removal of foreign bodies from the small bowel. ERCP may also be performed using deep enteroscopy techniques in patients with surgically modified anatomy [9–12]. The individual training in enteroscopy must develop a grasp of the nuances of the presentations and must develop an evidence-based clinical framework for using deep enteroscopy and/or its complements appropriately.

Bowel preparation and sedation for deep enteroscopy

Bowel preparation is unnecessary for most patients undergoing enteroscopy by the anterograde approach. Patients should be ideally nil per os for 10 hours prior to the procedure. In patients with profound motility disorders, a bowel prep can aid visualization in the proximal small intestine. On the other hand, a vigorous and complete bowel prep is necessary for all patient undergoing deep enteroscopy by the retrograde approach. A split dose preparation is ideal in these patients whenever possible.

Technical aspects of enteroscopy training

The pivotal skills for the trainee to master include all the skills necessary for upper endoscopy (EGD). In addition, they must learn judicious insufflation using standard air or carbon dioxide, duodenal intubation following reduction of gastric loops, ileal intubation during retrograde examinations, and endoscope navigation through the small bowel. The mechanics of navigating the small bowel will vary depending on the deep enteroscopy device chosen.

Equipment for deep enteroscopy

Endoscopes

There are two available endoscope platforms for deep enteroscopy. Overtube-assisted spiral enteroscopy may be performed with any of these two dedicated deep enteroscopy platforms.

Double-balloon enteroscopy was first described by Yamamoto in 2001 [13]. This system has evolved rapidly, and in its present form, there are currently three different Fujinon double-balloon enteroscopes [14]. The diagnostic enteroscope (EN450P5) has a 200-cm working length, a diameter of 8.5 mm, and an accessory channel of 2.2 mm. The therapeutic enteroscope (EN450T5) has a diameter of 9.4 mm and an accessory channel of 2.8 mm, making passage of accessories easier. The EC450BI5 has a working length of 1.52 m and a 2.8 mm accessory channel. The shorter length of this double-balloon enteroscope iteration allows the use of standard length ERCP accessories when this procedure is performed in patients with altered anatomy.

The Olympus *single-balloon system* [15] has a 9.2-mm diameter high-resolution video endoscope, the Olympus SIF-Q180 (Olympus Optical, Tokyo, Japan). This endoscope is 2 m long and has a 2.8-mm working channel. In contrast to the double-balloon enteroscopes, the single-balloon enteroscope does not have a balloon attached to its distal end. Spiral enteroscopy, in its present form, can be performed with any of these enteroscopes with exception of the EC450BI5 double-balloon enteroscope. Also, spiral enteroscopy cannot be performed with a pediatric colonoscope because the inner diameter of the overtube is too small, requiring the maximum endoscope diameter to be less than or equal to 9.5 mm.

Overtubes

The double-balloon endoscope is accompanied by a 145-cm polyurethane overtube that has an inflatable latex balloon. The inner surface of this tube is lubricated with water and the balloons on both the overtube and endoscope are controlled by an external balloon controller [16]. The single-balloon splinting tube is a 140-cm long tube made of silicone. The tube has an inner hydrophilic surface and is connected to a single balloon at its distal end. The balloon is connected to an external balloon controller that allows for sequential inflation and deflation of the balloon [17]. The overtube used in spiral enteroscopy is 118 cm long and 48 Fr in diameter with a 21-cm raised helical element at its distal end [18]. Clockwise rotation of the overtube coupled to a dedicated 9.1 to

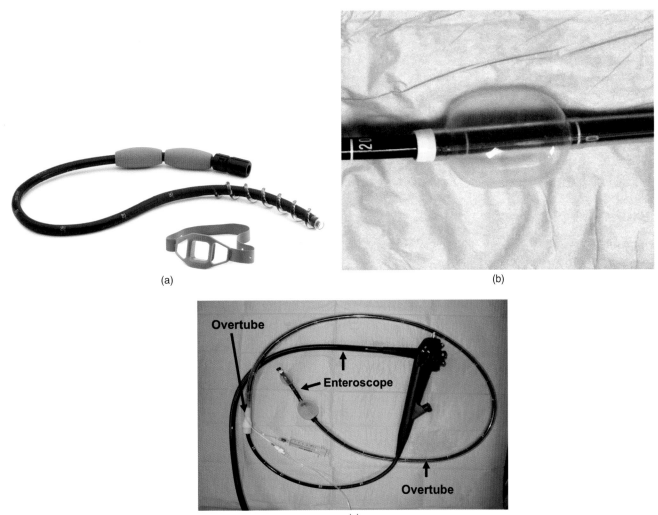

(a)

(b)

Overtube

← **Enteroscope**

Overtube

(c)

Figure 9.1 The Discovery SB overtube used in spiral enteroscopy is shown (a). Both the SBE overtube (b) and the DBE overtube (c) have a balloon incorporated at the distal tip of the device.

9.4 mm diameter enteroscope permits pleating of the small bowel, resulting in advancement through the small intestine (Figure 9.1).

Endoscopic accessories

Standard accessories for colonoscopy will suffice for deep enteroscopy through any of the enteroscope platforms with a 2.8 mm channel. Special length accessories are necessary to perform ERCP during enteroscopy except with the shorter double-balloon enteroscope. The trainee must be familiar with all the potentially useful accessories and how to successfully pass them through the enteroscope.

Diagnostic enteroscopy

Sedation

The use of propofol or general anesthesia is often necessary to perform anterograde device-assisted enteroscopy. The length and intricacy of these procedures lend to a wider acceptance of deeper forms of sedation. The trainee who will be performing enteroscopy should become familiar with the rudiments and nuances of deeper forms of sedation. General anesthesia is not a requirement for performing enteroscopy, and whenever feasible, the ability to form working relationships with anesthetists will help minimize cost overruns and excessive delays waiting for support. Conscious sedation is often adequate for performing retrograde enteroscopy. The use of glucagon or other antispasmodics during withdrawal should not be routine but may be helpful during withdrawal.

Other diagnostic considerations

The primary route of insertion should be chosen based on the clinical situation. In cases of obscure overt bleeding, the clinical presentation, i.e., anterograde examination to evaluate melena, is appropriate. In cases of suspected occult bleeding from the small bowel, CE may be helpful in determining the primary route of insertion [19]. The trainee must be able to review CE images [20] and liaison with referring doctors to develop the decision-making skills that presumably optimize the outcomes from enteroscopy. Since all forms of deep enteroscopy in the anterograde direction allow for reliable intubation of the distal jejunum or proximal ileum, it is reasonable to begin with a per os examination when evaluating abnormalities seen on CE within the initial 50% of total small-bowel transit time. For those lesions identified during the latter half of small-bowel transit time, or within the right lower quadrant, a more thoughtful approach towards route of insertion must be employed as the depth of retrograde enteroscope insertion (per rectum) is often less reliable and frequently limited to 200 cm or less.

All of the technical maneuvers germane to the performance of upper endoscopy and colonoscopy are necessary for the performance of enteroscopy. The trainee must be competent in both of these basic procedures and must be able to integrate them in addition to the push–pull and rotational maneuvers necessary to perform device-assisted enteroscopy. Esophageal intubation during anterograde enteroscopy is similar to standard upper endoscopy except for the bulk of the accompanying overtube.

The determination of the depth of insertion is a cardinal consideration during enteroscopy as there are no precise landmarks in the small bowel. The trainee must develop a working sense of the method described by May and others [21], where net advancement is recorded and collated at the conclusion of the procedure. This method, however, may be more difficult to use in rotational and single-balloon enteroscopy. Total enteroscopy is the most reliable way to evaluate the small bowel whenever necessary possible. It is difficult to achieve total enteroscopy via a single insertion route, and a combination of anterograde and retrograde enteroscopy is often necessary. The proper placement of a tattoo at the deepest site of insertion on the primary examination is a basic skill in enteroscopy—this makes the recognition of this site when the small bowel is examined from the opposite route [1,10,13,22]. Tattoo placement is also useful in marking the position of identified pathology to facilitate surgery or repeat intervention.

Fluoroscopy may be helpful during a trainee's initial experience with deep enteroscopy. It appears that with increasing experience, fluoroscopy is used less frequently [23,24]. Fluoroscopy is mandatory during deep enteroscopy when performing ERCP and often helpful in some instances of altered gastrointestinal anatomy.

Advancement technique(s)

Double-balloon enteroscopy is generally performed as a two-person procedure that requires an assistant to manage the overtube. A single operator method [25,26] has been also described. Anterograde double-balloon enteroscopy begins with securing the overtube to the shaft of the endoscope at its proximal end. The endoscope is passed in a manner similar to an upper endoscope and advanced to the pylorus. The overtube is then decoupled from the endoscope and is advanced to the 155 cm point on the endoscope. The endoscope is then advanced to a point beyond the ligament of Treitz. The endoscope balloon is then deployed to anchor the endoscope.

Following this, the overtube is advanced over the endoscope until it is distal to the duodenum. Both endoscope and overtube balloons are then inflated and withdrawn together to pleat the proximal small bowel. The overtube balloon is left inflated and used to hold the small bowel in place while the endoscope is advanced. This push–pull cycle of forward advancement and withdrawal is repeated until the pathology is reached, total enteroscopy is performed, or further advancement of the endoscope is no longer possible. Though this advancement technique appears repetitive and intuitive, structured training by an experienced operator is necessary to understand other accompanying nuances that facilitate advancement of the endoscope and overtube (Video 9.1).

Retrograde enteroscopy follows a carefully performed colonoscopy with minimal insufflation and careful attention to avoid loops. The cecum is collapsed and the IC valve is approached ideally in an almost *en-face* position. Ileal intubation may also be facilitated by passage of a stiffening wire of a dilating balloon into the ileum. Following ileal intubation, the endoscope is carefully manipulated to achieve a deeper position while avoiding the formation of a loop in the cecum that may flip the endoscope out of the distal ileum. Following deep intubation of the ileum, the overtube can follow into ileum and then push–pull maneuvers performed to achieve deep insertion.

Single-balloon enteroscopy is technically easier to perform and may be performed by a single operator. The system is inserted into the jejunum in a manner similar to the double-balloon enteroscope. Following jejunal intubation, the endoscope is held in place in the jejunum by a combination of endoscope tip angulation and suctioning. The overtube with a deflated balloon is the advanced to the scope tip. The overtube balloon is inflated and withdrawn along with the endoscope to pleat the small bowel. This cycle is repeated over and over to achieve deep intubation of the small bowel. Retrograde insertion is very similar to the technique used in double-balloon enteroscopy until deep ileal intubation is achieved. Advancement is then achieved by performing the same maneuvers as in anterograde insertion.

Spiral enteroscopy is performed as a two-person procedure, with an endoscopist keeping the lumen in view and the other operator maneuvering the spiral overtube. The overtube requires patience and a tactile understanding of its advancement characteristics. The use of a nonphysician assistant may make this procedure feasible in settings where it is impractical to have two physicians perform the procedure.

The overtube is first prepared by injecting the special prepackaged lubricant. The entire inner surface of the tube is coated and the endoscope is passed through the overtube and then coupled to the overtube, locking it to the 140 cm mark on the endoscope. The endoscope is inserted as usual into the upper esophagus. Advancement via the esophagus is then achieved by gentle clockwise rotation. After passage into the stomach, the endoscope is passed along the lesser curvature, avoiding forming any gastric loops. In the duodenum, it is often necessary to perform the Cantero maneuver, a shortening maneuver that is performed by clockwise rotation and simultaneous overtube withdrawal. Engagement is achieved by combination of very gentle forward pressure and clockwise rotation. Frequently, engagement after shortening of the overtube can be achieved by passage of an uncoupled endoscope beyond the ligament of Treitz followed by overtube advancement over the scope.

Once engaged in the jejunum, the view of the lumen is maintained by the endoscopist while rapid advancement is achieved by continued rotation of the overtube until a procedural end point is reached. Withdrawal is achieved by withdrawing the endoscope back to 130 cm mark and then gentle anticlockwise rotation to reverse advancement (Video 9.2).

A new retrograde overtube using a spiral overtube has also been described [27,28]. The technique is significantly different from anterograde advancement. This shorter overtube permits rotational pleating of the colon, allowing for deep intubation of the ileum using an uncoupled enteroscope.

Therapeutic maneuvers

Hemostasis

Most small-bowel bleeding sources can be treated using standard injection techniques or argon plasma coagulation. Hemoclips are also effective in treating angiodysplastic lesions with a Yano–Yamamoto classification 2 or greater [29], Forrest 1a and Forrest 2a lesions. Modification of the clips by desheathing greatly facilitates passage through the 2.8 mm channel.

Polyp resection

The trainee must be competent at lesion resection prior to attempting small-bowel polyp resection. Endoscopic maneuvering to present the lesion at the 6 o'clock position is necessary for most cases. Other requisite skills include submucosal injection and loop placement for polyps with a broad-based stalk. When there are multiple polyps in a single patient, retrieval of polyps after resection is a vexing problem. Multiple polyps can be retrieved by withdrawing the endoscope via the overtube anchored in place. The endoscope can be reinserted to return to the site of resection and then the procedure may continue.

Stricture dilation

Dilation of strictures within the small bowel is feasible and safe if the stricture is short and fibrostenotic. When the length of the stricture is not definable by endoscopic inspection, a selective enterocolysis can be performed. Strictures shorter than 1 cm are the most ideal for endoscopic treatment that can be easily achieved using a standard colon-length hydrostatic balloon with diameters up to and including 20 mm. In addition, similar to colonic dilation, fluoroscopy is often helpful during the dilation portion of the procedure itself.

ERCP/enteral stent placement in the setting of altered anatomy

ERCP in this setting can be performed in patients with altered anatomy. Device-assisted enteroscopy provides a stable small-bowel position to allow for cannulation of native papillae or choledochoenteric/pancreatoenteric anastomoses. Special-length accessories are necessary to perform ERCP during enteroscopy except with the EC450BI5 enteroscope. The trainee must have a detailed understanding of surgically altered anatomy and a demonstrated mastery of basic ERCP before pursuing training in this setting. Enteral stenting in the small bowel has been described for double-balloon enteroscopy [30] and spiral enteroscopy [31].

Ex vivo training models

Simulator-based training in enteroscopy has largely been conducted in *ex-vivo* animal models (Figure 9.2). At least two animal models have been described for teaching deep enteroscopy. Initially developed in 1992, the Erlangen Endo-Trainer consists of an *ex vivo* porcine organ package housed within a human-shaped dummy that has a transparent ventral shell [21]. The shell permits visualization of endoscope advancement. Insertion of the endoscope is realistic in this model and strategic fixation of the model at points facilitates simulation of device-assisted enteroscopy. Another *ex vivo* model has been modified to facilitate training in altered anatomy ERCP [32]. Finally, yet another *ex vivo* training model has been described for training in spiral enteroscopy [33]. The ASGE has conducted focused hands-on workshops incorporating *ex vivo* animal tissue models along with didactic instruction in deep enteroscopy. The objective benefits of attendance in such intensive training programs and the use of these simulators upon acquisition in skill in these procedures have not yet been determined. While such activities may improve the learning curve for trainees, at present they should be viewed as complementary educational tools that cannot replace supervised real patient training in deep enteroscopy.

Generally speaking, it appears that a measurable learning effect occurs after 5–10 cases when assessing expert endoscopists who are adding deep enteroscopy to their endoscopic skill set [2,23]. The learning curve for endoscopists in training is not well described and will vary among individuals depending on their prior experience. This learning effect can be demonstrated using both

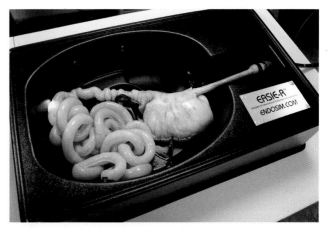

Figure 9.2 Small bowel adaptation of tabletop ex-vivo porcine model capable of hand-on instruction and practice in DBE, SBE, and spiral enteroscopy. [Courtesy of Dr. Kai Matthes].

procedural times and duration of fluoroscopy usage. A measurable decrease in both parameters appears to occur after the first 8–10 cases. Mastery, however, requires more procedures to achieve. In the United States multicenter study reported by Mehdizadeh et al., there was a significant negative correlation between procedural time and increasing experience for the centers studied [23]. Of note, these gains were not seen in patients undergoing retrograde enteroscopy by the double-balloon approach. Retrograde enteroscopy was not assessed in the spiral enteroscopy report by Buscaglia et al. [2]. Deep enteroscopy requires a commitment of both resources and effort to realize the gains afforded by experience in performing any of the aforementioned techniques

Recognition of complications

Complications in all forms of deep enteroscopy appear to be low. Therapeutic maneuvers, inflammatory enterides/collagen disorders, as well as altered anatomy appear to increase this low baseline risk. The trainee must be able to recognize complications directly, resulting from deep enteroscopy and those that may arise from deep sedation/anesthesia. The complication rate of diagnostic procedures is <1% [34] but may approach 3–4% in any of the aforementioned circumstances. Pancreatitis is infrequent but well reported with double-balloon enteroscopy [35–37]. The trainee must be able to recognize and manage the entire spectrum of potential complications.

Quality/performance assessment

While deep enteroscopy is still in its early stages of evolution, there is now a significant body of literature and at least two international consensus statements on the subject. Though formal quality indicators have not been described, adherence to established indications, depth of insertion, rate of total enteroscopy (when sought), and complication rates may all be useful indicators of performance and quality.

Conclusion

Deep enteroscopy is a rapidly evolving area of endoscopy. Deep endoluminal access to the small intestine had long eluded the endoscopist until the advent of these platforms. These platforms require a significant investment in terms of time and other resources. Proper training to ensure competence and mastery of these techniques is necessary in order to optimize outcomes.

Videos

Video 9.1 *Ex vivo* simulator demonstration of double balloon enteroscopy (DBE)
Video 9.2 Introduction and training in spiral overtube enteroscopy

References

1 Pohl J, Blancas JM, Cave D, et al.: Consensus report of the 2nd International Conference on double balloon endoscopy. *Endoscopy* 2008;**40**(2):156–160.

2 Buscaglia JM, Dunbar KB, Okolo PI, 3rd, et al.: The spiral enteroscopy training initiative: results of a prospective study evaluating the Discovery SB overtube device during small bowel enteroscopy (with video). *Endoscopy* 2009;**41**(3):194–199.

3 Gross SA, Stark ME: Initial experience with double-balloon enteroscopy at a U.S. center. *Gastrointest Endosc* 2008;**67**(6):890–897.

4 Ell C, May A: Mid-gastrointestinal bleeding: capsule endoscopy and push-and-pull enteroscopy give rise to a new medical term. *Endoscopy* 2006;**38**(1):73–75.

5 Zuckerman G, Benitez J: A prospective study of bidirectional endoscopy (colonoscopy and upper endoscopy) in the evaluation of patients with occult gastrointestinal bleeding. *Am J Gastroenterol* 1992;**87**(1): 62–66.

6 Raju GS, Gerson L, Das A, Lewis B: American Gastroenterological Association (AGA) Institute medical position statement on obscure gastrointestinal bleeding. *Gastroenterology* 2007;**133**(5):1694–1696.

7 Lin S, Rockey DC: Obscure gastrointestinal bleeding. *Gastroenterol Clin North Am* 2005;**34**(4):679–698.

8 Zuckerman GR, Prakash C, Askin MP, Lewis BS: AGA technical review on the evaluation and management of occult and obscure gastrointestinal bleeding. *Gastroenterology* 2000;**118**(1):201–221.

9 Sidhu R, Sanders DS, Morris AJ, McAlindon ME: Guidelines on small bowel enteroscopy and capsule endoscopy in adults. *Gut* 2008;**57**(1):125–136.

10 Tanaka S, Mitsui K, Tatsuguchi A, et al.: Current status of double balloon endoscopy–indications, insertion route, sedation, complications, technical matters. *Gastrointest Endosc* 2007;**66**(Suppl 3):S30–S33.

11 Pohl J, Delvaux M, Ell C, et al.: European Society of Gastrointestinal Endoscopy (ESGE) Guidelines: flexible enteroscopy for diagnosis and treatment of small-bowel diseases. *Endoscopy* 2008;**40**(7):609–618.

12 Leighton JA, Goldstein J, Hirota W, et al.: Obscure gastrointestinal bleeding. *Gastrointest Endosc* 2003;**58**(5):650–655.

13 Yamamoto H, Sekine Y, Sato Y, et al. Total enteroscopy with a nonsurgical steerable double-balloon method. *Gastrointest Endosc* 2001;**53**(2):216–220.

14 Gerson LB, Flodin JT, Miyabayashi K: Balloon-assisted enteroscopy: technology and troubleshooting. *Gastrointest Endosc* 2008;**68**(6): 1158–1167.

15 Tsujikawa T, Saitoh Y, Andoh A, et al.: Novel single-balloon enteroscopy for diagnosis and treatment of the small intestine: preliminary experiences. *Endoscopy* 2008;**40**(1):11–15.

16 Yamamoto H, Ell C, Binmoeller KF: Double-balloon endoscopy. *Endoscopy* 2008;**40**(9):779–783.

17 Kobayashi K, Haruki S, Sada M, Katsumata T, Saigenji K: [Single-balloon enteroscopy]. [Article in Japanese.] *Nippon Rinsho* 2008;**66**(7):1371–1378.

18 Akerman PA, Agrawal D, Cantero D, Pangtay J: Spiral enteroscopy with the new DSB overtube: a novel technique for deep peroral small-bowel intubation. *Endoscopy* 2008;**40**(12):974–978.

19 Gay G, Delvaux M, Fassler I: Outcome of capsule endoscopy in determining indication and route for push-and-pull enteroscopy. *Endoscopy* 2006;**38**(1):49–58.

20 Faigel DO, Baron TH, Adler DG, et al.: ASGE guideline: guidelines for credentialing and granting privileges for capsule endoscopy. *Gastrointest Endosc* 2005;**61**(4):503–505.

21 May A, Nachbar L, Schneider M, Neumann M, Ell C. Push-and-pull enteroscopy using the double-balloon technique: method of assessing depth of insertion and training of the enteroscopy technique using the Erlangen Endo-Trainer. *Endoscopy* 2005;**37**(1):66–70.

22 Sugano K, Marcon N: The first international workshop on double balloon endoscopy: a consensus meeting report. *Gastrointest Endosc* 2007;**66**(3 Suppl):S7–S11.

23 Mehdizadeh S, Ross A, Gerson L, et al.: What is the learning curve associated with double-balloon enteroscopy? Technical details and early experience in 6 U.S. tertiary care centers. *Gastrointest Endosc* 2006;**64**(5):740–750.

24 Lo SK: Technical matters in double balloon enteroscopy. *Gastrointest Endosc* 2007;**66**(Suppl 3):S15–S18.

25 Araki A, Tsuchiya K, Okada E, et al.: Single-operator method for double-balloon endoscopy: a pilot study. *Endoscopy* 2008;**40**(11): 936–938.

26 Araki A, Tsuchiya K, Okada E, et al.: Single-operator double-balloon endoscopy (DBE) is as effective as dual-operator DBE. *J Gastroenterol Hepatol* 2009;**24**(5):770–775.

27 Akerman PA, Cantero D, Pangtay J, Demarco D: Retrograde small bowel enteroscopy using the Olympus SIF-140 260 cm enteroscope and the Vista-SB spiral overtube. *Gastrointest Endosc* 2009;**69**(5):AB201-AB. [DOI: 10.1016/j.gie.2009.03.443.]

28 Cantero D, Akerman PA, Pangtay J: Retrograde spiral enteroscopy using the Fujinon EN-450T5 and Olympus SIF-180 200 cm enteroscopes with the Discovery SB overtube. *Gastrointest Endosc* 2009;**69**(5):AB192. [DOI: 10.1016/j.gie.2009.03.410.]

29 Yano T, Yamamoto H, Sunada K, et al.: Endoscopic classification of vascular lesions of the small intestine (with videos). *Gastrointest Endosc* 2008;**67**(1):169–172.

30 Ross AS, Semrad C, Waxman I, Dye C: Enteral stent placement by double balloon enteroscopy for palliation of malignant small bowel obstruction. *Gastrointest Endosc* 2006;**64**(5):835–837.

31 Lennon AM, Chandrasekhara V, Shin EJ, Okolo PI, 3rd: Spiral-enteroscopy-assisted enteral stent placement for palliation of malignant small-bowel obstruction (with video). *Gastrointest Endosc* 2010;**71**(2):422–425.

32 Maiss J, Diebel H, Naegel A et al.: A novel model for training in ERCP with double-balloon enteroscopy after abdominal surgery. *Endoscopy* 2007;**39**(12):1072–1075.

33 Akerman PA, Cantero D, Bookwalter WH, Ailinger R: A new in vitro porcine model for spiral enteroscopy training: The Akerman enteroscopy trainer. *Gastrointest Endosc* 2008;**67**(5):AB264. [DOI: 10.1016/j.gie.2008.03.722.]

34 Lo SK: Techniques, tricks, and complications of enteroscopy. *Gastrointest Endosc Clin N Am* 2009;**19**(3):381–388.

35 Groenen MJ, Moreels TG, Orlent H, Haringsma J, Kuipers EJ: Acute pancreatitis after double-balloon enteroscopy: an old pathogenetic theory revisited as a result of using a new endoscopic tool. *Endoscopy* 2006;**38**(1):82–85.

36 Lo SK, Simpson PW: Pancreatitis associated with double-balloon enteroscopy: how common is it? *Gastrointest Endosc* 2007;**66**(6): 1139–1141.

37 Gerson LB, Tokar J, Chiorean M, et al.: Complications associated with double balloon enteroscopy at nine US centers. *Clin Gastroenterol Hepatol* 2009;**7**(11):1177–1182, 1182.e1-3.

10 Choledochoscopy and Pancreatoscopy

Jeffrey H. Lee[1] & Peter Kelsey[2]

[1] MD Anderson Cancer Center, Houston, TX, USA
[2] Harvard Medical School, Boston, MA, USA

Introduction

The prospect of visualizing the biliary tree during ERCP has allured gastroenterologists for decades [1]. Significant mechanical challenges have resulted in a design evolution of both rigid and flexible endoscopes employing fiber optic and video technology. The nomenclature has likewise evolved through a spectrum of descriptive terms, including cholangioscopy, choledochoscopy, duodenoscope-assisted cholangiopancreatoscopy, and peroral cholangioscopy. The duct can now be accessed through a variety of approaches: percutaneously through a transhepatic route, through a choledochotomy, or the cystic duct created intraoperatively, or through the papilla of vater via a duodenoscope. The transpapillary route uses a two-endoscope system; the supporting duodenoscope and the cholangioscope are often referred to as the mother scope and baby scope, respectively.

This chapter begins with a detailed overview of the key aspects of diagnostic and therapeutic procedures performed using these baby scopes that need to be mastered by trainees, hoping to gain skill in this area. It will then offer trainees and their instructors some guidance as to the prerequisites for training, the skill sets and knowledge areas they must acquire, the best methods for getting trained, and help in gauging competency. Much of the recommendations about training in choledochoscopy and pancreatoscopy necessarily are based upon expert opinion, as there has yet been scant scientific attention given to training in this area.

Technical and cognitive aspects

Technique

For many years, prototype cholangioscopes have been sited in various academic institutions around the world. Currently, in the United States, the limited assortment of cholangioscopes available for purchase is listed in Table 10.1. In general, the smaller the outer diameter of the cholangioscope, the greater the maneuverability within the bile duct. The smaller size, however, leaves less room for important features such as a sufficiently large working channel.

A variety of accessories are used during routine cholangioscopy. A special adapter is attached to the opening of the mother scope's instrument channel through which the cholangioscope is passed. This adapter is designed to prevent crimping of the baby scope as it is maneuvered during the procedure. Because copious flushing and suctioning are routine during cholangioscopy, some processors are equipped with irrigation and suctioning components. Otherwise, this is done manually using tubing and syringes. A variety of miniaturized accessories specific to cholangioscopy are available, such as cytology brushes, biopsy forceps, snares, photodynamic, and electrohydraulic lithotripsy probes.

Cholangioscopy traditionally has been performed using the two-operator technique whereby one physician manages the mother scope while the second physician controls the baby scope and all of its accessories. With the development the Spyglass System (Boston Scientific Marlborough, MA, USA), the single operator technique has become widespread and permits a single interventionalist to manage both endoscopes. The endoscopist's left hand is used to control the mother duodenoscope scope. The baby scope is secured to the handle of the mother scope (see Figure 10.1). The endoscopist's right hand is then free to manage the controls and accessories of both the baby scope as well as the mother scope (Video 10.1).

The single operator technique has several advantages over the dual operator technique. First, cholangioscopy requires a carefully choreographed coordination of movement between the two endoscopes to both successfully maneuver the baby scope and to minimize the likelihood of damage due to crimping at its insertion into the mother scope. Piggybacking of the two scopes together eliminates this problem. Since these baby scopes are not designed to tolerate torque, most of the steering and maneuvering of the baby scope actually comes from the mother scope. The cholangioscope functions more as a catheter than as a true endoscope; therefore, the baby scope handle remains essentially motionless during the cholangioscopy. Finally, experience has clearly shown that cholangioscopy can easily be performed by a single physician, obviating the need for an additional interventional endoscopist.

In almost all cases, the presence of a papillotomy greatly facilitates the ease of the exam. Cholangioscopy has been successfully performed following balloon ampullary dilation without papillotomy [2]. Likewise, the development of the ultrathin caliber

Successful Training in Gastrointestinal Endoscopy, First Edition. Edited by Jonathan Cohen.
© 2011 Blackwell Publishing Ltd. Published 2011 by Blackwell Publishing Ltd.

Table 10.1 Cholangioscopes available in the United States.

Feature	Olympus	Pentax	Pentax	Boston Scientific
Model	CHF BP 30	FCP—9N	FCP—8P	Spyglass
Working channel	1.2 mm	1.2	0.75	1.2 mm
Guide wire size	0.035 in	0.035	0.025	0.035
Outer diameter	3.4 mm	3.1	2.8	3.1
"Mother Scope" channel diameter	4.2 mm	4.2	3.8	4.2 mm
Field of view	90°	90°	90°	70°
Depth of field	1–50	1–50	1–50	
Tip deflection	160° up/130° down	160°/130°	160°/130°	
Working length	187 cm	190	190	230 cm

endoscopes permits scope passage through supporting catheters without the need for a sphincterotomy [3]. These ultrathin scopes, still not widely used, do not have an instrument channel for tissue sampling or for interventions. The papilla can, however, be dilated using either catheter or balloon dilators to permit passage of the larger cholangioscopes over a guide wire into the biliary tree. Balloon dilation of the papilla carries a defined risk of pancreatitis. A papillotomy is required in the management of choledocholithiasis to permit egress of the stone fragments.

Indications for choledochoscopy

The primary indications for cholangioscopy include the evaluation and management of biliary strictures, filling defects, and difficult choledocholithiasis (Table 10.2). Conventional ERCP has an excellent track record in the diagnosis and management of well-defined bile duct abnormalities such as choledocholithiasis and

bile leaks. This technique has fared less well in the accurate diagnosis of two, less-defined classes of bile duct lesions: filling defects and strictures. Though there is some overlap between these two findings, it is useful to consider them separately.

Biliary filling defect

A filling defect relates to the fluoroscopic appearance of something that actually lies within the bile duct lumen such as a stone or a polypoid tumor. It has now been clearly established that cholangioscopy can improve the accuracy in the diagnosis of biliary filling defects [4–6]. One recent experience examined the impact of cholangioscopy on the diagnostic accuracy of ERCP when there was uncertainty in the ERCP diagnosis [7]. Patients were excluded if they had obvious stone disease or classic biliary obstruction due to malignancy in the head of the pancreas. In this study, 91 consecutive patients were evaluated by ERCP supplemented by

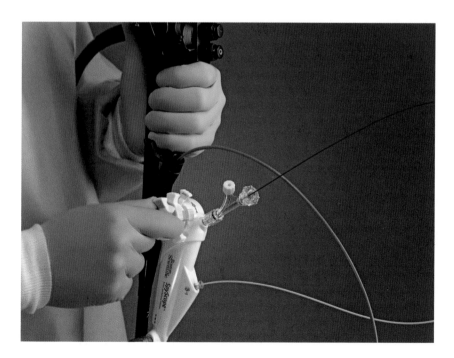

Figure 10.1 Close up of SpyScope™ as it is attached to the head of the mother scope.

Table 10.2 Indications for cholangioscopy.

ERCP diagnosis	Cholangioscopy offers
Strictures	Improved diagnostic accuracy
	Tissue acquisition under visualization
Filling defects	Improved diagnostic accuracy
	Definitive therapy
Stones, refractory	Visual guidance for EHL
	Confirm duct clearance
Mucosal lesions	Biliary candidiasis
	PSC related scarring

biopsy/brush cytology when indicated. There were 76 strictures and 21 filling defects in the study group. Of the patients with the 21 filling defects, ERCP with biopsy or brush cytology was able to correctly identify the eight malignant lesions and the nine benign tumors. ERCP did not, however, correctly diagnose the four cases of stone disease. In these patients, the stones were adherent to the bile duct wall and had the appearance of a mass. Cholangioscopy, on the other hand, was able to make the correct diagnosis using direct visualization alone in all 21 patients. The four patients with stone disease were easily identified and treated with stone removal.

Biliary stricture

A stricture implies a narrowing of the duct lumen due to either (a) wall thickening or (b) compression from extrinsic pathology. Stricture due to increased wall thickening can be intrinsic to the wall such as with a cholangiocarcinoma and might therefore have some associated mucosal defects that could be detected by direct visualization. Stricture due to compression from extrinsic disease, such as nodal metastasis, may result in a narrowing of the lumen, but in this case, the epithelial lining of the bile duct wall in the region of the stricture may retain a normal appearance. In some cases, cholangiocarcinoma can spread through the biliary tree in the submucosal layers, resulting in biliary stricture by compression; however, the overlying mucosa may have a completely unremarkable endoscopic appearance.

Differentiating malignant from benign biliary stricture

While the cholangioscopic differentiation between stone and tissue appears straightforward, the same is not true in the ability to differentiate malignant from benign strictures on the basis of direct visualization alone. Early cholangioscopic experience reported morphologic characteristics that claimed to distinguish malignant from benign tissue with an accuracy that approached 95% [8]. Several features were identified as being accurate predictors of malignancy, including tumor neovascularization, a dense papillary pattern, and friable nodularity. It was observed that bile duct adenocarcinomas had three classifications: nodular, papillary, and infiltrative.

1 Nodular-type lesions are bulky and eccentric with an overlying friable mucosa. There is often neovascularization with tissue friability and oozing.
2 Papillary type is identified by a high-density pattern of papilla or fish-egg type mucosa. There is often luminal mucin and blood obscuring the visual field (see Video 10.2).
3 Infiltrative type is the most difficult to diagnose because of the paucity of specific cholangioscopic characteristics. The overlying mucosa is bland and whitish with minimal neovascularization.

The authors described several other less common bile duct tumors, including biliary papillomatosis, mucin-hypersecreting cholangiocarcinoma, and biliary cyst adenocarcinoma. Biliary papillomatosis looks similar to the papillary adenocarcinoma except that it is a mutlifocal disease with areas of normal intervening mucosa. The mucin-hypersecreting cholangiocarcinoma is similar to the papillary-type adenocarcinoma except that according to the authors, the biliary ducts may be dilated and mucin filled.

These cholangioscopic criteria for malignancy were tested prospectively on 76 patients with biliary strictures of unknown type and compared to the accuracy of ERCP with biopsy alone. In this study, ERCP with tissue sampling had a sensitivity of 58% and a specificity of 100%. The addition of cholangioscopy to this group of patients did increase the sensitivity to 100% but dropped the specificity to 87%. The loss of specificity was due to the incorrect diagnosis of malignancy in five patients on the basis of the cholangioscopic appearance of neovascularization and the presence of a tumor vessel. These five false positives were found instead to have chronic pancreatitis in two patients and one patient each with primary sclerosing cholangitis, autoimmune pancreatitis, and a peribiliary cyst.

The potential advantage of cholangioscopy in the evaluation of biliary strictures for malignancy is in the opportunity to obtain pathologic material under direct observation. Brushings and biopsy forceps can be steered directly onto the area of suspicion and the sample obtained under visual guidance. Initial reports indicate a high sensitivity for the identification of malignancy in patients with suspicious appearing biliary strictures. In one study of 62 patients with indeterminate biliary strictures, cholangioscopy with and without biopsy detected malignancy with a sensitivity of 89%, specificity of 96%, positive predictive value of 89%, and negative predictive value of 96% [9]. Another study in patients with primary sclerosing cholangitis, comparing the accuracy of cholangioscopy directed biopsy to ERC alone, found cholangioscopy more accurate in the detection of malignancy in dominant biliary strictures [10]. A prospective study comparing biopsy and cytology tissue yield from indeterminate strictures obtained during ERCP versus cholangioscopy has not been published. Whether this approach actually increases the yield of correct diagnosis remains to be determined.

There are several reasons to account for difficulties in accurate tissue diagnosis of suspicious-appearing strictures. Negotiating angulated turns of the bifurcation and the small biliary radicals remain a challenge, given the limitation of maneuverability and steerability of the current choledochoscopes. It may not be feasible to deflect the scope tip to obtain a specimen from abnormal-appearing tissue off to one side. Finally, the cups on the biopsy forceps are quite small, approximately one millimeter (1 mm) in diameter and thus the tissue yield is likewise small and frequently insufficient when biopsying hard or fibrotic tissue. Brush cytology, however, is often feasible, and the yield may increase that of biopsying alone. In primary sclerosing cholangitis, difficulties come from not being able to traverse the strictures. As it is a risk for developing cholangiocarcinoma, performing targeted biopsy utilizing direct visualization would provide a better yield in tissue acquisition and increased sensitivity in obtaining diagnosis.

Managing filling defects with electrohydraulic lithotripsy

Fragmentation of giant or recalcitrant stones is one of the primary indications for interventional cholangioscopy. Candidate stones are usually too large to be trapped in a mechanical lithotripsy basket or are adherent to the bile duct wall and thus cannot be easily manipulated. In these circumstances, fragmentation using electrohydraulic lithotripsy (EHL) is an efficient and highly successful technique. Traditionally, endoscopists have been resigned to long-term stenting of large, recalcitrant stones. It has been demonstrated, however, that compared to stone removal using EHL, long-term stenting is associated with higher long-term complications such as cholangitis [11]. Thus, most patients with such stone burden should be considered for definitive fragmentation therapy.

EHL was originally designed as an industrial mining tool. The modification for endoscopy employs a fiber with two embedded electrodes. A power generator delivers a high-voltage electrical current, creating a spark across the two electrodes at the tip of the fiber. High frequency discharges cause rapid expansion of the fluid–stone interface, generating shock waves that fragment the stone. This technique has been successfully applied using percutaneous, surgical, and transampullary routes to the bile duct using either cholangioscopic or fluoroscopic guidance.

To perform EHL, the cholangioscope must first be positioned in front of the target stone. Achieving a satisfactory position is critical to the safe deployment of the probe. When the EHL probe projects from the cholangioscope, it must hit directly on the target stone and not touch or travel adjacent to the biliary epithelium. In addition, the contact interface between the probe and the stone must be in an aqueous environment for the shock wave to be transmitted and effect fragmentation (see Video 10.3).

In patients with a capacious bile duct and a generous papillotomy, the bile duct may drain too rapidly to perform EHL. The patient must then be rolled to place the biliary tree in a dependent orientation. Before firing, the probe tip should be in close apposition to the stone. The duct is lavaged to sweep away fragmented debris to maintain good visualization. The probe should be aimed at a single target on the stone, chipping away at a focus until the stone cleaves. Often the outer coating of a stone is more durable and requires more EHL pulses. Once chipped, continued firing at the same spot rapidly enlarges the defect and fragments the stone.

As the target stone mass is reduced in size, the choledochoscope is advanced up the duct to the next target. Fragmentation is then repeated until all of the target stones are fragmented or the visual field is obscured by debris. It is common to overestimate the degree of fragmentation that has occurred during a round of EHL discharges. With the cholangioscope removed from the bile duct, the stone fragments are swept out using standard balloon and basket techniques. Often, by simply fragmenting the lower stones in a packed duct, the remaining stones can then be more easily removed by standard maneuvers. The second round of EHL, if needed, proceeds more quickly as the duct is less tightly packed and there is more room to maneuver the cholangioscope. Once the bile duct has been cleared of debris and stones, the baby scope can be reintroduced into the bile duct to check for large retained fragments and for unsuspected strictures.

The success of EHL has been reported in a number of series [12–14]. In one large study, the power generator (Lithotripter Elgin, IL, USA) was configured at settings of 100 watts, a frequency of six shots per second and eight shots per pulse [14]. In the management of recalcitrant stone disease that has failed standard ERCP techniques, cholangioscopic directed EHL is 90–100% successful in complete stone eradication [15]. While the number of procedures required to achieve this success has ranged broadly from 1 to 13 exams, the experienced cholangioscopists can expect to achieve complete duct clearance in one exam of under 2 hours duration in the majority of patients [14].

Indications for cholangioscopy without fluoroscopy

Occasionally, urgent biliary exploration is indicated when fluoroscopy is either unavailable or not practical. The ability to examine the bile duct without fluoroscopy has proven useful in three clinical situations: (1) in morbidly obese patients whose features may not conform to standard fluoroscopy units, (2) in patients during their first trimester of pregnancy and (3) in those patients too critically ill to be transported to a fluoroscopy unit. This should be only considered when there is a clear need for endoscopic biliary intervention.

The technique of choledochoscopy without fluoroscopy requires few modifications from the technique described above. Routine biliary cannulation is performed using a papillotome and a wire. Once a duct has been deeply cannulated, the guide wire is removed. The observation of bile tracking up the lumen of the papillotome as the guide wire is withdrawn confirms the position of the papillotome in the bile duct. The guide wire is then advanced back up through the papillotome into the biliary system. Sphincterotomy is performed and the papillotome is removed, leaving the wire in the biliary tree. The cholangioscope is passed down through the mother scope over the guide wire and a wire-guided cannulation of the bile duct is performed. Once the baby scope is positioned in the region of the bifurcation, the guide wire is removed.

Cholangioscopy in therapy of malignant bile duct lesions

There is increasing interest in the targeting of therapy against a variety of malignant and premalignant bile duct lesions using cholangioscopic assistance. Photodynamic therapy of cholangiocarcinoma has been performed by both the percutaneous [16,17] and peroral route [18]. The technique appears safe with minimal complications but its long-term clinical effectiveness remains to be evaluated in multicentered trials. In general, these patients still require stenting to maintain duct patency and the goal of the PDT therapy is likely palliative rather than curative. Ortner et al. reported results of a randomized trial of cholangioscopically guided PDT with stenting versus stenting only for unresectable cholangiocarcinoma. The photodynamic therapy group had median survival to 493 days, while the stenting only group had median survival to 98 days ($p < 0.0001$). In this study, treatment with PDT and stenting provided less cholestasis and better quality of life compared with endoscopic stenting alone [19]. Biliary papillomatosis is an uncommon condition of multifocal papillary lesions of the bile duct. Patients can present with obstruction and may require transplantation. Transhepatic cholangioscopy using a variety of ablative therapies has been successful in controlling disease progression [20–22].

Cholangioscopy can be performed in most situations where ERCP is indicated. While there are no absolute contraindications to cholangioscopy, there are several noteworthy areas of caution:

1 Coagulopathic patients may not safely undergo sphincterotomy, thus preventing passage of many of the currently employed cholangioscopes. Also, their risk of bleeding due to EHL-induced tissue injury might be increased.

2 In patients with ascending cholangitis, the risk of inducing bacteremia during cholangioscopy might be increased.

Complications of cholangioscopy

The reported complications of cholangioscopy include
- Bacteremia
- Aspiration
- Bleeding
- Pancreatitis

Bacteremia, as determined by serial blood cultures in the minutes following cholangioscopy, can be demonstrated to occur in 15% of patients, but cholangitis is clinically relevant in only a minority of these situations [23]. Prophylactic antibiotics do not appear to be of benefit following cholangioscopy and stone removal in the surgical setting [24]. Bacteremia can result from over distention of the biliary tree during irrigation. This may be more likely if the ampulla forms a tight seal around the insertion tube of the cholangioscope, preventing the venting of excess irrigant into the duodenum. As a rule, irrigation can be safely performed with a volume equal to or less than the amount of bile aspirated from the obstructed ducal system. Patients suspected of having cholangitis should receive periprocedure antibiotics.

Aspiration occurs as a consequence of the irrigating fluid that accumulates in the stomach [25]. Aspiration of these contents can be prevented by frequent suctioning of the gastric contents.

The reported complications following EHL stone fragmentation during cholangioscopy include the following:
- Cholangitis
- Bleeding
- Pancreatitis [26]
- Perforation

Self-limited bleeding occurs when the EHL pulses are discharged in close apposition to the bile duct wall [27]. There are no reports of uncontrolled bleeding. Bile duct leaks due to EHL injury have been reported. Perforation can occur at either the papillotomy site or at the site of an errant EHL discharge.

Relative cost

There are no published cost comparisons between the technique of cholangioscopy and alternative techniques.

Peroral direct cholangioscopy

Peroral direct cholangioscopy (PDCS) is performed using an ultraslim scope that was originally designed for nasal endoscopy. It has an outer diameter of 5.0 mm with a working channel diameter of 2.0 mm. Most ultraslim scopes have only one dial as in baby scopes, allowing the tip deflection in only one plane: up and down movements. As it is a video-endoscope, the ultraslim endoscope provides much better images than a fiber-optic scope along with narrow band imaging (NBI). It has separate water and air channels. The large working channel of the scope allows not only passage of larger biopsy forceps, thus increasing diagnostic yield in tissue acquisition, but also therapeutic maneuvers including stone extraction, EHL, and others. As the outer diameter of the scope is wider than that of a baby scope, this requires either sphincterotomy and/or balloon dilation of the papilla for insertion into the bile duct. There are two ways to perform cholangioscopy using an ultraslim scope: (1) without using an anchoring device and (2) using a balloon anchor.

No balloon method

Using a duodenoscope, the bile duct is cannulated utilizing a sphincterotome (or a cannula) and a guide wire in traditional fashion. Then, the guide wire is advanced to a branch of the right hepatic duct (RHD) or the left hepatic duct (LHD). The duodenoscope is removed and the wire is back-loaded into the ultraslim scope. The ultraslim upper endoscope is advanced over the guide wire through the incised papilla into the bile duct by careful advancing and shortening the scope as a cecal intubation technique during colonoscopic examination. During this procedure, applying manual compression to the patient's abdomen may facilitate advancing the scope to the hilar area. Larghi et al. reported the direct cholangioscopy using an ultraslim scope added only 10–15 minutes to the procedure [28]. Perhaps, an overtube may be helpful to facilitate passage of the scope into the duodenum.

With balloon method

Using a duodenoscope, the bile duct is accessed and a guide wire is advanced into a branch of RHD or LHD. Next, a 5F balloon catheter with triple-lumens is advanced over the guide wire into the intrahepatic duct. The balloon is then inflated to anchor the wire in the duct. The scope is removed and the wire is retrofitted into the ultraslim scope. Under the fluoroscopic guidance, the ultraslim scope is advanced into the bile duct. As the scope is quite thin and flexible, advancing the scope through the stomach into the duodenum may be difficult. Careful negotiation and shortening of the endoscope will help avoid looping the scope in the stomach.

One study compared the two techniques; Moon et al. reported the success rate in wire-guided direct PDCS of 45.5% (5/11) compared with 95.2% (20/21) for intraductal balloon-guided direct POC [29].

Utilities of the ultraslim upper endoscope

Moon et al. reported successful biopsies using endobiliary forceps to establish histopathological analysis using ultraslim upper endoscopes. In four patients, PDCS was successful in removing difficult CBD stones by laser lithotripsy or EHL [30]. EHL can be performed using the ultraslim upper scope utilizing the same technique as in mother–baby scope system.

Park et al. reported successful ablation of a nodular mass in the right intrahepatic duct through an ultraslim upperscope. The patient presented with recurrent hepatoma obstructing the bile duct. Using an argon plasma coagulation (APC) system (VIO-300D; ERBE, Tubingen, Germany), APC was applied to the mass with a flow rate of 1 L/min and power setting of 60 W. After treatment with APC, the debridement of the ablated tissue was retrieved by a biopsy forceps [30].

Pancreatoscopy

Most pancreatic cancers are locally advanced or metastatic at the time of diagnosis, resulting in a poor 5-year survival rate of 4%. Current efforts to increase pancreatic cancer survival rate include progress in early-stage detection of pancreatic cancers, such as carcinoma *in situ*. Carcinoma *in situ* remains within the pancreatic ductal epithelium and has not yet invaded the parenchyma. As most pancreatic adenocarinomas are arising from the pancreatic duct, being able to visualize the duct during peroral pancreatoscopy (POPS) will theoretically increase the chance of finding the cancer early, thus improving 5-year survival rate.

In 1975, Takekoshi et al. first reported POPS through the accessory channel of a duodenal fiberscope [31]. Pancreatoscopes can be categorized into (1) those with a tip deflection mechanism and a suction/accessory channel and (2) ultrathin diameter instruments that have no deflection mechanism or suction/accessory channel.

Initially, the available pancreatoscopes were all fiber-optic scopes. Two of these common fiber optic pancreatoscopes include one with an outer diameter of 3.1–3.4 mm and the other, an ultrathin scope, with a diameter of 0.8 mm. During the past few years, we have observed emergence and applications of video pancreatoscopes [(CHF-B260); Olympus Medical Systems, Tokyo, Japan]. This video pancreatoscope has an outer diameter of 3.4 mm and a working-channel diameter of 1.2 mm. When the ultrathin fiber optic pancreatoscope is used, the pancreatic duct can be irrigated through the guiding catheter, but operation is still difficult as there is no tip-deflection mechanism. Also, as in fiber-optic scopes, there are issues with the durability and maneuverability of the video pancreatocoscopes. Electronic video pancreatoscopes provide high-quality images and are useful in finding subtle lesions in the pancreatic duct. Upon visualization, normal mucosa has a pinkish smooth surface with good vascularity. The reported abnormalities include coarse mucosa and submucosal tumor-like protrusions; in a study of 115 patients by Yamao K et al., findings in pancreatic cancer were coarse mucosa (59%), protrusion (27%), erythema(36%), friability(50%), tumor vessels(23%), and papillary tumor (14%) [32].

Peroral electronic pancreatoscopy

The peroral electronic pancreatoscopy (PEPS) device was developed with a 50,000-pixel interlined charge-coupled device (Matsushita Electronic Corporation, Osaka, Japan) in cooperation with the Olympus Optical Co. (Tokyo, Japan). The PEPS has an external diameter of 2.1 mm and has a forward-viewing optical system with a field view of 80° and a depth of field of 1–30 mm. It has a bidirectional angle function (up 120°, down 120°). Pancreatoscopy can possibly be carried out without sphincterotomy or balloon dilation of the papilla of vater. Kodama et al. reported that the rate of successful PEPS procedures was 90% (38 of 42), although the range of insertion varied (pancreatic head 17%, 7 of 42; body 26%, 11 of 42; tail 24%, 10 of 42; stenotic lesion 24%, 10 of 42) [33].

Sphincterotomy or not versus endoscopic sphincter dilation

There is some question as to whether endoscopic pancreatic sphincterotomy (EST) is necessary for pancreatoscopy. Jung et al. reported their experience of 20 pancreatoscopies in 18 patients with inconclusive ductal abnormalities that have been previously investigated by computed tomography (CT) scan, abdominal ultrasound, and ERCP. The endoscope (CHF-BP 30; Olympus Optical Co., Japan) had an outer diameter of 3.1 mm and an instrumentation channel of 1.2 mm. EST was carried out in every patient prior to insertion of the pancreatoscopy. One bleeding episode was noted after EST, but no other complications were observed [34].

On the other hand, Ueno et al. described endoscopic sphincter dilation (ESD) up to 6 mm to assist insertion of the endoscope in two patients with IPMN [35]. ESD has the advantage of preserving the sphincter function of the papilla. Authors observed significant hyperamylasemia after ESD and recommended temporary pancreatic ductal stenting. Considering the invasiveness and potential for complications of biliary and/or pancreatic sphincterotomy and/or dilation of the pancreatic duct, pancreatoscopy with a 3.5-mm diameter pancreatoscope should not be performed in patients with a normal papilla and a nondilated pancreatic duct.

However, with the development of ultrathin pancreatoscope, pancreatoscopy became feasible in patients with a normal papilla. Kodama et al. reported 42 pancreatosocpies using an electronic pancreatoscope with an outer diameter of 2.1 mm in 36 patients with chronic pancreatitis, without sphincterotomy or balloon dilation of the papilla of vater. As mentioned above, the insertion of the scope was successful in 38 of 42 procedures (90%) [33]. Therefore, the need for sphincterotomy and/or dilation depends on patient's anatomy and the diameter of the scopes used.

Pancreatoscopy with narrow-band imaging

Video pancreatoscopy makes it possible to use the NBI system. NBI is now widely used in distinguishing Barrett's mucosa, flat adenomas, or other subtle mucosal lesions. The NBI system (CV-260SL processor, CVL-260SL light source;Olympus) is based on narrowing the bandwidth of spectral transmittance of red–green–blue optical filters. The filters cut all illumination wavelengths, except two narrow wavelengths centered on 415 nm and 540 nm. The image is reproduced in the processor with information from the two illumination bands. The 415-nm centered band provides the most information on the capillary and pit patterns of the superficial mucosa and the 540-nm centered band provides information about thicker capillaries in slightly deeper tissues. Thus, NBI delivers accentuated images of the mucosal structures and mucosal microvessels [36].

In evaluation of the pancreatic duct with NBI, a conventional therapeutic duodenoscope (TJF 200;Olympus) with a working channel diameter of 4.2 mm is advanced to the duodenum. Then, a video pancreatoscope [(CHF-B260); Olympus Medical Systems, Tokyo, Japan] with an outer diameter of 3.4 mm and a working-channel diameter of 1.2 mm is advanced through the working channel of the duodenoscope into the pancreatic duct.

Biopsies of the lesions can be performed using a 3F ultrathin biopsy forceps (FB-44U-1;Olympus). The addition of NBI may aid in the diagnosis of the primary tumor and help in the determination of the extent of the tumor. Itoi et al. reported that pancreatoscopy with NBI allowed visualization of a skip-spreading lesion and a tumor in the pancreatic duct, not recognized by white light. The specimens obtained by biopsy at these lesions showed adenocarcinoma [37].

Pancreatoscopy for intraductal papillary mucinous neoplasm

Intraductal papillary mucinous neoplasm (IPMN) of the pancreas is generally classified as the main duct IPMN or side-branch IPMN. The main duct IPMN is characterized by dilatation of the main pancreatic duct, mucinous secretion, and papillary growth in the duct. Pancreatoscopy allows visualization of the pancreatic duct and even openings of the side branches.

Biopsy of a hypervascular area detected by pancreatoscopy with NBI may be helpful to distinguish benign from malignant IPMN. In an effort to detect the pancreatic cancer early, pancreatic juice analysis is often performed as well. Yamaguchi et al. reported the sensitivity for IPMN was 62.2% when pancreatic juice was collected via pancreatoscopy and was 38.2% when it was collected by using a catheter [38]. The authors could not explain the difference in sensitivity in two modalities. In aspiration of viscous fluid of IPMN, a larger working channel of a pancreatoscope would have theoretical benefit over thin caliber of a catheter. This difficulty in aspiration is also observed in endoscopic ultrasound-guided aspiration. Often, little amount of fluid is collected through a 22- or 25-gauge needles from suspected IPMN, especially when the fluid is viscous. Pancreatoscopy in 57 cases of IPMN revealed mucus (23%), coarse mucosa (4%), granular mucosa (16%), and papillary tumor (58%) [32].

Pancreatoscopy in chronic pancreatitis

Pancreatoscopy is of diagnostic value in the setting of chronic pancreatitis, poorly defined pancreatic lesions, and when assessing alterations of the ductal caliber without parenchymal lesions. In chronic pancreatitis, one can see protein plugs of various shapes coexisting with turbid pancreatic juice, calculi, and obstruction of side-branches by calcified pancreatic stones [33]. The mucosal surface appears pinkish-white in normal patients but is whitish in chronic pancreatitis. There are alterations in blood vessels with a visible vascular network with changes such as disruption, stenosis, irregularity, rearrangement, and stretching.

Intraoperative pancreatoscopy

Intraoperative pancreatoscopy can also be performed using the ultrathin pancreatoscope. For intraductal papillary mucinous tumors, it is necessary for not only making the diagnosis, but also for defining the extent of tumor involvement in the duct. In a study by Kaneko et al., intraoperative pancreatoscopy detected 10 cases of IPMN lesions that could not be detected by endoscopic ultrasonography or endoscopic retrograde pancreatography. In three cases, additional pancreatic resection was performed after intraoperative pancreatoscopy. For diagnosis of IPMN lesions, the sensitivity, specificity, and overall accuracy of intraoperative pancreatoscopy were all 100% [39].

Complications of pancreatoscopy

The reported complication rate is 1.8–5% with the main complications being bleeding and pancreatitis [34,35,37,40,41]. Mild pancreatitis has been reported in 2 of 52 (3.8%) after pancreatoscopy using an ultrathin pancreatoscope [41]. Howell et al. reported no complications due to the EHL procedure, immediately following any of the nine treatment sessions for six patients with pancreatic stones. One patient experienced increased abdominal pain for several days without biochemical evidence of pancreatitis. In Japan, drugs (gabexate mesilate, nafamostat mesilate, and ulinastatin) that inhibit the activation of pancreatic enzymes are used to reduce the risk of pancreatitis [37].

Training and development of competency

Trainee prerequisites

A trainee first needs to be proficient in performing diagnostic and therapeutic upper endoscopy as well as in performing therapeutic ERCP. In addition, a trainee needs to have a fund of knowledge in the anatomy of the hepatobiliary and pancreatic system, their pathophysiology, and related diseases.

Trainer and facility prerequisites

A trainer should be an expert in ERCP and a training facility should be a high-volume center with various cases of therapeutic ERCP. The training facility must be equipped and the trainer, staff, and trainee should be familiar with the equipment such as duodenoscope, fluoroscopy, choledochoscope for two people operation, Spyglass for one person operation, and electorhydraulic lithotripsy. The staff also needs to be familiar with accessory devices that can travel through the therapeutic channels of the choledochoscopes and pancreatoscopes in addition to the standard ERCP accessories, including the generator and grounding pads.

Skills to master

There are several advanced endoscopic skills to master in choledochoscopy and pancreatoscopy. As aforementioned, choledocoscopy can be performed as two endoscopist technique or one endoscopist technique (Spyglass peroral cholangiopancreatoscopy). Two endoscopist technique requires that both endoscopists be familiar with characteristics of the mother and baby scopes. It also requires a fluid coordination and teamwork between the two operators. With the advent of ultraslim upper endoscopes, now we are able to perform direct peroral cholangioscopy using these scopes. Direct peroral cholangioscopy can be performed with or without an anchoring device, such as a special balloon inflated in the biliary system.

Steps to learn

First, a trainee will review all aspects of therapeutic ERCP. This includes reviewing indications of ERCP, biliary and pancreatic cannulation, sphincterotomy, dilation, and stenting. In addition, a trainee will also review the indications, risks, and possible complications of cholangioscopy and pancreatoscopy. Before starting a case, a trainee will be familiar with the specifications of the scopes involved, mother scopes, baby scopes, therapeutic channels, and outer diameters of each scope. A trainee will then learn the techniques of how to maneuver the choledochoscopes and pancreatoscopes. Until recently, all such training was possible only in the course of actual cases at the home institution. Recent advances in ex-vivo and inanimate simulators have made possible the inclusion of choledochoscopy hands-on training; such opportunities have been featured at the NYSGE annuall course in 2009 and 2010 and at the ASGE inaugural Endofest training course in 2010. The impact of such training methods has yet to be determined, though given the limitation in case volume at many institutions, this is a promising development.

Competency

At the end of the training period, competency can be measured in two aspects: knowledge base and technical proficiency. In terms of knowledge base, a graduate is expected to know the specifications of the equipment and accessories used in cholangioscopy and pancreatoscopy, the anatomy and diseases of the hepato-biliary and pancreatic systems. From technical aspect, a graduate is expected to be proficient in diagnostic and therapeutic ERCP, choledochoscopy, and pancreatoscopy. There is no data published which describes how many supervised cases a trainee should perform in order to develop enough proficiency to competently do cases independently.

In order to maintain proficiency, we recommend to perform a minimum of 200 ERCPs and 10 choledochoscopies (or pancreatoscopy) per year.

Summary

Cholangioscopy and pancreatoscopy are important adjuncts to interventional ERCP. This technique of optical visualization of biliary and pancreatic ducts improves the diagnostic accuracy in the assessment of biliary and pancreatic strictures. Therapeutic maneuvers such as EHL can be performed through cholangioscopy assisting eradication of stones refractory to standard interventional ERCP techniques. There are few complications. With continuing developments of new technologies, we look forward to seeing novel applications of cholangiopancreatoscopy. Training to perform these emerging techniques requires mastery of many of the cognitive and technical skills required to perform standard ERCP interventions and is best obtained at high-volume ERCP centers under the direct supervision of expert instructors.

Videos

Video 10.1 Spyglass: techniques in direct biliary visualization
Video 10.2 Choledoschoscopy revealing papillary tumor of the bile duct
Video 10.3 Electrohydraulic lithotripsy through a cholangioscope
Video 7.14 Spincterotomy and cholangioscopy
Video 25.2 Through-the-scope mechanical lithotripsy
Video 25.3 Importance of continuous irrigation and proper probe positioning in EHL and laser lithotripsy
Video 25.4 Laser lithotripsy with the Freddy laser
Video 25.5 Holmium laser lithotripsy of pancreatic duct stone
Video 25.6 Giant bile duct stone removal

References

1 Kozarek RA: Direct cholangioscopy and pancreatoscopy at time of endoscopic retrograde cholangiopancreatography. *Am J Gastroenterol* 1988;**83**:55–57.

2 Minami A, Nakatsu T, Uchida N, et al.: Papillary dilation vs. sphincterotomy in endoscopic removal of bile duct stones. A randomized trial with manometric function. *Dig Dis Sci* 1995;**40**:2550–2554.

3 Soda K, Shitou K, Yoshida Y, Yamanaka T, Kashii A, Miyata M: Peroral cholangioscopy using new fine-caliber flexible scope for detailed examination without papillotomy. *Gastrointest Endosc* 1996;**43**:233–238.

4 Siddique I, Galati J, Ankoma-Sey V, et al.: The role of choledochoscopy in the diagnosis and management of biliary tract diseases. *Gastrointest Endosc* 1999;**50**:67–73.

5 Seo DW, Kim MH, Lee SK, et al.: Usefulness of cholangioscopy in patients with focal stricture of the intrahepatic duct unrelated to intrahepatic stones. *Gastrointest Endosc* 1999;**49**:204–209.

6 Seo DW, Lee SK, Yoo KS, et al.: Cholangioscopic findings in bile duct tumors. *Gastrointest Endosc* 2000;**52**:630–634.

7 Fukuda Y, Tsuyuguchi T, Sakai Y, Tsuchiya S, Saisyo H: Diagnostic utility of peroral cholangioscopy for various bile-duct lesions. *Gastrointest Endosc* 2005;**62**:374–382.

8 Nimura Y, Kamiya J, Hayakawa N, Shionoya S: Cholangioscopic differentiation of biliary strictures and polyps. *Endoscopy* 1989;**21**(Suppl 1):351–356.

9 Shah RJ, Langer DA, Antillon MR, Chen YK: Cholangioscopy and cholangioscopic forceps biopsy in patients with indeterminate pancreaticobiliary patholgy. *Clin Gastroenterol Hepatol* 2006;**4**(2):219–225.

10 Tischendorf JJ, Krüger M, Trautwein C, et al.: Cholangioscopic characterization of dominant bile duct stenoses in patients with primary sclerosing cholangitis. *Endoscopy* 2006;**38**(7):665–669.

11 Hui CK, Lai KC, Ng M, et al.: Retained common bile duct stones: a comparison between biliary stenting and complete clearance of stones by electrohydraulic lithotripsy. *Aliment Pharmacol Ther* 2003;**17**:289–296.

12 Adamek HE, Maier M, Jakobs R, Wessbecher FR, Neuhauser T, Riemann JF: Management of retained bile duct stones: a prospective open trial comparing extracorporeal and intracorporeal lithotripsy. *Gastrointest Endosc* 1996;**44**:40–47.

13 Binmoeller KF, Bruckner M, Thonke F, Soehendra N: Treatment of difficult bile duct stones using mechanical, electrohydraulic and extracorporeal shock wave lithotripsy. *Endoscopy* 1993;**25**:201–206.

14 Farrell JJ, Bounds BC, Al-Shalabi S, et al.: Single-operator duodenoscope-assisted cholangioscopy is an effective alternative in the management of choledocholithiasis not removed by conventional methods, including mechanical lithotripsy. *Endoscopy* 2005;**37**: 542–547.

15 Arya N, Nelles SE, Haber GB, Kim YI, Kortan PK: Electrohydraulic lithotripsy in 111 patients: a safe and effective therapy for difficult bile duct stones. *Am J Gastroenterol* 2004;**99**:2330–2334.

16 Shim CS, Moon JH, Cho YD, et al.: The role of extracorporeal shock wave lithotripsy combined with endoscopic management of impacted cystic duct stones in patients with high surgical risk. *Hepatogastroenterology* 2005;**52**:1026–1029.

17 Wiedmann MW, Caca K: General principles of photodynamic therapy (PDT) and gastrointestinal applications. *Curr Pharm Biotechnol* 2004;**5**:397–408.

18 Harewood GC, Baron TH, Rumalla A, et al.: Pilot study to assess patient outcomes following endoscopic application of photodynamic therapy for advanced cholangiocarcinoma. *J Gastroenterol Hepatol* 2005;**20**:415 420.

19 Ortner ME, Caca K, Berr F, et al.: Successful photodynamic therapy for nonresectable cholangiocarcinoma: a randomized prospective study. *Gastroenterology* 2003;**125**:1355–1363.

20 Bechmann LP, Hilgard P, Frilling A, et al.: Successful photodynamic therapy for biliary papillomatosis: a case report. *World J Gastroenterol* 2008;**14**(26):4234–4237.

21 Gunven P, Gorsetman J, Ohlsen H, Ruden BI, Lundell G, Skoog L: Six-year recurrence free survival after intraluminal iridium-192 therapy of human bilobar biliary papillomatosis. A case report. *Cancer* 2000;**89**:69–73.

22 Meng WC, Lau WY, Choi CL, Li AK: Laser therapy for multiple biliary papillomatosis via choledochoscopy. *Aust N Z J Surg* 1997;**67**:664–666.

23 Chen MF, Jan YY: Bacteremia following postoperative choledochofiberscopy—a prospective study. *Hepatogastroenterology* 1996;**43**:586–589.

24 Sheen-Chen SM, Chou FF: Postoperative choledochoscopy: is routine antibiotic prophylaxis necessary? A prospective randomized study. *Surgery* 1994;**115**:170–175.

25 Schebesta AG, Sporr D, O'Leary J, Moulton J: Gastric aspiration associated with operative choledochoscopy. *Anaesth Intensive Care* 1983;**11**:257–258.

26 Sheen-Chen SM, Eng HL: Acute pancreatitis following choledochoscopic stone extraction for hepatolithiasis. *Med Sci Monit* 2003;**9**:CS13–CS15.

27 Fan S, Choi T, Wong J: Electrohydraulic lithotripsy for biliary stones. *Aust NZ J Surg* 1989;**59**:217–221.

28 Larghi A, Waxman I: Endoscopic direct cholangioscopy by using an ultra-slim upper endoscope: a feasibility study. *Gastrointest Endosc* 2006;**63**(6):853–857.

29 Moon JH, Ko BM, Choi JH, et al.: Intraductal balloon-guided direct peroral cholangioscopy with an ultraslim upper endoscope. *Gastrointest Endosc* 2009: **70**; 297–302.

30 Park DH, Park BW, Lee HS, et al.: Peroral direct cholangioscopic argon plasma coagulation by using an ultraslim upper endoscope for recurrent hepatoma with intraductal nodular tumor growth. *Gastrointest Endosc* 2007;**66**:201–203.

31 Takekoshi T, Maruyama M, Sugiyama N, et al.: Retrograde pancreatocholangioscopy. *Gastroenterol Endosc* 1975;**17**:678–683.

32 Yamao K, Ohashi K, Nakamura T, et al.: Efficacy of peroral pancreatoscopy in the diagnosis of pancreatic diseases. *Gastrointest Endosc* 2003;**57**:205–209.

33 Kodama T, Imamura Y, Sato H, et al.: Feasibility study using a new small electronic pancreatoscope: description of findings in chronic pancreatitis. *Endoscopy* 2003;**35**(4):305–310.

34 Jung M, Zipf A, Schooonbroodt D, et al.: Is pancreatoscopy of any benefit in clarifying the diagnosis of pancreatic duct lesions? *Endoscopy* 1998;**30**(3):273–280.

35 Ueno N, Ozawa Y, Aizawa T, et al.: Pancreotoscopy assisted by endoscopic sphincter dilation. *J Gastroenterol* 2003;**38**(3):283–287.

36 Gono K, Yamazaki K, Doguchi N, et al.: Endoscopic observation of tissue by narrowband illumination. *Opt Rev* 2003;**10**:211–215.

37 Itoi T, Sofuni A, Itokawa F, et al.: Initial experience of peroral pancreatoscopy combined with narrow-band imaging in the diagnosis of intraductal papillary mucinous neoplasms of the pancreas (with videos). *Gastrointest Endosc* 2007;**66**(4):793–797.

38 Yamaguchi T, Shirai Y, Ishihara T, et al.: Pancreatic juice cytology in the diagnosis of intraductal papillary mucinous neoplasm of the pancreas: significance of sampling by peroral pancreatoscopy. *Cancer* 2005;**104**(12):2830–2836.

39 Kaneko T, Nakao A, Nomoto S, et al.: Intra-operative pancreatoscopy with the ultra-thin pancreatoscope for mucin-producing tumors of the pancreas. *Arch Surg* 1998;**133**(3):263–267.

40 Tajiri H, Kobayashi M, Niwa H, et al.: Clinical application of an ultra-thin pancreatoscope using a sequential video converter. *Gastrointest Endosc* 1993;**39**:371–374.

41 Howell DA, Dy RM, Hanson BL, et al.: Endoscopic treatment of pancreatic duct stones using a 10-F pancreatoscope and electrohydraulic lithotripsy. *Gastrointest Endosc* 1999;**50**:829–833.

11 Principles of Electrosurgery

David L. Carr-Locke[1] & John Day[2]

[1] Beth Israel Medical Center, New York, NY, USA
[2] ERBE USA Inc., Marietta, GA, USA

Learn and understand electrosurgery
It is potentially the most dangerous tool we use in endoscopy

Introduction

Electrosurgery is the medical harnessing of electricity to create various thermal tissue effects during clinical applications requiring resection, incision, hemostasis, and devitalization of target tissue. Electrocautery is often used interchangeably with electrosurgery but is a misnomer since it merely represents the ability to 'burn' (coagulate) with electricity and not cut or perform a combination of both cutting and coagulation tissue effects.

Electrosurgery was introduced in Europe in 1923 by ERBE Elektromedizin GmbH and in 1926 (Figure 11.1) in the United States by William Bovie and Harvey Cushing (Figure 11.2) [1]. Grant Ward, a well-known surgeon of his time, recognized early in 1932, how dangerous electrosurgery could be when used by an untrained individual. He stated: *"An adequate surgical training is a prerequisite to the adoption of electrosurgery... It little behooves the novice to take up such a powerful weapon—dangerous in the hands of the unskilled"* [2]. The surgeon JL Glover wrote about the use of thermal knives compared to other modalities in 1978, shortly after the arrival of modern isolated generators. He opined: *"There is no group of instruments in the surgical armamentarium that is used as frequently and understood as poorly as electrosurgery units..."* [3]. In the 1960s and 1970s, electrosurgical units (ESUs) were an absolute mainstay in medical care, but few among medical professionals had formal education regarding their use. The Journal of the Association of Operating Room Nurses, The Journal of the American Medical Association, and The American Journal of Surgery and Cancer all carried articles in the late 60s and 70s about injuries to patients from electrosurgery.

Before the newer "isolated system" safety features were developed in electrosurgery in the late 1960s, there were some catastrophic injuries surrounding the use of electrosurgery. The alternate site burn was usually caused by electrical energy taking the path of least resistance via an EKG electrode. This burn could be deep, even charring tissue down to bone. Another example was the return plate site burn resulting from the consequences of turning up power without first checking the status of the patient plate. It could have been incorrectly placed over a bony prominence, incorrectly oriented for the procedure being performed, be dehydrated when applied, or not adherent well to the skin. Electrosurgery was developing a "bad name," but these were all preventable errors. While burns cannot ever be totally eliminated when using ESUs, the current "isolated systems" work with safety systems in the generator to help prevent injuries such as these.

Multiple elements contribute to the skill of the art and science of using electrosurgery as depicted in Figure 11.3. Successful training in the use of electrosurgery therefore requires understanding of
1 The basics of electricity
2 The difference between monopolar and bipolar devices
3 Safety measures in electrosurgery
4 Tissue effects of electrosurgery in endoscopy
5 Clinical applications of electrosurgery in endoscopy.

Basics of electricity as applied to electrosurgery

There are some basic rules regarding all electrical circuits, which also apply to clinical use:
1 Electricity always takes the path of least resistance
2 Electricity always seeks ground
3 There must be a complete circuit for electricity to flow.
Basic terminology is important since generators vary and the user must understand how to adjust their controls in order to achieve the desired clinical effect safely: *Current* is the flow of electrons and is measured in amperes or amps. *Resistance* or *impedance* represents the obstacle to the flow of current and is measured in ohms. *Voltage* is the driving force pushing current through the resistance and is measured in volts. *Energy* is a basic universal concept in physics and applies to many systems where forces are applied or transferred and is measured in joules. *Power* is the rate of transfer of energy and is measured in watts. One watt is a rate of one joule per second. *Frequency* is the rate at which the electromagnetic wave (such as an alternating electric current)

Successful Training in Gastrointestinal Endoscopy, First Edition. Edited by Jonathan Cohen.
© 2011 Blackwell Publishing Ltd. Published 2011 by Blackwell Publishing Ltd.

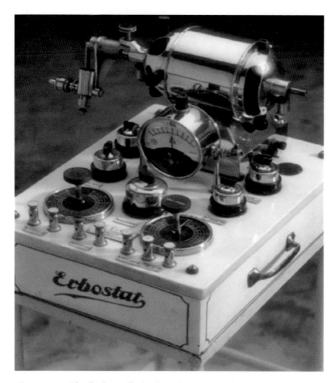

Figure 11.1 The "Erbostat": the first electrosurgical generator produced by ERBE Elektromedizin GmbH in 1923.

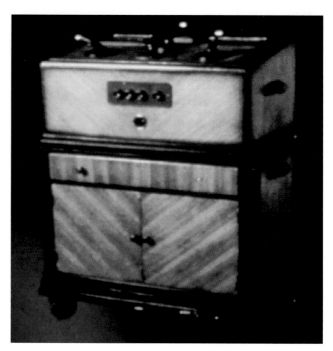

Figure 11.2 The first "Bovie" generator designed by Bovie and Cushing in 1926.

changes direction and is measured in hertz (abbreviated to Hz). One hertz is equivalent to one cycle per second.

The behavior of electricity is governed by the laws of physics and its principles are predictable. Four variables are present in its equations: resistance (R), voltage (V), current (I), and power (P). They are associated through the equations $V = I \times R$ and $P = V \times$

I. When any one of the variables changes, the others are affected. All three properties are present in an electrical circuit or pathway when used in electrosurgery.

Parts of the human body have electrical characteristics that can be represented by variations in impedance as shown in Figure 11.4. Materials that are good carriers of electrosurgery are "conductors," meaning that they have a low level of resistance. Materials that have a high level of impedance are called "insulators."

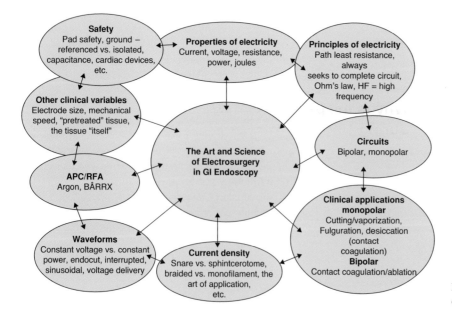

Figure 11.3 The integration of art and science in eletrosurgery.

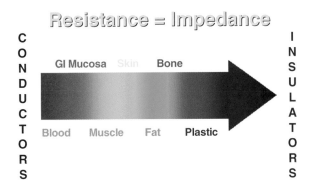

Figure 11.4 The spectrum of impedance of human tissue.

Tissue resistance depends to a large extent on its vascularity and water content. As tissue dries out or is desiccated electrosurgically, its resistance increases greatly and the current flowing through it decreases if the voltage is kept constant. Blood and the lining of the gastrointestinal tract are good conductors of electrosurgical energy. Muscle, skin, and fat are also conductors but have increasing levels of impedance in that order. Bone has a high level of impedance and plastic is an insulator. Gloves insulate us from the electrosurgical instruments.

Other than electrical differences between different tissues, patients are also different "electrically" from each other. Factors such as age, local and systemic disease processes, body build, air resistance in the electrical pathway, and hydration all play a role. The ESU must overcome all of these barriers and provide safe thermal tissue effects without unnecessary damage to the tissue being treated or elsewhere.

One of the most common questions about electrosurgery is "Why can the current from a wall socket kill you, but the energy from an electrosurgical generator plugged into the wall will not?" The answer is frequency. A low frequency alternating current of 60 Hz, as used in a domestic electricity supply, will cause nerve stimulation, muscle stimulation, pain, and potentially cardiac arrest since it mimics the frequency at which nerves fire. Much higher frequencies as emitted by an ESU generator operate significantly above body frequency, which allows for delivery of energy

without interference with the nervous system. For electrosurgery, electrical current from a wall outlet (60 Hz) is passed run through a transformer, which converts the energy to a high radio frequency (350,000–3,000,000 Hz).

This high-frequency alternating current produces thermal tissue effects, resulting in cutting and/or coagulation without neuromuscular stimulation. Figure 11.5 illustrates the spectrum of electromagnetic waves from household current at 60 Hz through 100,000 Hz or 100 kHz, which is the approximate threshold at which the body stops feeling electrical stimulation. ESUs operate at over three times this frequency between 350 kHz and 3 MHz similar to radio waves, which is why such outputs are often referred to as "radiofrequency" or "RF." Television waves operate at even higher frequencies usually above 50 MHz.

Monopolar and bipolar circuits

Generators typically deliver thermal effects via two types of circuit—monopolar and bipolar (Figure 11.6a,b). Monopolar modes use the patient's body to complete the circuit between the generator through the active electrode to the grounding pad or patient plate and back to the generator. The benefit of a monopolar circuit is the ability to achieve high levels of thermal effect from a device as well as versatility in regards to cutting and coagulation. Examples of the monopolar mode in endoscopy are the polypectomy snare, sphincterotome, needle-knife, and argon plasma coagulation. The bipolar or multipolar mode does not require a grounding pad because the circuit is completed between two points on the active electrode. The thermal effect is localized only to the tissue in direct contact with the target electrode. Two examples of bipolar/multipolar devices used in endoscopic intervention are the Gold Probe™ (Boston Scientific, Marlboro, MA, USA) used for hemostasis and the HALO™ devices (BÅRRX Medical, Sunnyvale, CA, USA) used for tissue devitalization. The instruments are designed to deliver the power and also return it to the generator using only target tissue as the "circuit." The advantage of this mode is the precise delivery of intense energy into a small space.

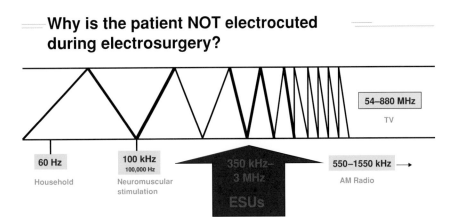

Figure 11.5 The spectrum of frequencies of electromagnetic waves.

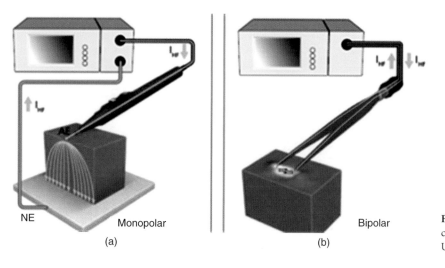

NE   Monopolar

(a)

Bipolar

(b)

Figure 11.6 (a) Monopolar circuit. (b) Bipolar circuit. (Reproduced with permission from ERBE USA Inc.)

Safety measures in electrosurgery

The return electrode

In monopolar circuits, the return plate, dispersive pad, grounding pad, or neutral electrode collects the electrosurgical energy from the patient and returns it safely to the generator. The energy is returned through a low current density interface between the skin and the pad (see below for an explanation of current density) so that there is no thermal effect to the patient's skin. Electricity must complete a circuit, or it will not flow. The grounded ESU is still available from several manufacturers and found usually in the Ambulatory Endoscopy Center or office setting. Occasionally, older units are still found in hospitals and users must be aware of the differences from modern ESUs and their potential dangers. The electrical energy must be able to return to "ground" (its place of origin). In these older units, the energy flows from the generator to the patient via the active electrode, through the patient, exits through the dispersive pad, and returns to the grounded generator. The problem with these generators is that the electricity can also seek an alternative path and result in burns. The guidelines from professional organizations maintain that all removable external metal should be removed in order to minimize the possibility of the circuit being completed through a path of least resistance via, e.g., an endoscopy table or IV pole.

Modern ESUs are "isolated" and keep current flow within the contained circuit and through the return pad, but electricity still adheres to the two principles: it seeks ground and follows the path of least resistance. If the circuit is broken, no current will flow at any point within the system. An isolated ESU has a transformer that causes the current to return only to the generator and not use alternate pathways to return to its source. If this is not possible, the generator will shut down. An isolated ESU prevents alternate site burns, but not patient return electrode burns.

Correct placement of the return electrode is essential to avoid problems with the circuit. The skin surface area must be adequate

to disperse the current so that the current density cannot be high enough in one spot to cause a burn. This is why the patient plate is many times larger than the active electrode tip. High current density in the active tip is needed to achieve the thermal effect for coagulation or cutting, but we need to avoid creating high current density at the return plate in order to prevent a burn. The safest types of return electrodes are split models that allow comparison of current flow (and therefore resistance) from the two sides. The generator safety system can detect disparities between the two sections and warn the user if current density is focused on a small area of the plate becoming unsafe. A pad monitoring system allows the ESU to monitor the level of pad to patient contact continuously and sound an alarm or interrupt the circuit if an unsafe condition is detected.

There are four basic rules of return pad placement safety:

1 The area should be clean, dry, and devoid of significant hair since hair is an insulator

2 There should be good musculature and vascularity beneath the pad

3 Avoid bony prominences and scar tissue

4 Placement should be as close to operative site as possible.

In endoscopy, the optimum area is the flank or overlying the kidney on the latissimus dorsi muscle, if possible. An active electrode in the colon usually has an improved response with this short distance to complete the circuit. Other common alternatives are the anterior thigh or upper arm, but both increase the circuit length. On the flank, the long side of a rectangular plate goes toward the spinal area. On the thigh and arm, the long side is facing the head.

Always use the correct size pad for the patient and never cut a pad to fit. Ensure that the pad is applied evenly with no "tenting." Also, make sure that the cord is oriented toward the machine. This reduces the risk that any movement of the patient could cause the pad to peel back.

If the endoscopist is calling for more power because the tissue effect is not as expected, this should be a "red flag." Electricity will not flow if it cannot complete the circuit. If the pad is in poor contact or the electricity is leaving the body through an alternate site (on a nonmonitored pad system), the endoscopist may not be getting all the power needed. Always recheck the pad site first.

Pacemakers

The use of RF current may damage older pacemakers but modern types are safe and do not need to be adjusted. Bipolar circuits are completely safe, but when using a monopolar circuit, placing the return pad well away from a pacemaker is also sufficient. ICDs (implanted cardiac defibrillators), however, require temporary deactivation by placing a magnet over them so that the electrosurgical current will not be detected and the ICD stimulated to fire erroneously. Removing the magnet allows immediate reactivation of the ICD after the procedure. This can be safely accomplished by the endoscopy staff after an initial training session with the appropriate cardiology personnel.

Neuromuscular stimulation

A well-sedated patient that suddenly jumps during use of electrosurgery may have experienced neuromuscular stimulation. This can be caused by any number of faults within the circuit such as inadequate connections, poor insulation, broken wire bundles under insulation, or defective/broken adapters. All are suspect for allowing demodulation of the current frequency to below the 100 kHz threshold.

Explosion risk

Poor bowel preparation poses a risk of explosion when combined with any electrosurgery. The risk is from trapped gases, such as hydrogen or methane, in the colon that are temporarily protected from insufflation and suction, allowing an explosive mixture to be ignited from the electrical spark at the active electrode.

Precautions can be taken to avoid this hazard before using electrosurgery (usually for polypectomy) such as water lavage of the colon clear during the colonoscopy if possible, exchange of the colonic gas with air or carbon dioxide from the colonoscope several times, strict avoidance of mannitol preparation which produces hydrogen, use of "cold snare" (without electrosurgery) technique for small polyps and use of alternative nonthermal methods for hemostasis such as clips.

Current leaks

RF leakage currents are those that find alternate paths back to the ESU generator. These leakage currents take away from functional power that should be delivered to the operative site and can cause alternate site burns to the patient or user. The accessory cables from the ESU should not be routed with other cables. They should be kept separated in order to avoid the phenomenon of capacitive coupling. This is a natural phenomenon that can be compounded when using electrosurgical accessories through endoscopes. Capacitive coupling or leakage from the active electrode within the endoscope channel to surrounding metal structures of the endoscope can occur. The escape of secondary currents can thus cause inadvertent burns away from the target site and loss of power at the active electrode.

Tissue effects of electrosurgery in endoscopy

Electrosurgery is the central component of many endoscopic procedures. It is imperative that the endoscopist gains an understanding of how the desired tissue effects are achieved in order to use and adjust different devices and different generators while treating different disease states.

Various processes take place in tissue during heating (thermal effect). They are primarily determined by the temperature achieved (Table 11.1). Most important for electrosurgery are denaturation of proteins, starting at about 60°C (coagulation) and vaporization of the tissue fluid at 100°C. How fast and how fully these processes occur depends on the speed of the heating and the effective duration of the increased temperature, which are determined by the amount and time-course of the power delivered to the tissue. The local effect also depends on the current density, which is a function of the tissue resistance. There are thus a number of influencing factors on the electrosurgical effect. The type and shape of the active electrode and the size of the contact area influences the current density. Small contact areas between the electrode and tissue can generate quick, intense heating due to the high current density, e.g., needle-knife, sphincterotome, and closed snare. At the same power but with a larger contact area, the current density is lower and the heating is slower and weaker, e.g., open snare, hemostatic probe, and coagulating forceps. The duration of the contact between the electrode and the tissue influences how rapidly the temperature is achieved and its effective duration. The contact area can be changed through the electrode's movement, e.g., deeper insertion of a sphincterotome and closing of a snare. Different types of tissue, such as muscle, fat, or vessels, can be heated to varying degrees due to their electrical and thermal properties but can also respond differently to heating. What

Table 11.1 Thermal effects on human tissue [1].

Temperature	Effect
≤40°C	None
40–50°C	Hyperthermia: Changes in the cell membrane and internal cellular structures depending on the duration of the necrosis
~60°C	Coagulation (denaturation) of the cellular proteins Devitalization
~80°C	Coagulation of the extracellular collagen Destruction of cell membranes
~100°C	Vaporization of tissue fluid depending on vaporization speed Desiccation and attrition Incision due to mechanical rupture of the tissue
>150°C	Carbonization
>300°C	Vaporization

is important here is that the electrical resistance depends greatly on the water content of the tissue, which differs depending on the type of tissue (Figure 11.4). The resistance rises quickly when desiccation is initiated through vaporization of the tissue fluid. This can lead to more intense heating of desiccated tissue areas. Current and voltage depend primarily on the tissue properties, the size of the contact area, and the properties of the generator in the electrosurgical unit.

With so many variables, a reproducible effect is difficult to achieve manually although that is how it was done in endoscopy for more than two decades. The introduction of regulated electrosurgery in the 1980s by the ERBE Company (ERBE Elektromedizin GmbH, Tuebingen, Germany) was a significant advance. Modern ESUs continuously monitor current and voltage, calculate parameters such as power and tissue resistance from this, and analyze these findings in milliseconds. Depending on the desired effect, such generators can keep the operating parameters constant or change them in a targeted manner through modulation. This enables the ESU to balance out differences between different types of tissue, react to changes in tissue properties, e.g., due to desiccation, and guarantee that the electrosurgical effect can be reproduced.

Cutting

In order to incise tissue, it must be quickly heated to over 100°C, so that the tissue fluid abruptly vaporizes and the tissue structure ruptures. The current density required for this achieves cutting by producing short electric arcs (sparks), which occur at peak voltages starting at around 200 V between the electrode and tissue (Figure 11.7). These sparks are essential for the cutting to be rapid and effective. Generators that do not achieve this "spark mode" quickly at initiation of the circuit are less effective than those that do so. In endoscopy, the cutting electrode is typically a thin wire, e.g., snare, sphincterotome, or needle-knife, with a linear leading edge. It does not directly touch the tissue during the cutting process because it is surrounded by a steam barrier

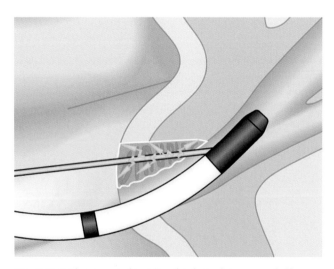

Figure 11.7 Electrosurgical incision: the electrode is surrounded by a layer of vapor and the current is transferred by electric arcs. (Reproduced with permission from ERBE USA Inc.)

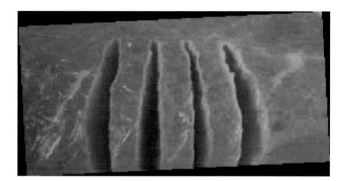

Figure 11.8 Four incisions in *ex vivo* muscle produced with increasing current density and voltage from left to right showing increasing coagulation effect (whitening) at the edges of the incision. (Reproduced with permission from ERBE USA Inc.)

of vaporized intracellular fluid. The microelectric arcs preferably occur on the leading edge between electrode's surface and the respective target tissue. This quickly vaporizes tissue at the leading edges, thus creating an electrosurgical incision. The electrode can be advanced through the tissue without mechanical force. If the voltage is increased deliberately or inadvertently, the intensity of the arcs also increases and a higher current flows than would be necessary for a simple incision. This can lead to the vaporization of more fluid and to more intense heating of the neighboring tissue. The result is an increased concurrent thermal insult or excessive coagulation along the incision plane (Figure 11.8). In the event of intense heating, undesired carbonization can also occur. The nature of the incision, especially the size of the coagulation zone at the edge of the incision, is also known as the incision quality. The desired incision quality depends on the application. The incision quality can be influenced by the user through the incision speed—a faster incision means less coagulation—and by the device through regulation of the operating parameters such as voltage regulation, arc regulation, and current modulation.

An adequate electrical voltage is necessary for the formation of microelectric arcs required for electrosurgical cutting. Together with the electric resistance of the tissue and multiple other circuit impedance variables, the voltage determines the current flow and thus the delivered energy of the microelectric arcing occurring between the electrode and target tissue. Therefore, a voltage that is kept constant creates a constant incision quality that is independent of the incision depth. However, the incision quality depends on the incision speed, surface area of the electrode, and the tissue type (as well other clinical variables). For example, because of its low resistance, lower voltages are required to cut muscle tissue than fatty tissue. This helps promote a reproducible incision in the presence of constant tissue properties. The intensity of the arcs or sparks is a measure of the incision effect. Modern ESUs can measure this intensity and keep it constant by setting the voltage correspondingly. Arc regulation enables constant incision quality independent of the tissue type, cutting speed, and type of electrode. Higher peak voltage is required for incisions requiring more intensive coagulation. Conversely, in order to prevent an excessive thermal insult during incision, the mean power must

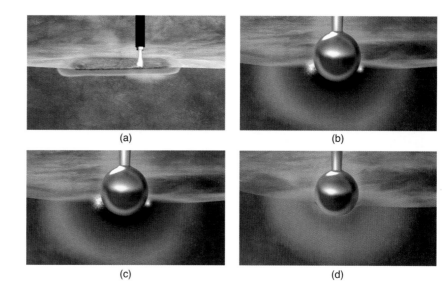

Figure 11.9 (a) Contact coagulation with low voltage. (b) Contact coagulation with high, modulated voltage. (c) Noncontact coagulation (fulguration). (d) Argon plasma coagulation. (Reproduced with permission from ERBE USA Inc.)

be decreased. This is achieved by modulating the alternating current, i.e., its peak value is varied with time. A frequent type of modulation is the "interstitial modulation," whereby the current stream is interrupted in very brief (microseconds) time intervals. As a rule, modulation takes place so quickly that the user only notices the changed tissue effect.

Coagulation

With sufficiently slow heating of bleeding tissue, the proteins in the tissue and extravasated blood coagulate first. The tissue atrophies and dries out due to the fluid vaporization, which then occurs. The shrinkage and coagulation of blood closes blood vessels and the bleeding stops. Coagulation can be performed in direct contact with the tissue (contact coagulation) or without contact (noncontact coagulation) (Figure 11.9a–d). Contact coagulation is primarily suitable for coagulation of localized bleeding such as a spurting artery. An additional benefit of using a contact method is the ability to apply pressure with a probe at a specific site, such as a spurting artery or visible vessel, in order to achieve "coaptive coagulation." This uses either low voltages or modulated forms of voltage with a higher peak values. The higher voltages enable faster work but can be associated with nonprecise arcing and carbonization. In general, the degree of coagulation obtained with a bipolar contact device correlates with the duration and force of application for a given set of power settings (Table 11.2a). This is because the probe delivers similar amounts of total energy (power over time) to overcome the tissue impedance, which increases more rapidly with higher power settings compared to lower power settings [4].

In noncontact coagulation, the current is transmitted by electrical arcs under high voltages of several thousand volts. In contrast to the incision, the arcs are generally distributed over a large area so that a coagulation zone is created. This way superficial, diffuse bleeding can be efficiently coagulated. The conventional procedure by arcing through an air gap to target tissue is described as fulguration. A more even and controllable result is provided by argon plasma coagulation (APC). This is a monopolar noncontact modality in which current is transmitted by electric arcs through ionized (i.e., electrically conductive) argon gas—an argon plasma. APC is used for the coagulation of diffuse bleeding, for superficial devitalization of tissue, and for volume reduction through vaporization and shrinkage. An important advantage of APC is that adhesion of an instrument and the resulting avulsion of coagulated tissue is avoided. The plasma also has a slight tendency to seek out not yet coagulated and therefore more conductive areas.

Table 11.2 Generic correlation between power and duration of application of a coagulating current using bipolar contact and monopolar noncontact methods. Caution in extrapolating these data to human use is needed since there are many other variables not taken into account—tissue type, degree of tissue hydration, generator type (constant voltage or constant power), generator software, device type, etc.

(a) Power/time comparisons of *ex vivo* tissue (meat) effects with contact coagulation using a 7 French diameter multipolar probe with a force of application of 75 g [4].

Power (W)	10	15	20
Depth of coagulation @ 2 s (mm)	0.07	0.59	0.63
Depth of coagulation @ 10 s (mm)	0.86	0.87	0.84

(b) Power/time comparisons of *ex vivo* tissue (meat) effects with argon plasma coagulation [1].

Power (W)	20	40	60	100
Depth of coagulation @ 1 s (mm)	0.5	0.75	1.0	1.5
Depth of coagulation @ 5 s (mm)	1.0	2.5	4.0	5.0

With the corresponding low power setting, this produces a relatively even superficial coagulation with low penetration depth. Deeper coagulation can also be achieved with increased power and time intervals as shown in Table 11.2b. Note that there are many "APC" generators commercially available and a technical and clinical understanding is needed prior to their application. Some have been studied *ex vivo* and *in vivo* and coagulation effects (depth, diameter, etc.) have been published as guidelines, thus giving guidance to the various modes by manufacturers.

Combination cutting and coagulation

There are many clinical situations in endoscopy where a simultaneous or sequential combination of cutting and coagulation is desirable. Different manufacturers have approached this need differently from many types of "blended" current to a proprietary modulated output of alternating cutting and coagulation. Nearly all modern generators allow some degree of customization by alteration of the control parameters. This can vary, however, from simply changing the proportions of cutting and coagulation current to the more complicated manipulation of detailed components of the current, such as power, duration, and interval of a pulsed output. Manufacturers' specifications need to be followed carefully if the default settings are to be altered.

Clinical applications of electrosurgery in endoscopy

Resection techniques

The removal of mucosal tumors using electrosurgery encompasses a variety of techniques ranging from snare polypectomy through a polyp pedicle or stalk to resection of the papilla (papillectomy) to endoscopic mucosal resection (EMR) and endoscopic submucosal dissection (ESD) of sessile polyps Figure 11.10. With the exception of ESD, which requires special devices, polypectomy, papillectomy, and EMR are performed with a snare with or without the addition of fluid injected into the submucosa.

Either a pure coagulating current or a modulated blend such as the "ENDOCUT™" mode invented by ERBE is used. A "pure" coagulation current delivering sufficient power can be used for polypectomy since the cutting is achieved mechanically by the snare wire once the tissue has been desiccated. It is important to understand how the principle of current density affects the snare's performance. As the area of the snare loop is made smaller during closure of the snare handle, the current density increases exponentially and the tissue effect is enhanced. The rate at which the snare loop is closed must be appropriate for the polyp being resected in order to avoid, at one extreme, mechanical avulsion

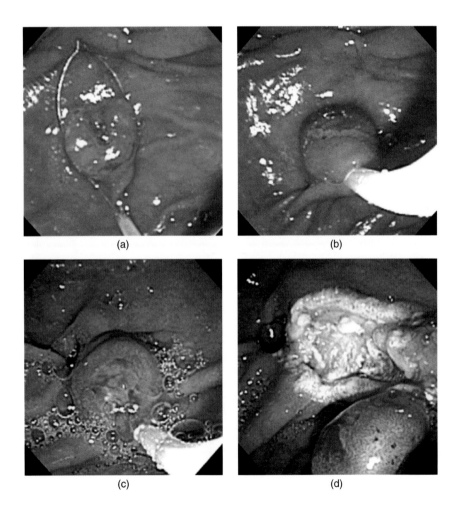

(a)   (b)

(c)   (d)

Figure 11.10 Snare resection of a benign adenoma of the major papilla in the duodenum (papillectomy): (a) snare loop being placed around the lesion, (b) snare loop closed, (c) current applied and the tumor changes color as its vascular supply is interrupted, and (d) immediate postresection appearance.

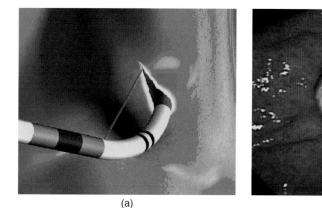

(a)   (b)

Figure 11.11 (a) Cartoon of sphincterotome in papilla and sphincterotomy incision with white coagulated edges. (Reproduced with permission from ERBE USA Inc.) (b) Actual sphincterotomy.

without sufficient coagulation and, at the other, over-desiccation (carbonization) preventing mechanical cutting. If a modulated or blended cutting/coagulating mode is used, the snare closure technique is different (slower) because the tissue is being cut electrically.

Incision techniques

Examples of the need for an incision without resection are biliary and pancreatic sphincterotomy (Figure 11.11), access (precut) papillotomy, cystgastrostomy and cystduodenostomy for pseudocyst drainage, and mucomyotomy for Zenker's diverticulum. All employ the principle of a very thin wire to which is usually applied a form of blended or modulated current since the objective is to achieve cutting without bleeding. The thin wire achieves a very high current density at the point of tissue contact and it becomes an electrical knife.

Bipolar techniques

There are specific bipolar accessories for hemostasis (e.g., Gold Probe™ by Boston Scientific Endoscopy), devitalization of Barrett's epithelium (BarrX), and intracorporeal electrohydraulic lithotripsy for biliary and pancreatic stones. All use the bipolar principle of active and return electrodes on the therapeutic device. These modalities require very different power needs and each has its own dedicated generator. In the case of hemostatic probes, however, the bipolar functions on a standard generator may be used.

Argon plasma coagulation (APC) (Figure 11.12)

As already described, APC is a noncontact monopolar system that has the unique property of surface coagulation, which makes it ideal for treating vascular ectasias (isolated, gastric antral vascular ectasia, radiation telangiectasia), tumor destruction (polyp, ampullary adenoma, cancer, Barrett's), hemostasis (postpolypectomy, ulcer, Dieulafoy), and other more novel applications (metal stent cosmetics, fistula closure).

Incorporation of electrosurgical principles into endoscopy training

What is the best way to ensure that endoscopy trainees gain a thorough understanding of these principles? Ideally, this would begin with inclusion of didactic teaching of the concepts detailed above into the introductory curriculum for gastroenterology fellows and surgical residents alike. Effort is needed to ensure that the individuals charged with teaching endoscopy understand these electrosurgical principles well enough to reinforce the didactic material during the ensuing apprenticeship teaching.

The growing availability of *ex vivo* animal tissue model hands-on workshops is detailed elsewhere in this book. While there are limitations in the simulation of electrosurgery due to the absence of real blood flow, these experiences may provide useful opportunities to learn about the accessories, generators, and the parameters suited to specific applications. Despite this, there is no substitute for the expertise gained by direct experience with coagulation

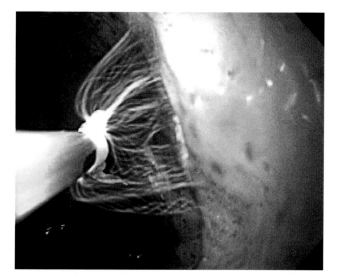

Figure 11.12 Current flowing through an argon plasma during treatment of GAVE.

and cutting of live tissue in supervised clinical practice. There are currently no specific tests of competency in electrosurgery, but assessment of trainees by their teachers during observation of their endoscopic skills must include this as an integral part of endoscopic education.

References

1 ERBE Elektromedizin GmbH, Tuebingen, Germany, and ERBE USA, Inc, Marietta, GA.

2 Kelly HA, Ward GE: *Electrosurgery*. Philadelphia: W.B. Saunders Company, 1932.

3 Glover JL, Bendick PJ, Link WJ: The use of thermal knives in surgery: electrosurgery, lasers, plasma scalpel. *Curr Probl Surg* 1978;**15**:1–78.

4 Laine L, Long GL, Bakos GJ, Vakharia OJ, Cunningham C: Optimizing bipolar electrociagulation for endoscopic hemostasis: assessment of factors influencing energy delivery and coagulation. *Gastrointest Endosc* 2008;**67**:502–508.

12 The Use of Fluoroscopy for Gastrointestinal Endoscopy

Douglas G. Adler

University of Utah School of Medicine, Huntsman Cancer Center, Salt Lake City, UT, USA

Introduction

Fluoroscopy plays a critical role in many endoscopic procedures and is a mainstay of most therapeutic endoscopic procedures such as ERCP, enteral stenting, pseudocyst drainage, etc. The proper use of fluoroscopy equipment and the ability to interpret fluoroscopic images correctly are core skills for gastroenterologists. Unfortunately, many GI fellows receive no formal instruction in the proper use of fluoroscopy and are left to learn about this technology independently, which often results in significant gaps in knowledge. This chapter will review the fundamentals of fluoroscopic technique as it is used in gastrointestinal endoscopy.

Training in fluoroscopy

While formal training in the use of fluoroscopy may be uncommon, all GI fellows have several potential routes to receive instruction in the proper use of fluoroscopy as it relates to the practice of clinical gastroenterology. Elective rotations in radiology, available to most GI fellows, allows direct experience working with radiologists and, perhaps more importantly, radiology technicians. These can be deep sources of knowledge regarding the use of fluoroscopy in general, the operation of fluoroscopic hardware, and the interpretation of fluoroscopic images. Outside of a formal elective, fellows requesting procedures on patients that require fluoroscopy should be encouraged to not simply order the test and read the radiologists report, but rather to attend the procedure itself and, if possible, be present for the radiologic interpretation of the images obtained. Lastly, when learning advanced procedures such as enteral stenting, ERCP, etc., fellows should also actively develop a good working understanding of how to generate and interpret adequate fluoroscopic images.

Hardware basics

Although gastroenterologists are infrequently called upon to directly operate a fluoroscope themselves, an understanding of how fluoroscopic hardware operates is very important. Many different types of fluoroscopy units are available, including portable C-arm units, fixed table models, and dedicated interventional units. All of these devices operate under the same set of principles. Generally, the X-ray beam passes from the X-ray source (the cathode), usually located below the table and above the floor, upwards through the patient and the examination table. Most people assume the beam passes in the opposite direction, but this is not the case.

The beam then is received by the image intensifier/receiver unit, which is typically suspended above the patient. As the X-ray beam passes through the table and the patient, there is always some degree of scatter. As X-rays encounter matter (such as the patient, the table, etc.) some of these rays are deflected from their initial direction of travel. In addition, scatter increases proportionally with the patient's BMI (adipose tissue scatters X-rays), which can make generation of adequate images difficult in obese patients [1].

The image intensifier should be placed as close to the patient as possible (within 1–2 inches). This will allow the procedure to be accomplished with less radiation usage overall and result in the generation of sharper, and often brighter, images. Placing the image intensifier further away from the patient will result in a darker, grainer, and more magnified image and is generally not preferable. An image that has been too greatly magnified will limit the field of view and will be of lower resolution.

Protective garments

Radiation exposure to the patient and medical staff should be minimized and adhere to the ALARA principle (as low as reasonable achievable). Personnel should always wear appropriate protective garments such as lead vests, skirts, aprons, as well as thyroid shields. Patients of reproductive age should also have their pelvis shielded, and all female patients of child-bearing age should undergo a pregnancy test prior to procedures if possible. Protective garments should fit properly and not be too large or too small for the wearer. Leaded eyewear is available as well to protect against the development of cataracts, but many find such eyeglasses to be unacceptably heavy and/or uncomfortable, and they are not

Successful Training in Gastrointestinal Endoscopy, First Edition. Edited by Jonathan Cohen.
© 2011 Blackwell Publishing Ltd. Published 2011 by Blackwell Publishing Ltd.

universally used. Radiation badges, which can monitor a person's exposure over a given time period, should be worn if they are available. The badge should be worn on the part of the body that is closest to the fluoroscope. If available, additional shielding in the form of leaded glass partitions should be placed between personnel and the fluoroscopy beam. These shields can be supported by an armature from the ceiling or can be stand-alone objects that can be wheeled into place [2,3].

Most modern fluoroscope units are digital in design. These units are able to generate clear, high contrast images using lower radiation doses when compared to older, analog units. Modern fluoroscopy units have two monitors. One monitor shows a "live" image when the fluoroscope is activated and often continues to display the last image captured once the fluoroscopy beam in deactivated. A second monitor is generally used as a reference monitor, upon which images previously obtained during the current or prior procedures may be recalled for study or comparison.

Most digital fluoroscopes can operate between 1 and 24 frames per second (fps). Radiation exposure can be significantly minimized by reducing the number of images per second (frame rate) that are generated. A common mistake is to set the frame rate too high, in the generally false assumption that this will allow better visualization. This results in excessive radiation exposure to the patient and personnel and often adds little to the procedure. With time and experience, almost all interventional GI procedures can be performed at very low frame rates. Often, no more than three frames per second are required to produce excellent visualization.

Clear, unambiguous communication between physicians and radiology technicians and support staff is important as it avoids confusion and can effectively serve to reduce radiation exposure. The use of phrases, such as "spot film" (a brief exposure to check position), "fluoroscopy on," "fluoroscopy off," and "full exposure" (to obtain an image that will be permanently saved) are very helpful for the fluoroscope operator.

All institutions should have a radiation safety officer, who maintains records of radiation exposure as measured by radiation badges. All personnel should wear radiation badges and have their exposure tracked to ensure they do not exceed annual and lifetime exposure limits. Fluoroscopy exposure can vary markedly between procedures with some straightforward cases accomplished with less than 60 seconds of exposure. More complex cases in patients with difficult anatomy may require significant exposure in excess of 15–20 minutes.

With some machines, the fluoroscopy time for a given procedure can be recorded as it provides a rough estimate of the total exposure, but this figure should be adjusted for the frame rate (i.e., 3 minutes of fluoroscopy at three frames per second may be less total exposure than 1 minute of fluoroscopy at a higher frame rate). The recording of the total fluoroscopy time and/or radiation dose is not mandatory, but many institutions do this as a means of assessing quality control.

Scout films

Prior to any fluoroscopic procedure, a baseline X-ray image of the area to be intervened upon should be obtained. Such an image is

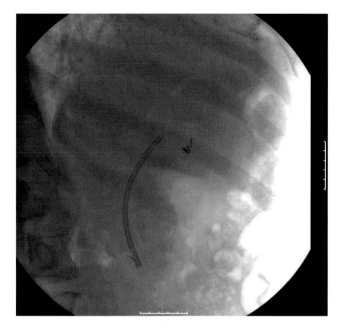

Figure 12.1 Representative scout film obtained prior to ERCP. Note presence of right upper quadrant cholecystectomy clips, previously paced plastic biliary stent, and partial air cholangiogram. Air is also seen in the stomach and small bowel.

known as a "scout film" (Figure 12.1). The scout film allows assessment of many features, including the presence of prior gastrointestinal contrast, the bowel gas pattern, the presence of any intraabdominal prostheses (feeding tubes, stents, drainage catheters, IVC filters, etc.), and the location of any air-filled structures (the stomach, the airways, etc.). Scout films also allow for jewelry or inappropriately placed EKG leads, both of which may obscure areas of interest, to be removed or adjusted. The scout film can also be used as a baseline reference during a procedure to evaluate landmarks and to look for evidence of complications such as a perforation (which may manifest as extraluminal air or contrast). In the case of ERCP, the trainee should note the presence or absence of surgical clips and pneumobilia, which provide important information as to prior biliary interventions and patency in the event of prior placed stents.

ERCP

Of all procedures in gastroenterology, none is as closely linked to the use of fluoroscopy as ERCP. While rare reports of ERCP being performed without X-rays exist, these are generally in unusual situations, such as in pregnant patients requiring urgent management of bile duct stones. For all intents and purposes, ERCP cannot be properly performed without the use of fluoroscopy.

While in theory imaging and intervening upon the pancreatic and bile ducts via ERCP is straightforward, in practice it remains the most involved and complicated of all GI procedures. Pancreaticobiliary anatomy tends to be highly individualized with many variations. Distorted anatomies, either due to surgery, inflammation, or neoplastic processes, are commonly encountered. Trainees should be taught to routinely review prior operative notes and radiologic imaging such as CT scans and MRCPs to best plan the procedure and understand how to interpret the fluoroscopic images seen. This will lead to shortening the procedure time and likely reducing the fluoroscopy exposure for the patient and staff. Furthermore, ERCP involves the use of a very wide range of endoscopic accessories, each of which has a specific fluoroscopic appearance and specialized radio-opaque markers that the operator must become familiar with.

With regards to fluoroscopy, ERCP is most commonly performed with a mobile C-arm but some facilities use dedicated fixed-table units or even more costly dedicated interventional fluoroscopes (of the kind more commonly used by interventional radiologists). In general, mobile C-arms are the simplest to use but generate images of lesser quality while fixed table units and interventional fluoroscopes generate higher quality images but at a higher financial cost.

ERCP is usually performed with patients in the prone position. Dye injected into the pancreaticobiliary tree produces pancreatograms and cholangiograms. Having the fluoroscope arranged vertically over the patient is often adequate to evaluate most pancreatograms given the anatomy of the pancreas. The biliary tree often has a more complex, three-dimensional shape and rotation of the fluoroscope ("rainbowing") is often required to fully interpret cholangiograms. Ducts may overlap (especially at or near the hepatic hilum) and rotation of the fluoroscope can help to image individual ducts more clearly. The biliary tree is also situated in a larger organ (the liver) than is the pancreas and as such requires more contrast to fully opacify. Dependent ducts will fill first and antidependent ducts may require additional contrast or patient manipulation to be fully visualized.

Fluoroscopy and enteral stents

Enteral stents (those deployed in the esophagus, small bowel, and colon) are universally designed to be deployed under fluoroscopic guidance. Small- and large-bowel stents are usually deployed under combined endoscopic and fluoroscopic guidance as they utilize through-the-scope (TTS) technology, whereas esophageal stents are generally deployed using only fluoroscopic guidance. Esophageal stents utilize delivery catheters that are too thick to pass through the working channel of even a therapeutic endoscope [4,5].

Fluoroscopy is critical for the proper and safe placement of enteral stents in several respects. Prior to stenting a luminal stenosis, fluoroscopy aids in the assessment of the stenosis beyond what can be seen endoscopically. Injection of radio-opaque contrast dye, usually through biliary catheters, provides valuable data regarding the length and geometry of the stricture and simplifies stent selection with regards to both length and diameter. Fluoroscopy allows precise localization of stents before, during, and after deployment. Most modern enteral stent delivery catheters, as well as the stents themselves, have built-in radio-opaque markers for better visualization under fluoroscopy.

Esophageal stents

All modern esophageal stents utilize relatively thick, semirigid delivery systems. None of these systems utilize TTS technology. Endoscopy is performed prior to stent placement to evaluate the stricture directly, obtain tissue as needed, or to perform other evaluations such as endoscopic ultrasound (to stage esophageal cancers) [6]. Esophageal stents are generally deployed placed under fluoroscopy and without endoscopic guidance. In cases where very precise control over stent deployment is needed, and the use of fluoroscopy alone is felt to be inadequate, an upper endoscopy may be advanced alongside the esophageal stent delivery catheter to provide direct visual assessment.

All esophageal stents are deployed over a central guide wire. The guide wire must be advanced across the stricture, typically into the stomach, to help ensure that the stent is deployed within the lumen and to reduce the risk of a perforation. Guide wires that are readily visible under fluoroscopy (Savary wires or wires used for ERCP) work best, and in general, stiffer wires are more commonly used. However, some endoscopists prefer floppy wires. Once a guide wire is in proper position, fluoroscopy can be used to make sure that the wire does not inadvertently migrate proximally or distally during the remainder of the procedure.

There is no universal agreement as to how best to position patients on the fluoroscopy table for esophageal stent placement. Left lateral decubitus is often more comfortable for the patient, but may make fluoroscopy more difficult if the fluoroscope itself cannot rotate ("rainbow") around the patient. If the fluoroscopic view is a lateral one, relevant structures such as the trachea and the diaphragm may be more difficult to discern than if an anterior–posterior (AP) view is obtained. The supine position allows for more *en face* fluoroscopic views to be obtained, but is a less comfortable position for the physician. The decision of how best to position the patient is often made based on the available fluoroscopy unit and the patient and physician preference.

When placing an esophageal stent, the endoscopists should take time to identify several key landmarks. These include the trachea and the bifurcation of the respiratory carina as well as the level of the diaphragm and the expected location of the esophageal stent after placement (Figure 12.2). In patients with esophageal tumors, the relationship between the tumor and the trachea is critical as airway compression due to esophageal stent expansion can occur. This is a rare event but has been reported. Most patients can have placement of an esophageal stent next to the airway without difficulty, but the physician should be aware of the relationship between these structures. For distal tumors, an understanding of the location of the diaphragm is important as these lesions typically extend to the gastroesophageal junction. In these cases, the distal end of the stent may need to be placed into the gastric fundus to ensure complete luminal patency [7–9]. The gastric lumen often contains air as well and can easily allow demarcation of the esophagogastric junction. Lastly, the inferior lung borders and the diaphragm are often visible on fluoroscopy and can serve as another rough marker for the level of the esophagogastric junction.

Prior to deployment of an esophageal stent, fluoroscopic markers may be used to help localize the proximal and distal extent of

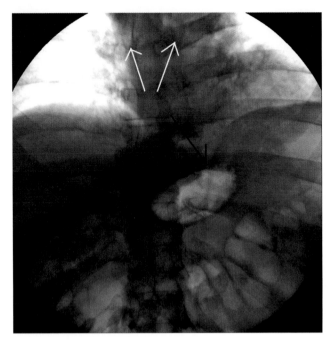

Figure 12.2 Fluoroscopic image in a patient with a mid-to-distal esophageal adenocarcinoma. The image reveals the left and right mainstem bronchi (white arrows) and the diaphragm with air in the gastric lumen (black arrow). The film demonstrates that the airways are far from the expected location of the stent and that airway compression is unlikely to develop.

the stenosis to ensure proper stent placement. Several techniques to mark these locations have been developed [10].

If the lumen through the stenosis is wide enough to allow passage of a standard gastroscope, it is possible to mark both the proximal and distal portion of the esophagus to be stented. Endoscope passage through the stricture also allows accurate measurement of the length of the stricture and, along with information obtained via contrast injection, assists in the selection of an appropriately sized stent. The proximal and distal portion of the stricture can be fluoroscopically marked or labeled in several ways.

Submucosal radiocontrast dye injection

Using a standard needle catheter, contrast dye can be injected into the submucosal space above and below the stricture. One to two milliliters of contrast dye are usually adequate. This technique is inexpensive and simple to do. The primary disadvantage of this technique is that the submucosal radiocontrast dye is absorbed into the surrounding tissues in several minutes, limiting the time between injection and stent deployment. Lopiodol, a radio-opaque poppyseed oil-based contrast agent, has also been used in this context as it takes longer to dissipate, but most GI labs do not routinely stock this agent as there are safety issues associated with it that limit its usage. If the endoscope cannot pass through the stenosis, then the proximal end alone can be marked. This marker, along with the known length of the stenosis obtained via contrast injection, is often adequate for stent placement.

Endoscopic clips as markers

Endoscopic clips, which are made of metal and thus easy to see fluoroscopically, can be placed at the proximal and distal margins of the obstruction. This technique also requires endoscopic advancement through the stenosis if a distal marker is desired. An advantage of this technique is that, once placed, the clips remain in position and the need to rapidly place the stent (as is the case with submucosal dye injection) is obviated. A disadvantage is that clip placement in the esophagus, especially at the distal margin of the stenosis, may be challenging.

External markings

Another method for marking the proximal and distal end of an esophageal stenosis involves attaching, usually with tape, radio-opaque markers (paperclips or other metal objects) to the patient at the margins of the tumor as determined by fluoroscopy using contrast injection or evaluation of endoscope position. This technique is easy to do and inexpensive.

Gastroduodenal stents

Gastroduodenal stents are usually placed in patients with malignant gastric outlet obstruction (GOO). Malignant GOO almost exclusively occurs in patients with unresectable disease. All currently available gastroduodenal stents are TTS devices and as deployed under both endoscopic and fluoroscopic guidance. As a rule, patients with clinical signs of GOO often present late in their clinical course and typically have high grade obstruction. In many/most patients with GOO, endoscope passage through the obstructed segment is not possible and access to the distal small bowel must be obtained using catheters and guide wires, emphasizing the role of fluoroscopy [11,12].

Patients can be positioned on the fluoroscopy table in several ways. The left lateral position is easier and more comfortable for patients and endoscopists, but often provided an "end-on" view of the gastroduodenum, and will likely require rotation of the fluoroscope. Placing patients in the prone position with the head turned to the patient's right (the same position used during ERCP procedures) allows an AP view to be generated with the image intensifier in the vertical position and is also commonly used.

When obtaining a scout film and after endoscope insertion, air present in the stomach and/or the small bowel may provide valuable information regarding the location of the stenosis. The air-filled stomach and small bowel will appear bright on fluoroscopy, while the site of the obstruction will be airless. Only the proximal end of the stenosis may be visible using this technique as in some patients the bowel distal to the obstruction may be decompressed.

If possible, it is helpful to obtain an upper GI series to prior to gastroduodenal stenting to assess the location, length, severity, and geometry of the stenosis. In practice, such studies are rarely obtained prior to endoscopy. As with esophageal stents, injection of radiocontrast medium across the stricture under fluoroscopy will provide a "stricture-gram" that will help guide stent selection. Contrast can sometimes be followed fluoroscopically as it flows into the distal small bowel. Patients with malignant GOO can sometimes develop peritoneal carcinomatosis and have multiple small-bowel stenoses. If multiple stenoses are present, enteral stenting is relatively contraindicated as it will not provide long-lasting relief. Unfortunately, sometimes no other stenosis are apparent even with adequate imaging studies, and after a gastroduodenal stent is placed, it becomes apparent that other, more distal, strictures exist. Dilated small bowel beyond a stricture may also be an indirect sign of downstream small-bowel stenoses.

As with all stents, placement of a guide wire through the stenosis and into the nonobstructed lumen beyond is essential for proper stent placement and minimizes the risk of complications. Guide wire passage into the distal small bowel should be confirmed fluoroscopically prior to stent advancement over the guide wire. Rarely, the guide wire can perforate the small bowel wall distal to the site of obstruction. If this occurs and the endoscopist does not recognize this, the stent could be mistakenly be advanced and subsequently deployed across and/or through the perforation.

Stent deployment is carried out under combined endoscopic and fluoroscopic guidance. Neither endoscopy nor fluoroscopy alone can provide the operator with a complete picture of what is occurring during deployment and careful evaluation of both monitors simultaneously can help to assure satisfactory placement and deployment of the stent. Careful assessment and reassessment of the positions of the stenosis, the guide wire, the stent, and the endoscope during deployment are critical. Once the stent has been fully deployed, fluoroscopy can also be helpful to evaluate for signs of any complications including misdeployment, migration, or perforation. Referencing the previously obtained scout film can be helpful when ruling out a perforation as free air in the abdomen should be absent prior to the procedure. Injection of radiocontrast dye through the deployed stent can be used as a means of definitively confirming the restoration of bowel patency.

Late complications, such as migration, can also be identified fluoroscopically, but other complications such as tumor ingrowth and tumor overgrowth are best diagnosed endoscopically.

Colon stents

Colonic stents are most commonly indicated in patients with malignant large-bowel obstruction (LBO). Benign indications for colonic stents include diverticular strictures and anastomotic strictures, although these are far less common and constitute off-label usage. Unlike patients with malignant dysphagia or malignant GOO (which are chronic problems), malignant LBO can sometimes present acutely and constitute a medical emergency. Chronic partial LBO can also occur. If untreated, acute malignant LBO can result in respiratory compromise (due to limited diaphragmatic movement above a distended abdomen), colonic perforation, sepsis, and death. Historically, most patients with malignant LBO were treated surgically with a diverting colostomy or, less commonly, a resection with an internal anastomosis. The rise of colonic stenting has made such operations in this context relatively uncommon. Many of these patients have advanced colorectal cancer and are poor candidates for surgery [13,14].

Fluoroscopy is essential when placing stents in the large bowel. The scout film will provide clues as to the site of LBO as the colon proximal to the blockage is often quite dilated and filled with a mixture of air and stool. As with esophageal and gastroduodenal

stents, contrast injection and guide wire advancement should be performed under fluoroscopy.

The proximal colon above the level of the obstruction is often friable and distended. As such, patients with malignant LBO are likely at a greater risk for perforation during stent placement than are patients with gastroduodenal obstruction (where the bowel beyond the obstruction is more likely to be normal). Perforations can arise due to inappropriate catheter, guide wire, or stent placement or from excessive air passing above the level of obstruction into the distended colon. Fluoroscopy can provide information about the diameter and air content of the proximal colon and be used to watch for any signs of perforation such as free air.

With regards to positioning, patients can be placed in either the left lateral decubitus position or in the supine position for an *en face* fluoroscopic view.

Currently available colonic stents can come on relatively large deployment catheters that cannot pass through the working channel of an endoscope (similar to esophageal stents) or as TTS devices (similar to gastroduodenal stents). For non-TTS stents, fluoroscopy alone is often adequate to provide visualization during deployment. If desired, an endoscope can be advanced alongside the catheter as well. TTS stents are deployed under combined endoscopic and fluoroscopic guidance.

The proximal and distal ends of colonic obstruction are rarely marked and predeployment injection of radiocontrast through the obstruction allows the creation of a "stricture-gram" as has been described above for esophageal and gastroduodenal stents (Figures 12.3 and 12.4).

Clinical improvement (manifested by decompression of stool and gas) after colonic stent placement typically occurs rapidly.

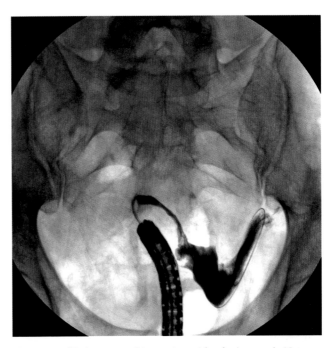

Figure 12.3 "Stricture-gram" in a patient with colonic stenosis. Note narrowed areas in the colorectum just above the endoscope with contrast passing into the more normal appearing large bowel above the stenosis.

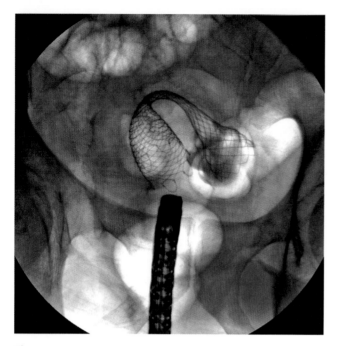

Figure 12.4 Same patient as in Figure 12.3, following colonic stent placement over a guide wire.

As described above with esophageal and gastroduodenal stenting, fluoroscopy should be used following deployment to watch for any postprocedure complications and to make final assessments regarding the adequacy of stent placement.

Enteroscopy

Enteroscopy using dedicated push enteroscopes, single-balloon enteroscopes, or double-balloon enteroscopes may be performed with or without the use of fluoroscopy. Fluoroscopy can be used to look for (and help eliminate) the formation of loops in the endoscope that would otherwise retard forward motion, assess progress, and evaluate the position of the enteroscope in the abdomen. Some patients with postsurgical anatomy require the use of an enteroscope to undergo ERCP (most commonly patients who have undergone a Roux-en-Y gastric bypass); fluoroscopy can be used to help maneuver the enteroscope into the afferent limb and to the right upper quadrant of the abdomen. No optimal patient position for fluoroscopy can be recommended. The prone, supine, and left lateral positions are all viable options. The author favors prone position for enteroscopy as it minimizes the need for fluoroscope rotation and may be technically easier for the endoscopist.

Push enteroscopy

Push enteroscopy describes the use of a dedicated enteroscope to evaluate patients with known or suspected gastrointestinal pathology to approximate the level of the mid to distal jejunum. Push enteroscopy involves the use of dedicated push enteroscopes,

which have an insertion tube of 240–250 cm in length (depending on the manufacturer). Patients who undergo upper endoscopic evaluation with a pediatric colonoscope inserted *per os* are not undergoing a true enteroscopy, given the limited insertion tube length of these instruments. In general, the advancement of longer instruments into the upper GI tract can be difficult as loops tend to form, most commonly along the greater curvature of the stomach, which can significantly reduce the maximum depth of intubation obtained. Looped sections of endoscopes are typically perceived as painful by the patient. It is critical to minimize looping to the maximum extent allowable and to keep the endoscope as "straight" as possible. A straight endoscope also will allow easier forward motion, better control during movement and endoscopic maneuvers such as polypectomy, etc., and during endoscopic withdrawal at the end of the case.

Overtubes can be used to minimize looping in the stomach. Overtubes have been shown to reduce the frequency and severity of loop formation and to increase the depth of endoscope insertion [15,16].

Fluoroscopy is not universally used during enteroscopy procedures, although the author often performs enteroscopy with fluoroscopic assistance. Fluoroscopic monitoring of the position of the endoscope can minimize the formation of loops. Even experienced endoscopists may be fooled into thinking they have a "straight" endoscope and may be unaware of the presence of loops and, as such, stand to benefit from the use of fluoroscopy. Fluoroscopy can also be used during endoscopic withdrawals to avoid recoil, which would limit endoscopic evaluation of the small intestine.

Single- and double-balloon enteroscopy

Single-balloon enteroscopy (SBE) and double-balloon enteroscopy (DBE) are techniques that potentially allow visualization of the entire small bowel during a single endoscopic procedure. DBE (Fujinon America, Wayne, NJ, USA) requires the use of a dedicated forward viewing enteroscope with a specialized overtube. This device has a 200 cm insertion tube and an overtube with a length of 135 cm [http://www.fujinonendoscopy.com/]. The end of the overtube and the enteroscope are each equipped with special balloons that, when inflated, generate sufficient friction between the balloon surface and the small bowel to temporarily hold the enteroscope, the overtube, or both devices in position during advancements and withdrawals. These techniques reduce (but does not eliminate) looping and allow pleating of the bowel around the endoscope/overtube system during forward advancement.

The overtube and endoscope balloons are inflated and deflated separately or in tandem by controls on a pressure-controlled pump system. By inflating the balloon attached to the overtube, the overtube becomes relatively "fixed" at a specific location in the small bowel. The endoscope can then be advanced through the overtube and forward motion though the small bowel is achieved. The presence of the overtube reduces, but does not eliminate, the rate of formation of endoscopic loops.

Once the endoscope has been advanced through the overtube to its maximum extent, the balloon located on the tip of the endoscope is then inflated to hold the endoscope in position, and the balloon affixed to the overtube is deflated. The overtube is then advanced over the endoscope to a point just proximal the balloon on the tip of the endoscope. At this point, the overtube balloon is inflated again, fixing both the endoscope and the overtube positions simultaneously, and the entire endoscope/overtube complex is withdrawn. This allows removal of any loops that may have formed during advancement and maintains the depth of endoscope insertion already obtained. This process is repeated as many times as needed to allow very deep intubation of the small bowel, often to the level of the ileum. DBE can also be performed retrograde as well, with the system first passing through the entire colon to access the terminal ileum from below, although in general this is more difficult and more time consuming [17–19].

SBE utilizes a dedicated enteroscope/overtube system manufactured by Olympus Endoscopy (Center Valley, Pennsylvania, USA). The system is similar to DBE except for the fact that only the overtube itself has a balloon attached. The advancement and withdrawal cycles of the system are simplified in that the balloon is inflated just prior to shortening of the joint enteroscope/overtube system and deflated to allow the overtube to advance over the enteroscope.

Balloon enteroscopy (SBE or DBE) is generally performed with the aid of fluoroscopy. These procedures can be time consuming, often requiring more than 60 minutes per procedure. Many cycles of staged balloon inflations and deflations with their pared endoscopic maneuvers are required to achieve access to the distal small bowel. In some patients, the distal small bowel can be reached without any significant looping, but in others, loops may still form despite the use of these overtube/balloon systems (Figure 12.5).

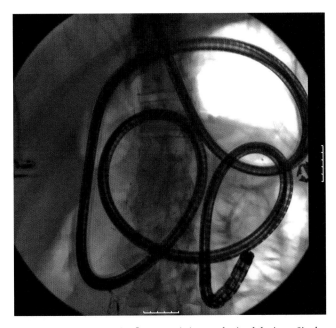

Figure 12.5 Representative fluoroscopic image obtained during a Single Balloon Enteroscopy procedure. Note multiple loops formed during advancement of the enteroscope.

Fluoroscopy is useful during endoscope and overtube advancements as well as during the combined endoscope/overtube withdrawals to visualize the extent to which loops previously created have been reduced. Fluoroscopy during endoscopic advancement is extremely helpful as the operator can get a very immediate understanding of how far the endoscope is actually moving and if loops are or are not being simultaneously formed. A typical cycle of advancement will result in 10–50 cm of advancement. Progress can be tracked via fluoroscopy in a way that may be difficult using just endoscopic views.

Conclusion

Fluoroscopy represents one of the most powerful tools in the gastrointestinal physician's armamentarium and plays a role in almost all realms of interventional endoscopy. Gastroenterologists should understand the principles of fluoroscopy and have a working knowledge of the operation of fluoroscopic hardware. ERCP, enteral stenting, and all manner of enteroscopy utilize fluoroscopy to maximize success and minimize complications. Judicious use of fluoroscopy can provide extensive information during a procedure while keeping radiation exposure to both patients and staff at a minimum.

Videos

Video 24.1 Esophageal stent placement procedure
Video 24.2 Duodenal stent placement procedure
Video 24.3 Through-the-scope colonic stent placement procdure
Video 25.4 Laser lithotripsy with the Freddy laser
Video 28.1 Pancreatic pseudocyst drainage

References

1 Chida K, Saito H, Otani H, et al.: Relationship between fluoroscopic time, dose-area product, body weight, and maximum radiation skin dose in cardiac interventional procedures. *Am J Roentgenol* 2006;**186**(3):774–778.

2 Heyd RL, Kopecky KK, Sherman S, Lehman GA, Stockberger SM: Radiation exposure to patients and personnel during interventional ERCP at a teaching institution. *Gastrointest Endosc* 1996;**44**(3):287–292.

3 Johlin FC, Pelsang RE, Greenleaf M: Phantom study to determine radiation exposure to medical personnel involved in ERCP fluoroscopy and its reduction through equipment and behavior modifications. *Am J Gastroenterol* 2002;**97**(4):893–897.

4 Austin AS, Khan Z, Cole AT, Freeman JG: Placement of esophageal self-expanding metallic stents without fluoroscopy. *Gastrointest Endosc* 2001;**54**(3):357–359.

5 Rathore OI, Coss A, Patchett SE, Mulcahy HE: Direct-vision stenting: the way forward for malignant oesophageal obstruction. *Endoscopy* 2006;**38**(4):382–384.

6 Adler DG, Fang J, Wong R, Wills J, Hilden K: Placement of Polyflex stents in patients with locally advanced esophageal cancer is safe and

improves dysphagia during neoadjuvant therapy. *Gastrointest Endosc* 2009 [Epub ahead of print].

7 De Olabozal J, Roberts J, Hoeltgen T, Berkelhammer C: Double stenting to prevent airway compression in proximal malignant esophageal strictures. *Am J Gastroenterol* 2001;**96**(9):2800–2801.

8 Rasiah K, Keogh G: Tracheal obstruction after insertion of a self-expanding oesophageal stent. *Aust N Z J Surg* 1999;**69**(1):77–78.

9 Farivar AS, Vallieres E, Kowdley KV, Wood DE, Mulligan MS: Airway obstruction complicating esophageal stent placement in two post-pneumonectomy patients. *Ann Thorac Surg* 2004;**78**(2):e22–e23.

10 Merenger K, Kozarek RA: Stenting of the gastrointestinal tract. *Dig Dis* 2002;**20**(2):173–181.

11 Adler DG, Baron TH: Endoscopic palliation of malignant gastric outlet obstruction using self-expanding metal stents: experience in 36 patients. *Am J Gastroenterol* 2002;**97**(1):72–78.

12 Dormann A, Meisner S, Verin N, Wenk Lang A: Self-expanding metal stents for gastroduodenal malignancies: systematic review of their clinical effectiveness. *Endoscopy* 2004;**36**: 543–550.

13 Adler DG, Merwat S. Endoscopic approaches for palliation of luminal gastrointestinal obstruction. *Gastroenterol Clin North Am* 2006;**35**(1):65–82.

14 Adler DG, Baron TH. Stents and lasers for colonoscopic lesions. *Curr Gastroenterol Rep* 2000;**2**(5):399–405.

15 Benz C, Jakobs R, Riemann JF: Do we need the overtube for push-enteroscopy? *Endoscopy* 2001;**33**(8):658–661.

16 Taylor AC, Chen RY, Desmond PV: Use of an overtube for enteroscopy—does it increase depth of insertion? A prospective study of enteroscopy with and without an overtube. *Endoscopy* 2001;**33**(3):227–230.

17 Yamamoto H, Sugano K: A new method of enteroscopy—the double-balloon method. *Can J Gastroenterol* 2003;**17**(4):273–274.

18 May A, Nachbar L, Ell C: Double-balloon enteroscopy (push-and-pull enteroscopy) of the small bowel: feasibility and diagnostic and therapeutic yield in patients with suspected small bowel disease. *Gastrointest Endosc* 2005;**62**(1):62–70.

19 May A, Ell C: European experiences with push-and-pull enteroscopy in double-balloon technique (double-balloon enteroscopy). *Gastrointest Endosc Clin N Am* 2006;**16**(2):377–382

13 Pediatric Endoscopy

Michael A. Manfredi[1,2] & Jenifer R. Lightdale[1,2]

[1]Harvard Medical School, Boston, MA, USA
[2]Children's Hospital Boston, Boston, MA, USA

Introduction

The history of pediatric endoscopy dates back to the 1970s, when the diameter of endoscopes became small enough to allow investigation in children [1]. In the 1980s, endoscopes were designed specifically for pediatric use, thereby cementing their role in clinical practice. Today, the diagnosis of gastrointestinal diseases in children is often based on direct visualization of tissue and targeted tissue biopsies. In addition, therapeutic endoscopy has allowed for safe minimally invasive treatments that were once only performed by open surgical techniques with longer recovery periods.

Achieving competence in endoscopy is a fundamental component of fellowship training in pediatric gastroenterology. As with endoscopy in adults, pediatric endoscopy requires both cognitive and technical expertise to diagnose and treat disorders of the gastrointestinal tract. There are many similarities in endoscopy training for adults and children. However, there are also fundamental differences that must be respected if endoscopic procedures are to be successfully performed safely, effectively, and efficiently in children. In this chapter, we will highlight those aspects unique to endoscopic training in pediatric gastroenterology.

Training program requirements

The North American Society for Pediatric Gastroenterology, Hepatology, and Nutrition (NASPGHAN) has stipulated that training programs in endoscopy have the following educational components [2]:

1 Exposure to clinical care and problem-solving in pediatric patients with gastrointestinal disorders, including the provision of didactic sessions regarding endoscopic procedures.

2 The opportunity to learn appropriate technical and cognitive endoscopy skills from competent instructors.

3 A proper training environment for endoscopy and related procedures. This includes appropriately trained ancillary personnel (e.g., endoscopy nurses or technicians), functioning and well-maintained age-specific equipment, and trained personnel to perform cardiopulmonary resuscitation in pediatric patients.

4 Access to services provided by certified specialists in pediatric intensive care, pediatric surgery, pediatric anesthesia, pediatric radiology (including experts in interventional radiology), pathology (with expertise in pediatric gastrointestinal histology), and subspecialists to provide interactive exposure and teaching in these disciplines. These services must be available as a backup for pediatric patients who experience complications during or after procedures.

5 Availability of endoscopic teaching materials (e.g., books, atlases, DVDs, digital, or online libraries) to enhance training and exposure.

6 Opportunities for trainees to work with "hands on models" or endoscopic simulators to learn and practice endoscopic techniques.

7 Procedures in place to periodically and formally review the progress of trainees.

8 Periodic reviews and updates of training methods, as well as the ability to monitor the quality of training in an endoscopy unit.

Esophagogastroduodenoscopy and colonoscopy

Expertise in pediatric endoscopic procedures requires technical, diagnostic, and therapeutic competence. Trainees should perform endoscopic procedures with pediatric gastroenterologists primarily. They must also learn the indications for and the technique of performing each procedure, document the results, and understand the clinical significance of endoscopic findings. It is also vital that all pediatric endoscopists respect the potential for complications associated with the procedure, including risks of bleeding, infection, and bowel perforation. Trainees must be able to weigh those risks and determine if the procedure is warranted.

Patient assessment

To optimally prepare for pediatric gastrointestinal procedures, trainees in pediatric endoscopy should learn to obtain a careful medical history, perform a complete physical exam, and

Successful Training in Gastrointestinal Endoscopy, First Edition. Edited by Jonathan Cohen.
© 2011 Blackwell Publishing Ltd. Published 2011 by Blackwell Publishing Ltd.

review appropriate laboratory tests before sedation is administered. Patient risk factors that may affect pediatric endoscopy are myriad and include presence of sepsis, shock or dehydration, and electrolyte imbalance; acute and chronic respiratory conditions; underlying cardiovascular diseases, especially cyanotic congenital heart disease; acute and chronic neurological conditions, including seizure disorders; and liver or renal dysfunction. The physical exam should focus on the heart, circulation, lungs, head, neck, and airway. Laboratory tests are not required in the preprocedure assessment. However, trainees should recognize clinical indications where obtaining blood work would be useful for either pre-procedure or pre-anesthesia planning.

Informed consent

The process of obtaining informed consent to perform procedures in children mandates the endoscopist to interact not only with the patient, but also with the parents or guardians, who in the majority of the cases will be providing informed consent. If the patient is an adolescent, it may be appropriate to obtain informed assent. Trainees must learn to recognize that the pre-procedure period is a stressful time for both patients and families. In turn, they must develop interpersonal and communication skills that reflect both professionalism and compassion.

Sedation

To achieve optimal sedation for endoscopy in their young patients, pediatric gastroenterologists must be trained to consider many factors, including patient age, medical history, clinical status, anxiety level, as well as targeted sedation level to select the appropriate methods and agents [3]. The two primary types of sedation are endoscopist-administered intravenous (IV) sedation and anesthesiologist-administered general anesthesia. General anesthesia involves the depression of a child's respiratory drive and requires the presence and expertise of an anesthesiologist. IV sedation maintains the child's ability to breathe spontaneously and protect his/her own airway. In mastering procedural sedation skills, trainees in pediatric gastroenterology must learn to perform simultaneous tasks of administering sedation while performing the procedure.

Trainees must also learn the wisdom of carefully assessing children as to their level of cooperation both prior to scheduling and again on the day of the procedure [4]. Personality and psychosocial development stages may vary widely and greatly impact children's reactions to sedative medications in both the rapidity and the depth of sedation achieved. Infants under 6 months of age have little anxiety and sedate easily. Infants greater than 6 months who have developed "stranger anxiety" may sedate more easily if parents remain next to them during induction. School-aged children may be surprisingly difficult to sedate, belying higher anxiety levels than may be appreciated. Adolescents may be composed during preprocedure preparations, and then become disinhibited and exhibit strong anxiety with initial doses of sedatives.

Sedation for pediatric endoscopy procedures: When not to use it

Trainees must learn that certain pediatric gastrointestinal procedures may not require sedation. In particular, flexible sigmoidoscopy, percutaneous liver biopsy, changes or removals of percutaneous endoscopically placed gastrostomy (PEG) tubes, and placement of pH or impedence probes can generally be performed without sedation. The use of no sedation also allows children an almost immediate return to normal functioning after a procedure, including the ability to eat and return to school. However, by not sedating patients, endoscopists incur the risk of not completing procedures in a satisfactory way for both the doctor and the child.

Cognitive aspects of training in sedation

Once the decision to employ sedation during a procedure has been made, trainees must learn to judge the best sedation option targeted to the appropriate level. If IV sedation is used, pediatric endoscopists must be prepared for children to become agitated, adding to stress for both patients and clinical staff. General anesthesia provides the advantage of complete patient immobility, but increased costs and utilization of hospital resources.

It is our opinion that trainees in pediatric endoscopy should master skills involved in both working with anesthesiologists, in addition to skills in administering IV sedation without anesthesiology assistance, as part of their standard training program. Indeed, there may be vast institutional differences regarding access to anesthesiologists, as well as operating room time, that may impact the ease with which general anesthesia can be scheduled for pediatric gastrointestinal procedures. Graduates of programs that do not use endoscopist-administered IV sedation may find themselves learning a completely new skill upon starting a new position in an institution with limited access to anesthesia. Within institutions, there may be tremendous variation in care between anesthesiologists, who may employ a variety of inhalational and intravenous agents [5]. Pediatric endoscopists should understand the various risks and side effects of various anesthesia regimens so as to best advocate for their patients.

Technical aspects of training in sedation

The choice of which type of sedation and which specific medications to employ in sedating pediatric and adolescent patients for gastrointestinal procedures should be tailored to the procedure and the patient. The two most common classes of sedatives used in pediatric endoscopy units are benzodiazepines and narcotics. However, trainees should gain an understanding of all classes of drugs that may be used for pediatric procedures. Table 13.1 lists different sedation agents and recommended doses.

Topical agents

In children undergoing upper endoscopy, there may be some benefit derived from applying a topical anesthetic spray to the posterior pharynx, such as cetacaine or lidocaine. Mastering the skill of

Table 13.1 Recommendations for dosages of drugs commonly used for IV sedation for pediatric gastrointestinal procedures.

Drug	Route	Maximum dose (mg/kg)	Time to onset (min)	Duration of action (min)
Benzodiazepines				
Diazepam	IV	0.1–0.3	1–3	15–30
	Rectal	0.2–0.3	2–10	15–30
Midazolam	Oral	0.5–0.75	15–30	60–90
	IV	0.05–0.15	2–3	45–60
	Rectal	0.5–0.75	10–30	60–90
Opioids				
Meperidine	IV	1–3	<5	2–4
	IM	1–3	10–15	2–3
Fentanyl	IV	0.001–0.005	2–3	30–60
		(1–5 µg/kg in 0.5–1.0 µg/kg increments)		
Ketamine	IV	1–3	1	15–60
	IM	2–10	3–5	15–150

topical drug delivery for children requires depression of the tongue and elicitation of a gag reflex with a tongue blade during spraying. This may be highly unpleasant for children, and trainees may be taught to perform this after some light sedation has been administered. Trainees should also learn about specific drug risks associated with the use of topical anesthetics, including systemic absorption and methemoglobinemia, which is treated with methylene blue [6].

Benzodiazepines

As a class of sedatives, benzodiazepines are generally safe and fast-acting, with high therapeutic indexes. They are well known for their anxiolytic and amnestic effects and may be combined with narcotics for added analgesia and sedation. In turn, respiratory depression is unusual when benzodiazepines are used alone, but quite common when used in conjunction with narcotics. To date, it is recommended that all benzodiazepines be administered to children in small serial increments, with close clinical monitoring to determine the level of sedation achieved with each dose. It is not recommended that benzodiazepines be given as bolus doses during pediatric endoscopy.

Narcotics

Narcotics are primarily analgesics, but have enhanced sedative effects when used in combination with benzodiazepines. Com-

mon side-effects of narcotics include pruritus and nausea. Many children may be anecdotally noted to scratch their noses after a narcotic is infused, and trainees must learn to avoid oversedating in response. Indeed, trainees must learn to appreciate that respiratory depression is very commonly seen with the use of narcotics alone, and especially in combination with benzodiazepines.

Ketamine

Trainees will also gain from learning about the pros and cons of ketamine, a derivative of phencyclidine that binds to opiate receptors and rapidly induces a trancelike cataleptic condition with significant analgesia [7]. The resulting dissociative state largely spares upper airway muscular tone and laryngeal reflexes. Thus, unlike most sedatives, ketamine can be used with high reliability to significantly immobilize children with minimal cardiac or respiratory risks. The main disadvantages to using ketamine include its association with hallucinogenic emergence reactions in some children, increased airway secretions, as well as an increased potential for laryngospasm.

Propofol

Use of anesthesiologist-administered propofol in pediatric endoscopy units has become very common in recent years, and trainees should gain an understanding of its properties [5]. Propofol is an ultra short-acting anesthetic that features a rapid onset of action and a short recovery time. It can be used to induce and maintain a spectrum of sedation levels, ranging from moderate to deep anesthesia. Propofol also confers excellent amnesia for the procedure in children. Nevertheless, a main disadvantage of propofol is its relatively narrow therapeutic range. In children, lower propofol dosages may be required to achieve adequate sedation when it is given in combination with midazolam and fentanyl.

Reversal agents for pediatric sedation

Trainees in pediatric endoscopy should become familiar with reversal agents for oversedation in children. In particular, they should understand that reversal effects are nearly always shorter than the effects of the drugs being reversed. As such, patients who receive a dose of a reversal agent should be monitored for an extended period and should be administered repeat doses if necessary. Reversal agents are available for benzodiazpines and narcotics and are listed in Table 13.2 with recommended dosages for children. Currently, there are no reversal agents for ketamine or propofol.

Table 13.2 Reversal agents for benzodiazepines and opioids and recommended dosages.

Drug	Class antagonist	Route	Dose	Time to onset (min)	Duration of action (min)
Flumazenil	Benzodiazepines	IV	0.01 mg/kg (max 3 mg/h)	1–2	<60
Naloxone	Narcotics	IV/IM	0.1 mg/kg	2–5	20–60

Table 13.3 Indications for upper endoscopy.

Procedure type	Clinical indication
Diagnostic	Abdominal pain with significant morbidity or signs of organic disease (weight loss, anemia, vomiting, fevers)
	Anemia (unexplained)
	Anorexia
	Caustic ingestion
	Diarrhea/malabsorption (chronic)
	Dysphagia
	Hematochezia
	Intractable or chronic GERD (including surveillance for Barrett's esophagus)
	Odynophagia
	Vomiting/hematemesis
	Weight loss/failure to thrive
Therapeutic	Dilation of esophageal and upper-GI strictures
	Esophageal varices eradication
	Foreign-body removal
	Upper-GI bleeding control

Upper endoscopy

Diagnostic esophagogastroduodenoscopy (EGD) is the most common procedure performed in pediatric gastroenterology. Before a trainee touches an endoscope, he or she must develop an understanding of the basic upper gastrointestinal tract anatomy, as well as the indications and contraindications of performing endoscopy. For a description of landmarks and anatomy for EGD, see Chapter 4.

The majority of EGDs in children are performed for diagnostic purposes. Indications for diagnostic and therapeutic upper endoscopy are listed in Table 13.3. There are relatively few contraindications to upper endoscopy in children. Size of the patient is rarely a contraindication and the procedure can be performed safely in neonates as small as 1.5–2 kg [8]. The only absolute contraindication for endoscopy is when bowel perforation is suspected.

Most other conditions that might give an endoscopist pause before obtaining consent for EGD in children represent relative contraindications and should be weighed in terms of whether the benefits of performing the procedure outweigh its risks. For example, coagulopathy is a relative contraindication for diagnostic endoscopy, although extra care is certainly required and biopsies would be contraindicated until the coagulopathy is corrected. Neutropenia is another relative contraindication. Cardiopulmonary issues may also preclude the performance of upper endoscopy, with the exceptional indication of therapeutic endoscopy for gastrointestinal hemorrhage. Even in these situations, the patient should be stabilized with initial resuscitation measures (i.e., administration of crystalloid and blood products) prior to performing the procedure.

Technical skills

The technical aspects of performing upper endoscopy are essentially the same in adults and in children. The main difference between the two lies in the choice of equipment. It is important to have an understanding and general knowledge of smaller endoscopy equipment required to scope the smaller anatomy of infants and young children.

Instruments

Pediatric endoscopes are commercially produced by Olympus USA (Center Valley, PA), Pentax USA (Montvale, NJ), and Fujinon Inc., (Wayne, NJ) and in general are similar in design to adult endoscopes, with only subtle differences. Today's modern pediatric gastroscopes have a fiberoptic light source, an instrument/suction channel, and an air/water nozzle. They have four-way directional tip control that ranges from 180° to 210° in the up direction, 90° to 120° in the down direction, and with 100° to 120° deflection in both the left and right direction. The technical aspects of these scopes can be found in Table 13.4. Most new modes of pediatric gastroscopes by all three major companies have comparable tip deflection when compared to standard adult scopes. Older model gastroscopes have less tip deflection, which can limit visibility somewhat.

Endoscope diameter in gastroscopes range from 5.4 to 6 mm in diameter (Figure 13.1a). There is also an ultraslim 4.9 to 5.1 mm two-directional control endoscope designed for transnasal endoscopy in adults that can be used for oral insertion in infants. The main limiting factor with all pediatric endoscopes is the 2.0 mm working channel, which is considerably smaller than the working channel in adult endoscopes. The small working

Table 13.4 Pediatric gastrocopes.

	Olympus	Pentax	Fujinon
Model name	GIF-N180	EG-1580K	EG-530NP
Distal end diameter	4.9 mm	5.1 mm	4.9 mm
Bending capability			
Up/down	210°/120°	210°/120°	210°/120°
Left/right	–	–	–
Forcep channel diameter	2.0 mm	2.0 mm	2.0 mm
Field of view	120°	140°	120°
Model name	GIF-XP180N	EG-1690K	EG-530N
Distal end diameter	5.5 mm	5.4 mm	5.9 mm
Bending capability			
Up/down	210°/90°	210°/120°	210°/90°
Left/right	100°/100°	120°/120°	100°/100°
Forcep channel diameter	2.0 mm	2.0 mm	2.0 mm
Field of view	120°	120°	120°

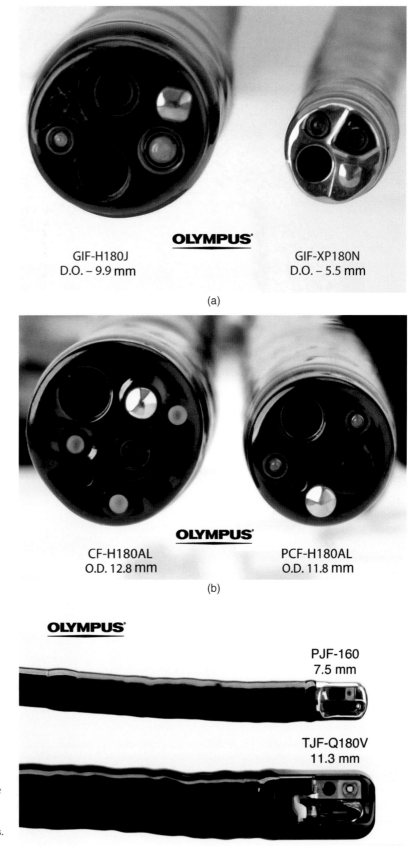

Figure 13.1 These images illustrate the diameter of the standard pediatric endoscopes relative to the corresponding adult model instrument. (a) gastroscopes, (b) colonoscopes, and (c) duodenoscopes. (Images courtesy of Olympus America, Corp. Center Valley, PA, USA.)

Table 13.5 Equipment compatible with pediatric endoscope (2 mm channel).

- Small biopsy forcep
- Small polyp snare
- Pediatric Rothnet
- Small alligator forcep
- Small rat-tooth forcep
- Small injection needle
- Small APC probe
- 2-prong grasper

channel makes suctioning more difficult and limits the ability to use pediatric endoscopes for therapeutic maneuvers, as less equipment is available in small enough sizes to pass through. The pediatric endoscopy trainee should have full working knowledge of the size of the endoscope being used as well as what equipment can be used to perform their procedure. Table 13.5 lists equipment that can be used in small pediatric endoscopes with a single small working channel.

Colonoscopy

Pediatric colonoscopy is a technically challenging procedure when compared to upper endoscopy and generally requires more exposure to achieve competency [9]. The main indication for colonoscopy in children is to rule out inflammatory mucosal processes, such as Crohn's disease. There is no pediatric colon cancer screening guideline. Therefore, patient volume of pediatric colonoscopies at the population level is far less than that of adults, who are uniformly recommended to undergo colonoscopy after age 50. Because of limited case volume at many pediatric training programs, fellows are partnered with adult gastroenterologists for periods of time in order to increase their experience to the procedure.

Cognitive skills

Generally speaking, endoscopy trainees must have a fundamental understanding of colonic anatomy with respect to anatomic landmarks. In addition, it is important for trainees to appreciate the colon's segmental connections to the mesentery. Please refer to Chapter 5 for more in-depth description.

Two obvious differences between pediatric and adult colons are their length and diameter. The colon is a tubular structure that is approximately 60 cm in length in the newborn and reaches up to 150 cm in adults. Therefore, pediatric endoscopists must keep the patient's age in mind when looking at how much scope they have inserted. The indications for diagnostic and therapeutic colonoscopy are listed in Table 13.6.

The main indications for performing colonoscopy in children are to look for evidence of colitis, ileitis, and intestinal polyps. Symptoms associated with these conditions, such as rectal bleed-

Table 13.6 Indications for colonoscopy.

Procedure type	Clinical indication
Diagnostic	Abdominal pain (clinically significant)
	Anemia (unexplained)
	Diarrhea (chronic, clinically significant with weight loss, fevers, anemia)
	Failure to thrive/weight loss
	Hematochezia/melena
	Lower-GI tract lesions seen on imaging studies
	Polyposis syndrome (diagnosis and surveillance)
	Rejection of intestinal transplant
Therapeutic	Dilation of strictures
	Foreign-body removal
	Lower-GI bleeding control
	Polypectomy

ing and chronic diarrhea, warrant colonoscopy. Polypectomy and hemostasis represent standard colonoscopic therapeutic techniques that can be performed by endoscopists, and the training to perform these procedures is similar to that for adult patients.

As with upper endoscopy, there are relatively few contraindications to pediatric colonoscopy. The only absolute contraindication is again suspected intestinal perforation. Relative contraindications include severe fulminant colitis, which may place a patient at high risk for perforation. In addition, coagulopathy, neutropenia, and cardiopulmonary issues may increase procedural and anesthetic risks. As always, the endoscopy trainee must learn to weigh the risks and benefits of the procedure.

Technical skills

The technical aspects of colonoscopy are similar in adults and children. One key difference is that the majority of pediatric colonoscopies require ileocecal intubation to screen for the diseases of interest. In terms of instrument choices, there are specialized pediatric colonoscopes that may be useful for achieving these procedures in children older than 4 years (>20 kg). However, pediatric colonoscopes, despite the moniker, may be too large for children younger than 4 years. In small patients, use of a gastroscope to perform the procedure may be more appropriate, based on size of the instrument. Here, it is necessary to recognize that gastroscopes are stiffer and have less tip angulation compared with colonoscopes. Trainees should gain experience using gastroscopes to perform colonoscopy and should develop an awareness of when this approach may be indicated. Please refer to Chapter 5 for in-depth description of procedural techniques in colonoscopy.

Instruments

Pediatric colonoscopes, like gastroscopes, are commercially made by Olympus USA (Center Valley, PA, USA),

Table 13.7 Pediatric colonoscopes.

	Olympus	Pentax	Fujinon
Model name	PCF-Q180AL/I	EC-3470LK	EC-450LP5
Distal end diameter	11.3 mm	11.6 mm	11.0 mm
Bending capability			
Up/down	180°/180°	180°/180°	180°/180°
Left/right	160°/160°	160°/160°	160°/160°
Forcep channel diameter	3.2 mm	3.8 mm	3.2 mm
Field of view	140°	140°	140°
Model name	PCF-H180AL/I*	EC-3490Li HD*	EC-450LS5*
Distal end diameter	11.7 mm	11.6 mm	11.5 mm
Bending capability			
Up/down	180°/180°	180°/180°	180°/180°
Left/right	160°/160°	160°/160	160°/160°
Forcep channel diameter	3.2 mm	3.2 mm	3.8 mm
Field of view	140°	140°	140°

*HD capable.

Pentax USA (Montvale, NJ, USA), and Fujinon Inc (Wayne, NJ, USA). Pediatric colonoscope outer diameter size can vary from 11.1 to 11.7 mm (Figure 13.1b). Like gastroscopes, pediatric colonoscopes have four-way directional tip control, with more range in all directions. In particular, they feature 180° deflection in the up and down direction and 160° in both the left and right direction. The enhanced tip mobility of colonoscopes allows passage throughout the colon and into the ileum.

The modern colonoscope is capable of producing high-definition quality images. These scopes have a fiberoptic light source, an instrument/suction channel that ranges in size from 3.2 to 3.8 mm in diameter, and an air/water nozzle. The Olympus colonoscopes also have a variable stiffness dial that increases the stiffness of the insertion tube and can be helpful in difficult looping colons. The technical aspects of pediatric colonoscopes scopes can be found in Table 13.7.

Diagnostic techniques in upper endoscopy and colonoscopy

A mainstay of diagnostic endoscopy in children consists of obtaining mucosal biopsies. If *Candida* or other fungal agents are suspected, cytology brushes are commonly used to send for culture. Suction traps can also be temporarily connected to the suction line and allow for sampling of bile, intestinal, and gastric secretions for microbiology, chemistry, or cytology.

The sizes of biopsies vary by forceps size, but in general are 0.5–2 mm in length. While some biopsy forceps can be used to obtain multiple biopsies, pediatric forceps can only be used to obtain single biopsies. The trainee must realize that the risks of biopsy are bleeding and perforation; fortunately, both are extremely rare. Pediatric endoscopists often err on the side of obtaining biopsies, even in the absence of gross abnormalities, as the risks of seda-

tion and performing repeat endoscopy may outweigh the risks of obtaining biopsies.

Identifying pathology

For the trainee, mastering the technical aspects of performing pediatric endoscopy represents only half the battle. The trainee must also be able to recognize, describe, and understand the endoscopic features of lesions they encounter to carry out proper clinical management. The identification of endoscopic pathology is a cognitive skill that develops during trainee and instructor interaction during actual cases. This should be augmented through the trainee's use of endoscopy atlases, as well as didactic sessions.

Therapeutics procedure in endoscopy

Foreign body

Foreign body removal is commonly required in children. Esophageal foreign bodies require urgent attention because of risk of perforation. There are three areas of normal physiologic esophageal narrowing where a foreign body can get lodged [10]. The first and most common location is the proximal esophagus at the level of the thoracic inlet. The second location is the mid-esophagus at the level of aortic arch, and the third location is the distal esophagus, slightly proximal to the gastroesophageal junction. Foreign bodies that pass through the esophagus will usually pass unimpeded. Other locations where objects can become lodged more distally are the pylorus, the distal duodenum, and the ileocecal valve.

It is generally recommended that foreign-body removal in children be done under general endotracheal anesthesia to protect the airway from aspiration. A common exception to this rule is a coin, which can be easily removed without risk of airway compromise. Emergent foreign body removal would include any symptomatic esophageal foreign body as well as asymptomatic esophageal button battery due to the high risk of esophageal tissue necrosis and risk of fistula formation.

Asymptomatic esophageal foreign bodies and gastric button batteries should be removed within 24 hours. Trainees must learn how to triage esophageal foreign bodies versus gastric foreign bodies, which may not require the same urgent approach. Gastric foreign bodies that should be endoscopically removed include large objects (with a diameter 20 mm or greater and or a length greater than or equal to 30 mm), sharp objects that are at risk of causing bleeding or perforation, and battery ingestion [10]. In most other instances, a conservative approach of observation for up to a month can be taken to see if the object passes before attempting endoscopic removal.

There are a variety of instruments to remove foreign bodies. These include retrieval nets, rat tooth and alligator forceps, polyp snares, wire baskets, and graspers. Trainees should strive to gain experience with each—either on live patients or during simulations. They should also learn the wisdom to searching for a similar object to the one ingested prior to starting the procedure in order to identify the ideal instrument to remove it.

Percutaneous endoscopic gastrostomy (PEG)

Trainees in pediatric gastroenterology should have an understanding of indications for gastrostomy tube placement in children, including the need for supplemental calories or an inability to eat by mouth. PEG tube placement is associated with faster recovery time and less pain than open gastrostomy procedures and is generally the preferred method in children [11]. Trainees in pediatric gastroenterology should strive to learn to place PEGs, as many institutions expect their gastroenterologists to perform this procedure.

PEG placement in children requires two physicians: one performing the endoscopy and the other acting as a surgical assistant. The first advances the endoscope into the stomach and a site is identified by transillumination of the skin by the endoscope light. The assistant indents the chosen spot with a finger, which is observed internally with the endoscope. The finger may be moved anywhere in the transilluminated region until an ideal location within the stomach is decided upon. Once the spot is identified and the area has been surgically cleansed and draped, an angiocatheter is inserted through the skin into the stomach, and a looped guide wire is inserted through the catheter. The guide wire is grasped using a snare or forceps and is pulled out through the mouth as the endoscope is withdrawn. In most children, a 12 or 16 Fr PEG represents the most appropriate size for placement. The gastrostomy tube is attached to the wire at the mouth and is then pulled down through the esophagus and out through the abdominal wall by the assistant. An inner disk or "bumper" prevents the tube from being accidentally pulled out, and a similar bolster is placed at the skin to prevent inner migration of the tube.

Table 13.8 Relative contraindications to PEG placement in children.

- Malrotation
- Heterotaxy
- Situs inversus
- Ascites
- Peritoneal dialysis catheter
- Prior abdominal surgery
- Hepatomegaly
- Splenomegaly
- Scoliosis
- Ventriculoperitoneal shunt
- Gastric varices

Contraindications

Relative contraindications for the procedure are listed in Table 13.8 and include congenital malformations, as well as patient size less than 2 kg. At our institution, we prefer to place PEGs in patients who weigh at least 2.5 kg, but the procedure has been performed successfully in patients who weigh less. Performance of PEGs in all neonates may be especially risky due to the technical need to insufflate air to distend the stomach, which may limit ventilation by impinging on the diaphragm. Absolute contraindications to PEG placement in children include inability to achieve successful transillumination of the stomach or to visualize the finger indentation, presumably for anatomical reasons, such as the presence of an overlying liver or colon.

Complications

It is imperative that all trainees learn the multitude of early and late complications that can occur with placement of PEGs. A rare late complication is the development of gastrocolocutaneous fistula due to placement of the PEG tube through the colon and stomach. Other more commonly encountered complications can include tube migration into the abdominal wall (buried bumper), intrahepatic placement, peritonitis, hemorrhage, necrotizing fasciitis, pneumoperitoneum, leakage around the g-tube, and wound infection. Trainees must learn to recognize the complications of PEG placement, as well as various approaches to clinical management.

Stricture dilation

Trainees in pediatric endoscopy may wish to become proficient in endoscopic dilation of esophageal strictures. The causes of esophageal strictures in children are usually benign and include narrow anastomoses after surgical repair of esophageal atresia, peptic injury, eosinophilic esophagitis, congenital lesions, Schatzki's rings, achalasia, and caustic injury. Strictures can also be found in the proximal or distal small bowel and colon related to Crohn's disease and previous surgical anastomoses.

Endoscopic dilation can be performed by through-the-scope (TTS) balloon dilation or by Savary–Gillard dilators. Trainees in this procedure should become familiar with the variety of available TTS balloon dilators, which are available in either single or multiple diameters. TTS dilators are not compatible with pediatric gastroscopes. In small children <10 kg, they can be advanced over a guide wire that has been placed endoscopically through the stricture. This procedure is usually done under fluoroscopic guidance, and the balloon is inflated with gastrograffin or water under pressure to a preset maximum diameter. The most serious complication of dilation is perforation, with a reported pediatric rate of 0.1–0.4%.

Management of GI bleeding

Trainees in pediatric gastroenterology require comprehensive exposure to the differential diagnosis of, diagnostic techniques for, and treatment of gastrointestinal hemorrhage, as well as a thorough understanding of its pathophysiology. Significant gastrointestinal bleeding in children is a rare event, but can be life threatening [12]. Trainees must be familiar with the differential diagnosis and diagnostic approach to the pediatric patient with subacute, intermittent, or chronic gastrointestinal bleeding from either an upper or lower tract source. This includes the appropriate use of upper endoscopy and/ or colonoscopy as both a diagnostic and therapeutic tool.

Trainees in pediatric gastroenterology should recognize and have sufficient training in the variety of endoscopic therapies that are available for the treatment of gastrointestinal bleeding. These include injection, thermal coagulation, band ligation, and mechanical clipping. There is little published pediatric experience with these different techniques. Therefore, the best technique for each type of bleeding has not yet been established in children.

Injection therapy

Injection therapy is a common treatment used to achieve hemostasis. Various chemical agents can be injected depending on the indication, and each has recommended aliquot volumes to administer and maximum doses (see Table 13.9). All sclerosing agents are administered via endoscopic needles. Endoscopic needles are available to fit through a 2.0 mm working channel of a pediatric gastroscope. Epinephrine in a 1:10000 dilution is the most commonly used agent. It has three major modes of action: local vasoconstriction, platelet aggregation, and mechanical tamponade. Epinephrine is not tissue-destructive, so relatively large volumes can be administered, even in children.

Sclerosing agents such as sodium tetradecyl sulfate and sodium morrhuate induce tissue destruction by causing local inflammation, thrombus formation, and scarring. These agents and others can be injected directly into varices for the treatment of variceal hemorrhage. Complications of sclerotherapy include stricture formation, tissue ulceration, bleeding, perforation, infection, and fistula formation. This mode of treatment has been replaced largely by band ligation, but is still useful in infants and small children in whom the band ligator is too large to pass through the oropharynx.

Thermal coagulation

Thermal coagulation can be divided into contact and noncontact devices. Examples of contact devices are bipolar coagulation probes and heater probes. Heater probes provide a constant temperature of 250°C and deliver a set programmed amount of energy. Bipolar probes transmit current between two electrodes in the probe, limiting the depth of tissue injury compared to monopolar probes, which are less commonly used. The goal of contact therapy (coaptive coagulation) is to provide steady heat to coagulate the local tissue and the bleeding vessel. This treatment is useful in bleeding ulcers and vascular lesions. Complications of coaptive coagulation include increased bleeding and deep tissue injury, including perforation. Trainees should be aware that bipolar and heater probes can only fit through a standard adult gastroscope. Argon plasma coagulation (APC) is a newer noncontact thermal modality that has the benefit of covering larger areas with less risk of deep tissue injury. This modality has probes that are small enough to fit through the 2.0 mm working channel of the pediatric gastroscope.

Mechanical therapy

Mechanical clips are devices that apply mechanical tamponade to a lesion. They are effective in closing mucosal defects as well as applying mechanical compression to a visible bleeding vessel. There are several types of clips commercially available and range in opening size from 9 to 11 mm. Some clips can open and close multiple times, while others are rotatable to facilitate accurate placement. Clip placement may be difficult depending on the location of the lesion. In addition, clips are not compatible with the pediatric gastroscopes and therefore not helpful for infants and young children.

Band ligation

Band ligation is a hemostatic approach used for varices. A band ligator consists of a cylindrical cap, preloaded with multiple elastic

Table 13.9 Common sclerosing agents and indications for therapeutic pediatric endoscopy.

Solution	Indications	Volumes per injection, maximum total dose
Epinephrine (1:10,000 concentration)	Bleeding ulcer	0.5–2 mL aliquots injected around bleeding site. Max total dose of 10 mL
Ethanol (98%)	Varices	0.1–0.2 mL aliquots surrounding bleeding site. Max total dose 0.6–1.2 mL
Sodium morrhuate 5%	Varices	0.5–1.0 cc aliquots, watching for effect. Max total dose 5–10 cc per session
Sodium tetradecyl sulfate 1–3%	Varices	0.5–1.0 mL aliquots, watching for effect. Max total dose 3–5 cc per session

bands, which is placed over the tip of the endoscope. The varix is sucked into the cap and a band is released onto the tissue. Band ligation has replaced sclerotheray in most instances since it causes less ulceration and stricturing, but may be difficult to perform in small children under 10–15 kg and also requires the use of a standard adult gastroscope.

The role of adult endoscopists in pediatrics

As our chapter highlights, pediatric endoscopy is a unique field that requires specialized training. We also acknowledge the collegial relationship pediatric gastroenterologists have shared with their adult counterparts and recognize that adult endoscopists are on occasion asked to perform endoscopic procedures in children. This may be particularly the case for difficult therapeutic procedures, such as endoscopic ultrasound (EUS), endoscopic retrograde cholangiopancreatography, and massive GI bleeding.

Even for full-trained adult endoscopists, performing procedures in small children will entail a steep learning curve. In most instances, it is important for adult gastroentoenterologists to work closely with their pediatric colleagues in both preprocedure and intraprocedural planning. It may be also important to enlist the help of a pediatric anesthesiologist. The pediatric team may have more familiarity with dosing of medications, size-appropriate instrument choices, as well as the pathophysiology of the patient. The pediatric endoscopist may also have a strong relationship with the patient and their family. In geographic regions of the country with limited access to pediatric gastroenterologists, it is very important for adult endoscopists to learn to work with the pediatric care team.

Defining and assessing procedural competency

Diagnostic endoscopic competence is the ability to recognize pathology and to understand the clinical significance as it applies to management of pediatric patients with gastrointestinal disorders [9]. Therapeutic competence is the ability to recognize when a therapeutic procedure is clinically indicated as well as the ability to perform that procedure safely and successfully in pediatric patients.

As per the new NASPGHAN guidelines, after completion of a training program in pediatric gastroenterology, trainees should be able to [2]
- recommend endoscopic procedures for pediatric patients based on evaluating specific indications, contraindications, and diagnostic and therapeutic alternatives;
- counsel the pediatric patient and family on bowel preparation and other supportive methods as indicated;
- select and apply appropriate sedation as indicated;
- identify age-, size-, and condition-appropriate endoscopy equipment;
- perform each indicated procedure safely, completely, independently, and expeditiously;
- interpret and describe endoscopic findings accurately;

- integrate endoscopic findings or therapy into the management plan;
- understand the inherent risks of endoscopic procedures and counsel the patient and family on the expected risks, benefits, and alternatives of various procedures;
- recognize personal and procedural (including equipment) limitations and know when to request assistance;
- be able to recognize and manage complications including requesting assistance from colleagues in related disciplines such as pediatric anesthesia, critical care, pediatric surgery, or adult gastroenterology as required;
- clean and maintain endoscopic equipment and be familiar with Joint Commission of American Hospital Organization (JCAHO) and institutional standards for quality improvement, infection control, sedation, and monitoring; and
- understand how an endoscopy unit is run, including how the unit interfaces with the inpatient and outpatient gastroenterology practice and other services including pediatric anesthesiology.

Assessing competency

There is little known about endoscopic skill learning curves among pediatric gastroenterologists. Assessing competency in pediatric endoscopy has in the past always been based around procedure numbers. For example, national guidelines have traditionally recommended minimum threshold numbers of 100 upper endoscopies and 100 colonoscopies to achieve competency in these procedures [13]. And although the more procedures completed will undoubtedly lead to the development of better basic motor skills, procedural numbers do not in themselves determine competency. As with many aspects of training there must be both formal and informal feedback by instructors. This may be best accomplished using a validated assessment tool, such as the Global Assessment of Gastrointestinal Endoscopic Skills (GAGES), which was recently validated for both adult and pediatric endoscopy [14] (Figures 13.2 and 13.3). Of note, NASPGHAN is currently in the process of developing and validating a pediatric-specific metric, which may help with the assessment of trainee competence in performing endoscopy in children.

Simulation in pediatric endoscopy

Simulation may represent an important tool for training in pediatric gastroenterology. Generally speaking, small patient size may increase the level of technical difficulty involved in performing pediatric endoscopy, while young patient age often leads to increased protectiveness by parents and staff endoscopists. Both of these may in turn detract from the training experience, and fellows in pediatric gastroenterology.

In recent years, hands-on courses in pediatric endoscopy have been developed that have featured *ex vivo* model simulators. Computer-based endoscopic simulators (CBES) have also been demonstrated to be effective for pediatric trainees for gaining technical skills and confidence, while maintaining patient safety. They

Intubation of the Esophagus Reflects patient management, understanding of anatomy, and sedation	Score ☐
5 – Able to independently (successfully) intubate esophagus without patient discomfort 4 3 – Requires detailed prompting and cues 2 1 – Unable to properly intubate, requiring take over	

Scope Navigation Reflects navigation of the GI tract using tip deflection, advancement/withdrawal, and torque	Score ☐
5 – Expertly able to manipulate the scope in the upper GI tract autonomously 4 3 – Requires verbal guidance to completely navigate the upper GI tract 2 1 – Not able to achieve goals despite verbal cues, requiring take over	

Ability to Keep a Clear Endoscopic Field Utilization of insufflation, suction, and/or irrigation to maximize mucosal evaluation	Score ☐
5 – Use insufflation, suction, and irrigation optimally to maintain clear view of endoscopic field 4 3 – Requires moderate prompting to maintain clear view 2 1 – Inability to maintain view despite extensive verbal cues	

Instrumentation (if applicable; leave blank if not applicable) Random biopsy: targeting is assessed by asking the endoscopist to take another biopsy from the identical site. Targeted instrumentation: evaluation is based on ability to direct the instrument to the target.	Score ☐
5 – Expertly directs instrument to desired target 4 3 – Requires some guidance and/or multiple attempts to direct instrument to target 2 1 – Unable to direct instrument to target despite coaching	

Quality of Examination Reflects attention to patient comfort, efficiency, and completeness of mucosal evaluation	Score ☐
5 – Expertly completes the exam efficiently and comfortably 4 3 – Requires moderate assistant to accomplish a complete and comfortable exam 2 1 – Could not perform a satisfactory exam	

Figure 13.2 GAGES (global assessment of gastrointestinal endoscopic skills)—upper GI endoscopy scoresheet.

have also been shown to have face validity for pediatrics, despite the fact that most CBES are modeled on adults [15]. This finding is important as pediatric endoscopy programs can take advantage of commercially available simulators, which may enhance the education of trainees.

Full-scale simulation of pediatric endoscopy may also be helpful for training physicians in more comprehensive technical and teamwork skills necessary for endoscopy. As an example, our endoscopy unit regularly stages full scale simulations of crisis scenarios, which allows our physicians, our trainees, and our nurses

to practice handling high stakes adverse events, which fortunately occur extremely infrequently in our unit. Full-scale simulation also allows trainees to simulate the simultaneous tasks involved in performing procedures while administering and supervising IV sedation. Of course, whether incorporating part-task CBES or full-scale simulation into training programs, it must be recognized that pediatric GI fellows are often very busy. Accordingly, they must have scheduled times for simulation training built into their educational program, if simulation is to be optimally offered as an educational tool.

Scope Navigation Reflects navigation of the GI tract using tip deflection, advancement/withdrawal, and torque	Score ☐

5 – Expertly able to manipulate the scope in the GI tract autonomously 4 3 – Requires verbal guidance to completely navigate the lower GI tract 2 1 – Not able to achieve goals despite verbal cues, requiring take over

Use of Strategies Examines use of patient positions, abdominal pressure, insufflation, suction, and loop reduction to comfortably complete the procedure	Score ☐

5 – Expert use of appropriate strategies for advancement of the scope while optimizing patient comfort 4 3 – Use of some strategies appropriately, but requires moderate verbal guidance 2 1 – Unable to utilize appropriate strategies for scope advancement despite verbal assistance

Ability to Keep a Clear Endoscopic Field Utilization of insufflation, suction, and/or irrigation to maximize mucosal evaluation	Score ☐

5 – Use insufflation, suction, and irrigation optimally to maintain clear view of endoscopic field 4 3 – Requires moderate prompting to maintain clear view 2 1 – Inability to maintain view despite extensive verbal cues

Instrumentation (if applicable; leave blank if not applicable) Random biopsy: targeting is assessed by asking the endoscopist to take another biopsy from the identical site. Targeted instrumentation: evaluation is based on ability to direct the instrument to the target.	Score ☐

5 – Expertly directs instrument to desired target 4 3 – Requires some guidance and/or multiple attempts to direct instrument to target 2 1 – Unable to direct instrument to target despite coaching

Quality of Examination Reflects attention to patient comfort, efficiency, and completeness of mucosal evaluation	Score ☐

5 – Expertly completes the exam efficiently and comfortably 4 3 – Requires moderate assistant to accomplish a complete and comfortable exam 2 1 – Could not perform a satisfactory exam

Figure 13.3 GAGES (global assessment of gastrointestinal endoscopic skills)—colonoscopy scoresheet.

Advanced procedures

A relatively new phenomenon in the field of pediatric endoscopy is the pursuit of advanced training in therapeutic techniques, including ERCP and EUS. The technical aspects of both procedures in pediatrics are very similar to that in adults. The major differences are in the approach to sedation and equipment available in pediatrics.

Endoscopic retrograde cholangiopancreatography (ERCP)

ERCP involves the passage of a side-viewing endoscope into the second portion of the duodenum and cannulation of the major duodenal papilla. Biliary indications for pediatric ERCP include choledocholithiasis, evaluation of primary sclerosing cholangitis, choledochal cyst, biliary strictures, bile plug syndrome, intra- or extrahepatic ductal dilation, and bile leak after liver transplantation or cholecystectomy [16]. Pancreatic indications for ERCP include persistent acute pancreatitis, recurrent episodes of acute pancreatitis, chronic pancreatitis, pancreatic divisum, annular pancreas, and pancreatic trauma.

As a rule, most pediatric endoscopist prefer to perform pediatric ERCP cases under general anesthesia rather than sedation, which ensures safer airway management and allows better patient comfort for potentially lengthy difficult procedures. In terms of equipment, standard adult duodenoscopes can generally be used in children 2 years of age and older. These scopes may also be utilized in younger children, albeit with more technical challenges, and carry the benefit of allowing the passage of most equipment through working channels, including stents up to 7 Fr in diameter.

The main limiting factor to Pediatric ERCP lies in the lack of adequate equipment intended for use in infants and young children. In infants <1 year of age, it is necessary to use a smaller endoscope, such as the Olympus PJF 160, which has a tip diameter of 7.5 mm with a single 2.0 mm working channel (Figure 13.1c]. This scope is capable of therapeutic procedures such as sphincterotomy, stone extraction, and stenting. However, there are fewer devices available to fit through the small 2.0 mm working channel.

As with all trainees in ERCP, trainees in pediatric ERCP must strive to achieve selective duct cannulation in >90% of the cases to be declared competent. The American Society for Gastrointestinal Endoscopy (ASGE) recommends that trainees have to perform 180–200 ERCP procedures with at least half being therapeutic [17]. For pediatric trainees seeking advanced training in ERCP, it may be imperative to receive supplemental training with adult patients. For a more in-depth discussion on competency in ERCP, please review Chapter 7.

Endoscopic ultrasound

EUS utilizes an ultrasound transducer attached to the endoscope to obtain high resolution images of the GI tract layers, submucosal lesions, liver, bile ducts, and pancreas, as well as extraluminal masses and lymph nodes in the mediastinum and peritoneal cavity. A miniprobe has been developed that can be passed through conventional endoscopes and has increased the potential for this procedure in children. EUS is particularly useful for assessment of submucosal lesions, and its indications include cancer staging, pancreatic and biliary disease, and anorectal malformations [18]. Needle aspiration of cystic lesions can be accomplished via EUS, and chronic pancreatitis and autoimmune pancreatitis can be diagnosed. Since the incidence of esophageal, gastric, biliary, and pancreatic cancer is low in children, pediatric EUS is typically performed with the help of adult gastroenterologists. Pediatric trainees who wish to develop independent skills in EUS must be prepared to meet the same competence requirements as adult endoscopists.

Wireless video capsule endoscopy

Wireless video capsule endoscopy has emerged in the last 5 years as a noninvasive technology that can also provide diagnostic imaging of the small intestine. Indications for capsule endoscopy in children include looking for an obscure source of gastrointestinal bleeding, suspected Crohn's disease, celiac disease, and polyps in patients with hereditary polyposis syndromes. Capsule endoscopy is FDA approved for children 10 years of age and older and have been reported in children as young as 2 [19]. Young patients who cannot swallow the capsule can have it placed endoscopically using a delivery device. The main risk associated with capsule endoscopy is capsule retention, which is clinically significant in less than 1% of patients. The ASGE recommends completion of a gastrointestinal endoscopy training program that included training in the recognition and management of small intestinal diseases [20].

Trainees in capsule endoscopy should have privileges to perform EGD and colonoscopy and have familiarity with the hardware and software systems. In addition, they must have either (1) formal training during GI fellowship or (2) completion of a hands-on course endorsed by a national or international GI or surgical society, in addition to review of their first 10 capsule studies by a credentialed capsule endoscopist. Currently, most pediatric gastroenterology programs do not have formal training programs for learning capsule endoscopy. Therefore, pediatric trainees need to seek experience through CME courses. In order to achieve competency in wireless capsule endoscopy in pediatrics, trainees should have experience in reading capsules, as well as in their endoscopic placement.

References

1 Gilger MA: Gastroenterologic endoscopy in children: past, present, and future. *Curr Opin Pediatr* 2001;**13**:429–434.

2 Kay M, Piccoli DA, Barth B, Nowicki M, Gilger MA: NASPGHAN guideline for training in endoscopy and related procedures. *J Pediatr Gastroenterol Nutr.* (in press.)

3 Gilger MA: Sedation for pediatric GI endoscopy. *Gastrointest Endosc* 2007;**65**:211–212.

4 Mahoney LB, Lightdale JR: Sedation of the pediatric and adolescent patient for GI procedures. *Curr Treat Options Gastroenterol* 2007;**10**:412–421.

5 Lightdale JR, Mahoney LB, Schwarz SM, Liacouras CA: Methods of sedation in pediatric endoscopy: A survey of NASPGHAN members. *J Pediatr Gastroenterol Nutr* 2007;**45**:500–502.

6 Dahshan A, Donovan GK: Severe methemoglobinemia complicating topical benzocaine use during endoscopy in a toddler: a case report and review of the literature. *Pediatrics* 2006;**117**:e806–e809.

7 Kirberg A, Sagredo R, Montalva G, Flores E: Ketamine for pediatric endoscopic procedures and as a sedation complement for adult patients. *Gastrointest Endosc* 2005;**61**:501–502.

8 Fox V: Pediatric endoscopy. In: Classen M, Tytgat G, Lightdale CJ (eds). *Gastroenterological Endoscopy*. New York: Thieme, 2002: 720–748.

9 Fox VL: Clinical competency in pediatric endoscopy. *J Pediatr Gastroenterol Nutr* 1998;**26**:200–204.

10 Kay M, Wyllie R: Pediatric foreign bodies and their management. *Curr Gastroenterol Rep* 2005;**7**:212–218.

11 Avitsland TL, Kristensen C, Emblem R, Veenstra M, Mala T, Bjornland K: Percutaneous endoscopic gastrostomy in children: a safe technique with major symptom relief and high parental satisfaction. *J Pediatr Gastroenterol Nutr* 2006;**43**:624–628.

12 Boyle JT: Gastrointestinal bleeding in infants and children. *Pediatr Rev* 2008;**29**:39–52.

13 Rudolph CD, Winter HS: NASPGN guidelines for training in pediatric gastroenterology. NASPGN Executive Council, NASPGN Training and Education Committee. *J Pediatr Gastroenterol Nutr* 1999;**29**(Suppl 1):S1–S26.

14 Vassiliou MC, Kaneva PA, Poulose BK, et al.: Global Assessment of Gastrointestinal Endoscopic Skills (GAGES): a valid measurement tool for technical skills in flexible endoscopy. *Surg Endosc* 2010;**24**:1834–1841.

15 Lightdale JR, Newburg AR, Mahoney LB, Fredette ME, Fishman LN: Fellow perceptions of training using computer-based endoscopic simulators. *Gastrointest Endosc* 2010;**72**:13–18.

16 Cheng CL, Fogel EL, Sherman S, et al.: Diagnostic and therapeutic endoscopic retrograde cholangiopancreatography in children: a large series report. *J Pediatr Gastroenterol Nutr* 2005;**41**:445–453.

17 Spier BJ, Benson M, Pfau PR, Nelligan G, Lucey MR, Gaumnitz EA: Colonoscopy training in gastroenterology fellowships: determining competence. *Gastrointest Endosc* 2010;**71**:319–324.

18 Fox VL: Gastrointestinal endosonography. In: Kleinman RE, Sanderson IR, Goulet O, Sherman PM, Mieli-Vergani G, Shneider BL (eds), *Walker's Pediatric Gastrointestinal Disease*. Hamilton, ON: B.C. Decker, Inc., 2008: 1321–1328.

19 Fritscher-Ravens A, Scherbakov P, Bufler P, et al.: The feasibility of wireless capsule endoscopy in detecting small intestinal pathology in children under the age of 8 years: a multicentre European study. *Gut* 2009;**58**:1467–1472.

20 Faigel DO, Baron TH, Adler DG, et al. ASGE guideline: guidelines for credentialing and granting privileges for capsule endoscopy. *Gastrointest Endosc* 2005;**61**:503–505.

III Training in Specific Techniques

14 Contrast-Enhanced Endoscopy—Chromo and Optical Contrast Techniques

Anna M. Buchner[1], Prateek Sharma[2], & Michael B. Wallace[3]

[1] University of Pennsylvania School of Medicine, Philadelphia, PA, USA
[2] Veterans Affairs Medical Center, University of Kansas School of Medicine, Kansas City, KS, USA
[3] Mayo Clinic, Jacksonville, FL, USA

Introduction

Over the last decade, a major role of digestive endoscopy has become the early detection and prevention of gastrointestinal malignancies. This has been achieved through accurate detection of precursor lesions, including the most subtle and minute ones and their subsequent resection. Therefore, the current diagnostic endoscopy aims at detection and characterization of all lesions and confirmation of their neoplastic potential. The current advances in endoscopy have provided endoscopists with novel modalities to reach those goals. Digestive endoscopy has evolved from standard endoscopy to contrast-enhanced endoscopy. Conventional white-light video endoscopy, which has been used initially as a primary diagnostic modality, was found to be associated with a disproportionate miss rate for subtle lesions (e.g., flat adenomas). Numerous studies have demonstrated that even experienced gastroenterologists miss up to 6% of advanced adenomas and 30% of all adenomas [1,2]. Since subtle dysplastic and early neoplastic lesions remain often too small, flat, or depressed to be detected during regular standard white-light endoscopy, new contrast-enhanced endoscopic technologies have been introduced to maximize the detection of subtle GI lesions. In experienced hands, these methods truly represent a significant advance in endoscopy practice and may improve the diagnostic yield of significant lesions, decrease the burden of insignificant biopsies, and lead to appropriate on-table decisions, such as endoscopic resection of malignant lesion versus leaving lesions in situ if they are benign. The training in contrast-enhanced endoscopic technologies has become a critically important issue, and it has to be undertaken in order to maximize the clinical usefulness of these new technologies.

Overview of contrast (image)-enhancement techniques: chromoendoscopy and other optical techniques

Contrast-enhanced endoscopy includes the image-enhanced endoscopy (IEE) technologies such as dye-based IEE, with chromoendoscopy, and equipment- based IEE with NBI, electronic-based IEE with spectral estimation technologies such as NBI, MBI, and iScan, and confocal laser endomicroscopy (CLE) as well as autofluorescence (AFI) [3]. These technologies are used in conjunction with recently developed high-resolution and high-definition endoscopes. High-resolution endoscopes (HRE) with high-density couple-charged device (CCD) (600,000–1,000,000 pixels per CCD) produce high-resolution images with increased spatial resolution for the detection of minute abnormalities in mucosal glandular and vascular structures. In conjunction with a movable lens for magnification endoscopy, the focal distance may be controlled to allow detailed examination of the mucosal surface at close range (<3 mm). This new generation of endoscopes can provide enlargement of the image up to 115× as compared with 30× with standard endoscopes and can be used in conjunction with contrast-enhancement technologies such as chromoendoscopy/NBI techniques in diagnosing neoplastic and nonneoplastic lesions, detection of flat and subtle lesions, and evaluating the depth of malignant lesions. Some of these techniques can provide in vivo microscopic evaluation of the GI mucosa known as optical biopsy obtained in real time.

Chromoendoscopy

The use of HRE has been combined with chromendoscopy (dye staining) in an attempt to improve detection of mucosal

---

Successful Training in Gastrointestinal Endoscopy, First Edition. Edited by Jonathan Cohen.
© 2011 Blackwell Publishing Ltd. Published 2011 by Blackwell Publishing Ltd.

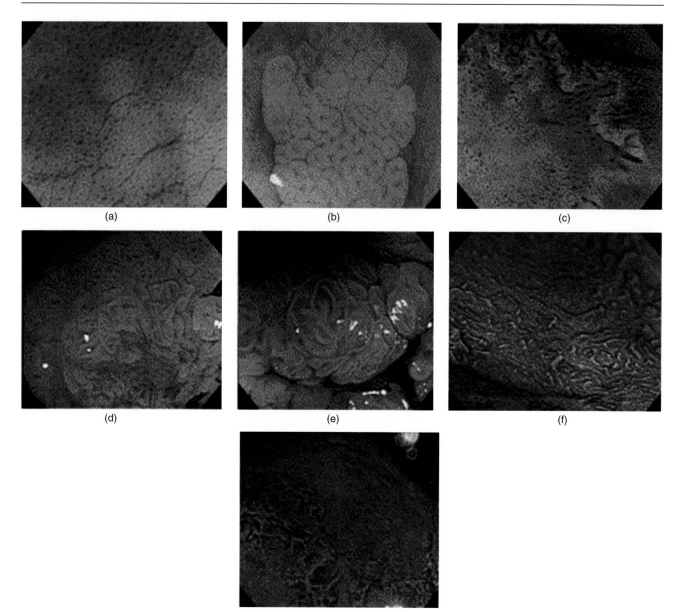

Figure 14.1 Pit pattern classification. (a) Type I: normal roundish pits. (b) Type II: large star-shaped pits. (c) Type IIIs: small roundish pits. (d) Type IIIl: long tubular pits. (e) Type IV: branched pits. (f) Type Vi: irregular pits. (g) Type Vn: nonstructural pit pattern. Types I and II are non-neoplastic pit patterns. Types IIIs, IIIl, and IV are adenomatous pit patterns. Types Vi and Vn are cancerous pit patterns. (Reproduced from Kudo S, Tamura S, Nakajima T, Yamano H, Kusaka H, Watanabe H. Diagnosis of colorectal tumorous lesions by magnifying endoscopy. *Gastrointest Endosc* 1996;**44**:8–14, with permission from Elsevier.)

abnormalities. The key point in chromoendoscopy is applying various dyes to visualize subtle GI lesions and to define surface-staining patterns, with subsequent targeted biopsies of those lesions. Kudo pit pattern classification for colonic lesions became widely adopted and it allows to distinguish five types of staining pattern of the mucosa [4]. Type 1 with round pits and type 2 with stellate pits represent nonneoplastic lesions, whereas type 3 tubular pits, type 4 gyrus-like pits, and type 5 irregular pits correspond to neoplastic lesions (Figure 14.1).

Various studies showed that chromoendoscopy with methylene blue-targeted biopsies increased the diagnostic yield for dysplastic lesions, including flat lesions in patients with ulcerative colitis as opposed to using standard colonoscopy [5–7]. Therefore, chromoendoscopy has become a part of some surveillance guidelines in patients with long standing ulcerative colitis [8,9].

Both traditional chromoendoscopy with 2% Lugol's iodine [10] and virtual chromoendoscopy methods such as NBI [11] have been shown to improve detection of squamous-cell neoplasia in the esophagus. The methods for Lugol's application are similar to other chromoscopy techniques, but are contraindicated in individuals with iodine allergy. Lugol's is a negative stain for squamous dysplasia, thus normal epithelium stains dark brown, whereas

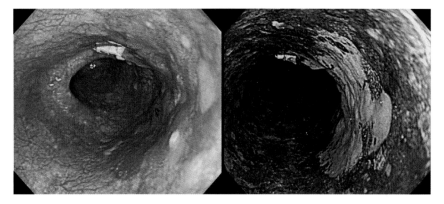

Figure 14.2 Lugol's iodine of squamous dysplasia showing white light on left, and lugols on right with the negative stained area representing dysplasia. (Reproduced from Dawsey SM, Fleischer DE, Wang GQ, Zhou B, Kidwell JA, Lu N, Lewin KJ, Roth MJ, Tio TL, Taylor PR. Mucosal iodine staining improves endoscopic visualization of squamous dysplasia and squamous cell carcinoma of the esophagus in Linxian, China. *Cancer* 1998;**83**:220–231.)

dysplasia does not stain (Figure 14.2). In NBI, the key pattern is development of increased and distorted intrapapillary capillary loops (IPCLs) (Figure 14.3).

Several investigators reported the improved detection of intestinal metaplasia and dysplasia in Barrett's esophagus using dye-based chromoendoscopy methods compared with a random biopsy protocol [12–18]. Sharma et al. described three mucosal patterns visualized with indigo carmine and magnification endoscopy in patients with Barrett's esophagus (ridged/villous, circular, irregular/distorted) with the ridged or villous patterns found be associated with intestinal metaplasia while the irregular or distorted pattern with Barrett's high grade dysplasia or superficial adenocarcinoma [19]. The presence of the ridged or villous pattern had high sensitivity, specificity, and positive predictive value (97%, 76%, and 92%, respectively) for detecting Barrett's metaplasia [19]. However, some studies using methylene blue spraying have failed to demonstrate a detection benefit for either Barrett's metaplasia or dysplasia [12,18]. There has also been a report that raises the issue of DNA damage resulting from

methylene blue staining and white light illumination [20]. Similar conflicting results have been found with studies using acetic acid (a mucolytic agent that alters cellular protein structure) and crystal violet staining [21–23]. Therefore, the initial enthusiastic results have been found later to vary, possibly due to differences in technique, operator experience, and the prevalence of Barrett's esophagus within the particular patient population under investigation [24,25].

Further use of the chromoendoscopy techniques was also described in other upper GI pathologies, including gastric cancer and esophageal cancer [26,27].

The main value of those techniques, however, appears to be detection for small and flat lesions not seen by conventional colonoscopy and furthermore distinction between neoplastic and nonneoplastic lesions [28–30]. A recent study by Soetikno confirmed [30] the high prevalence of flat, nonpolypoid colorectal lesions detected with the use of dye-based chromoendoscopy.

However, despite its potential for colonic diseases, chromoendoscopy has not been widely adopted into clinical practice in

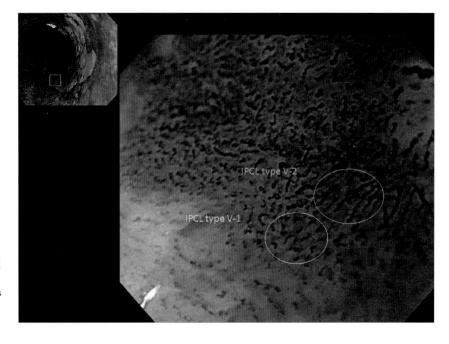

Figure 14.3 Squamous neoplasia in the esophagus demonstrating irregular dilated intrapapillary capillary loops (IPCL). (Reproduced with permission from Shibuya K, Hoshino H, Chiyo M, et al. High magnification bronchovideoscopy combined with narrow band imaging could detect capillary loops of angiogenic squamous dysplasia in heavy smokers at high risk for lung cancer. *Thorax* 2003;**58**:989–995.)

the United States because of difficulty in standardization of techniques, requirement for specialized disposable equipment, and increased procedure time [31,32].

A simpler chromoendoscopy method that could be widely implemented is to mix powdered indigo carmine (2.0 g) with 1 L of sterile normal solution and use this as part of a powered washing device connected to the colonoscope. This method allows rapid, convenient pan chromoendoscopy concurrent with standard washing of the colon wall (see Video 14.1).

Despite the well-established benefits of dye-based chromoendoscopy, the limited application in Western countries has led to efforts to develop so-called virtual chromendoscopy with no requirements of the use of topical stains.

Narrow band imaging

The NBI is a commercially available method of optical chromendoscopy that improves detection of mucosal abnormalities without the messy, time-consuming problems associated with vital dye staining chromoendoscopy. This is currently the best studied advanced endoscopic imaging technique for the detection of Barrett's dysplasia and detection and characterization of colorectal polyps. While conventional white-light endoscopy uses the full visible wavelength range (400–700 nm) to produce a red green blue image, NBI in combination with magnification endoscopy illuminates the tissue surface using special filters that narrow the red–green–blue bands and simultaneously increase the relative intensity of the blue band.

Various studies have demonstrated the value of this technology in the evaluation of patients with upper GI lesions, including Barrett's esophagus dysplasia and gastric lesions [33,34]. Wolfsen et al. [35] demonstrated that in patients evaluated for Barrett's esophagus with dysplasia, NBI detected significantly more patients with dysplasia and higher grades of dysplasia with fewer biopsy samples compared with standard resolution endoscopy (Figure 14.4 and Video 14.2).

A recent systematic review by Curvers et al. [36] summarized the promising performance and clinical utility of narrow band imaging (NBI) in upper GI endoscopy with a focus on the primary detection of premalignant lesions and the differentiation between neoplastic and nonneoplastic lesions.

NBI techniques seem to be also a useful tool in the detection of colorectal lesions as well [37–41] although a few recent studies revealed conflicting results with no improvement of adenoma detection rates with the use of this novel technique as compared to traditional dye-based chromoendoscopy [42–44]. Adler et al. [43] demonstrated the increased adenoma detection rates only in the initial phase of the study, but not in the second phase of the study, suggesting that exposure to NBI (and perhaps the awareness that small, flat adenomas are common) leads to increased adenoma detection with both white light and enhanced methods. The study by Rex et al. further supports this concept since they observed that both high-definition white light and NBI led to nearly doubling of the adenoma detection rate compared to their own well-documented historical controls [40]. Results of another prospective randomized back-to-back trial comparing NBI to conventional colonoscopy for adenoma detection demonstrates that the miss-rate for polyps, and for adenomas, is lower with HD-NBI than for standard colonoscopy [45].

The use of NBI for the detection of dysplasia in long-term standing ulcerative colitis has not led to improvement of neoplasia detection [44]. On the other hand, East et al. [46] demonstrated that NBI could play a role in adenoma detection in high-risk group patients. The investigators found that a second additional examination with NBI use doubled the total number of adenomas detected in 62 patients with hereditary nonpolyposis colorectal cancer [44].

In a recent systematic review, summarized data on the performance and clinical utility of NBI during colonoscopy did not show a significant improvement in adenoma detection with the use of NBI, but it confirmed the value of NBI for differentiation neoplastic from nonneoplastic colon polyps when used by experts [47] (see Video 14.3).

Therefore, in spite of existing controversy on the role of NBI in adenoma detection, the NBI system has been showed to have a relatively high sensitivity 90–95% and specificity 80–85% for differentiation neoplastic from nonneoplastic lesions using microvascular features [48]. This level of accuracy is comparable to that of expert chromoendoscopist based on the available studies [31,49,50]; thus, potentially the time-consuming chromoendoscopy may, in time, be replaced by NBI. At the current time, the ability to

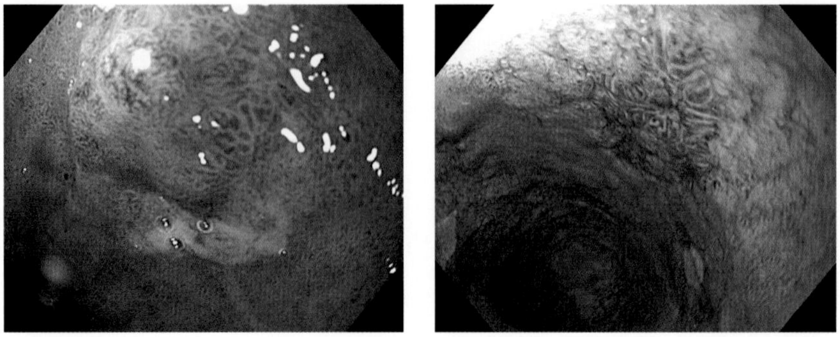

Figure 14.4 Narrow band images of Barrett's esophagus. (a) A nodular dysplasia with irregular dilated vessels in Barrett's. (Image courtesy of Herbert Wolfsen, MD.) (b) Flat-depressed dysplasia in Barrett's esophagus with focal areas of irregular mucosa and vessels (arrow) surrounded by nondysplastic areas. (Image courtesy of Herbert Wolfsen, MD.)

(a)   (b)

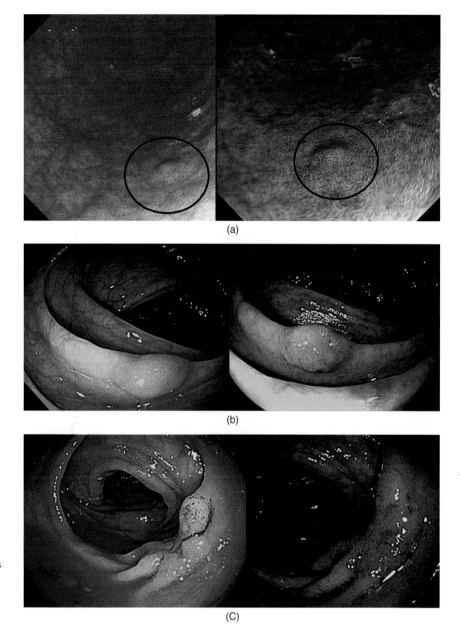

Figure 14.5 (a) Hyperplastic polyp white light (left) and NBI (right); tubular adenoma with 1s morphology. (b) Sessile tubular adenoma with white light and NBI. (c) High-grade intraepithelial neoplasia in a flat-depressed (Kudo 2a/c) colon lesion.

differentiate between adenomas and hyperplastic polyps appears to be the important clinical utility of NBI (Figure 14.5).

MBI and iScan

While NBI system depends on optical filters within the light source, the new MBI system, introduced by Fujinon, is based on a computed spectral estimation technology that processes the reflected photons to reconstruct virtual images with a choice of different wavelengths. A similar system called iScan has been also developed by Pentax. Both systems are based on the same physical principle as NBI, but they are not dependent on optical filters. These systems lead to enhancement of the tissue microvasculature as a result of the differential optical absorption of light by hemoglobin in the

mucosa. These abnormal areas can be defined by the magnification [51–55].

MBI systems used in esophageal neoplasia demonstrated improvement in detection of early neoplasia [54]. The application of MBI system in detection and classification of colorectal lesions has been also currently investigated. Pohl et al. [37] in their prospective trial compared computed virtual chromoendoscopy system (MBI) with other modalities such as standard colonoscopy, conventional chromoendoscopy with indigo carmine in low- and high-magnification modes for determination of colonic lesions histology. On the basis of this study, MBI was able to identify morphological details that efficiently predict adenomatous histology and was superior to standard colonoscopy and equivalent to conventional chromoendoscopy. Investigators have also been able to show that computed virtual chromoendoscopy is a helpful adjunct for surveillance of Barrett's esophagus and it appears to be as accurate as traditional chromoendoscopy in the detection of HGIN/early cancer [54].

Hoffman et al. showed also that high-definition endoscopy combined with iScan system is significantly superior in detecting colorectal neoplasia as compared to standard video colonoscopy, and it allows prediction of histology of the identified lesions and surface enhancement [56,57]. The application of iScan system has been also demonstrated in upper GI lesions such as minimal changes of esophagitis [58].

While these techniques of NBI, MBI, and iScan are very promising, further studies are needed to evaluate their final application, efficiency, and cost-effectiveness in both detection and characterization of gastrointestinal lesions, including various forms of GI malignancy from subtle dysplastic lesions to early cancer.

Fluorescence imaging

Fluorescence imaging endoscopy is primarily based on autofluorescence imaging techniques that differentiate tissue types based on their differences in fluorescence emission. Once the tissue is exposed to short wavelength light, endogenous fluorophores are excited, leading to emission of fluorescent light of a longer wavelength (autofluorescence imaging AFI). Because of changes of endogenous fluorophores in normal, dysplastic, and neoplastic mucosa, the altered autofluorescence is reflected by a pseudocolored image of normal mucosa (green color) and dysplasia/neoplasia with varying tones of red/purple color. AFI has been incorporated into multimodality imaging endoscopes that combine HRE and virtual chromoendoscopy with NBI system.

In a prospective randomized study, AFI significantly increased the diagnostic yield of surveillance endoscopy to detect intraepithelial neoplasia in high-risk patients with ulcerative colitis [59]. However, AFI has not been demonstrated to enhance the diagnostic yield of screening colonoscopy in a tandem colonoscopy trial by the same group [60].

Curvers et al. [61] published the results of four expert endoscopy centers using tri-modal imaging for the evaluation of 84 patients with Barrett's dysplasia. The use of AFI increased the number of patients found to have HGD from 53 to 90%. On the other hand, the use of NBI reduced the false-positive rate of AFI from 81 to 26%. Thus far, the experience with systems combining AFI, HRE, and NBI is based on the expert endoscopists evaluating the use for detection dysplasia and carcinoma. The application of this technology has not been fully studied in other practice settings yet.

Confocal laser endomicroscopy

CLE allows high-resolution imaging of cellular and subcellular tissue when optical slices of mucosal surface created by detecting reflected light and tissue autofluorescence enhances through the administration of fluorescent contrast agent.

It has been used along with chromoendoscopy techniques in evaluation of various GI lesions, including colorectal lesions enabling visualization of the gastrointestinal tract at a cellular level [62–69]. Currently, there are two CLE systems available: one

in which miniaturized confocal scanner has been integrated into the distal tip of a flexible endoscope (eCLE, Pentax, Fort Wayne, NJ, USA) and the other with a probe-based confocal endomicroscopy (pCLE, Cellvizio, Mauna Kea Technologies, Paris, France). Both systems have been demonstrated to improve the accuracy of diagnosing colorectal neoplasia [62,70,71] (see Video 14.4).

Kiesslich et al. [62] published the first report of the use of confocal endomicroscopy in 42 patients during ongoing colonoscopy in diagnosing intraepithelial neoplasia and colorectal cancer. A total of 134 small lesions (mean size 4 mm) were identified during colonoscopy after staining with methylene blue. With the help of the confocal endoscope, intraepithelial neoplasia could be predicted with a sensitivity of 97% and a specificity of 99% (accuracy, 99%). Preliminary results from the Mayo clinic have demonstrated the role of confocal endomicroscopy in accurate differentiation between neoplastic and nonneoplastic lesions (see Video 14.4) as well as detection of recurrence of neoplastic tissue following endoscopic mucosal resection of large colon polyps [72,73].

The potential applications of this technology extend beyond the discrimination of neoplastic and nonneoplastic (hyperplastic) polyps, to detection of other pathologies such as Barrett's esophagus, esophagitis, gastritis, celiac disease, etc. [62,63,74]. In a study of 63 patients with Barrett's esophagus using fluorescein-aided endomicroscopy, Kiesslich et al. [66] predicted BE with a sensitivity of 98% and specificity of 94% (see Video 14.5).

Molecular imaging

In vivo, molecular imaging with the fluorescent labeling of cells by their molecular features has been introduced recently, and it represents the true development in contrast-enhanced endoscopic technologies. Prior various animal studies demonstrated its applicability. As an example in a melanoma mouse model, cancer cells were visualized with the injection of FITC-labeled antibodies when a handheld CLE probe was used [75]. In humans, the targeted labeling of malignant crypts using identified specific heptapeptide sequence, VRPMPLQ, conjugated with fluorescein, has become possible during colonoscopy with sensitivities and specificities of diagnosing neoplastic lesions exceeding 80% [76]. Further studies are on the way, and it will likely provide a powerful set of tools with the potential to improve the early detection of cancer.

Methods for training in contrast-enhanced endoscopy techniques

The clinical application of the contrast-enhanced endoscopy technologies depends on the adequate training of the endoscopists who plan to use these technologies in everyday practice.

The primary methods of training include traditional self-learning by doing procedures and by studying endoscopic videos and textbooks prior to it. Critical to this process is the feedback derived from comparing the pathology reports with the endoscopist's histologic predictions based on image interpretation at the time of endoscopy. Though this method has been certainly applied by many image expert pioneers who had to use this self-taught method, it has some limitations. It may be time-consuming with a prolonged learning curve. It does not offer immediate feedback and thus can delay further learning. Mahmood et al. [77] clearly showed that the lack of feedback negatively impacts learning of a new procedure. The other disadvantage could be the high costs of new contrast image methods and delicate equipment, which when used by inexperienced user may have an overall limited use due to a lack of adequate handling.

Thus, learning by self-teaching is overall less acceptable. Therefore, alternative methods to teach image enhancement technologies and gain procedural experience have been developed.

Since expert instructions at academic centers have become available, the most adequate method of learning could be a special mentoring training from the expert endoscopists in the academic centers or designated learning centers setting.

A common option would be to allocate part of the current GI fellowship to acquire image-enhancement knowledge as part of training under the supervision of an expert endoscopist with one-to-one instructions. Traditional standard teaching would include hands-on, supervised one-to-one instructions as the mainstay of contrast enhancement technologies during the learning of traditional endoscopic procedures.

Part of the training would also include the review of the appropriate indications for the use of these new technologies based on the available clinical studies, providing evidence that these new systems have shown to have a clear improvement in clinical practice. The introduction of various atlases written by image experts and available both as a book and online, devoted to each contrast-enhanced technology has been also very beneficial [78,79]. Fellowship training is best suited for teaching the next generation of endoscopic imaging experts and teachers, but is time consuming with a slow (3-year fellowship) rate of integration into practice.

For already practicing gastroenterologists, a specifically designed mentored training could be introduced with comprehensive seminars with hands-on experience, live demonstrations, lectures, hands-on practice, plus advanced image interpretation in designed centers. The disadvantage of this approach is that it requires the physical presence of participants and this may be logistically challenging and cost-prohibitive. The rate of learning new techniques will likely to vary for different applications; for example, Rogart et al. from Yale established that four experienced endoscopists increased their accuracy in small polyp optical histology assessment to 87% over the course of 1 year with an average of 30 cases each. This group did not undergo a formal training program [80].

In both instances, the trainees would also be required to undergo a special training session for image interpretation by reviewing teaching sets of typical patterns of various lesions visualized by various technologies prior to learning the technical aspects of the utilization of these technologies.

This teaching set would provide training physicians with a wide variety of pathologies, then easily recognized during the technical part of learning of these technologies. This could be followed by training set of unknown lesions in which testing of acquired interpretation skill would take place. This could also allow determination of learning curves patterns for learning specific technologies and help in designing special training requirements.

Table 14.1 Methods of training in contrast-enhanced endoscopy.

Training in contrast-enhanced endoscopy
Video and text supplements
Mentored training
CME courses
Tutorials and short courses
Fellowships
Web-based education programs

In addition, over the last decade, there has been an expansion of the number of tools available to enhance the new techniques and medical education in general through Web-based structures. Table 14.1 summarized these various techniques of training in contrast-enhanced endoscopy extending from CME and tutorial course available through Web-based education. These include courses and tutorials offered by national gastrointestinal societies and gastrointestinal journals online. With the wide spread availability of Internet resources, building Web-based systems for training various contrast-enhancement methods could play an important role.

Evidence for effect of training

A recent study by Dinis-Ribeiro et al. [81] evaluated the use of Web-based technologies in assessment of learning curve and reproducibility of a simplified version of gastric magnification chromoendoscopy (MC). As part of a multicenter study, the training of endoscopists and teaching of a new classification was planned using a Web-based system. Endoscopists from various centers were asked to evaluate ten endoscopic videos within an interval of at least 3 days. Over time, the interobserver agreement on the MC classification increased from moderate to excellent. This led to the conclusion that the MC classification is easily explainable and learnable based on the achieved excellent intra- and interobserver agreements in the late phase of the study.

De Lange et al. [82] in their study recorded 2,084 assessments of endoscopic still images and 35 assessments of video. The reliability of the Internet interface was confirmed by adequate repeatability and intraobserver agreement of the assessments. Video running from a DVD were successfully shown on the Internet interface. The investigators concluded that the present Internet-based tool is functional, efficient, and reliable for high-volume assessment of endoscopic images and video.

Furthermore, Web methods permit the inclusion of a large number of participants worldwide, making it an optimal model for teaching the new contrast-enhancement methods and for assessing their general applications.

The introduction of Kudo pit patterns based on various chromoendoscopy methods through various representative images used in expert opinion texts, reviews, and studies is another example of training endoscopists.

Togashi et al. [83] described the learning curve for the correct identification of pit patterns. On the basis of their results, experience with approximately 200 lesions was needed to overcome the learning phase and to maintain sensitivity at the level above 90% with the average sensitivity after 200 lesions of 94.5%. This classification has been broadly investigated in various studies, which showed consistently good sensitivity though with various specificities [4,84]. Its reproducibility has been demonstrated when used among experienced endoscopists [85]. A study by Huang et al. evaluated intra- and interobserver agreement of experienced endoscopists in the assessment of colonic pit patterns when using the Kudo classification. A total of 220 magnification chromoendoscopic pictures of colonic lesions were randomly displayed twice to six experienced endoscopists 1 week apart. Each picture was assessed for predominant pit pattern by using the classification of Kudo. Histopathologic diagnosis also was predicted based on the pit pattern diagnosis. The mean inter- and intraobserver kappa values for experienced endoscopists were very good with values 0.716 and 0.810, respectively. For prediction of histopathology according to the pit pattern diagnosis, the mean inter- and intraobserver kappa values were also very good at 0.776 ($p = 0.001$) and 0.862 (0.069) ($p = 0.028$), respectively.

On the other hand, Meining et al. demonstrated a low interobserver agreement among experts for intestinal metaplasia classifications [86] using magnification endoscopy after contrast enhancement with acetic acid or staining with methylene blue. In that study, four expert gastrointestinal endoscopists in Europe separately analyzed magnification chromendoscopy images of Barrett's esophagus using acetic acid or methylene blue. The interobserver agreement was only fair (kappa = 0.40) for all parameters studied, including the mucosal patterns, methylene blue positive staining, and the presence of specialized intestinal metaplasia. These inconsistencies, along with safety issues, increased cost, and procedure time, have prevented the widespread use of vital dye-staining chromoendoscopy techniques [87].

Interobserver agreement for the classification of mucosal morphology in Barrett's esophagus has also been assessed using NBI among experts and nonexperts. Curvers et al. evaluated the interobserver agreement for the proposed mucosal morphology classification of BE [88,89]. In that study, the interobserver agreement was moderate and did not significantly differ between expert and nonexpert endoscopist (see Video 14.6).

Van den Broek el al. [60] evaluated a combined algorithm of advanced technologies with AFI and NBI for the differentiation of adenomas from nonneoplastic colon polyps among experienced and nonexperienced endoscopists. Still images of 50 polyps were randomly distributed to three experienced and four nonexperienced endoscopists. All images were scored for Kudo classification and AFI images for color. Nonexperienced endoscopist were found to have better interobserver agreement and better accuracy for AFI than for NBI, indicating then AFI may be easier to use for polyp differentiation in nonexperienced setting.

The learning curve for the use of NBI and in particular differentiation of polyps needs to be further established. In the multi-endoscopists study by Adler [43], NBI appeared to increase adenoma detection in the initial phase of the study compared with the white light, but the white light detection has also improved in the later phase of the study, suggesting a possible learning effect of NBI and improved visualization in white-light endoscopy as well.

The learning curves for interpretation of CLE images have been also described in the preliminary reports. Dunbar et al. reported that that highly accurate, efficient in vivo prediction of BE could be achieved after approximately 100 independently performed esophageal CLE procedures [90]. The Mayo group demonstrated the learning curve for interpretation of confocal images of colorectal lesions appeared to be rapid among new users achieving an accuracy of above 80% after only 60 cases [91]. A key difference in these studies was the provision of structured teaching sets of images and immediate one-by-one feedback of the reference standard diagnosis, which may accelerate learning.

The high accuracy and interobserver agreement of pCLE for the detection of Barrett's esophagus with high-grade dysplasia was demonstrated in a recent multicenter pilot study [92].

Summary

Although contrast-enhanced imagining modalities truly represent milestone technologies that may assist in the detection of precursor malignant lesions during endoscopy, they are not yet widely established in the GI community. Chromoendoscopy used in surveillance of high-risk patients may be potentially replaced by virtual chromoendoscopy techniques in view of their easier use. CLE with endoscope-based (eCLE) system or probe-based system (pCLE) can provide instantaneous histopathology in vivo, and this directs further therapeutic decisions.

It is important for these technologies to be further developed and used; however, the requirements for education and training need to be developed simultaneously as well. Large, international, multicenter trails to determine learning curve of each contrast-enhancement technology would be in particular helpful in setting these training requirements. In addition, following the training of these technologies in academic centers by experts, some competency process would need to be established in order to show the full ability of a trainee to detect, characterize lesion, as well as obtain high-quality images using these new technologies. The final applications of these technologies also need to be further formulated based on evidence-based studies.

Videos

Video 14.1 Chromoendoscopy using indigo carmine during surveillance colonoscopy in a patient with long-standing ulcerative colitis

Video 14.2 High definition white light and NBI examination for Barrett's dysplasia

Video 14.3 In vivo polyp classification

Video 14.4 High-resolution endoscopy combined with confocal imaging (pCLE) in assessment of benign colon polyp

Video 14.5 NBI combined with pCLE of low grade dysplasia in Barrett's esophagus with targeted band EMR

Video 14.6 NBI detection of focal dysplasia in Barrett's esophagus using cap examination

References

1 Rex DK, Cutler CS, Lemmel GT, et al.: Colonoscopic miss rates of adenomas determined by back-to-back colonoscopies. *Gastroenterology* 1997;**112**:24–28.

2 Postic G LD, Bickerstaff C, Wallace MB: Colonoscopic miss rates determined by direct comparison of colonoscopy with colon resection specimens. *Am J Gastroenterol* 2002;**97**:3182–3185.

3 Kaltenbach T, Sano Y, Friedland S, Soetikno R: American Gastroenterological Association (AGA) Institute technology assessment on image-enhanced endoscopy. *Gastroenterology* 2008;**134**:327–340.

4 Kudo S, Tamura S, Nakajima T, Yamano H, Kusaka H, Watanabe H: Diagnosis of colorectal tumorous lesions by magnifying endoscopy. *Gastrointest Endosc* 1996;**44**:8–14.

5 Hurlstone DP, McAlindon ME, Sanders DS, Koegh R, Lobo AJ, Cross SS: Further validation of high-magnification chromoscopic-colonoscopy for the detection of intraepithelial neoplasia and colon cancer in ulcerative colitis. *Gastroenterology* 2004;**126**:376–378.

6 Rutter MD, Saunders BP, Schofield G, Forbes A, Price AB, Talbot IC: Pancolonic indigo carmine dye spraying for the detection of dysplasia in ulcerative colitis. *Gut* 2004;**53**:256–260.

7 Kiesslich R, Fritsch J, Holtmann M, et al.: Methylene blue-aided chromoendoscopy for the detection of intraepithelial neoplasia and colon cancer in ulcerative colitis. *Gastroenterology* 2003;**124**:880–888.

8 Itzkowitz SH, Yio X: Inflammation and cancer IV. Colorectal cancer in inflammatory bowel disease: the role of inflammation. *Am J Physiol Gastrointest Liver Physiol* 2004;**287**:G7–G17.

9 Kiesslich R, Neurath MF: Surveillance colonoscopy in ulcerative colitis: magnifying chromoendoscopy in the spotlight. *Gut* 2004;**53**:165–167.

10 Dawsey SM, Fleischer DE, Wang GQ, et al.: Mucosal iodine staining improves endoscopic visualization of squamous dysplasia and squamous cell carcinoma of the esophagus in Linxian, China. *Cancer* 1998;**83**:220–231.

11 Shibuya K, Hoshino H, Chiyo M, et al.: High magnification bronchovideoscopy combined with narrow band imaging could detect capillary loops of angiogenic squamous dysplasia in heavy smokers at high risk for lung cancer. *Thorax* 2003;**58**:989–995.

12 Lim CH, Rotimi O, Dexter SP, Axon AT: Randomized crossover study that used methylene blue or random 4-quadrant biopsy for the diagnosis of dysplasia in Barrett's esophagus. *Gastrointest Endosc* 2006;**64**:195–199.

13 Canto MI, Setrakian S, Petras RE, Blades E, Chak A, Sivak MV, Jr.: Methylene blue selectively stains intestinal metaplasia in Barrett's esophagus. *Gastrointest Endosc* 1996;**44**:1–7.

14 Canto MI, Setrakian S, Willis J, et al.: Methylene blue-directed biopsies improve detection of intestinal metaplasia and dysplasia in Barrett's esophagus. *Gastrointest Endosc* 2000;**51**:560–568.

15 Canto MI, Setrakian S, Willis JE, Chak A, Petras RE, Sivak MV: Methylene blue staining of dysplastic and nondysplastic Barrett's esophagus: an in vivo and ex vivo study. *Endoscopy* 2001;**33**:391–400.

16 Rey JF, Inoue H, Guelrud M: Magnification endoscopy with acetic acid for Barrett's esophagus. *Endoscopy* 2005;**37**:583–586.

17 Fortun PJ, Anagnostopoulos GK, Kaye P, et al.: Acetic acid-enhanced magnification endoscopy in the diagnosis of specialized intestinal metaplasia, dysplasia and early cancer in Barrett's oesophagus. *Aliment Pharmacol Ther* 2006;**23**:735–742.

18 Wo JM, Ray MB, Mayfield-Stokes S, et al.: Comparison of methylene blue-directed biopsies and conventional biopsies in the detection of intestinal metaplasia and dysplasia in Barrett's esophagus: a preliminary study. *Gastrointest Endosc* 2001;**54**:294–301.

19 Sharma P, Weston AP, Topalovski M, Cherian R, Bhattacharyya A, Sampliner RE: Magnification chromoendoscopy for the detection of intestinal metaplasia and dysplasia in Barrett's oesophagus. *Gut* 2003;**52**:24–27.

20 Olliver JR, Wild CP, Sahay P, Dexter S, Hardie LJ: Chromoendoscopy with methylene blue and associated DNA damage in Barrett's oesophagus. *Lancet* 2003;**362**:373–374.

21 Ferguson DD, DeVault KR, Krishna M, Loeb DS, Wolfsen HC, Wallace MB: Enhanced magnification-directed biopsies do not increase the detection of intestinal metaplasia in patients with GERD. *Am J Gastroenterol* 2006;**101**:1611–1616.

22 Amano Y, Kushiyama Y, Ishihara S, et al.: Crystal violet chromoendoscopy with mucosal pit pattern diagnosis is useful for surveillance of short-segment Barrett's esophagus. *Am J Gastroenterol* 2005;**100**:21–26.

23 Hoffman A, Kiesslich R, Bender A, et al.: Acetic acid-guided biopsies after magnifying endoscopy compared with random biopsies in the detection of Barrett's esophagus: a prospective randomized trial with crossover design. *Gastrointest Endosc* 2006;**64**:1–8.

24 Canto MI: Chromoendoscopy and magnifying endoscopy for Barrett's esophagus. *Clin Gastroenterol Hepatol* 2005;**3**:S12–S15.

25 Armstrong D: Review article: towards consistency in the endoscopic diagnosis of Barrett's oesophagus and columnar metaplasia. *Aliment Pharmacol Ther* 2004;**20**(Suppl 5):40–47; discussion 61–62.

26 Yagi K, Aruga Y, Nakamura A, Sekine A, Umezu H: The study of dynamic chemical magnifying endoscopy in gastric neoplasia. *Gastrointest Endosc* 2005;**62**:963–969.

27 Yokoyama A, Ohmori T, Makuuchi H, et al.: Successful screening for early esophageal cancer in alcoholics using endoscopy and mucosa iodine staining. *Cancer* 1995;**76**:928–934.

28 Rembacken BJ, Fujii T, Cairns A, et al.: Flat and depressed colonic neoplasms: a prospective study of 1000 colonoscopies in the UK. *Lancet* 2000;**355**:1211–1214.

29 Kiesslich R, von Bergh M, Hahn M, Hermann G, Jung M: Chromoendoscopy with indigocarmine improves the detection of adenomatous and nonadenomatous lesions in the colon. *Endoscopy* 2001;**33**:1001–1006.

30 Soetikno RM, Kaltenbach T, Rouse RV, et al.: Prevalence of nonpolypoid (flat and depressed) colorectal neoplasms in asymptomatic and symptomatic adults. *JAMA* 2008;**299**:1027–1035.

31 Chiu HM, Chang CY, Chen CC, et al.: A prospective comparative study of narrow-band imaging, chromoendoscopy, and conventional colonoscopy in the diagnosis of colorectal neoplasia. *Gut* 2007;**56**:373–379.

32 Helbig C: Chromoendoscopy and its alternatives for colonoscopy: useful in the United States? *Rev Gastroenterol Disord* 2006;**6**:209–220.

33 Kara MA, Peters FP, Rosmolen WD, et al.: High-resolution endoscopy plus chromoendoscopy or narrow-band imaging in Barrett's esophagus: a prospective randomized crossover study. *Endoscopy* 2005;**37**:929–936.

34 Gono K, Obi T, Yamaguchi M, et al.: Appearance of enhanced tissue features in narrow-band endoscopic imaging. *J Biomed Opt* 2004;**9**:568–577.

35 Wolfsen HC, Crook JE, Krishna M, et al.: Prospective, controlled tandem endoscopy study of narrow band imaging for dysplasia detection in Barrett's esophagus. *Gastroenterology* 2008;**135**:24–31.

36 Curvers WL, van den Broek FJ, Reitsma JB, Dekker E, Bergman JJ: Systematic review of narrow-band imaging for the detection and differentiation of abnormalities in the esophagus and stomach (with video). *Gastrointest Endosc* 2009;**69**:307–317.

37 Pohl J, Nguyen-Tat M, Pech O, May A, Rabenstein T, Ell C: Computed virtual chromoendoscopy for classification of small colorectal lesions: a prospective comparative study. *Am J Gastroenterol* 2008;**103**:562–569.

38 Pohl J, May A, Rabenstein T, Pech O, Ell C: Computed virtual chromoendoscopy: a new tool for enhancing tissue surface structures. *Endoscopy* 2007;**39**:80–83.

39 Lapalus MG, Helbert T, Napoleon B, Rey JF, Houcke P, Ponchon T: Does chromoendoscopy with structure enhancement improve the colonoscopic adenoma detection rate? *Endoscopy* 2006;**38**:444–448.

40 Hirata M, Tanaka S, Oka S, et al.: Magnifying endoscopy with narrow band imaging for diagnosis of colorectal tumors. *Gastrointest Endosc* 2007;**65**:988–995.

41 Su MY, Hsu CM, Ho YP, Chen PC, Lin CJ, Chiu CT: Comparative study of conventional colonoscopy, chromoendoscopy, and narrow-band imaging systems in differential diagnosis of neoplastic and non-neoplastic colonic polyps. *Am J Gastroenterol* 2006;**101**:2711–2716.

42 Rex DK, Helbig CC: High yields of small and flat adenomas with high-definition colonoscopes using either white light or narrow band imaging. *Gastroenterology* 2007;**133**:42–47.

43 Adler A, Pohl H, Papanikolaou IS, et al.: A prospective randomised study on narrow-band imaging versus conventional colonoscopy for adenoma detection: does narrow-band imaging induce a learning effect? *Gut* 2008;**57**:59–64.

44 Dekker E, van den Broek FJ, Reitsma JB, et al.: Narrow-band imaging compared with conventional colonoscopy for the detection of dysplasia in patients with longstanding ulcerative colitis. *Endoscopy* 2007;**39**:216–221.

45 Gress S, Buchner A, Cangemi J, et al.: A prospective randomized back-to-back trial comparing narrow band imaging to conventional colonoscopy for adenoma detection. *Gastroenterology* 2008;**134**:A47–A48.

46 East JE, Suzuki N, Stavrinidis M, Guenther T, Thomas HJ, Saunders BP: Narrow band imaging for colonoscopic surveillance in hereditary non-polyposis colorectal cancer. *Gut* 2008;**57**:65–70.

47 van den Broek FJ, Reitsma JB, Curvers WL, Fockens P, Dekker E: Systematic review of narrow-band imaging for the detection and differentiation of neoplastic and nonneoplastic lesions in the colon (with videos). *Gastrointest Endosc* 2009;**69**:124–135.

48 East JE, Saunders BP: Narrow band imaging at colonoscopy: seeing through a glass darkly or the light of a new dawn? *Expert Rev Gastroenterol Hepatol* 2008;**2**:1–4.

49 Machida H, Sano Y, Hamamoto Y, et al.: Narrow-band imaging in the diagnosis of colorectal mucosal lesions: a pilot study. *Endoscopy* 2004;**36**:1094–1098.

50 East JE, Suzuki N, Saunders BP: Comparison of magnified pit pattern interpretation with narrow band imaging versus chromoendoscopy for diminutive colonic polyps: a pilot study. *Gastrointest Endosc* 2007;**66**:310–316.

51 DaCosta RS, Andersson H, Cirocco M, Marcon NE, Wilson BC. Autofluorescence characterisation of isolated whole crypts and primary cultured human epithelial cells from normal, hyperplastic, and adenomatous colonic mucosa. *J Clin Pathol* 2005;**58**:766–774.

52 DaCosta RS, Wilson BC, Marcon NE: Optical techniques for the endoscopic detection of dysplastic colonic lesions. *Curr Opin Gastroenterol* 2005;**21**:70–79.

53 Wallace M: Advances in endoscopic imaging of Barrett's esophagus. *Gastroenterology* 2006;**131**:699–700.

54 Pohl J, May A, Rabenstein T, et al.: Comparison of computed virtual chromoendoscopy and conventional chromoendoscopy with acetic acid for detection of neoplasia in Barrett's esophagus. *Endoscopy* 2007;**39**:594–598.

55 Pohl J, Nguyen-Tat M, Pech O, May A, Rabenstein T, Ell C: Computed virtual chromoendoscopy for classification of small colorectal lesions: a prospective comparative study. *Am J Gastroenterol* 2008;**103**:562–569.

56 Hoffman A: High definition Plys Colonoscopy combined with I-scan is superior in the detection and characterization of colorectal neoplasia compared to standard videocolonoscopy. A prospective randomized trial. *Gastrointest Endosc* 2009;**69**:AB132.

57 Hoffman A, Kagel C, Goetz M, et al.: Recognition and characterization of small colonic neoplasia with high-definition colonoscopy using i-Scan is as precise as chromoendoscopy. *Dig Liver Dis* 2010;**42**(1):45–50.

58 Hoffman A: High-definition endoscopy (HD+) in conjunction with iScan and chromoednoscopy reliably define minimal change esophagitis in NERD and asymptomatic patients. *Gastrointest Endosc* 2009;**69**:AB344.

59 van den Broek FJ, Fockens P, van Eeden S, et al.: Endoscopic trimodal imaging for surveillance in ulcerative colitis: randomised comparison of high-resolution endoscopy and autofluorescence imaging for neoplasia detection; and evaluation of narrow-band imaging for classification of lesions. *Gut* 2008;**57**:1083–1089.

60 van den Broek FJ, Fockens P, Van Eeden S, et al.: Clinical evaluation of endoscopic trimodal imaging for the detection and differentiation of colonic polyps. *Clin Gastroenterol Hepatol* 2009;**7**:288–295.

61 Curvers WL, Singh R, Song LM, et al.: Endoscopic tri-modal imaging for detection of early neoplasia in Barrett's oesophagus: a multi-centre feasibility study using high-resolution endoscopy, autofluorescence imaging and narrow band imaging incorporated in one endoscopy system. *Gut* 2008;**57**:167–172.

62 Kiesslich R, Burg J, Vieth M, et al.: Confocal laser endoscopy for diagnosing intraepithelial neoplasias and colorectal cancer in vivo. *Gastroenterology* 2004;**127**:706–713.

63 Sakashita M, Inoue H, Kashida H, et al.: Virtual histology of colorectal lesions using laser-scanning confocal microscopy. *Endoscopy* 2003;**35**:1033–1038.

64 Polglase AL, McLaren WJ, Skinner SA, Kiesslich R, Neurath MF, Delaney PM: A fluorescence confocal endomicroscope for in vivo microscopy of the upper- and the lower-GI tract. *Gastrointest Endosc* 2005;**62**:686–695.

65 Kiesslich R, Goetz M, Lammersdorf K, et al.: Chromoscopy-guided endomicroscopy increases the diagnostic yield of intraepithelial neoplasia in ulcerative colitis. *Gastroenterology* 2007;**132**:874–882.

66 Kiesslich R, Gossner L, Goetz M, et al.: In vivo histology of Barrett's esophagus and associated neoplasia by confocal laser endomicroscopy. *Clin Gastroenterol Hepatol* 2006;**4**:979–987.

67 Kiesslich R, Hoffman A, Goetz M, et al.: In vivo diagnosis of collagenous colitis by confocal endomicroscopy. *Gut* 2006;**55**:591–592.

68 Kiesslich R, Goetz M, Burg J, et al.: Diagnosing *Helicobacter pylori* in vivo by confocal laser endoscopy. *Gastroenterology* 2005;**128**:2119–2123.

69 Becker V, Vercauteren T, von Weyhern CH, Prinz C, Schmid RM, Meining A: High-resolution miniprobe-based confocal microscopy in

combination with video mosaicing (with video). *Gastrointest Endosc* 2007;**66**:1001–1007.

70 Meining A, Saur D, Bajbouj M, et al.: In vivo histopathology for detection of gastrointestinal neoplasia with a portable, confocal miniprobe: an examiner blinded analysis. *Clin Gastroenterol Hepatol* 2007;**5**:1261–1267.

71 Hurlstone DP, Tiffin N, Brown SR, Baraza W, Thomson M, Cross SS: In vivo confocal laser scanning chromo-endomicroscopy of colorectal neoplasia: changing the technological paradigm. *Histopathology* 2008;**52**:417–426.

72 Buchner AM, Ghabril MS, Krishna M, Wolfsen HC, Wallace MB: High resolution confocal endomicroscopy probe system for in vivo diagnosis of colorectal neoplasia. *Gastroenterology* 2009;**135**:295.

73 Buchner AM, Shahid MW, Van Den Broek FL, et al.: Probe based confocal laser endomicroscopy (pCLE) in predicting recurrence of colorectal neoplasia after endoscopic mucosal resection. *Gastrointest Endosc* 2009;**69**(5):AB367.

74 Dhar A, Johnson KS, Novelli MR, et al.: Elastic scattering spectroscopy for the diagnosis of colonic lesions: initial results of a novel optical biopsy technique. *Gastrointest Endosc* 2006;**63**:257–261.

75 Goetz M, Fottner C, Schirrmacher E, et al.: In-vivo confocal real-time mini-microscopy in animal models of human inflammatory and neoplastic diseases. *Endoscopy* 2007;**39**:350–356.

76 Hsiung PL, Hardy J, Friedland S, et al.: Detection of colonic dysplasia in vivo using a targeted heptapeptide and confocal microendoscopy. *Nat Med* 2008;**14**:454–458.

77 Mahmood T, Darzi A: The learning curve for a colonoscopy simulator in the absence of any feedback: no feedback, no learning. *Surg Endosc* 2004;**18**:1224–1230.

78 Kiesslich R, Galle PR, Neurath MF (eds): *Atlas of Endomicroscopy.* Heidelberg: Springer, 2008.

79 Cohen J: *Advanced Digestive Endoscopy: Comprehensive Atlas of High resolution Endoscopy and Narrowband Imaging.* Wiley-Blackwell, 2007.

80 Rogart JN, Siddiqui UD, Jamidar PA, Aslanian HR: Fellow involvement may increase adenoma detection rates during colonoscopy. *Am J Gastroenterol* 2008;**103**:2841–2846.

81 Dinis-Ribeiro M, Correia R, Santos C, et al.: Web-based system for training and dissemination of a magnification chromoendoscopy classification. *World J Gastroenterol* 2008;**14**:7086–7092.

82 de Lange T, Svensen AM, Larsen S, Aabakken L: The functionality and reliability of an Internet interface for assessments of endoscopic still images and video clips: distributed research in gastroenterology. *Gastrointest Endosc* 2006;**63**:445–452.

83 Togashi K, Konishi F, Ishizuka T, Sato T, Senba S, Kanazawa K: Efficacy of magnifying endoscopy in the differential diagnosis of neoplastic and non-neoplastic polyps of the large bowel. *Dis Colon Rectum* 1999;**42**:1602–1608.

84 Tung SY, Wu CS, Su MY: Magnifying colonoscopy in differentiating neoplastic from nonneoplastic colorectal lesions. *Am J Gastroenterol* 2001;**96**:2628–2632.

85 Huang Q, Fukami N, Kashida H, et al.: Interobserver and intra-observer consistency in the endoscopic assessment of colonic pit patterns. *Gastrointest Endosc* 2004;**60**:520–526.

86 Meining A, Rosch T, Kiesslich R, Muders M, Sax F, Heldwein W: Inter- and intra-observer variability of magnification chromoendoscopy for detecting specialized intestinal metaplasia at the gastroesophageal junction. *Endoscopy* 2004;**36**:160–164.

87 Canto MI, Kalloo A: Chromoendoscopy for Barrett's esophagus in the twenty-first century: to stain or not to stain? *Gastrointest Endosc* 2006;**64**:200–205.

88 Kara MA, Ennahachi M, Fockens P, ten Kate FJ, Bergman JJ: Detection and classification of the mucosal and vascular patterns (mucosal morphology) in Barrett's esophagus by using narrow band imaging. *Gastrointest Endosc* 2006;**64**:155–166.

89 Curvers WL, Bohmer CJ, Mallant-Hent RC, et al.: Mucosal morphology in Barrett's esophagus: interobserver agreement and role of narrow band imaging. *Endoscopy* 2008;**40**:799–805.

90 Dunbar K, Montgomery E, Canto M: The learning curve for in vivo confocal laser endomicroscopy for prediction of Barrett's esophagus. *Gastroenterology* 2008;**134**:A62–A63.

91 Buchner AM, Gomez V, Gill KR, et al.: The learning curve for in vivo probe based confocal laser endomicroscopy (pCLE) for prediction of colorectal neoplasia. *Gastrointest Endosc* 2009;**69**:AB364.

92 Wallace MB: Accuracy and inter-observer agreement of experts for probe based confocal laser endomicroscopy detection of dysplasia in Barrett's Esophagus. *Gastrointest Endosc* 2009;**69**:AB351.

15 GI Hemostasis

Brian J. Dunkin[1], Kai Matthes[2], & Dennis M. Jensen[3]

[1] The Methodist Hospital, Houston, TX, USA
[2] Beth Israel Deaconess Medical Center, Harvard Medical School, Boston, MA, USA
[3] David Geffen School of Medicine at UCLA, Los Angeles, CA, USA

Introduction

Acute gastrointestinal (GI) bleeding requiring emergency endoscopic intervention is an example of a low frequency, high-risk medical event. The traditional apprentice model of training for such events is often inadequate because of their unpredictable frequency, common occurrence off hours, and high stakes for patient outcome. Similar problems occur in other specialties in medicine such as the management of cardiac rhythm disturbances or traumatic injury. This has led to the development of the Advanced Cardiac Life Support (ACLS) and Advanced Trauma Life Support (ATLS) programs to help health care professionals better prepare for these infrequent events. Both programs allow learners to rehearse resuscitation scenarios outside of the clinical environment until proper management is learned. A similar type of program would be useful for training in the management of acute GI bleeding.

When learning about the endoscopic management of GI bleeding, the number of disease processes and potential sources seems daunting. However, if these disease processes are categorized by general anatomy, location, type of blood supply, and focality, similarities in endoscopic treatments become apparent and the list becomes less extensive (Table 15.1). Further focus can be gained by concentrating on the available endoscopic management strategies for GI bleeding, which fall into only three categories—injection, thermal, and mechanical. The trainee should concentrate their efforts first on understanding the lesions that bleed and their type of blood supply and then on these three management strategies.

This chapter focuses on defining the processes and techniques of learning the skills required to successfully achieve endoscopic GI hemostasis. It does not explore indications for the procedures or efficacy as this material is typically covered in a general textbook of gastroenterology. Instead, the chapter describes how one trains in endoscopic hemostatic techniques by outlining both the prerequisite and necessary knowledge and technical skills required to become proficient. The appropriate setting to learn hemostatic strategies is also discussed as are the benefits and limitations of simulators, current hemostasis guidelines, and use of additional learning tools and aids. Finally, assessment of competency in endoscopic hemostasis and maintenance of skills is reviewed.

Hemostasis as defined in this chapter is the cessation of active bleeding and prevention of rebleeding with an endoscopic intervention. The medical management of GI bleeding, while critically important, is not the focus of this discussion.

Prerequisite cognitive knowledge required prior to learning endoscopic hemostatic techniques

The first step to becoming proficient in endoscopic hemostasis begins with acquiring a solid knowledge base about the pathophysiology and clinical presentation of GI bleeding. This knowledge is gained through reading textbooks of gastroenterology, reviewing pertinent literature, and participating in postgraduate medical training focused on diseases of the GI tract. Such knowledge is critical so that the endoscopist embarking on endoscopically gaining GI hemostasis can generate a differential diagnosis that will guide the therapeutic plan. The following examples illustrate the importance of this differential:

Example 1: A 55-year-old cirrhotic patient presents with hematemesis and melena.

A knowledgeable endoscopist should suspect this patient to have a lesion related to portal hypertension, such as esophageal or gastric varices, or a Mallory Weiss tear [1]. He or she will further know that bleeding from these lesions is venous and therefore band ligation, sclerotherapy, or injection of glue (cyanoacrylate) may be necessary (Table 15.2). The GI team can thus be instructed to equip the endoscopy cart with the proper supplies and be prepared to use them. The endoscopist will also realize that airway protection strategies are important to prevent aspiration of blood and that there may be a large amount of blood and clot encountered during the procedure that will require various strategies to remove so the bleeding source can be identified. He or she may consequently elect to perform the procedure in the ICU with tracheal intubation and the GI team might want to bring special endoscopes, irrigators, or accessory devices to remove blood clot. Finally, once the procedure is underway, the endoscopist must communicate closely with the

Successful Training in Gastrointestinal Endoscopy, First Edition. Edited by Jonathan Cohen.
© 2011 Blackwell Publishing Ltd. Published 2011 by Blackwell Publishing Ltd.

Table 15.1 Sources of GI hemorrhage categorized by location.

Esophagus	Varices
	Mallory–Weiss tear
	Esophagitis
	Ulcer
	Mass
	Postsurgical
	Postendoscopic intervention
Stomach	Varices
	Ulcer
	Dieulafoy
	Mass
	Arteriovenous malformation
	Postsurgical
	Postendoscopic intervention
Duodenum	Ulcer
	Arteriovenous malformation
	Mass
	Postsurgical
	Postendoscopic intervention
Small bowel	Ulcer
	Arteriovenous malformation
	Mass
	Postsurgical
Colon	Diverticulum
	Mass
	Arteriovenous malformation
	Hemorrhoids
	Postendoscopic intervention
	Postsurgical

GI team to ensure proper use of sedation and accurate application of hemostatic devices.

Example 2: A 65-year-old patient with multiple comorbidities presents with painless melena, hypotension, and severe anemia while on aspirin and clopidogrel.

The knowledgeable endoscopist will know that the most likely diagnosis is an aspirin-induced ulcer and will expect to find some stigmata of recent hemorrhage (SRH) during the procedure. He or she will further understand that the method of hemostasis used and the likelihood of rebleeding after the procedure are guided by these SRH, which might include active arterial bleeding, a non-bleeding visible vessel (NBVV), an adherent clot, oozing bleeding without other SRH, or a flat spot [2]. It is much less likely that this patient has a UGI cancer, varices, an angioma syndrome, or a diffuse lesion such as esophagitis. The endoscopist must be prepared to perform emergency endoscopy with a therapeutic gastroscope that has a large accessory channel to control active bleeding and prevent rebleeding. He or she will further understand that the source of bleeding is likely arterial and that combination therapy beginning with injection of dilute epinephrine (1:20,000 dilution in saline) followed by thermal coagulation or hemoclipping is the most effective way to gain hemostasis (Table 15.2) [2,3,4].

Example 3: A 70-year-old patient presents with severe hematochezia, hypotension, and anemia.

A knowledgeable endoscopist knows that an urgent colonoscopy after purge is recommended [5,6]. An UGI source should be considered for those patients with cirrhosis, a history of hematemesis or melena, a positive nasogastric aspirate, and for all patients who develop severe hematochezia as inpatients [5,6]. In contrast, for the elderly patient who started to have hematochezia while out of the hospital, the more likely location of the lesion is the colon and the differential diagnosis of lesions includes, in descending order of prevalence, diverticulosis, ischemia, internal hemorrhoids, rectal ulcers, colitis, delayed postpolypectomy ulcer (if recent polypectomy), or an angioma syndrome [5–7]. Urgent colonoscopy and treatment of focal lesions is recommended after thorough cleansing of the colon with purge to remove all clots, blood, and stool. Lesions that are amenable to colonoscopic hemostasis include those with underlying arteries and SRH (definitive diverticular bleeds and ulcers of any type), angioma syndromes (radiation or angiodysplasia), or venous-type bleeding (internal hemorrhoids). The three general types of endoscopic accessories that will be required for treatment of this spectrum of colon lesions are thermal probes, hemoclips with or without epinephrine injection, or banding (for bleeding internal hemorrhoids).

These examples illustrate the in-depth knowledge base required to generate an accurate differential diagnosis for GI bleeding and to prepare the proper equipment and team to successfully manage the problem. Obtaining this knowledge is a prerequisite to embarking on learning the technical aspects of endoscopically controlling GI hemorrhage.

Prerequisite technical knowledge and skills required to learn endoscopic hemostatic techniques

Emergency endoscopic hemostasis is an advanced procedure and should not be attempted by a novice endoscopist. Once the cognitive aspects about sources of bleeding discussed above are mastered, substantial technical knowledge and skill related to the procedure are still required. Requisite knowledge includes understanding the proper setup and function of the endoscopic equipment, such as a standard gastroscope, therapeutic gastroscope (single and double channel), duodenoscope, and colonoscope. A thorough knowledge of proper strategies for the safe administration of moderate sedation is also required, including careful airway management to prevent aspiration. Finally, at least a basic understanding of the principles of electrosurgery is assumed, although a more thorough review is critical to successful and safe hemostatic technique.

Prerequisite technical skills include the safe administration of moderate sedation and the ability to not only minimize the risk of aspiration, but also to apply airway rescue management strategies such as the use of oral airway adjuncts and the ability to bag ventilate and intubate a patient if necessary. Mastery of basic endoscopic manipulation is also required. This can be better understood if the

Table 15.2 CURE hemostasis group basic guide to anatomy, type of blood supply, and location of hemostasis.

General anatomy	Type of blood supply	Usual locations	Usual stigmata of recent hemorrhage (SRH)	Treatment
Ulcers (peptic, ischemic, infections, postsurgical, post-EMR)	Arterial	All GI	Any SRH	Combo
Dieulafoy's lesion	Arterial	UGI	Spurting, NBVV	Combo
Mallory–Weiss tears	Arterial (unless with portal hypertension)	GEJ	Ooze, spurt, clot, or clean	HC if no PHTN, RBL/sclero if PHTN
Ulcerated polyps or PPIUs	Arterial	All GI	Any SRH	Resect polyp; Combo—PPIU
Varices	Venous	UGI (colon, anastomoses)	Spurting, clot, NBVV, or none	RBL or Sclero Rx
Internal hemorrhoids	Venous	Rectum	Ooze or none	RBL
Angioma Syndromes (OWR, WMS, XRT, angiodysplasia, and idiopathic angiomas)	AVM	All GI	Oozing, clot, spot, or clean lesions	Thermal—MPEC, HP, or APC
Cancers—ulcerated	Neovascularity	All GI	Oozing	Possible hemoclipping and tattooing, surgery
Inflammatory lesions (esophagitis, celiac disease, or colitis)	Capillaries	All GI	Oozing	Medical
Infections	Capillaries	All GI	Oozing	Medical

Abbreviations: SRH, stigmata of recent hemorrhage; NBVV, nonbleeding visible vessel; EMR, endoscopic mucosal resection; RBL, rubber band ligation; HP, heater probe; Combo, combination injection of epinephrine and either MPEC/HP or hemoclipping; PPIU, postpolypectomy induced ulcer; AVM, arteriovenous malformation; GEJ, gastroesophageal junction; PHTN, portal hypertension; OWR, Osler Weber Rendu syndrome; WMS, watermelon stomach or gastric vascular ectasia (GAVE); XRT, radiation telangiectasia.

skill is deconstructed into component steps. Both upper and lower endoscopy requires a common skill set that includes the ability to provide scope traversal, four-way tip deflection, and torque to deliver the endoscope to the desired location. It also requires the correct use of insufflation to properly identify lesions and access various areas of the GI tract. Targeting is another critical skill that enables the practitioner to deliver the endoscopic tool to the lesion of interest with proper orientation (see Video 15.1). Upper endoscopy requires the additional skill of being able to traverse a sphincter. Finally, an endoscopist must be able to communicate well with the rest of the endoscopic team in order to provide advanced therapies.

Any practitioner who is embarking on a training program to learn endoscopic hemostasis is assumed to have all of the above technical knowledge and skills.

Required technical knowledge and skills to be proficient in endoscopic hemostasis

While the knowledge required to understand the pathophysiology of all causes of GI bleeding and the proper medical management is rather broad, the knowledge and skills required to actually perform endoscopic hemostatic maneuvers is rather concentrated into particular areas. It is easiest to understand these areas if the tasks are broken down into their component parts with common strategies. Each of these strategies requires a specific fund of knowledge and technical skill to be properly applied.

Common knowledge and skills for all hemostatic strategies

Knowledge

No matter what hemostatic strategy is to be applied or what source of GI bleeding treated, there is a common knowledge base required to perform endoscopic hemostasis. This certainly begins with a thorough understanding of the most common GI lesions, their anatomy, and their vascular supply (Table 15.2), but also includes a familiarity with the endoscopic devices [8]. It is not adequate to rely on the endoscopic assistant for an understanding of the proper use, deployment, or manufacturing differences of the various devices used for endoscopic hemostasis. An expert endoscopist should understand the proper use of all devices better than anyone else on the endoscopy team. They should also examine new technologies as these are developed and continuously survey the literature to keep up to date on the efficacy and safety of devices and strategies. In addition, trainees must develop the pattern recognition skills to correctly identify the SRH for the various etiologies and locations of bleeding within the GI tract and understand both the prognostic significance and the appropriate management decisions for each one that is encountered (Figure 15.1).

Skill

Common skills sets for endoscopic hemostasis include those described in the prerequisites above. In addition, an ability to

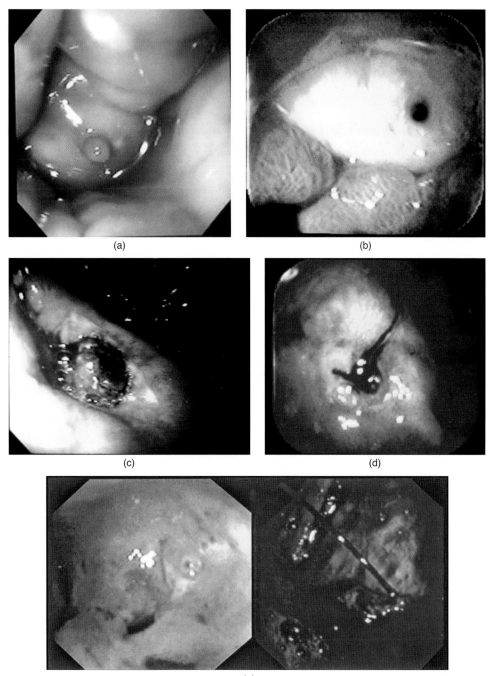

Figure 15.1 Stigmata of recent hemorrhage. (a) "Nipple sign" platelet plug on esophageal varix. (b) Ulcer with flat black spot. (c) Ulcer with adherent clot. (d) Ulcer with active oozing. (e) Ulcer with pearly clear visible vessel in the 2:00 position with subsequent spurting observed 3 days later after failure to recognize and coagulate this stigmata of recent hemorrhage (SRH). Trainees must learn to recognize, correctly identify, and understand how properly to respond to stigmata that have been associated with particular prognostic implications for various GI bleeding lesions.

use different strategies to clear the endoscopic field of blood is essential. Such strategies include use of power irrigation systems and endoscopes with large bore accessory channels. A standard upper endoscope typically has a 2.8 mm accessory channel, whereas a therapeutic upper endoscope will have a 3.7 mm or 3.8 mm accessory channel depending on the manufacturer. An

adult colonoscope typically has a 3.7–3.8 mm accessory channel but can increase to 4.2 mm. Modern therapeutic duodenoscopes have a 4.2 mm accessory channel. The larger channel therapeutic upper endoscopes and colonoscopes also have a separate port for water jet irrigation operated by a pump and separate foot pedal. Use of a snare to remove an adherent clot is another skill required

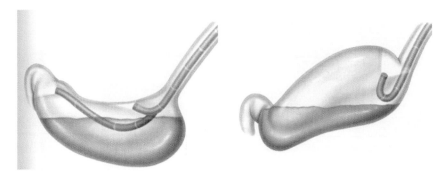

Figure 15.2 Effect of changing patient position on gastric liquid. On the left is the stomach with fluid for the patient in the left-side down position. The fundus and upper stomach are obscured by blood or fluid. Rotation of the patient to the right-side down position after protection of the airway by intubation or an endoscopic overtube usually moves blood, fluid, and clots to the antrum. This allows the endoscopist to visualize and treat bleeding lesions such as gastric varices, ulcers, or Dieulafoy's lesions in the upper stomach [2].

for gaining endoscopic hemostasis. Also, changing patient position can aid in the examination of different areas of the GI tract. When performing upper endoscopy in the standard left lateral position, gastric fluid will pool in the fundus and possibly obscure the cardia. By rolling the patient into right lateral position, the fluid and clots will usually move toward the antrum, leaving a clearer view of the fundus and cardia (Figure 15.2). Elevation of the thorax to 45° or more and protection of the airway with an over tube or intubation beforehand are recommended prior to such maneuvering to prevent aspiration. This simple strategy can be very effective in identifying a bleeding source in the stomach during emergency endoscopy.

The ability to effectively communicate with the rest of the endoscopy team is also critical in the successful endoscopic management of GI bleeding, particularly during emergency procedures. Proper use of the endoscopic accessories requires coordination with the assistant while the patient's nurse carefully monitors sedation and airway protection. A pre-brief of the management plan is extremely helpful prior to introducing the endoscope and a rehearsal use of equipment that is unfamiliar to the team is also critical before starting the procedure. As a rule of thumb, such pre-procedure planning will involve making sure that sufficient supplies will be available and that the team is prepared for the use of more than one hemostasis modality in the event that a back-up plan is needed.

Specific hemostatic strategies

Injection

Knowledge

The most common method of gaining initial hemostasis is by injection of a drug (e.g., vasoactive or sclerosant) with a sclerotherapy needle (Figure 15.3). Understanding what substance to inject for different lesions, where to inject it (e.g., intravariceal or paravariceal), and the complications of injection is critical. One common example is the use of epinephrine—the most common substance injected for nonvariceal bleeding. It is typically used at 1:10,000 or 1:20,000 concentrations, but may be diluted more with saline if lower concentrations are desired. It is injected into the submucosal layer or directly into the base of the ulcer around the SRH, typically in four quadrants. Common side effects are transient tachycardia and hypertension. Table 15.3 lists substances used for injection into bleeding lesions [48].

Skill

One of the reasons injection therapy is so common is that it is technically easy to perform with little chance for an adverse event, at least with dilute epinephrine or other vasoactive injectants. The skills required to perform sclerotherapy include an ability to pass the device down the working channel, deliver it to the target, and

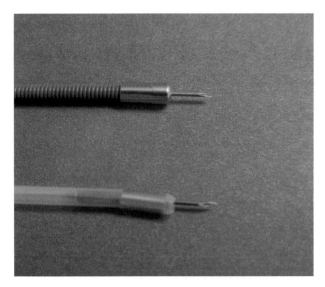

Figure 15.3 Sclerotherapy needle. A type of injector needle for nonvariceal hemostasis or variceal sclerotherapy.

Table 15.3 Injectables for endoscopic hemostasis.

	Nonvariceal lesions with SRH	Varices
Epinephrine (1:10,000 or more dilute)	Yes	No
Ethanol 99.5%	Yes	Yes
Hypertonic (50%) dextrose	Yes	No
Plidochanol 0.5–3%	Yes	Yes
Ethanolamine oleate 5%	No	Yes
Sodium morrhuate 5%	No	Yes
Sodium tetradecyl sulfate 1% or 3%	No	Yes

insert the needle into the desired tissue plane. Communication with the assistant for deployment of the needle and injection of the sclerosant is critical (see Video 15.2).

Thermal

Knowledge

Applying thermal energy to a bleeding lesion either alone or in combination with epinephrine injection therapy is another common strategy for endoscopic hemostasis [2]. A thorough knowledge of the principles of electrosurgery is critical for this technique. A comprehensive review of this topic is beyond the scope of this chapter and included in a separate chapter in this book, but a basic understanding of the types of electrosurgical energy will be reviewed.

Cauterizing a lesion with electromechanical energy (electrocautery) can be achieved by applying an alternating electrical current via a device to the target tissue. Patients are not "shocked" by this energy the way they would be by coming into contact with a common wall outlet because it is delivered at a very high frequency in the radio wave spectrum (radiofrequency). All electrocautery requires a complete circuit to be delivered to the desired tissue. There are essentially two ways to complete this circuit. Monopolar electrocautery completes the circuit by the electrical current passing through the patient to a grounding pad or plate and back to the generator (Figure 15.4). Bipolar or multipolar electrocautery (MPEC) passes through the effected tissue only (Figure 15.5).

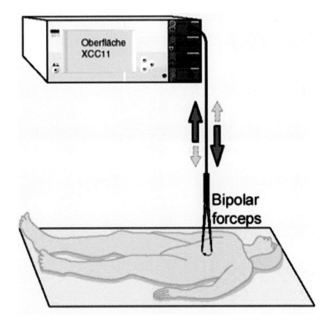

Figure 15.5 Bipolar or multipolar electrocautery. Current passes around the tip of the probe or (forceps) from one plate (or jaw) to the other and back to the generator. A grounding pad is not required and superficial coagulation results. (Reproduced with permission from ERBE USA Inc.)

Monopolar electrocautery can penetrate deeply into tissues and is effective for hemostasis, but risks deep thermal injury and possible perforation in thin-walled structures. Bipolar energy does not penetrate as deeply, but may be less effective in gaining hemostasis, unless pressure is applied [2]. A thorough knowledge of these principles along with proper energy settings on the generator used for electrocautery is critical for the safe application of this technology (see Tables 15.6–15.8).

Argon plasma coagulation (APC) is a special version of monopolar electrocautery that requires additional understanding. Argon gas, when "electrified," converts to plasma that will conduct monopolar current. APC is very useful in situations where it is desirable to apply electrocautery to large surface areas without touching the tissue. This prevents build up of debrides on the probe tip and allows for the expeditious "painting" of large areas, such as in watermelon stomach or angiodysplasia (Figure 15.6). Understanding the unique energy settings and argon gas flow rates for operating an APC probe is essential. Being mindful to constantly aspirate the argon gas from the GI tract is also important. Limitations of APC for GI hemostasis must also be understood. For example, touching the electrode tip directly to the tissue results in monopolar coagulation and risks deep tissue injury. In addition, coaptive coagulation (applying pressure with the electrocautery probe to collapse the walls of the bleeding vessel together for sealing) is not possible with APC, which limits its hemostasis application to AVMs or oozing bleeding from very small arteries [2].

Another method of applying thermal energy to tissue in the GI tract is with a heater probe. This device heats up rapidly and transfers a preselected amount of heat across a Teflon-tipped probe to the tissue. The heater probe does not apply electrocautery to the

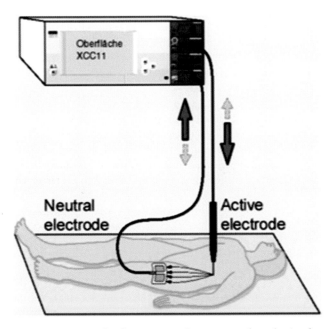

Figure 15.4 Monopolar electrocautery. Current passes from the tip of the electrode, through the patient, to the grounding pad and back to the grounded generator. A grounding pad is required and deep tissue injury may occur. This is also the type of radiofrequency monopolar generator and current for APC. (Reproduced with permission from ERBE USA Inc.)

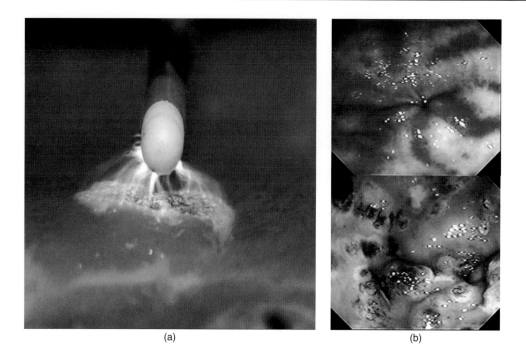

(a)   (b)

Figure 15.6 (a) Argon plasma coagulation (APC). Non-touch technique with APC. Refer also to Figure 15.4. A grounding pad is required and, if tissue is touched with the tip of the catheter, monopolar coagulation (which may be deep) occurs. (b) Gastric antral vascular ectasia (GAVE) pre- and post-APC treatment painting all visible stripes with noncontact thermal coagulation (see Videos 15.6 and 15.7).

tissue, but cauterizes it by generating heat at its tip. Deep tissue injury is possible if repeated pulses are applied. Understanding the energy settings for different types of lesions, the size of probe to use, methods of irrigation, and conformity of the tip are all important (Table 15.6).

Skill

Application of a heater probe or electrocautery device by touching the probe tip to the tissue is called contact coagulation. When using these devices in the upper GI tract for hemostasis, it is best to apply the principle of coaptive coagulation (Figure 15.7) (see Video 15.3). This technique requires applying the thermal device directly on the actively bleeding site or SRH with enough pressure to stop the bleeding by interrupting blood flow in the underlying vessel and collapsing its walls against each other [2]. When the heat or electrocautery is applied, the vessel walls seal together and hemostasis is achieved. Having the skill to deliver the thermal device to the target with the proper angle and force is a necessary skill for effective thermal hemostasis and coaptive coagulation [2]. To do this requires the ability to keep the endoscope in a stable position with the probe tip close to the endoscope tip to maximize the ability to apply firm and steady pressure.

Mechanical

Knowledge

The third general method of gaining endoscopic hemostasis is mechanical ligation. This is done with an endoscopic hemoclip, banding device, or ligating loop. There are different manufactur-

ers for these devices, so it is essential to become familiar with the design and function of each (see Video 15.4). In addition, the knowledge required to place endoscopic clips includes the principle of working distal to proximal on a lesion so as not to cross clips that have already been applied and risk dislodging them, and a desire to apply the clip as perpendicular to the target as possible. A successful strategy in applying hemoclips to nonvariceal lesions with underlying arteries (see Table 15.2) is to place one hemoclip well into the submucosa at 45–75° on each side of the SRH [2]. This has been shown by Doppler ultrasound probe (DUP) and clinical outcomes studies to substantially reduce rebleeding [3,10].

The required knowledge for proper endoscopic band placement on esophageal varices is similar with a distal to proximal application and knowledge of stigmata of recent variceal hemorrhage that will aid in directing where to apply the bands most effectively.

Skill

The skill set required to place an endoscopic clip includes proper introduction into the working channel without dislodging the clip and proper application to the target by changing the angle of both the endoscope and clip so as to be as perpendicular to the target as possible (see Video 15.5). Endoscopic bands are usually applied using a device capable of delivering multiple bands without reintroduction of the endoscope (see Videos 15.8 and 15.9). All banding devices fit over the tip of the endoscope, extending beyond the tip by 1–1$^1/_2$ cm and resulting in "tunnel vision." As a result, an additional skill required for endoscopic banding is the ability to pass the endoscope with the banding device attached through the oropharynx and upper esophageal sphincter safely.

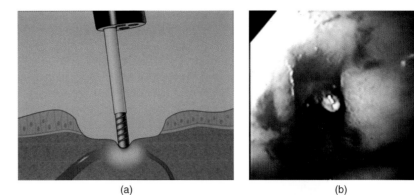

(a)   (b)

(c)

Figure 15.7 (a) Coaptive coagulation. Firm pressure (tamponade) to stop active bleeding and interrupt the blood flow of the underlying artery is first applied. Then coagulation (MPEC) or heat (heater probe) for long pulse duration. Utilizing the large thermal probes (heater or MPEC probes) will coagulate tissue and can weld the walls of underlying arteries as large as 2 mm together (Reproduced from Jensen DM, Machicado GA: Endoscopic hemostasis of ulcer hemorrhage with injection, thermal, or combination methods. Tech Gastrointest Endosc 2005;7:124131, with permission from Elsevier.). (b) Visible vessel pre-coaptive and (c) post-coaptive coagulation with bipolar probe.

Ligating loops, which may be utilized for bleeding from polypectomy stalks or areas of endoscopic mucosal resection (EMR), work similar to a polypectomy snare. The skill set required for proper application is an ability to deliver the device around the tissue of interest. Good communication with the assistant is mandatory for proper application of loops so that it is closed snuggly around the lesion while taking great care to not overtighten and cause accidental cold guillotine or transection.

Simulators to learn and practice endoscopic hemostasis

GI and surgical endoscopy fellows typically acquire knowledge in endoscopic hemostasis by performing clinical cases under the supervision of their endoscopy teacher. This mode of education does not always allow for learning in a calm, controlled environment or the opportunity to obtain timely and comprehensive feedback. In critical clinical situations, patient instability may require the supervising physician to take over the procedure. The frequency of exposure to patients with acute GI hemorrhage may also vary significantly from one training institution to another. With the development of more realistic simulator technology, intensive hands-on instruction in hemostasis techniques using a simulated environment may overcome some of these limitations of standard bedside training.

The initial introduction of videoendoscopy to replace fiberoptic systems has been an important aid in clinical teaching, enabling the entire team to see what the endoscopist sees [9]. Use of this technology to provide live endoscopy courses, interactive teaching programs, and video tapes can help trainees to better recognize pathology and understand the appropriate application of therapeutic techniques. However, such passive activities cannot replace the performance of actual procedures with real-time personal feedback from an experienced tutor. This is especially applicable when new techniques are practiced for the first time [11,12].

Simulation of GI hemorrhage provides the opportunity to practice endoscopic hemostasis without the risk of patient harm and free from time limitations. Various models have been developed to simulate an acute bleeding source in the UGI tract in order to evaluate the feasibility of new endoscopic devices or to practice interventional techniques in a calm and controlled environment.

Available models of endoscopic hemostasis

Virtual reality simulators

Computer simulators may play an important role in the early phase of endoscopic training, especially for first steps in colonoscopy [13–24]. However, for the close-to-reality training of complex therapeutic interventions, such as endoscopic hemostasis techniques, computer simulators still require improvement. In addition, virtual instruments differ considerably from real ones. The GI mentor II (Simbionix USA Inc., Cleveland, OH, USA) includes ten cases of upper GI hemorrhage. The Accu Touch Simulator (CAE, Montreal, Quebec, Canada) provides a simulated case of postpolypectomy bleeding. There is currently no reported scientific data about the use of virtual reality simulation for endoscopic hemostasis. In the future, computer- and Web-based simulator technology has the potential to reinforce the cognitive instruction about image interpretation, accessories, and generator settings, as well as review management approaches to particular scenarios using interactive quizzes integrated with multimedia displays. At present, such opportunities are essentially limited to direct interaction with a live mentor.

In vivo large animal models of upper GI hemorrhage

While large animal porcine and canine models have been used to train interventional endoscopic retrograde cholangiopancreatography (ERCP) and endoscopic ultrasound (EUS) [25–27], these in vivo models have had limited utility for the simulation of GI hemorrhage. Such live animal models do not afford the ability to reproduce desired pathological lesions or SRH. While certain basic techniques such as application of electrocautery devices and clipping of normal tissue can be performed, the cost and ethical concerns of utilizing live animals solely for hemostasis training mitigate against this practice when comparable education may now be achieved using other simulators. For these reasons, live animal models in hemostasis are currently used in research studies to evaluate the efficacy of new devices and pharmaceutical agents, rather than for the purpose of training in interventional endoscopy.

Ex vivo models of GI hemorrhage

Because of the limitations of live animal models described above, *ex vivo* models for the simulation of esophageal varices and nonvariceal hemorrhage have been developed. The Erlangen active training simulator for interventional endoscopy (EASIE, CompactEASIE® (Erlangen, Germany), the EASIE-R (Endosim LLC, Berlin, MA, USA), Endo X Trainer™ (Medical Innovations International, Rochester, MN, USA), and Endo Eddie (Delegge Medical, Mount Pleasant, SC, USA) are four related models prepared from explanted porcine organs for teaching endoscopic hemostasis [28–32]. In these models, porcine UGI organ packages including esophagus, stomach, and duodenum are cleaned thoroughly and placed into a special simulator mold. A perfusion system is used to simulate arterial bleeding by sewing a conduit (portion of splenic artery or latex or polyvinylchloride tubing) into the wall of the stomach and connecting this to an artificial blood circuit (Figure 15.8). While this roller pump mechanism can simulate pulsatile arterial bleeding, a simplified model can be made by manual injection of "virtual blood" using saline with red food coloring. Artificial (nonbleeding) varices in this model are created by longitudinal submucosal injection of stained saline with a 23-gauge needle. Several of these *ex vivo* models are available commercially for purchase or rental, and tissue packages can be shipped for local use.

Artificial tissue models

The artificial tissue models developed by Grund and colleagues at the University of Tübingen have been utilized for the specific hemostasis technique of APC. Theoretically, the method of incorporating artificial arteries using the method described above in *ex vivo* animal tissue models is possible with this model to simulate arterial bleeding. The Grund model is not available commercially and there have been no published data validating its use in training for hemostasis.

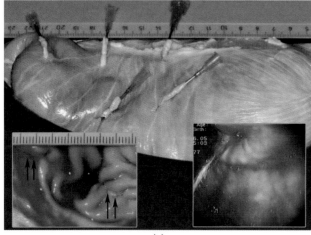

(a)

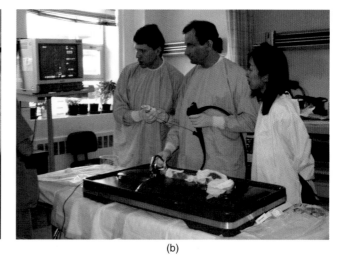

(b)

Figure 15.8 (a) Compact EASIE simulator hemostasis setup with rubber tubing sutured into the anterior stomach wall and connected to a 60 mL Luer-lock syringe to deliver artificial blood. Image of the porcine *ex vivo* specimen for the training of endoscopic hemostasis in the EASIE® model. Shown are sewn-in vessels from outside as well as from inside (detailed pictures). The left lower image displays the orifice of the vessels. The right image shows the endoscopic view of a bleeding simulation before treatment. This resembles a Dieulafoy's lesion, in soft, nonulcerated tissue. (b) *Ex vivo* hemostasis workshop sponsored by the NYSGE. Trainee practices clip application on simulator in concert with assistant in relaxed environment. This allows repetitive risk-free practice in communication as well as technical skills with opportunity for expert feedback and instruction.

Teaching in endoscopic hemostasis

Key components of hemostasis to teach

The EASIE team training concept for hemostasis was first described by Hochberger et al. in 2001 [33]. It consists of a four-block sequence. First, trainees are evaluated individually on the model to assess their baseline hemostasis skills. This allows detection of both deficiencies in theoretical knowledge as well as practical skills in order to adjust the workshop according to the skill level of the trainees. The second block is the workshop itself, which consists of expert demonstration on the model of correct technique, followed by hands-on practice and feedback from experienced endoscopy instructors. This takes approximately 30–45 minutes per fellow per technique. The third block is the post-training evaluation on the simulator to assess the improvement of performance after training. The final block consists of post-evaluation feedback from the instructor with final recommendations about common mistakes observed during the post-training evaluation. Trainees benefit particularly from this last section of constructive criticism and recommendations relevant to their clinical application of hemostasis techniques. An essential element of this training program is the hands-on instruction and individual critique of technique coupled with significant time for practice on the simulator [33].

Data supporting the role of hemostasis training on simulators

Two studies have been done evaluating the role of simulation in GI hemostasis training—one in New York and the other in France. Each used *ex vivo* simulation in the curriculum of GI endoscopy fellows, with the study group receiving intense *ex vivo* simulation training in UGI hemorrhage and the control group having no *ex vivo* simulation experience [34,35].

The data in the New York study demonstrated that even a single 1-day EASIE®-training session significantly improved the performance on the simulator of four important hemostasis techniques. The results of the final evaluation revealed that three full-day EASIE®-workshops during a 7-month period allowed the members of the intensive training group to develop hemostasis skills, as assessed on the model, that were significantly better than their baseline abilities. In contrast, the fellows in the control group, who received only conventional endoscopy education at their home hospitals, did not improve significantly over the 7-month period, except for their performance of variceal band ligation [34].

The analysis of actual clinical performance in clinical bleeding cases of 50% of the participants from the control group and 69% from the intensive training group in the New York study supported the finding that fellows with access to intensive simulator training performed better on clinical cases. In terms of overall clinical performance, intensive group fellows had significantly higher hemostasis success rates and fewer complications. This limited amount of postsimulator work outcome data remains the only prospective demonstration of the benefit of simulator hemostasis training on real clinical performance.

In the French study [35], the intensive EASIE training group improved significantly over baseline in all training subjects ($p < 0.001$), whereas the control group showed interval improvement in only two disciplines (manuals skills $p = 0.02$, injection/coagulation $p = 0.013$). In this study, a direct skills comparison between simulator-trained and control groups at the end of the study showed that the simulator group performed significantly better than their control group peers in all disciplines ($p < 0.001$). The results of both studies are shown in Table 15.4.

Learning progress in endoscopic hemostasis

Both the New York and French studies provided valuable insight into learning patterns of endoscopic hemostasis by GI fellows.

Table 15.4 Comparison of longitudinal progress of simulator-trained GI-fellows in French and American training projects.

		American study			French study		
		(a) Baseline evaluation ($n = 14$)*	(b) Final (blinded) evaluation ($n = 13$)*	(a)–(b) p-value[†]	(c) Baseline evaluation ($n = 12$)*	(d) Final (blinded) evaluation ($n = 12$)*	(c)–(d) p-value[†]
Manual skills	Overall score*[‡]	4.5 (3.0−6.25)	8.0 (7.0−9.0)	0.004	4.0 (2.75−6.0)	8.00 (5.25−8.0)	0.004
Injection and coagulation	Overall score*[‡]	4.3 (3.6−5.2)	7.0 (6.0−7.7)	0.002	4.6 (3.2−4.95)	8.1 (7.05−8.55)	0.002
	Successful hemostasis	8/14 (57%)	12/13 (92%)	0.102	1/12 (8%)	12/12 (100%)	0.001
Clip application	Overall score*[‡]	1.0 (1.0−1.0)	7.6 (6.0−8.4)	0.001	4.6 (3.25−5.06)	6.80 (5.75−7.95)	0.001
	Successful hemostasis	0/14 (0%)	8/13 (62%)	0.005	1/12 (8%)	9/12 (75%)	0.005
Variceal ligation	Overall score*[‡]	1.0 (1.0−1.0)	8.3 (7.9−8.8)	0.002	5.67 (4.33− 6.5)	9.50 (8.33−10.0)	0.002
	Successful hemostasis	3/14 (21%)	13/13 (92%)	0.007	8/12 (63%)	10/12 (83%)	0.180

*Median and interquartile range, [†]Wilcoxon test, [‡]ordinary scale: 1, worst performance; 10, best performance.

Both groups showed comparable learning curves and learning progress despite the differences in the educational systems and endoscopic background [34,35]. The New York fellows had no clinical experience in hemoclip application and variceal ligation, whereas the French fellows had varying clinical experience in these two techniques before the studies began. Despite these differences, participants of both groups showed significant improvements in clip application and injection/coagulation at the end of the first training, which improved further until the end of both studies. However, in variceal ligation, French and American GI fellows achieved maximum overall scores after only one training workshop and this level was sustained until the end of both projects. This fact emphasizes that training programs require adaptation to the complexity of various endoscopic techniques. More complex techniques (e.g., reusable clip loading and application) require repeated training sessions to produce a steady state level of skill, whereas easier techniques (e.g., band ligation) may be taught effectively even in a single training workshop. Simulators like the Compact EASIE® may prove most beneficial as a training tool for those interventional skills that require repetitive practice and larger procedure volumes than may occur naturally during the course of standard GI endoscopy training.

Concept of integrating simulator work into standard endoscopy training

Similar to the simulator education of commercial pilots, which occurs both before and during their actual flight experience, these validation studies for the CompactEASIE workshops were completely integrated into the fellows' standard experience with supervised clinical endoscopy. The studies demonstrated that the fellows enrolled in the New York study were able to achieve a significantly better hemostasis rate with fewer complications in comparison to the control group receiving solely clinical education in endoscopic hemostasis [34]. In general, the benefit of EASIE training is viewed primarily as an adjunct to actual supervised hemostasis experience and not as a substitute for it.

More data are needed to confirm that hands-on simulator training improves outcomes on clinical endoscopic performances in GI hemostasis, as well as to better characterize the influence of such simulator work on subsequent endoscopic practice (i.e., attempted hemostasis, choice of therapeutic modalities).

Maintaining skills in endoscopic hemostasis

There is little doubt that the knowledge learned from hands-on courses decreases with time. Little is known about the volume of hemostasis cases needed to maintain technical skills and continue to achieve good outcomes.

Experience in endoscopic hemostasis and exposure to clinical cases varies significantly from program to program and may be limited especially for gastroenterologists with predominantly outpatient practices. The logs of clinical hemostasis cases by fellows in the Hochberger study illustrate this great variability [34]. For example, while fellows in the simulator training group performed a median of 14.0 hemostasis cases over 7 months, there was a wide interquartile range of 7.5–25.0.

The hemostasis skills of practicing gastroenterologists without repetitive training in this technique may be insufficient to maintain competency. While simulator training has the potential to facilitate skills maintenance in hemostasis for individuals already in practice as well as to teach individuals in practice how to use new devices, there are no data yet that confirm this benefit or describe how often such refresher courses are needed.

Additional teaching aides for learning GI hemostasis

In training programs for GI fellows, surgical endoscopists, and new faculty, additional aides are recommended to teach about the diagnosis and treatment of GI bleeding. These include atlases, case videos, and lectures by members of an experienced GI bleeding team on diagnosis, techniques, adjunctive management (medical, surgical, and/or interventional radiology (IR)), and outcomes. Table 15.5 contains a more comprehensive list of other adjuncts to the teaching of lesion-specific diagnosis and hemostasis.

Having skilled GI attendings present with trainees on every diagnostic and therapeutic case to provide one-on-one teaching is the best way to learn and master GI techniques, especially management of GI hemostasis emergencies. Learning centers and workshops on accessories and techniques at GI meetings now include models and endoscopic simulators for endoscopists to practice new techniques. These are an important adjunct to bedside teaching of both GI endoscopists and staff who assist them. A recent example is the introduction of new endoscopic hemoclips into clinical practice. Local, regional, and national hands-on practice in learning centers, such as that of the American Society for Gastrointestinal Endoscopy (ASGE), have been helpful to introduce endoscopists to this new technology.

Atlases focused on GI bleeding can facilitate teaching of GI fellows, new faculty, or GI assistants about specific lesions and their underlying type of vasculature (e.g., vein, artery, AVM, or neovascularity). When actual case examples are included, illustrated, and explained with labels and text, each hemostasis technique can be more readily understood. Although few such detailed atlases are available, the CURE (Center for Ulcer Research and Education) Hemostasis Group has recently produced one on hemoclipping and a more expansive version is in preparation [36].

Treatment guidelines generated through studies or by consensus from medical societies can be helpful in guiding the novice endoscopist in management of GI hemorrhage. Specific treatment guidelines have been developed and tested clinically by a few groups. Two examples are for thermal coagulation and

Table 15.5 Teaching aides for hemostasis and their usefulness.

What	Goals and utility
+ GI hemostasis team attending	+ Bedside teaching of trainees on every case by skilled experts
+ Learning centers and workshops on hemostasis accessories (Local, ASGE, GI models and simulators)	+ Familiarize trainees, endoscopists, and staff with new techniques or accessories
+ Atlas on GI bleeding (such as CURE-BSC Hemoclipping Atlas)	+ Teach anatomy and diagnosis, such as SRH
+ Treatment guidelines (such as CURE Group guidelines on accessory probe or generator settings for nonvariceal GI bleeding)	+ Help standardize treatments and potentially improve outcomes
+ Participation in GI hemostasis research studies or electives in GI hemostasis	+ Learn techniques under expert guidance, define new guidelines, and improve outcomes
+ Attend live therapeutic endoscopy courses	+ Although GI bleeding emergency cases are uncommonly included, new techniques for elective cases may be taught by an expert

hemoclipping (Tables 15.6–15.8). The CURE Hemostasis Group guidelines were based upon prospective bench to bedside published results in animal models, clinical pilot and feasibility studies, cohort studies, and randomized controlled trials (RCTs). These guidelines are useful for guiding treatment of specific bleeding GI lesions based upon the underlying type of blood flow and visual SRH.

Participation in GI hemostasis research studies or clinical electives or rotations by trainees and staff, and elective rotations in GI hemostasis during GI fellowship are both ways to increase the number and kind of experience for GI fellows or new GI faculty

in management of GI bleeding. This is particularly important for new members of a GI bleeding team.

Attending live video therapeutic endoscopy courses may help experienced endoscopists polish and refine their own techniques. Watching experts will also help some to learn about the effectiveness and limitations of GI hemostasis techniques. True emergency cases of GI bleeding are rare in live courses because of the inability to schedule such emergencies for daytime viewing. Supplementation of such teaching by prerecorded videos of emergency hemostasis cases is a helpful alternative. Such video cases are also part of the ASGE learning center (www.asge.org) and available

Table 15.6 CURE MPEC settings for nonvariceal UGI hemostasis.

Multipolar coagulation (Gold probe)	Peptic ulcer			Dieulafoy's lesion		Mallory–Weiss tear
	Active bleeding	Nonbleeding visible vessel	Adherent clot	Active bleeding	Nonbleeding visible vessel	Active bleeding
Probe size	Large	Large	Large	Large	Large	Large or small
Pressure	Very firm	Very firm	Firm	Firm	Firm	Moderate
Power setting (watts)	12–16	12–16	12–16	12–16	12–16	12–14
Pulse duration	10	10	10	10	10	2
End point	Bleeding stops, vessel flat and white; DUP	Visible vessel flat and white; DUP	NBVV or clot remnant flat and white; DUP	Bleeding stops, vessel flat and white; DUP	Visible vessel flat and white; DUP	Bleeding stops, vessel flat and white; DUP

Settings and guidelines for ulcer, Dieulafoy's lesion, and Mallory–Weiss tear (without portal hypertension) treatment

This table summarizes the guidelines for endoscopic hemostasis of nonvariceal UGI lesions for control of active bleeding or prevention of rebleeding with multipolar probe coagulation (MPEC).

The guidelines are based upon randomized laboratory study results and clinical prospective studies of bleeding UGI ulcers and other nonvariceal lesions.

For chronic ulcers and large lesions, large MPEC probes (e.g., 10 Fr size) yield better hemostatic results than small probes (7 Fr).

For coaptive coagulation of chronic ulcers with major stigmata of hemorrhage, moderate tamponade directly on the stigmata of recent hemorrhage—SRH (such as an NBVV) to interrupt arterial blood flow prior to coagulation, at a low power setting (about 12 W) and long duration pulses (i.e., 7–10 s), will control active bleeding, and prevent rebleeding in most patients with severe UGI bleeding.

If available, utilize a Doppler ultrasound probe (DUP) before endoscopic hemostasis of SRH, and if positive at baseline, recheck to confirm absence of arterial flow under the SRH after standard endoscopic hemostasis. This will reduce rebleeding.

Table 15.7 CURE guidelines for hemoclipping with or without injection of nonvariceal UGI lesions.*

Lesions	Ulcers	Dieulafoy's				PPIU	MW tear[†]
Stigmata[‡]	Spurting	NBVV	Adherent Clot[§]	Oozing		Flat spot	Active bleed
Preinject epi[¶]	Yes	If coagulopathy	Yes and shave down	No		No	If severe bleeding
Other prep**	Target wash	DUP	DUP	Wash, use DUP		Rx if +DUP	No
Where HC[††]	Across spurter	Across NBVV	Across 2–4 mm pedicle	Across oozer		Across spot	Across MW tear
HCs	≥2	1–2	≥2	1–2		1–2	2–4
End point(s)[‡‡]	Control bleeding, DUP	HC NBVV, DUP and no rebleed	HC pedicle or NBVV DUP	Stop ooze DUP		DUP	Stop bleed, zipper close MW tear
Med Rx[§§]	High-dose IV PPI	High-dose IV PPI	High-dose IV PPI	BID PPI		BID PPI	Antiemetic and PPI BID

*In this table are the CURE Hemostasis Group's guidelines with hemoclips (HC) for hemostasis of nonvariceal UGI lesions including ulcers, Dieulafoy's lesion, postpolypectomy induced ulcers (PPIUs), and Mallory–Weiss (MW) tears (without portal hypertension).

[†]For MW tears, only active bleeding is an indication for endoscopic treatment, because the bleeding stops, unless the patient has portal hypertension and esophageal varices.

[‡]The specific stigmata of recent hemorrhage (SRH), which are indications for endoscopic hemostasis, are for all lesions except MW tears include spurting, nonbleeding visible vessel (NBVV), adherent clot, and oozing as well as flat spots if Doppler ultrasound probe (DUP) indicates blood flow underneath.

[§]Target washing with a water jet is recommended to clear the lesion of blood or clots and verify the SRH.

[¶]Preinjection with epinephrine is recommended for spurting and adherent clot. This should also be considered with other stigmata, if severe coagulopathy is present. Shave down adherent clots with a cold, rotatable snare after preinjection with epinephrine.

**Recheck SRH with DUP for blood flow after initial endoscopic hemostasis. If there is still blood flow, further hemoclipping with or without epinephrine injection is warranted

[††]Hemoclips are placed across the focal spurter, NBVV, or pedicle of the clot (after shaving it down with a rotatable snare).

[‡‡]The endpoints of endoscopic hemostasis are control of active bleeding and placement of 1–2 hemoclips across the SRH to prevent rebleeding and obliterate blood flow as monitored by DUP.

[§§]Medical therapy is high-dose PPIs for all SRH except oozing and flat spots.

online through the DAVE Project (Digital Atlas of Video Education, www.daveproject.org).

Limitations of GI endoscopy for diagnosis and hemostasis of GI bleeding: teaching pearls for troubleshooting and challenges for the future

Table 15.9 itemizes some of the current problem areas for all GI endoscopists who perform emergency or elective hemostasis. New GI endoscopists should be instructed about the limitations and potential solutions now and in the future. In most cases, simulators have not been applied to help in development of potential solutions to these problems, but rather are limited to introducing endoscopists to new accessories and their potential clinical applications. Recent examples of the latter include training for use of the BioVac™ direct suction device (US Endoscopy, Mentor, OH, USA) for removal of liquid clots by bypassing the suction channel in the umbilicus of the endoscope and draining directly into a suction canister, a combination injector and snare (iSnare®, US Endoscopy, Mentor, OH, USA) for combination injection and cold guillotining of adherent clots or treatment of polyps; the injection-MPEC probe for combination treatments of ulcers with SRH (Injection Gold Probe™, Boston Scientific Corp., Boston,

MA, USA); and the rotatable snare for shaving down adherent clots on GI lesions after epinephrine preinjection with a separate needle catheter.

A particularly vexing problem for all endoscopists who manage GI bleeding is the evacuation of blood clot that is obscuring the bleeding site, particularly in the fundus of the stomach. Various clot removal techniques are available, but none are consistently successful. Older methods include the use of large orogastric tubes (e.g., Ewald tube) or simply changing the patient's position to move the clot out of the way (Figure 15.1). Newer techniques include use of a therapeutic endoscope with a large suction channel (e.g., Olympus gastroscope "Clot buster") or double channel therapeutic gastroscopes (from Olympus or Pentax), the BioVac™ direct suction device, and an over-the-endoscope rail system for introduction of high volume irrigation and supplemental suctioning (Clear Path™, EasyGlide, Ltd., Kfar Truman, Israel). The Clear Path™ and BioVac™ devices are still being evaluated and are not yet standard of care.

There is a need for better promotility drugs than erythromycin or metaclopramide to help empty the foregut of clots. Erythromycin and metaclopramide have been studied and have mixed results on improving visualization, but none have reported improvement in clinical outcomes of UGI bleeding [37,38].

Table 15.8 CURE settings and guidelines for MPEC hemostasis of bleeding colonic lesions*

Multipolar coagulation (Gold probe)	Angiomas or radiation telangiectasia		Postpolypectomy, diverticulosis, focal ulcer, or solitary rectal ulcer		
	Active bleeding[†]	Nonbleeding	Active bleeding[†]	Nonbleeding visible vessel (NBVV)	Adherent clot[†]
Probe size[‡§]	Large	Large or small	Large	Large	Large
Pressure[¶]	Light	Light	Moderate	Moderate	Moderate
Power setting (watts)*	10–14	10–14	12–16	12–16	12–16
Pulse duration (s)	1	1	1–2	1–2	1–2
End points**	Bleeding stops; DUP	White coagulum; DUP	Bleeding stops, vessel flat; DUP	Flatten NBVV; DUP	Flatten and whiten vessel; DUP

*These are general guidelines that were developed from laboratory and clinical prospective studies. Power, pressure, and pulse duration should be reduced for small or deep colonic lesions. Repeated coagulation on the same point of a flat lesion such as an angioma will cause transmural coagulation and increase the risk of perforation. The CURE Hemostasis Research Group recommends checking probes for heating or coagulation prior to endoscopic application.

[†]Preinjection with 1:10,000 epinephrine in four quadrants around the actively bleeding lesion or clot pedicle is recommended, then cold guillotine off the clot to shave it down to 2–4 mm above attachment before multipolar coagulation.

[‡]Small diameter colonoscopes with a large diameter suction channel (3.7–3.8 mm) are recommended for all colonoscopies on patients with severe lower GI hemorrhage. These facilitate suctioning and allow the endoscopist to pass a large diameter coagulation probe (3.2 mm diameter). Large diameter probes are recommended for treatment of all actively bleeding lesions and for treatment of angioma or radiation telangiectasia >3 mm in diameter.

[§]Small diameter thermal probes (~2.4 mm diameter) have less washing capacity, have less volume of coagulation, and are more likely to bend with passage through a colonoscope. These are recommended for coagulation of small angiomata or radiation telangiectasia.

[¶]Pressure can be exerted en face or tangentially directly on the bleeding or nonbleeding lesion. In the colon, firm tamponade with the coagulation probes and colonic distension should be avoided, because these will increase the risk of complications related to transmural coagulation.

**The end point for actively bleeding lesions is acute hemostasis. However, repeated coagulation to the same point to control oozing from angiomas and to achieve a totally dry field may be unnecessary and will increase the risk of transmural injury. Check stigmata of recent hemorrhage (SRH) with Doppler ultrasound probe (DUP) at baseline and after initial hemostasis. After initial endoscopic hemostasis based on visual cues, apply hemoclips or further thermal if arterial blood flow is still detected under the SRH by DUP. This will significantly reduce rebleeding.

For patients with severe hematochezia and clots in the colon, the best technique is to pre-emptively cleanse the colon and to remove all clots, blood, and stool by rapid purge before performing urgent colonoscopy [5–7]. A practical recommendation is to check the rectal effluent at the bedside to confirm that it is clear before starting the procedure. If it is not clear, then give more purge (and if needed for nausea metoclopramide IV) before the colonoscopy [5–7]. Bedside instruction is currently the only way to teach endoscopic treatment of lower GI bleeding as no adequate models yet exist to mimic clinically severe hematochezia. *Ex vivo* simulators developed for training in colonoscopic therapeutic techniques are described later in this volume and have the potential to reproduce the problem of a colonic lumen obscured by blood.

Adherent clots on lesions obscuring the underlying SRH have recently been simulated in a new endoscopic model created by industry (US Endoscopy, Mentor, OH, USA) and is being used in national and international workshops. Techniques for safe clot removal can now be practiced by experienced or new endoscopists for this common SRH.

CURE guidelines for the endoscopic management of adherent clots have been validated in RCTs [2,39,40]. The CURE Hemostasis Group's recommendation is to first inject epinephrine (1:20,000 dilution), then cold snare guillotining of the clot to shave it down (without cautery), and finally treatment of the underlying pedicle

or SRH with hemoclipping or thermal coagulation (Table 15.7). Two recent US RCTs have documented the effectiveness, safety, and improvement in clinical outcomes by utilizing this type of combination treatment for adherent clots and SRH with severe ulcer hemorrhage [39,40]. As a further modification of diagnosis and treatment, a new DUP [2,7] can also be utilized to detect blood flow under the clot. This device can be used before deciding to treat (e.g., for risk stratification) and during endoscopic treatment to confirm and complete successful hemostasis (e.g., obliteration of underlying blood flow). For ulcer hemorrhage where high-dose PPIs are an alternative to endoscopic treatment, this is feasible [41] if underlying blood flow is negative [42]. Further RCTs of DUP for risk stratification and as an adjunct to treatment of lesions with clots or other SRH are warranted.

It is often difficult to find or target bleeding lesions in the GI tract because of awkward location. Gaining adequate access may require a different endoscope, such as a side viewing duodenoscope or a newer oblique viewing endoscope (prototypes by Olympus and Pentax). These endoscopes have "elevators" that can change the direction of attack of the accessory as it exits the working channel and thus facilitate targeted treatments in difficult-to-approach lesions. Visualization and targeting may also be disrupted because of hypermotility of the bowel or brisk bleeding. Glucagon will slow gut peristalsis. A large channel therapeutic endoscope with

Table 15.9 Challenges for GI hemostasis and potential solutions.

Problem	Potential solutions
Clots	
Large placental clots and blood	Large channel endoscopes, BioVac and Clear Path "rail"-type suction; better promotility agents; liquefy clots, change position of patient, and clot
Adherent clot on lesion	Epi injection, cold guillotine, and treat pedicle; I-snare; DUP to risk stratify first
Access to lesion	
Preparation endoscope	Oblique endoscopes with elevators
	Large volume irrigation
Failures of hemostasis	
Initial	Combination therapies
	Newer hemoclips
	DUP to confirm hemostasis
	Cyanoacrylate or detachable loops and sclerosants (for gastric varices)
Rebleeding	Epinephrine and hemoclipping
	Suturing devices
	Bear claw
Role of IR	Need RCT to assess for treatment of failures of endoscopic hemostasis or severe rebleeds
New adjunctive medical therapies (high-risk patients)	Foregut-IV PPI infusion and/or octreotide Colon need nanoparticles or adhesives to prevent delayed bleeding
Anticoagulants for comorbidities (Warfarin, aspirin, clopidogrel)	Need RCT of lesion closure (to promote healing) after successful endoscopic hemostasis or new healing

Abbreviations: DUP, Doppler ultrasound probe; Epi, epinephrine; bear claw, a toothed device that can be used endoscopically to clamp bleeding ulcers or nonvariceal lesions; IR, interventional radiology; RCT, randomized controlled trials; IV PPI, intravenous proton pump inhibitor; BioVac™ direct suction device (US Endoscopy, Mentor, OH), a suction device that bypasses umbilical cord of endoscope to facilitate suctioning of clots, blood, and fluids; iSnare® (US Endoscopy, Mentor, OH), combined retractable needle injector and snare.

water jet irrigation and injection of lesions with dilute (1:20,000 in saline) epinephrine (for nonvariceal lesions) or sclerosant injection (such as ethanolamine oleate with or without ethanol for varices) will improve visualization in cases of active arterial ulcer bleeding or active variceal bleeding.

While instruments and accessories can be demonstrated in workshops and practiced in models, most of these clinical access problems and potential solutions require actual clinical cases.

Bleeding gastric varices can be difficult to manage endoscopically. Cyanoacrylate glue has been used for large bleeding gastric varices, but is not FDA approved and subsequently not com-

monly used in the United States. What may facilitate endoscopic hemostasis and more widespread treatment of gastric varices in US centers is a detachable loop for initial tamponade of bleeding and stoppage of venous inflow and outflow, and then injection of a sclerosant to obliterate the GV [43]. Definitive hemostasis could be monitored by DUP, and obliteration of varix blood flow documented at endoscopy [44]. These techniques are experimental and further endoscopic improvements are warranted.

The role of IR in nonvariceal hemostasis requires a reassessment. This is particularly applicable to lesions with large arteries such as posterior duodenal ulcers, tumors, and Dieulafoy's lesions, either after failure of initial endoscopic hemostasis or with severe rebleeding from these endoscopically documented and treated lesions. Although a large RCT from Hong Kong established the superiority of repeat endoscopic hemostasis rather than emergency surgery for severe ulcer rebleeding [45], similar clinical trials have never been reported for IR when severe bleeding from ulcers or other nonvariceal lesions cannot be controlled endoscopically. With the aging of the population, increasing prevalence of serious comorbidities, and higher risks for emergency surgery, alternatives such as emergency IR performed by skilled radiologists are often recommended, but supportive outcomes data on relative effectiveness, safety, and cost are not yet available. Clinical experience and RCTs will be required to advance our knowledge about IR for rebleeding or refractory bleeding.

Definition of minimal thresholds for determining competency in endoscopic hemostasis

More than 30 years ago, an ASGE task force on endoscopic training directed by Jack Vennes, MD, investigated and formulated guidelines for competency of different GI procedures, including elective and emergency GI hemostasis [46]. These guidelines were based on "expert opinion" and standard practice at the time, but not on objective data nor prospective studies or RCTs. Observation data based upon teaching endoscopic hemostasis in large animals to trained, experienced endoscopists was also incorporated. The guidelines were advanced by the ASGE and since then have been utilized as minimal thresholds in some GI fellowship training programs. They are also often used by GI Quality Insurance (QI) Committees of hospitals and practices for initial credentialing. These guidelines have been supplemented and updated over the years as new procedures have been developed. However, none of them have ever been validated as confirming "competency," clinical effectiveness, or safety; nor have they been investigated for accurately measuring these qualities in new trainees; or for assessing competency for "recredentialing."

The UCLA QI adaptations of the ASGE guidelines of minimal thresholds for assessing competence in GI hemostasis cases are shown in Table 15.10 [46]. These attending supervised cases are usually performed during GI or surgical endoscopy fellowship, are documented in endoscopic training logbooks, and are reviewed and confirmed by fellowship directors. Letters of recommendation and confirmation of training, as well as safety issues

Table 15.10 Current UCLA guidelines for minimal thresholds for assessing competence of faculty for GI hemostasis procedures.

GI hemostasis procedure	Number of supervised cases required
Hemorrhoid ablation	15
Elective hemostasis	
Angiomas or polyp	15
Thermal coagulation	
Emergency and elective UGI hemostasis	
Variceal	15 with 5 emergencies
Ulcers, Mallory–Weiss tears, Dieulafoy's	15 with 5 emergencies
Colon GI hemostasis	15 with 5 emergencies

Source: Adapted from ASGE and modified by the UCLA QI Committee [46].

and complications (if any) are typically reviewed by the Hospital Chief of Staff's office and GI QI committees prior to granting GI procedure privileges. Proctoring of selected cases may be required of new GI endoscopists (including new faculty), prior to granting full privileges to perform GI hemostasis cases. Prior to granting these procedures, the new faculty or GI endoscopist must have documented competency to perform routine and emergency colonoscopy, upper endoscopy, push enteroscopy, flexible sigmoidoscopy, and anoscopy.

In July 2007, the American College of Graduate Medical Education (ACGME) published similar guidelines for GI hemostasis fellowship training as "General Program Requirements for Fellowship Education in Gastroenterology" [47]. What they mandated to satisfy ACGME requirements for training in GI hemostasis during GI fellowship was supervised training for 25 (elective or emergency) nonvariceal GI hemorrhage cases (UGI or Colon) with any hemostasis modality, including ten cases with "active bleeding." This includes oozing GI bleeding, which is not a high-risk SRH [1,2]. For variceal hemorrhage, 20 supervised cases of variceal hemostasis are required, including five with active variceal bleeding. There are no documented requirements by the ACGME for urgent colonoscopy, colonoscopic hemostasis, hemorrhoid ablation, nor push enteroscopy with or without endoscopic hemostasis [47]. The ACGME reportedly will establish new guidelines in 2011, which will depend more on certification of "competency" of the GI fellow by GI fellowship or endoscopy training director rather than quantitative minimal thresholds for assessing competency. New, non-quantitative standards for competency will present a major challenge for GI QI committees in assessing the true competency of newly graduated GI fellows who are applying for GI hemostasis privileges from different institutions.

To date there have been no systematic, prospective, or randomized studies to document whether any published minimal thresholds for assessing competency are adequate or accurate enough to measure true competency and safety in GI hemostasis. Nor are there studies that document whether training on simulators reduces the numbers of clinical cases to reach competency.

These standards have depended upon "expert opinion" rather than objective measures to estimate minimal thresholds of assessing competency in GI hemostasis [46,47]. The development and assessment of new standards and instruments to measure individual competency in performing GI hemostasis procedures are strongly recommended.

Requirements to maintain endoscopic hemostasis skills

There are no validated standards on what the minimal requirements should be to maintain endoscopic hemostasis skills. Common practice and hospital credentialing depend upon GI QI committees to set such minimal standards. These vary regionally and with the type of hospital. At the Ronald Reagan UCLA Medical Center, endoscopists must renew their privileges every 2 years. The criteria for renewal are maintenance of active hospital admitting and attending staff privileges, attending on and performance of these GI procedures regularly in their GI practice, and performing independently a minimum of 12 sedated cases per year in the UCLA medical procedure units or hospital intensive care units. To maintain emergency GI hemostasis privileges, the physician must document performance of at least five such cases per year at UCLA and/or the affiliated hospitals. If the GI endoscopist applies for new GI hemostasis privileges, they must document their training and experience, including their safe and effective performance of the minimal number of cases to assess competency (see Table 15.10). Proctoring by another faculty member of the GI hemostasis team for each type of new hemostasis procedure is then required. The ASGE has a document that outlines key elements of how such a proctoring program may facilitate the credentialing process (www.asge.org), although it is uncertain how many institutions take advantage of these guidelines.

Similar to initial determination of competency for elective and emergency GI hemostasis procedures, further studies are warranted to determine the best methods to measure and document continued competency. This is particularly an area of controversy for GI endoscopists who infrequently perform emergency GI hemostasis procedures, but want to move to a different practice setting in the same hospital where these are required. For example, those who were previously trained but were away from clinical GI procedures for a few years and desire to renew their GI endoscopy privileges pose a common problem to GI QI committees. Practice on simulators of new or current GI hemostasis techniques (such as hemoclipping) and enrolling in a GI hemostasis elective or rotation to cover emergencies may be necessary for them to renew and improve their skills, as well as to demonstrate competency. Subsequent proctoring by other experienced endoscopists will assure fair peer review and satisfy GI QI requirements.

Summary

Endoscopic management of GI bleeding is an advanced procedure that may seem daunting to the novice. However, with proper preparation and a systematic categorization of both the source of bleeding and the techniques used to control it, the necessary knowledge base and technical skills can be mastered. Various simulation platforms, particularly using explanted tissue, can be helpful in gaining this mastery, although validated criteria for obtaining and maintaining procedural competence in this area are still lacking.

Videos

Video 15.1 Manual skills

Video 15.2 Simulation and teaching of endoscopic hemostasis

Video 15.3 Demonstration of the principle of blood vessel coaptation to achieve hemostasis endoscopically

Video 15.4 Simulation-based demonstration of available clips and their proper deployment

Video 15.5 Tips for clips: demonstrating proper technique and common errors on the EASIE *ex vivo* model

Video 15.6 Principle and technique of APC demonstrated on the Tübingen Phantom Model Live Broadcast from NYSGE Annual Course

Video 15.7 Radiation telengiectasias: treatment with APC

Video 15.8 Multiband ligation: steps of set-up and deployment

Video 15.9 Demonstration of multiband ligation of internal hemorrhoids

Video 1.1 The EASIE hemostasis ex vivo training workshop

Video 7.13 Pancreatic wire-assisted cannulation

Video 14.5 NBI combined with pCLE of low grade dysplasia in Barrett's esophagus with targeted band EMR

Video 30.1 Ampullectomy

Video 30.3 ES bleed

Video 30.4 Management of immediate bleeding during cap EMR

Video 33.1 Endofest 2010

References

1 Kovacs TOG, Jensen DM: Endoscopic treatment of acute esophageal variceal bleeding. *Drugs Today* 2000;**36**:339–353.

2 Jensen DM, Machicado GA: Endoscopic hemostasis of ulcer hemorrhage with injection, thermal, or combination methods. *Tech Gastrointest Endosc* 2005;**7**:124–131.

3 Jensen DM, Kovacs TOG, Ohning GV, Jutabha R, Machicado GA, Dulai GS: Hemostasis of very high risk patients with severe non-variceal UGI hemorrhage comparing injection-hemoclipping with injection-MPEC. *Gastrointest Endosc* 2008;**67**;AB106:882.

4 Jensen DM, Stuart R, Ahlbom H, et al.: Re-assessment of re-bleeding of Forrest IB (oozing) peptic ulcer bleeding (PUB). *Gut* **58**(Suppl 2):A92:OP439.

5 Jensen DM, Machicado GA: Colonoscopy and severe hematochezia. In: Waye JD, Rex DW, Williams CB (eds), *Colonoscopy—Principles and Practice*, 2 nd edn. London: Blackwell Sciences, 2009:631–645.

6 Kovacs TOG, Jensen DM: Upper or small bowel hemorrhage presenting as hematochezia. *Tech Gastrointest Endosc* 2001;**3**:206–215.

7 Jensen DM, Machicado GA: Colonoscopy for diagnosis and treatment of severe lower gastrointestinal bleeding: routine outcomes and cost analysis. *Gastrointest Endosc Clin N Am* 1997;**7**:477–498.

8 Nelson DB, Barkun AN, Block KP, et al.: ASGE technology status evaluation report: endoscopic hemostatic devices. *Gastrointest Endosc* 2001;**54**:833–840.

9 Carr-Locke DL: Videoendoscopy in clinical application. Impact on teaching. *Endoscopy* 1990;**22**(Suppl 1):19–21.

10 Jensen DM, Ohning G, Kovacs TOG, Jutabha R, Machicado GA, Dulai G: Doppler ultrasound probe (DUP) for risk stratification and endoscopic hemostasis of bleeding colonic lesions. *Gastrointest Endosc* 2009;**69**:AB289 (T1411).

11 Carr-Locke DL, Gostout CJ, Van Dam J: A guideline for live endoscopy courses: an ASGE white paper. *Gastrointest Endosc* 2001;**53**:685–688.

12 Deviere J, Hochberger J, Neuhaus H, et al.: Recommendations of the ESGE workshop on ethical, clinical, and economic dilemmas arising from the implementation of new techniques. First European symposium on ethics in gastroenterology and digestive endoscopy, Kos, Greece, June 2003. *Endoscopy* 2003;**35**:768–771.

13 Sedlack RE, Kolars JC: Computer simulator training enhances the competency of gastroenterology fellows at colonoscopy: results of a pilot study. *Am J Gastroenterol* 2004;**99**:33–37.

14 Dunkin BJ: Flexible endoscopy simulators. *Semin Laparosc Surg* 2003;**10**:29–35.

15 MacDonald J, Ketchum J, Williams RG, Rogers LQ: A lay person versus a trained endoscopist: can the preop endoscopy simulator detect a difference? *Surg Endosc* 2003;**17**:896–898.

16 Ladas SD, Malfertheiner P, Axon A: An introductory course for training in endoscopy. *Dig Dis* 2002;**20**:242–245.

17 Bar-Meir S: A new endoscopic simulator. *Endoscopy* 2000;**32**:898–900.

18 Aabakken L, Adamsen S, Kruse A: Performance of a colonoscopy simulator: experience from a hands-on endoscopy course. *Endoscopy* 2000;**32**:911–913.

19 Ferlitsch A, Glauninger P, Gupper A, et al.: Evaluation of a virtual endoscopy simulator for training in gastrointestinal endoscopy. *Endoscopy* 2002;**34**:698–702.

20 Datta V, Mandalia M, Mackay S, Darzi A: The PreOp flexible sigmoidoscopy trainer. Validation and early evaluation of a virtual reality based system. *Surg Endosc* 2002;**16**:1459–1463.

21 Gerson LB, Van Dam J: The future of simulators in GI endoscopy: an unlikely possibility or a virtual reality? *Gastrointest Endosc* 2002;**55**:608–611.

22 Williams CB, Saunders BP, Bladen JS: Development of colonoscopy teaching simulation. *Endoscopy* 2000;**32**:901–905.

23 Noar MD, Soehendra N: Endoscopy simulation training devices. *Endoscopy* 1992;**24**:159–166.

24 Baillie J, Jowell P, Evangelou H, Bickel W, Cotton P: Teaching by endoscopy simulation. *Endoscopy* 1991;**23**:239–240.

25 Noar MD: An established porcine model for animate training in diagnostic and therapeutic ERCP. *Endoscopy* 1995;**27**:77–80.

26 Gholson CF, Provenza JM, Doyle JT, Bacon BR: Endoscopic retrograde sphincterotomy in swine. *Dig Dis Sci* 1991;**36**:1406–1409.

27 Bhutani MS, Aveyard M, Stills HF, Jr.: Improved model for teaching interventional EUS. *Gastrointest Endosc* 2000;**52**:400–403.

28 Hochberger J, Neumann M, Hohenberger W, Hahn EG: Neuer Endoskopie-Trainer für die therapeutische flexible Endoskopie. *Z Gastroenterol* 1997;**35**:722–723.

29 Hochberger J, Neumann M, Maiss J, Bayer J, Nägel A, Hahn EG: Erlanger Ausbildungssimulator für die interventionelle Endoskopie

(EASIE)—Eine neue Perspektive für die qualitätsorientierte praktische Ausbildung. *Endoskopie heute* 1998;**4**:23–25.

30 Hochberger J, Neumann M, Maiss J, Hohenberger W, Hahn EG: EASIE (Erlangen active simulator for interventional endoscopy)—A new biosimulation model: first experiences gained in training workshops. *Gastrointest Endosc* 1998;**47**:AB116.

31 Neumann M, Hochberger J, Felzmann T, Ell C, Hohenberger W: Part 1. The Erlanger endo-trainer. *Endoscopy* 2001;**33**:887–890.

32 Neumann M, Stangl T, Auenhammer G, Horbach T, Hohenberger W, Schneider I: [Laparoscopic cholecystectomy. Training on a bio-simulation model with learning success documented using scorecards]. *Chirurg* 2003;**74**:208–213.

33 Hochberger J, Maiss J, Magdeburg B, Cohen J, Hahn EG: Training simulators and education in gastrointestinal endoscopy: current status and perspectives in 2001. *Endoscopy* 2001;**33**:541–549.

34 Hochberger J, Matthes K, Maiss J, Koebnick C, Hahn EG, Cohen J: Training with the compactEASIE biologic endoscopy simulator significantly improves hemostatic technical skill of gastroenterology fellows: a randomized controlled comparison with clinical endoscopy training alone. *Gastrointest Endosc* 2005;**61**:204–215.

35 Maiss J, Wiesnet J, Proeschel A, et al.: Objective benefit of a 1-day training course in endoscopic hemostasis using the "compactEASIE" endoscopy simulator. *Endoscopy* 2005;**37**:552–558.

36 Dennis M. Jensen, MD. *CURE Atlas*, 2009, Personal communications.

37 Barkun A, Bardou M, Kuipers E, Sung J, Martel M, Sinclair P, and International Consensus, Upper GI Bleeding, Conference Group: International consensus recommendations on the management of patients with non-variceal upper gastrointestinal bleeding (ICON-UGIB). *Ann Intern Med* 2010;**152**(2):101–113.

38 Savides TS, Jensen DM: GI bleeding. In: Feldman M, Friedman LS, Brandt LJ (eds) *Sleisenger and Fordtran's Gastrointestinal and Liver Disease. Pathophysiology/Diagnosis/Management*, 8th edn. Philadelphia: Saunders Elsevier, 2010:285–322.

39 Bleau BL, Gostout CJ, Sherman KE, et al.: Recurrent bleeding from peptic ulcer associated with adherent clot: a randomized study comparing endoscopic treatment with medical therapy. *Gastrointest Endosc* 2002;**56**:1–6.

40 Jensen DM, Kovacs TOG, Jutabha R, et al.: Randomized, controlled trial of medical therapy compared to endoscopic therapy for prevention of recurrent ulcer hemorrhage in patients with non-bleeding adherent clots. *Gastroenterology* 2002;**123**:407–413.

41 Sung JJ, Chan FK, Lau JY, et al. The effect of endoscopic therapy in patients receiving omeprazole for bleeding ulcers with nonbleeding visible vessels or adherent clots: a randomized comparison. *Ann Intern Med* 2003;**139**:237–243.

42 Jensen DM, Ohning GV, Kovacs TOG, Jutabha R, Machicado GA, Dulai GS: Doppler ultrasound probe (DUP) as a guide to endoscopic hemostasis of ulcers with stigmata of recent hemorrhage (SRH). *Gastrointest Endosc* 2010;**75**(5):AB113.

43 Jensen DM, Machicado GA, Hirabayashi K: Randomized controlled study of detachable loop compared to control, cyanoacrylate, or sclerosant for hemostasis of bleeding canine gastric varices. *Gastrointest Endosc* 2007;**65**; AB275:T1498.

44 Jensen DM: Endoscopic hemostasis and tumor palliation—experimental results and techniques. In: Jensen DM, Brunetaud JM (eds), *Medical Laser Endoscopy*. Dordrecht, The Netherlands: Kluwer Academic Publishers, 1990: 45–70.

45 Lau JY, Sung JJ, Lam YH, et al.: Endoscopic retreatment compared with surgery in patients with recurrent bleeding after initial endoscopic control of bleeding ulcers. *N Engl J Med* 1999;**340**:751–756.

46 Jensen DM, Personal communications.

47 American College of Graduate Medical Education (ACGME). General Program Requirements for Fellowship Education in Gastroenterology. Available: ACGME.org (accessed July 1, 2007).

48 Croffie J, Somogyi L, Chuttani R, et al.: ASGE technology status evaluation report: Sclerosing agents for use in GI endoscopy. *Gastrointest Endosc* 2007;**66**:1–6.

16 Luminal Dilation Techniques (Strictures, Achalasia, Anastomotic, IBD)

Syed M. Abbas Fehmi[1] & Michael L. Kochman[2]

[1] University of California San Diego, San Diego, CA, USA
[2] University of Pennsylvania Health System, Philadelphia, PA, USA

Introduction

"Dilation" when mentioned by a gastroenterologist refers to widening or opening an intraluminal stricture in a segment of the gastrointestinal tract. A stricture is an abnormal narrowing or constriction of the luminal GI tract, which may be in the form of an intraluminal, intrinsic mural, or extramural process.

The focus of this chapter will be on the technique of performing effective and safe dilation in the luminal gastrointestinal tract. We will comment on the skill set required to perform this procedure, how to best acquire this skill set, pearls on mastering the technique, and propose some measures to assess the proficiency of an endoscopist in performing dilation. We will concentrate on making the concepts of dilation clear rather than focusing on any specific device type. The small differences that exist between similar devices manufactured by different companies and between the categories of devices are always changing, and as long as the technique is understood, one can easily adapt to new technology device iterations. Lastly, we shall not be covering dilation of pancreatico–biliary system as this is discussed in a separate chapter. Likewise, discussion regarding the efficacy data of different techniques and other available treatments for stricture management other than dilation and the management of complications is beyond the scope of this chapter.

Before reviewing the technique of dilation, it is essential to be familiar with the equipment utilized for the procedure. The devices mentioned in this chapter will be limited to those that are FDA-approved and utilized in routine practice in the United States.

Equipment

Dilators can be divided into two basic types: semi-rigid fixed-diameter push-type "Bougie" dilators and the through-the-scope balloon dilators.

Fixed-diameter push-type or "Bougie" dilators

The polyvinyl wire guided dilators are available from various manufacturers. An excellent summary of different designs can be found in the technology status evaluation report from the ASGE [1]. The differences between manufacturers are not of substantive importance, but familiarity is needed. These differences include the length of the dilator (usually 70 cm to 100 cm), the length of the distal taper, the size measured in either mm or Fr, and the cost. The radio-opaque markers may be either focally embedded (the proximal marker usually marking the site of maximal diameter) or with barium impregnation throughout the entire dilator. The length of the bougie dilators is measured in two different ways, and both are marked on some dilators: the American system measures the distance from the distal tip of dilator, while the European measures from the point of maximal diameter (size) of the dilator. The wire (available separately and in different sizes) used with these dilators should be marked for distance (usually one mark every 20 cm) and kept kink-free.

The traditional nonwired-guided bougie dilators include the liquid metal-filled Maloney dilators. Given the concerns of mercury contamination and the clear limited life of this type of dilator, most have been replaced by tungsten-filled Maloney dilators of much the same feel. These nonwired-guided push-type dilators are quite flexible, tend to easily curl at the tip during use, and have a higher complication rate when used by physicians in complex strictures. They are overall used less frequently and are now primarily used in the setting of low-risk dilation of Schatzki's rings and by nonsedated patients for self-dilation.

Balloon dilators

These may also be referred to as "through-the-scope" (TTS) dilators with the exception of those that are primarily used for dilation in patients with achalasia and are not passed through the working channel of the endoscope. Balloon dilators are also available from various manufacturers. A summary of the various designs can be found in the technology status evaluation report from the

Successful Training in Gastrointestinal Endoscopy, First Edition. Edited by Jonathan Cohen.
© 2011 Blackwell Publishing Ltd. Published 2011 by Blackwell Publishing Ltd.

ASGE [1]. The differences between manufacturers include wire or nonwire-guided forms, cost, a single fixed or multidiameter balloon, the balloon length, the channel size of endoscope required, the catheter size, and the different pressures required for achieving the marked nominal size. These may be filled with saline or with contrast for improved fluoroscopic visualization.

Differences between fixed-diameter push-type and balloon dilators

Push-type dilators can be reprocessed, while most balloon dilators are single-use only. Cost-effectiveness ultimately depends upon local reprocessing costs and the acquisition costs of the dilators from the vendors. Balloon dilators do not have the "tactile feel" that fixed-diameter push-type dilators do, though the push-type dilators require experience to be able to recognize the contribution of the stricture resistance. Balloon dilators do allow real-time visualization of stricture dilation under fluoroscopic control of the dilation if filled with contrast. Some feel that the availability of multidiameter balloon dilators can make the dilation process more time-effective. These also provide the ability to perform the "continuous access technique" (see the technique section for detail), which can be extremely helpful under certain conditions (traversing malignant obstructions, etc.). Multidiameter balloons have been shown to compare favorably with fixed diameter balloons with regard to diameter consistency and dilating force [2]. Both types of dilators are most commonly used in the esophagus and current data does not suggest any difference in technical success or perforation rates between various types of dilators [3–8]. The exception to the above is the use of blind nonwire-guided dilators (Maloney-type dilators) in the setting of complex strictures that are associated with a higher complication rate [9].

Ancillary devices

These are typically devices used during biliary endoscopy (biliary guide wires, catheters, and dilators). Their rare application in luminal dilation is in order to facilitate traversing and dilating tight complex strictures. These will be discussed throughout the chapter.

Endoscope key points to remember

Endoscopists should be familiar with the endoscope outer diameter/tip diameter and channel size to best plan the dilation procedure and the type and size of dilator selected. Representative information for the Olympus series as available at their Website is shown. Similar information for the Pentax or Fujinon endoscopes can be found on their representative Websites. Occasionally the adjunctive use of bronchoscopes may be helpful (Table 16.1).

Fluoroscopy

This is not required for all dilations but is extremely useful in selected cases, especially when dilation is initially being performed in the setting of a complex non-traversed stricture. When there is angulation, luminal irregularity, or a compromised lumen that may preclude passage of endoscope, the use of fluoroscopy can help the endoscopist overcome these issues. Without fluoroscopy, safe passage of a guide wire or dilator can be extremely difficult, if not impossible. Fluoroscopy can also help in successful intubation of the esophagus when strictures are located proximally, making adequate visualization difficult. The esophagus is easily visualized on fluoroscopic images as an air column immediately posterior to the trachea and anterior to the spine. Fluoroscopy can also help affirm that the push-type dilator's maximal diameter has traversed the stricture. It can help in positioning of a balloon dilator; to check if a "waist" is present and to document relief of the stricture during the procedure. In a tertiary care referral center with referral for complex strictures, fluoroscopy may be used in up to 33% of all dilation procedures [10]. Fluoroscopy benefits are well established when using Maloney bougies, where fluoroscopy reduced the risk of perforation [11–13]. The topic of training in the use of fluoroscopy is addressed in more detail in another chapter in this volume.

Mechanism of dilation

All dilators use radial force to dilate the stricture zone. This concept is easy to understand especially when using the multidiameter balloon dilators with fluoroscopy. The Maloney and polyvinyl dilators

Table 16.1 Endoscope outer diameter and channel size.

	Outer diameter	Channel size
Olympus GIF-H180 (standard upper endoscope)	9.8 mm	2.8 mm
Olympus TJF-160VF (therapeutic ERCP scope)	11.3 mm	4.2 mm
Olympus PCF-Q180 (pediatric colonoscope)	11.3 mm	3.2 mm
Olympus CF-Q180 (adult colonoscope)	12.8 mm (tip 13.2 mm)	3.7 mm
Olympus GF-UE160 (radial echoendoscope)	11.8 mm (tip 13.8 mm)	2.2 mm
Olympus GIF-XP160 (pediatric upper endoscope)	5.9 mm	2.0 mm
Olympus GIF-N180 (transnasal endoscope)	4.9 mm	2.0 mm

are inserted with a longitudinal pushing force that is converted to radial expansible force by the slope of the distal ramp. This is relatively inefficient, and one can actually push a stricture distally (and potentially perforate proximal to the stricture) if the resistance of the stricture in the radial vector is greater than the resistance of the esophagus to movement in the longitudinal vector (shear force). Nonwire-guided bougie dilators may curl proximal to a stricture and not actually engage it, potentially causing a more proximal perforation.

Terminology

It is important to have a good understanding of terms used to describe strictures as they will be used throughout this chapter [3,9,14–16].

Simple stricture

These are symmetric or concentric, straight, short, and allow passage of a diagnostic upper endoscope or visualization of the distal lumen.

Complex stricture

Analogously, these are asymmetric, there is an inability to pass diagnostic upper endoscope, length greater than 2 cm, multiple strictures, angulated, or accompanied by a significant hiatal hernia or esophageal diverticulum.

Refractory or recurrent stricture (esophagus)

We have proposed and published the following definition, which is being utilized in current clinical studies: "an anatomic restriction because of cicatricial luminal compromise or fibrosis that results in the clinical symptom of dysphagia in the absence of endoscopic evidence of inflammation. This may occur as the result of either an inability to successfully remediate the anatomic problem to a diameter of 14 mm over 5 sessions at 2-week intervals (refractory) or as a result of an inability to maintain a satisfactory luminal diameter for 4 weeks once the target diameter of 14 mm has been achieved (recurrent). This definition is not meant to include those patients with an inflammatory stricture (which will not resolve successfully until the inflammation subsides) or those with a satisfactory diameter who have dysphagia on the basis of neuromuscular dysfunction (e.g., those with postoperative and postradiation therapy dysphagia)" [17].

Technique of dilation

Strictures are most commonly encountered in the esophagus and as such the video illustrating the technique of dilation also features a prototypical esophageal stricture. The technique and concepts are applicable to all strictures in the gastrointestinal luminal tract unless otherwise indicated in the text and discussed separately (e.g., achalasia). Once it has been confirmed that luminal dilation is required (after review of history and all imaging studies available) and there are no contraindications, dilation of the stricture is performed with preliminary notion as to whether it is a simple or complex stricture. As mentioned previously, the push-type or balloon dilators may be utilized.

Fixed-diameter push-type or "Bougie" dilation

These dilators (the commonly ones used are American or Savary-Gillard) have a central lumen to accommodate a soft spring tip guide wire. The use of the guide-wire technique (whether rigid or balloon dilators) allows for both proximal and distal control of the stricture, which is felt to decrease the likelihood of a perforation. The first step is to position the tip of guide wire distal to the stricture, in the case of esophageal stricture preferably in the gastric antrum. If the stricture allows the passage of regular upper endoscope, this can be performed under direct visual guidance. However, if the endoscope cannot traverse the stricture, fluoroscopy can be used to direct passage of the guide wire tip into the stomach. The spring tip should remain straight and not be allowed to coil and there should not be significant resistance felt to the passage of wire. As the wire passes the GE junction and the diaphragm into the gastric body, the passage of wire along the greater curve of the stomach can be visualized under fluoroscopy as confirmation of wire placement intraluminally into the gastric body.

Step two is removal of the endoscope while maintaining wire position in the stomach. If fluoroscopy is being used, the wire position can be confirmed fluoroscopically as well. The assistant should be poised at the mouth to hold the wire in place. Care must be taken that the sharp proximal tip of the guide wire does not hit the assistant, patient, or physician, as the endoscope is removed. Before completely removing the endoscope, the endoscopist should affirm optimal positioning of the wire by checking the marks on the guide wire that indicate its location. Each mark represents 20 cm of the wire. Three marks are typically seen at the incisors, which would indicate 60 cm of wire in esophagus and stomach.

Step three is passing bougie dilator over the wire after the endoscope has been removed. The physician should check the size on the dilator to make sure it is what was requested. When using the commonly used push-type Savary-Gillard (size shown in mm) or American Dilation System (size shown in Fr) dilators, there may be two sets of markings on the dilator. The American system measures the distance from the tip of dilator, while the European measures from the point of maximal diameter of the dilator. Optimal patient position during this part of the procedure is very important. The patient should be left lateral with neck slightly hyper extended in the "sword swallowing position." Physician stance is important, feet shoulder width apart with position at the level of the head or slightly above with the right hand holding the wire stably against the physician's hip or chest and the dilator being grasped with the fingers of the left hand and advanced gently. A small amount of lubrication on the dilator may help. A stable position should be maintained on the guide-wire with the right hand held against the physician's body so that it is stable and does not migrate distally. If fluoroscopy was being used, this can confirm a stable position of wire and additionally document traversing of the stricture with the dilator.

Removal of dilator to allow the passage of additional dilators over the wire is analogous to the removal of the endoscope. If no further dilation is being performed, gently withdraw the wire through the dilator until the tip gently impacts the tip of dilator and then withdraw as a unit.

"Rule of Threes": After moderate resistance is felt on the dilator, it is often stated that the size of dilator should not be increased more than two additional consecutive dilators for a total of three dilators.

One has to be careful with the application of the above rule. If a total loss of resistance is felt after moderate resistance was first appreciated, resistance at the subsequent larger diameter dilator will not be felt, giving a false impression to continue dilations; the earlier sudden loss of resistance may represent a tear in the muscularis propria layer and further dilation should not be performed. The patient may need to be closely monitored and examined for crepitus and perforation ruled out.

TTS balloon dilation

These dilators can be easily passed through the working channel of the standard upper endoscope and some are designed with both wire- and nonwire-guided forms. Step one is to place the balloon dilator in optimal position (if wire placement is not necessary). However, if the endoscope cannot traverse the stricture (e.g., tight esophageal stricture), fluoroscopy can be used for safe passage of guide wire tip into the stomach (using the same technique as explained above for push-type dilators) and the balloon dilator can then be advanced through the scope over the wire. The balloon can then also be inflated slightly in the stomach and the dilator pulled back to locate the distal aspect of the stricture to assess the length of the stricture. Occasionally, when the endoscope itself cannot be passed through a stricture, the endoscopist can forgo fluoroscopic assistance if the stricture is known to be short or the distal lumen is easily visualized. In these instances, it is endoscopically confirmed that the tip of the dilator) is safely intraluminal.

Step two: Once the balloon has been positioned such that inflation would position the stenosis in the center of the balloon (if fluoroscopy is being used a waist may be seen), inflation of the balloon can be performed. However, before inflation of the balloon, the left hand should be used to anchor the shaft of the balloon catheter against the endoscope to prevent movement of the dilating balloon (either distally into or proximally out of the stricture, leading to ineffective dilation), and the right hand should be on the endoscope with the fingers against the bite block to stabilize the endoscope against either distal or proximal migration of the endoscope and catheter during balloon insufflation.

Step three: If a multidiameter controlled radial expansion balloon dilator is being used (e.g., 10 mm for the 10–12 mm balloon), once the dilating balloon is inflated to the first stage position, it is maintained for 30 seconds (the authors' preference) before going to the next larger size (if needed). The published literature is quite variable for duration of inflation, ranging from instantaneous deflation to maintenance of inflation for 2 minutes at each size. At each step, obliteration of the waist may be checked on fluoroscopy (Figure 16.1). Since the rule of threes does not apply to TTS dilators, the endoscopist can attempt to move the dilator minimally

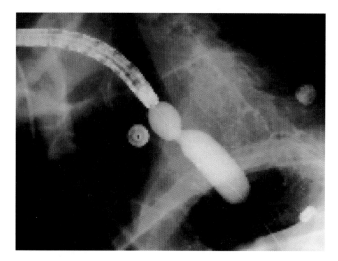

Figure 16.1 Demonstration of a TTS balloon in good position as verified by fluoroscopy with the waist caused by the stricture in the midpart of the balloon. (Reprinted from Kochman ML: Minimization of risks of esophageal dilation. *Gastrointest Endosc Clin N Am* 2007;**17**(1), with permission from Elsevier.)

in a to-and-fro motion within the stricture. If this cannot be performed easily, it may be a surrogate marker to stop if 2–3 diameters have been utilized or if significant mucosal tearing is noted (see accompanying Video 16.1).

Continuous access technique

Once the balloon is inflated to the maximal diameter for dilation session, at a size that is slightly larger than the endoscope being utilized, prior to deflation the balloon may be snugged up to the tip of the endoscope and simultaneously with the balloon deflation, the endoscope and balloon advanced as one unit through the stricture while maintaining constant pressure and fluoroscopic control (Figure 16.2). This technique may aid in traversing a stricture that

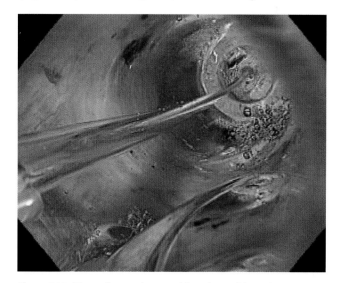

Figure 16.2 Picture from endoscopy video of one of the patients, showing balloon optimally placed, resulting in good visualization through the balloon of real-time stricture dilation.

is angulated or that may have slightly obscured field due to edema or blood. Care should be taken to prevent injury from the tip of the deflated balloon or wire and once the endoscope has traversed the stricture, the endoscopist should wait for the dilating balloon to be completely deflated and pulled into the endoscope prior to further distal insertion of the endoscope. This maneuver should only be performed if the endoscopist is reasonably certain that the lumen beyond the stricture will allow unimpeded passage of the balloon and endoscope (see accompanying Video 16.2).

Maloney dilators

It is our current practice that their use is limited to patients for self-dilation. Given the variety of endoscopically placed dilators and the relative safety of wire-guided and balloon dilators, the use of Maloney dilators in sedated patients or those who are undergoing endoscopy is antiquated and potentially dangerous. Self-bougienage is performed unsedated, and without topical anesthesia, with the goal of decreasing the number of hospital visits for frequent recurrence of dysphagia for a refractory stricture. By the performance of self-dilation daily and then gradually decreasing the frequency over a 3–4 month period, luminal patency may be maintained, as the inflammatory process resolves and the stricture heals.

Dilator selection

The dilator size should be similar or slightly smaller than the estimated diameter of the stricture when performing the initial dilation. One can never start the dilation process with a dilator that is "too small." Conversely, starting with "too large" a dilator may have the potential for disastrous consequences. Subsequently, if using the bougie-type dilators, the rule of three should be followed. If using the balloon dilators, one can gauge need for further dilation as discussed above.

The type of dilator being used is usually based on training, tradition, and one's own experience. Wire-guided dilators (either balloon or push-type) are the preferred choice for complex strictures, proximal strictures, or when the endoscope has not been able to be passed beyond the stricture. Wire-guided balloon dilators are preferred in our practice when performing dilation in the setting of indwelling tracheo–esophageal speech prosthetic or esophageal endoprosthetic, in the setting of epidermolysis bullosa, a complex stricture not previously dilated and/or not well characterized, or when the subsequent passage of endoscope is desired. For subsequent dilations, once the characteristics of the stricture are known, either push-type or balloon dilators may be utilized.

Goal

Dilation goal: Most strictures in the esophagus when dilated to 12–14 mm will give patients relief from dysphagia in >90% of the cases [18]. Long-term benefits of dilation appear greatest when a luminal diameter of greater than 12 mm is achieved for benign esophageal stricture [19]. Recurrent dilation is needed in anywhere from 12% to 60% of the cases. With the increasing use of PPI therapy, repeat dilation procedures are decreasing, especially in the subgroup with a peptic etiology.

Ancillary techniques

When complex strictures cannot be safely dilated using the above-mentioned techniques, ancillary techniques may be used. Advanced endoscopists, who tend to be familiar with the range of tools used in pancreatico–biliary endoscopy, usually undertake these dilations.

An ERCP catheter may be used to facilitate passage through difficult strictures under fluoroscopy with passage of an ERCP guide wire to the gastric lumen (e.g., esophageal stricture) and subsequent dilation is performed using standard wire-guided techniques. The ERCP catheter may also be used to inject contrast proximal to stricture. This can provide intraprocedural anatomic detail of stricture anatomy (length, angulation, etc.) and thereby help guide the wire. Care should be taken to minimize the risk of aspiration of the hyperosmotic contrast.

Our practice is to optimize all factors when dealing with complex strictures and to ensure that the patient is on a PPI to facilitate healing, and to remove suture material/surgical staples when present at the stricture site (these can cause an inflammatory reaction and decrease the effectiveness of dilation).

Another useful technique in the setting of tight strictures is to use a narrow diameter endoscope (pediatric upper endoscope or bronchoscope) that can facilitate identification of residual lumen and help advance the guide wire over which sequential dilation may be performed. The use of these smaller diameter endoscopes is particularly helpful when fluoroscopy is not available or when there is marked anatomic distortion or angulations.

When antegrade dilation with ancillary technique is not successful, as may be the case with long-standing radiation-induced strictures in the setting of head and neck cancer, retrograde dilation can be performed [20]. This is best performed with a mature gastrostomy tract. The gastrostomy tube is removed and a guide wire introduced and the intragastric location is confirmed with fluoroscopy. Dilation of this tract may be performed to facilitate passage of the endoscope into the gastric lumen. Once the GE junction is identified, the esophagus is entered under direct visualization. The stricture is then identified and a guide wire may be passed in retrograde fashion into the oropharynx. A polyvinyl or balloon dilator may then be passed. The wire can subsequently be double-exchanged to perform antegrade dilation in a standard fashion.

Contraindications

There are not many absolute contraindications to performing dilation beyond those that apply to standard endoscopic procedures. Absolute contraindications would include those for standard endoscopy as well as acute or incompletely healed perforations. Relative contraindications may include coagulopathy, unstable pulmonary or cardiac disease, and thoracic aortic aneurysm.

Complications

The most serious and frequent complication of dilation is perforation [3,10]. Overall incidence of perforation ranges from 0.1% to 0.4% [9]. Bleeding, up to approximately 0.2%, and aspiration (mostly chemical) are other rare, but recognized complications.

Postprocedure follow-up for the early detection of complications is helpful. Patient complaints of pain or worse dysphagia should be appropriately evaluated with a low threshold for admission and obtaining an imaging study to aid in ruling-out a perforation. The initial imaging is best performed by esophagram obtained with water-soluble contrast.

Some key points

• There is no best technique that is applicable for all strictures. One should be familiar with the various techniques and technologies. The techniques discussed may be used for the dilation of malignant and benign strictures throughout the luminal digestive tract with minor modifications, except when otherwise indicated (e.g., achalasia).

• Dilation technique and experience for achalasia is quite different from that already discussed (see below).

• Benign strictures of the gastro-duodenum and small bowel (especially postsurgical strictures in the setting of bariatric procedures, Whipple, pyloric stenosis, inflammatory lesions) can be managed with TTS balloon dilators (our preference is using the standard technique described above) if one can achieve endoscopic access to the area of interest [21–23]. Benign colorectal strictures (IBD, diverticulitis, NSAIDs, or radiation) can also be successfully managed using the standard techniques mentioned above [24–30].

• Strictures in the setting of Crohn's disease have usually been treated with TTS balloon dilators up to 25 mm in diameter. In most series, the balloon is left inflated for 1–4 minutes.

• Biopsies can be performed during the session when dilation is being performed.

• Dilation can be done during radiation therapy, though dilation in the setting of radiation therapy may carry a slightly increased risk of complication. The exact timing needs to be weighed against the potential for nutritional decline of the patient and worsening of the stricture, which may be caused by a delay to the endoscopic therapy [31].

• For Schatzki's ring, the effective therapy is one-time dilation to at least 18 mm (polyvinyl dilator over the wire preferred) as the goal is to achieve rupture of the ring [32]. If a lower esophageal ring cannot be distinguished from a short peptic stricture, then a graded stepwise dilation may be performed.

• Complex strictures have a higher incidence of complications and one needs to know the risk factors for complications (complex stricture, malignant stricture, prior radiation therapy, caustic ingestion, eosinophilic esophagitis, and esophageal pseudodiverticulosis) and are also likely increased in the settings of steroid use and altered anatomy [3].

• There is an increased risk of perforation for dilation performed in the setting of eosinophilic esophagitis. It is important for trainees to recognize the endoscopic features of this condition and to consider this diagnostic possibility before beginning the procedure [33–35] and weigh the benefits of medical therapy as the first-line therapy.

• For complex strictures, the use of wire-guided dilators and fluoroscopy are helpful when the endoscope has not traversed the stricture. Fluoroscopy is not required for all dilations.

• Be aware of the common presenting symptoms of complications and have a low threshold for investigations including water-soluble esophageal contrast exam and CT scan.

The occurrence of esophageal aortic-fistulae are not unusual in the natural history of squamous-cell carcinoma of esophagus and may present dramatically during dilation of esophageal stricture or occur intraprocedurally.

Achalasia

One should be aware of the classic clinical presenting symptoms, radiographic findings, and manometric findings of achalasia. It is important to assure that when dilation for achalasia is performed, that the diagnosis is as certain as possible due to the potential for complications and emergent surgical intervention. It is noteworthy that the risk of perforation during pneumatic dilation in the setting of achalasia is 3–4% with a mortality rate of <1% [15,36,37]. The literature suggests that early recognition and surgical repair of dilation-related perforations does not carry with it a worse clinical outcome than primary surgical remediation [38]. Pneumatic dilation is one of the treatment modalities for achalasia, and a complete discussion of the other treatment options is beyond the scope of this chapter.

Endoscopy and performance of pneumatic balloon dilation in achalasia

Characteristic resistance at the GE junction or lower esophageal sphincter (LES) is usually felt with a give or "pop" sensation felt at passing the GE junction with the endoscope. A stiff guide wire is passed and placed in the gastric antrum. Endoscope withdrawal is performed as for routine esophageal dilation. The dilating balloon is passed over the wire under fluoroscopy. Different balloons are available from various manufacturers and differ in cost, balloon length, catheter size, and balloon diameter. The usual starting diameter is based upon preference and experience and is usually 30 mm as smaller balloons are not as efficacious. An excellent summary is available in the recent ASGE technology status report [1]. The lubricated balloon should be tested outside the patient first to affirm proper functioning and then deflated completely. Balloon should then be passed into the esophagus and advanced to GE junction. A twisting pressure can help easily pass the balloon through LES to the optimal location (confirmed with fluoroscopy—usually 1–2 cm below diaphragmatic silhouette) so that the balloon is properly centered at the LES. The balloon is gently inflated such that the balloon has a waist in the center, confirming its positioning. The shaft of dilator is gripped firmly to prevent displacement. The most critical aspect is the actual balloon insufflation, and there are variations in the technique in the literature. Our practice is to inflate quickly (making sure we are well positioned with the waist in the center) and to deflate immediately as soon as waist obliteration is noted. The balloon is then completely deflated and the wire and balloon withdrawn as one unit. We do not usually repeat the dilation procedure in the same setting or hold the balloon insufflated (some physicians may do a second dilation or hold pressure for 60 seconds). Post-procedure, the patient is sent for a water-soluble contrast study to rule out a perforation. We usually discharge the patient on a restricted diet and inform them to contact us immediately for any complaints of pain. In our experience, this technique achieves the safest and most efficacious result. Rarely, if pneumatic balloon dilation does not result in a good response, we may consider the use of 35 mm or 40 mm balloon. As mentioned above, we like to use fluoroscopy for these procedures although there are balloons commercially available that do not necessarily require availability of fluoroscopy [39,40] and the procedure may be endoscopically controlled.

Suggested skill set to master and potential outcome measures to assess proficiency in performing luminal dilation

Skills to master

- Basic endoscopy skills as suggested per ASGE guidelines [15]
- Knowledge of equipment utilized during dilation as mentioned above [1]
- Indications for dilation and ability to recognize immediate or late complications and their avoidance [3]
- Ability to withdraw the endoscope while maintaining wire in antrum (for esophageal stricture)
- Smooth transition from wire being held at the mouth (for esophageal stricture) to endoscope removal over the wire and loading up of dilator (best if same method is used with gastrointestinal assistant familiar with the technique)
- Correct stance, angulations, and push force with patient in optimal position
- Ability to assess resistance and to maintain balloon in correct position without balloon movement
- Continuous access technique success >90% in appropriate setting

Measurable outcomes for instructor to assess while working with trainee

- Ability to differentiate simple, complex, and refractory or recurrent strictures
- Ability to gauge when it may be beneficial to use balloon dilators over push-type dilators
- Ability to select an appropriate size of dilator for initial dilation

For push-type dilation

- After placement of wire in antrum for esophageal stricture dilation, ability to withdraw endoscope by the trainee with maintained wire position in the antrum (this can be accurately assessed using fluoroscopy)
- When using fluoroscopy, confirmation that guide wire tip does not coil and its passage through the GE junction (passing the diaphragmatic into the stomach along the greater curve is obtained
- Maintenance of the guide wire in position without distal migration during the passage of bougie dilator (this can be accurately assessed using fluoroscopy)
- Confirmation that the maximal diameter of the dilator traverses the stricture (this can be accurately assessed using fluoroscopy)
- Following the guideline of "rule of threes"

For balloon dilation

- Initial placement of the balloon with stricture in the center portion of the balloon (this can be accurately assessed using fluoroscopy)
- Effective inflation of the balloon dilator without movement or need for deflation with repositioning (this can be accurately assessed without using fluoroscopy)
- Ability to successfully perform "continuous access technique"

For Achalasia

- Initial placement of the balloon with LES in the center portion of the balloon (this can be accurately assessed using fluoroscopy and identifying the diaphragm silhouette)
- Ability to deflate immediately as soon as waist obliteration is noted on fluoroscopy

Suggested skill level to perform dilation

The "Gastroenterology Core Curriculum" published in May 2007 divides endoscopic training into two levels. Level 1 (referred to as basic) includes gastroenterologists performing routine GI endoscopic and nonendoscopic procedures as a part of their daily practice. Level 2 (referred to as advanced) includes gastroenterologists who in addition to all or part of the above perform some or all advanced (both diagnostic and therapeutic) gastrointestinal endoscopy procedures including ERCP, EUS, etc. Per this curriculum, one must perform a minimum 130 EGDs and 20 dilations (guide wire and TTS) based on expert opinion. It is assumed that this number will be the threshold number of procedures performed before assessment of competency. Most trainees will require additional procedures to meet this threshold, and no trainee should be assessed with fewer procedures. Interesting data concerning operator experience and the risk of perforation has been published, indicating that 500 endoscopies seem to be a cut-off above which the risk of dilation-associated perforation decreases [41].

We agree that technical skills are acquired in sequential fashion and that proficiency develops incrementally through the performance of procedures under direct supervision with an increasing complexity of procedures and gradual acquisition of procedural independence. On the basis of the above document and experience, the following are the authors' suggestions.

Basic

This would be the level 1 endoscopist who has met the minimum criteria of endoscopic training. More importantly, he or she was assessed by an expert endoscopist to be competent in performing the procedure of dilation. In our opinion, gastroenterologists falling in this category should be able to perform dilation of simple strictures using standard technique not involving use of ancillary techniques. We feel that at least 50 procedures need to be performed under the supervision of an expert endoscopist before competency is achieved in performing these procedures independently. One should continue to perform at least 20 such procedures per year to maintain a fluent methodical sequence of performing this procedure.

Advanced

This would be the level-2 endoscopist who is proficient in advanced endoscopy and facile with the tools utilized during those procedures. He or she should be well aware of the ancillary techniques described above and should be performing them frequently enough to maintain skills. They should have expertise in the diagnosis and acute management of complications. The care for patients with perforations typically requires a multidisciplinary effort and the use of endoscopic closure devices and temporary endoprosthetic may be appropriate in selected patients. Most likely, these endoscopists are based in an academic or large referral center. In our opinion, gastroenterologists falling in this category will be performing dilation of most complex, refractory, or recurrent strictures. In addition, patients with increased risk of complication but with simple strictures may be referred to these gastroenterologists. For training, one needs to perform at least 75 such procedures (complex stricture dilation, use of fluoroscopy or ERCP devices during dilation, thin caliber endoscope, etc.) under the direct supervision of an expert endoscopist before gaining competency. One should continue to perform at least 20 such procedures a year to maintain the skill set. In some tertiary centers, achalasia-related dilations are performed by dedicated one or two physicians given its infrequency, also enabling them to be performing such procedure in numbers adequate to maintain their skill set.

Some gastroenterologists who are at the basic level but wish to seek advanced level training can occasionally seek 1–3 month sabbaticals at a tertiary care center working with an expert endoscopist gaining proficiency in advanced techniques for dilation and gaining some familiarity with ancillary tools. Data concerning operator experience and risk of dilation-associated perforation support the argument of dedicated supervised training to minimize complications [42].

Videos

Video 16.1 Esophageal balloon dilation technique
Video 16.2 Continuous access technique for esophageal dilation

References

1 Siersema PD: Therapeutic esophageal interventions for dysphagia and bleeding. *Curr Opin Gastroenterol* 2006;**22**:442–447.

2 Siersema PD: Endoscopic therapeutic esophageal interventions: something old, something new, something to be established. *Curr Opin Gastroenterol* 2004;**20**:397–403.

3 Ahlawat SK, Davidson BJ, Al-Kawas FH: Successful use of biliary accessories in antegrade dilation of complex upper esophageal stricture due to chemoradiation and surgery. *Dis Esophagus* 2008;**21**:86–89.

4 Singh D, Maley RH, Santucci T, et al.: Experience and technique of stapled mechanical cervical esophagogastric anastomosis. *Ann Thorac Surg* 2001;**71**:419–424.

5 Soehendra N, Kempeneers I, Eichfuss HP, Butzow GH, von Braun HH: Fiberscopic obliteration of esophageal varices (author's transl.). *Langenbecks Arch Chir* 1980;**351**:219–228.

6 Solt J, Moizs M, Orovica A, Gardos A, Battyanyi I, Bognear B: Postoperative ischemic jejunal stenosis treated with balloon catheter dilation and Wallstent implantation. *Endoscopy* 1997;**29**:409–412.

7 Standards of PC, Egan JV, Baron TH, et al.: Esophageal dilation. *Gastrointest Endosc* 2006;**63**:755–760.

8 Steele NP, Tokayer A, Smith RV: Retrograde endoscopic balloon dilation of chemotherapy- and radiation-induced esophageal stenosis under direct visualization. *Am J Otolaryngol* 2007;**28**:98–102.

9 Maciver RH, Sundaresan S, DeHoyos AL, Sisco M, Blum MG: Mucosal tube technique for creation of esophageal anastomosis after esophagectomy. *Ann Thorac Surg* 2009;**87**:1703–1707.

10 Al-Haddad M, Pungpapong S, Wallace MB, Raimondo M, Woodward TA: Antegrade and retrograde endoscopic approach in the establishment of a neo-esophagus: a novel technique. *Gastrointest Endosc* 2007;**65**:290–294.

11 Pereira-Lima JC, Ramires RP, Zamin I Jr., Cassal AP, Marroni CA, Mattos AA. Endoscopic dilation of benign esophageal strictures: report on 1043 procedures. *Am J Gastroenterol* 1999;**94**:1497–1501.

12 Sullivan CA, Jaklitsch MT, Haddad R, et al.: Endoscopic management of hypopharyngeal stenosis after organ sparing therapy for head and neck cancer. *Laryngoscope* 2004;**114**:1924–1931.

13 Takeo Y, Yoshida T, Shigemitu T, Yanai H, Hayashi N, Okita K: Endoscopic mucosal resection for early esophageal cancer and esophageal dysplasia. *Hepatogastroenterology* 2001;**48**:453–457.

14 Ament ME, Berquist WE, Vargas J, Perisic V: Fiberoptic upper intestinal endoscopy in infants and children. *Pediatr Clin N Am* 1988;**35**:141–155.

15 Tam PK, Sprigg A, Cudmore RE, Cook RC, Carty H: Endoscopy-guided balloon dilatation of esophageal strictures and anastomotic strictures after esophageal replacement in children. *J Pediatr Surg* 1991;**26**:1101–1103.

16 Tan HL, Roberts JP, Grattan-Smith D: Retrograde balloon dilation of ureteropelvic obstructions in infants and children: early results. *Urology* 1995;**46**:89–91.

17 Kochman ML, McClave SA, Boyce HW: The refractory and the recurrent esophageal stricture: a definition. *Gastrointest Endosc* 2005;**62**:474–475.

18 Tucker LE: The importance of fluoroscopic guidance for Maloney dilation. *Am J Gastroenterol* 1992;**87**:1709–1711.

19 Vaezi MF, Richter JE: Current therapies for achalasia: comparison and efficacy. *J Clin Gastroenterol* 1998;**27**:21–35.

20 Zerbib R, Sarfati E, Celerier M, Tran BH: Evaluation of 16 severe pharyngo-esophageal caustic stenoses. Value of the anterior approach in an ileo-colic transplant. *Ann Otolaryngol Chir Cervicofac* 1986;**103**:581–588.

21 Vicari JJ, Johanson JF, Frakes JT: Outcomes of acute esophageal food impaction: success of the push technique. *Gastrointest Endosc* 2001;**53**:178–181.

22 Villegas L, Rege RV, Jones DB: Laparoscopic Heller myotomy with bolstering partial posterior fundoplication for achalasia. *J Laparoendosc Adv Surg Tech A* 2003;**13**:1–4.

23 Ramirez FC, Grade AJ, Drewitz DJ, Shaukat MS: Diagnostic and therapeutic endoscopy through the gastrostomy site. *J Clin Gastroenterol* 1997;**24**:113–115.

24 Zentilin P, Savarino V, Mastracci L, et al.: Reassessment of the diagnostic value of histology in patients with GERD, using multiple biopsy sites and an appropriate control group. *Am J Gastroenterol* 2005;**100**:2299–2306.

25 Yi A, Shin JH, Song HY, et al.: Esophageal achalasia: comparison of fluoroscopically guided double vs. endoscopically guided single balloon dilation. *Abdom Imaging* 2008;**33**:177–182.

26 Yamamoto H, Hughes RW Jr., Schroeder KW, Viggiano TR, DiMagno EP: Treatment of benign esophageal stricture by Eder-Puestow or balloon dilators: a comparison between randomized and prospective nonrandomized trials. *Mayo Clin Proc* 1992;**67**:228–236.

27 Williams VA, Watson TJ, Zhovtis S, et al.: Endoscopic and symptomatic assessment of anastomotic strictures following esophagectomy and cervical esophagogastrostomy. *Surg Endosc* 2008;**22**:1470–1476.

28 Werre A, Mulder C, van Heteren C, Bilgen ES: Dilation of benign strictures following low anterior resection using Savary-Gilliard bougies. *Endoscopy* 2000;**32**:385–388.

29 Wehrmann T, Kokabpick H, Jacobi V, Seifert H, Lembcke B, Caspary WF: Long-term results of endoscopic injection of botulinum toxin in elderly achalasic patients with tortuous megaesophagus or epiphrenic diverticulum. *Endoscopy* 1999;**31**:352–358.

30 Webb WA: Technique of esophageal dilation. *Chest Surg Clin N Am* 1995;**5**:471–479.

31 Ng TM, Spencer GM, Sargeant IR, Thorpe SM, Bown SG: Management of strictures after radiotherapy for esophageal cancer. *Gastrointest Endosc* 1996;**43**:584–590.

32 Thomas-Gibson S, Brooker JC, Hayward CM, Shah SG, Williams CB, Saunders BP. Colonoscopic balloon dilation of Crohn's strictures: a review of long-term outcomes. *Eur J Gastroenterol Hepatol* 2003;**15**:485–488.

33 Cohen MS, Kaufman AB, Palazzo JP, et al.: An audit of endoscopic complications in adult eosinophilic esophagitis. *Clin Gastroenterol Hepatol* 2007;**5**:1149.

34 Vasilopoulos S, Murphy P, Auerbach A, et al.: The small-caliber esophagus: an unappreciated cause of dysphagia for solids in patients with eosinophilic esophagitis. *Gastrointest Endosc* 2002;**55**:99.

35 Straumann A, Rossi L, Simon HU, et al.: Fragility of the esophageal mucosa: a pathognomonic endoscopic sign of primary eosinophilic esophagitis? *Gastrointest Endosc* 2003;**57**:407–412.

36 Venkatesh KS, Ramanujam PS, McGee S: Hydrostatic balloon dilatation of benign colonic anastomotic strictures. *Dis Colon Rectum* 1992;**35**:789–791.

37 Velanovich V, Ben Menachem T: Laparoscopic Nissen fundoplication after failed endoscopic gastroplication. *J Laparoendosc Adv Surg Tech A* 2002;**12**:305–308.

38 Raju GS. Endoscopic management of gastrointestinal leaks. *Gastrointest Endoscopy Clin N Am* 2007;**17**:487–503.

39 Lambroza A, Schuman RW: Pneumatic dilation for achalasia without fluoroscopic guidance: safety and efficacy. *Am J Gastroenterol* 1995;**90**:1226–1229.

40 Rai RR, Shende A, Joshi A, et al.: Rigiflex pneumatic dilation of achalasia without fluoroscopy: a novel office procedure. *Gastrointest Endosc* 2005;**62**:427–431.

41 Quine MA, Bell GD, McCloy RF, et al.: Prospective audit of perforation rates following up per gastrointestinal endoscopy in two regions of England. *Br J Surg* 1995;**82**:530–533.

42 Zur KB, Putnam PE, Rutter MJ: Combined retrograde and anterograde hypopharyngeal puncture and dilatation in a child with complete hypopharyngeal stenosis. *Int J Pediatr Otorhinolaryngol* 2007;**71**:153–157.

17 Foreign Body Extraction

Gregory A. Coté[1], Steven A. Edmundowicz[2], & Sreenivasa S. Jonnalagadda[2]

[1]Indiana University School of Medicine, Indianapolis, IN, USA
[2]Washington University School of Medicine, St. Louis, MO, USA

Introduction

Foreign body (FB) ingestions often require emergent endoscopic intervention by a gastroenterologist. While these cases are often anxiety-provoking, a successful FB retrieval is instantly gratifying to the patient and their physician. Although 75–90% of FB ingestions pass spontaneously and without complication [1,2], most FBs retained in the GI tract are found in the esophagus [3,4]. Esophageal FBs have the highest mortality and morbidity due to the risk of perforation and associated complications such as mediastinitis, pnuemothorax, pericarditis, lung abscesses, and cardiac tamponade. Since retention times greater than 24 hours have the highest rates of complication [5], all esophageal FBs should be managed on an urgent basis. Fortunately, success rates for endoscopic management of esophageal FBs typically range from 90 to 100% [1,6–11]. FB retrieval is primarily achieved using standard or therapeutic gastroscopes, although iatrogenic FBs such as video capsules and enteral stents may require overtube-assisted enteroscopy or colonoscopy. Experienced endoscopists at high volume centers should perform these less commonly encountered cases.

Endoscopic retrieval of FBs ranges in complexity from the equivalent of a standard upper endoscopy with snare retrieval to more complex cases requiring an open toolbox performed by a gastroenterologist with more resources. A key principle in these cases is recognizing which patients require emergent intervention or those who should be referred to a high volume endoscopy center. Training and maintenance of competency in the endoscopic management of foreign bodies requires a combination of simulator-based preparation, experienced mentorship, and comprehensive exposure to standard endoscopic techniques. We will detail our recommended approach to patients with FB ingestions and outline the fundamental components of successful training in FB retrieval.

Training in FB extraction

The complexity of endoscopic retrieval of FBs is highly variable. As a result, competency in these cases is difficult to measure. For example, extraction of blunt, nontoxic objects in the stomach or proximal duodenum can be performed by a supervised trainee with modest experience in standard upper endoscopy. On the other hand, retrieval of self-expandable metallic stents (SEMS) is best performed by endoscopists who deploy them on a regular basis. The porcine model plays a particularly important role in FB extraction training, providing a unique opportunity for trainees to practice using a variety of retrieval instruments while attempting to extract sharp or dull FBs both large and small. This allows trainees to develop an understanding of how different retrieval instruments perform while grasping FBs of various shapes and sizes.

Although there are no standard criteria to measure competence in FB retrieval, trainees should not perform cases involving esophageal FBs until they are comfortable with esophageal intubation under direct endoscopic visualization. A traumatic intubation carries a particularly high risk of FB migration or perforation. With the exception of particularly advanced FB cases (sharp FBs, SEMS), an instructor can often guide a trainee through the procedure. We suggest five important landmarks that should be reached during each case (Table 17.1). An instructor may be able to guide their trainee through some or all of these steps. Once each step is completed, the instructor may elect to "pause" and elaborate on the sequence of maneuvers that should be performed in order to execute the next phase of the procedure. Ideally, instruction should begin with a thorough pre-procedure assessment, since many issues can be anticipated before endoscopic intubation. Instructors should recognize which factors increase the procedure's degree of difficulty: FBs lodged in the esophagus, sharp FBs, large FBs (>5 cm in greatest diameter), and potentially toxic FBs. In the body of this chapter, we present our approach to FB retrieval beginning with the pre-procedure assessment and concluding with post-endoscopic issues (Table 17.2).

Pre-procedure assessment

Before proceeding to endoscopy, the location of the FB (esophageal versus other) and its classification should be considered. FBs can be grouped into one of four categories: sharp foreign objects (e.g., fish bones), blunt foreign objects (e.g., coins, batteries), iatrogenic objects (e.g., stents, video capsules), and food boluses [12].

Successful Training in Gastrointestinal Endoscopy, First Edition. Edited by Jonathan Cohen.
© 2011 Blackwell Publishing Ltd. Published 2011 by Blackwell Publishing Ltd.

Table 17.1 Recommended steps for endoscopic retrieval of FBs.

- Confirm the location of the FB
- Grasp FB with appropriate retrieval instrument
- Use an overtube to reduce the risk of aspiration when appropriate
- Remove endoscope, instrument, and FB simultaneously, maintaining continuous visualization of the FB
- After removal, consider reintubating with the endoscope to evaluate the mucosal integrity and perform biopsies when appropriate
  - Delay endoscopic biopsies or dilation for at least one week if there is significant mucosal edema or tears

Emergent endoscopy is typically indicated for esophageal FBs and those involving sharp or potentially toxic items (i.e., batteries). One exception to this rule is contraband (e.g., cocaine, heroin) wrapped in plastic or latex condoms (aka "body packing"), often visible on plain radiographs or CT scan [13,14]. Endoscopic extraction and use of gastric lavage are not recommended since rupture and leakage of contents can be lethal [1,15,16].

While symptoms of esophageal FBs usually include dysphagia and odynophagia, nonesophageal FBs are likely to present without localizing symptoms [3,17]. Odynophagia may be due to persistent impaction of a FB but can also indicate mucosal injury by a FB that has already passed. Patients who cannot tolerate salivary secretions require emergent endoscopy to evaluate for complete esophageal obstruction.

Signs and symptoms of perforation or associated FB-related complications should be considered before endoscopic intervention. Notably, perforation at the level of the esophagogastric junction may occur distal to the diaphragmatic hiatus. Therefore, signs of peritonitis or bowel obstruction should be assessed, as these would preclude endoscopic management [15]. If a perforation is suspected, or to facilitate localization of ingested FBs, standard plain radiography or computed tomography (CT) can be performed before endoscopy. In the setting of esophageal FBs, radiographic evaluation of the chest and neck can locate most artificial objects, steak bones, and mediastinal or peritoneal free air [18]. Radiolucent objects include chicken or fish bones, plastic, wood, and most glass. Both anteroposterior and lateral views should be reviewed to differentiate an esophageal from a tracheal FB. Oral contrast studies should be limited to cases where the presence of an esophageal perforation is suspected by exam or plain film findings. CT scans have proven useful in identifying ingested bones lodged in the esophagus [19], and three-dimensional reconstruction may improve this technology [20]. A normal radiographic examination does not generally preclude the need for an endoscopy in a symptomatic patient.

Identify devices

Protective instruments

The endoscopy suite should be equipped with a broad array of devices that confer airway and mucosal protection, as well as facilitate FB retrieval. Protective devices include overtubes and

Table 17.2 Five-step approach to patients with FB ingestion.

Step	Description

1. Pre-procedure assessment	- Classify FB: sharp, dull, iatrogenic, food
	- Consider radiographic evaluation
	  - Evaluation for FB-related complication
	  - Localize FB

2. Identify device(s)	- Mucosal shields/protective instruments
	  - Transpharyngeal vs. transesophageal overtube
	  - Latex protector hood
	- Isolate retrieval instruments that may be useful for FB extraction
	  - Forceps: alligator, rat tooth
	  - Polypectomy snares
	  - Retrieval nets

3. Practice	- Using the same or similar FB, practice grasping and retrieving the FB outside the patient using a number of potential instruments
4. Endoscopic removal	- Endoscopically confirm location of FB - Use a protective overtube or hood with sharp objects or large food boluses - Consider referral to a high volume center for removal of SEMS
5. Post-procedure follow-up	- For food impactions, consider evaluation for underlying pathology (eosinophilic esophagitis) - Hospital observation if there is a clinical suspicion of bowel perforation - Repeat endoscopy after a short interval (1–4 weeks to confirm healing)

FB, Foreign body.

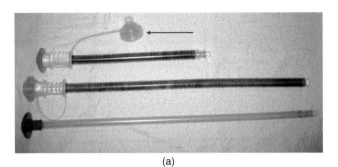

(a)

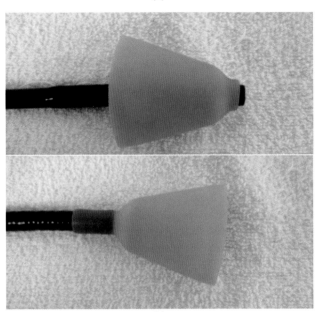

(b)

Figure 17.1 Protective devices. (a) Transpharyngeal (top) and transesophageal (bottom) overtubes. The transpharyngeal overtube is 25 cm in length, protecting the upper airway during FB extraction (top). The transesophageal overtube is 50 cm in length, conferring protection of the airway and gastroesophageal junction (middle). An inner tube with a tapered end is used to insert the overtube (bottom). This can be removed and replaced with an airseal (arrow), which allows insufflation during endoscopy. (b) Latex protective hood. The hood is retracted during insertion of the endoscope (top) and extended over the tip of the endoscope to protect the gastroesophageal junction during withdrawal (bottom).

protector hoods (Figure 17.1a,b). Overtubes are particularly useful for sharp objects and larger food impactions. Since the incidence of complications may be as high as 35% [14], endoscopic removal of sharp objects should be attempted if localized proximal to the duodenum.

Overtubes facilitate repeated endoscopic intubation, provide airway protection, and reduce the risk of mucosal lacerations during the removal of sharp objects (Video 17.1). However, overtubes also confer a risk of hypopharyngeal injury, particularly in the setting of very proximal FB obstructions or esophageal strictures. Short, transpharyngeal overtubes (25 cm length) provide airway protection and facilitate repeated endoscopic intubation, while

longer overtubes (50 cm length) confer additional protection for the distal esophagus and lower esophageal sphincter. While the latter is more cumbersome to use, this device is particularly helpful for the removal of sharp objects that are located in the stomach. Longer overtubes produce greater resistance and less maneuverability for flexible endoscopes.

The entire shaft of the endoscope and overtube should be adequately lubricated before preloading the overtube. Endoscopic intubation can be cumbersome while the overtube is retracted to the hub of the endoscope. After careful endoscopic intubation with direct visualization, the endoscope should be advanced well into the stomach prior to deploying a longer overtube or to the midesophagus before advancing a transpharyngeal overtube. The endoscope should be stabilized using your left hand to keep the shaft of the endoscope straight and slightly taut. Then, the overtube can be advanced over the shaft with minimal resistance until the proximal end of the overtube is close to the patient's mouth, or the distal end of the overtube is just proximal to the bending section of the endoscope. If necessary, an assistant can hold the overtube in place, allowing the endoscopist to return both hands to the control dials and shaft of the endoscope. Alternatively, the overtube can be preloaded onto a passage dilator for intubation. Once the overtube has been fully inserted, the dilator can be removed and the endoscope reinserted for retrieval of the FB [21].

FB protector hoods are less cumbersome than overtubes and particularly useful for removal of objects from the stomach that may injure the esophageal body or esophageal sphincters during extraction [22–24]. To further reduce the risk of mucosal lacerations with extraction, the blunt end of the object should be grasped so as to extract the object with the sharp-end trailing behind. For example, a safety pin can be grasped at its circular elbow using a rat tooth forceps and pulled to the tip of the endoscope, where the protector hood will shield the object as the endoscope is withdrawn (Video 17.2). The hood should be securely fitted to the tip of the endoscope, lightly lubricated, and then retracted before endoscopic intubation.

Retrieval instruments

The endoscopist should be comfortable using a variety of retrieval instruments, including rat tooth and alligator forceps, polypectomy snares, as well as retrieval baskets and nets (Figure 17.2) [15,25]. The optimal instrument for FB retrieval depends on the size, shape, and location of a FB. In general, snares and forceps are most useful for sharp objects, whereas retrieval nets and baskets are preferred for small, blunt objects [26,27]. Retrieval baskets and nets are now available in a variety of shapes and sizes. The endoscopist should be comfortable with each of these instruments and understand each of their unique properties.

Once the FB is securely grasped, the instrument should be pulled back into the working channel until the FB is abutting the tip of the endoscope. If an overtube has been used, the FB should be completely pulled into the overtube at this time. Then, the instrument sheath should be firmly grasped. The endoscope and overtube, if applicable, should be slowly withdrawn while keeping the retrieval instrument and FB against the tip of the endoscope. The entire

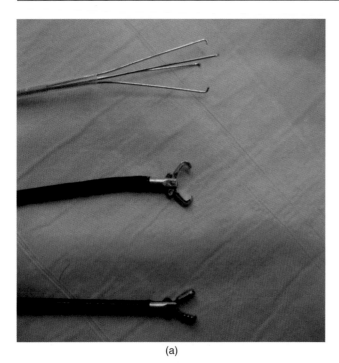

(a)

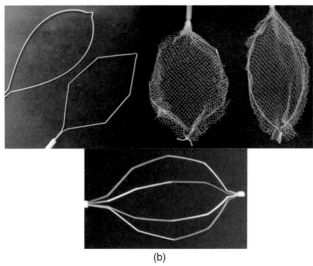

(b)

Figure 17.2 (a) Grasping instruments (top to bottom): four-prong grasper, rat-tooth forceps, alligator forceps. (b) Retrieval snares (top left), nets (top right), and basket (bottom)

apparatus should be removed simultaneously to minimize the risk of injury. As the endoscope is withdrawn, it will flip the protector hood from its retracted position, cover the tip of the endoscope and FB and protect the mucosa during withdrawal.

Anticipate the endoscopy

Practicing with a particular device prior to the procedure can help in choosing the best device for that specific case. This is particularly important for sharp objects and blunt items that may be caustic

to the mucosa after prolonged contact or if ruptured. A classic example is disk or button batteries, which can either pass spontaneously or induce liquefaction necrosis and perforation related to extrusion of concentrated potassium hydroxide. Pressure necrosis or low-voltage electrical burns may also lead to esophageal injury. The majority of reported cases can be managed without severe complications [28]. A total of nineteen cases of esophageal injury due to battery ingestion have been reported since 1979, all of which occurred with batteries >20 mm in diameter [29]. Since batteries are easily recovered with retrieval baskets or nets, endoscopic removal of all batteries lodged in the esophagus is recommended [15]. Avoid instruments that may pierce objects containing caustic material, such as rat tooth or grasping forceps.

Many FB cases now involve iatrogenic objects, including covered SEMS, intragastric balloons, as well as wireless pH and video capsules [30–32]. SEMS pose a unique problem due to the presence of overlying hyperplastic tissue or tumor ingrowth within the interstices of the stent. During attempted endoscopic extraction, the stent may become disrupted, causing sharp wires to protrude and increase the risk of bowel perforation. For this reason, removal of SEMS should be performed by endoscopists who have extensive experience in deploying and removing SEMS. Anecdotally, if a snare cannot be draped over the proximal aspect of the stent, we prefer using a double channel endoscope that permits grasping opposing sides of the SEMS with alligator forceps (Figure 17.3). Once a firm grip is acquired, the entire endoscope is withdrawn while simultaneously maintaining tension on both forceps (Video 17.3).

Video capsule devices, measuring approximately 11 mm × 26 mm, are now used to provide images of the esophagus and small bowel without the need for a traditional endoscope. On the

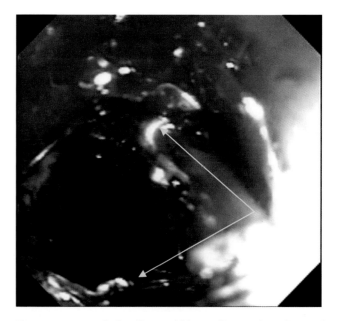

Figure 17.3 Removal of a self-expandable metallic stent (SEMS). Several attempts to remove the covered esophageal stent using a single alligator forceps were unsuccessful. Using a double channel gastroscope, the stent is grasped and extracted using two alligator forceps simultaneously.

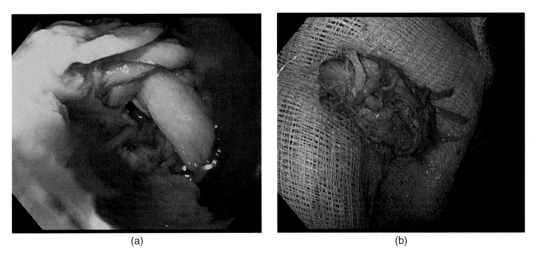

(a)   (b)

Figure 17.4 (a) Food bolus impaction. A partially chewed piece of chicken obstructs the esophageal lumen. (b) Extracted food bolus. The entire bolus was successfully grasped using a retrieval net and removed en bloc.

basis of the site of capsule impaction, standard or overtube-assisted enteroscopy can be performed to recover the retained device using standard retrieval nets (Video 17.4) [33–35].

Endoscopic removal

Endoscopic retrieval of FBs varies in complexity depending on its size, shape, and location within the gastrointestinal tract. In general, esophageal FBs are emergent cases that require advanced endoscopic training since the potential for FB-related and procedure-related complications are significant. Removal of sharp FBs can be technically demanding and should be limited to experienced endoscopists. When feasible, these particular cases should be referred to high-volume endoscopy centers.

Endoscopic management of acute esophageal food impactions represents a broad spectrum of complexity. Some cases can be safely performed by a supervised trainee, while others can challenge even the most experienced endoscopists. Also known as the "steakhouse syndrome," adults typically present minutes to hours after swallowing a bolus of food and feeling a FB sensation in the chest. Urgent treatment is indicated for patients with severe symptoms or those who are unable to swallow their own secretions. While patients with mild symptoms often resolve spontaneously, endoscopic intervention is indicated within 24 hours to reduce the risk of complications [1,5]. Uncomplicated cases may be successfully managed via the "push technique," provided the endoscopist has visualization of the distal lumen and can rule out an obstructing lesion such as a tumor or tight stricture. This involves advancing the bolus into the stomach using the blunt end of the endoscope [36]. The push technique is less effective and confers greater risk in the setting of proximal esophageal strictures or cases where the distal lumen is completely occluded. Despite these limitations, this approach was successful in 184 of 189 cases (97%) [9]. As an alternative to the push technique, a retained food bolus can be disrupted using snare or basket devices, thereby facilitat-

ing passage through an esophageal stricture. If this is not feasible, the bolus can be removed en bloc, similar to foreign objects, or piecemeal, utilizing the "pull" technique. Retrieval nets are the preferred device for food bolus extraction when the push technique is unsuccessful [27]. In many cases, a single piece of meat is the culprit (Figure 17.4a,b). An overtube should be employed to reduce the risk of mucosal laceration and aspiration when the food bolus cannot be completely retrieved with a net and several intubations appear necessary. A suction technique has been reported, where a cap attached to the tip of the endoscope facilitates trapping the food bolus prior to extraction [37].

Further evaluation

Esophageal lesions such as Type B (Schatzki's) esophageal rings, eosinophilic esophagitis (EoE), peptic strictures, webs, and extrinsic compression may be present in 75–100% of cases of acute food impactions [36,38,39]. Motility disorders such as nutcracker esophagus and esophageal malignancies less commonly present in this fashion [40–42].

EoE has now emerged as one of the most common causes of food impaction [43,44]. Among patients with an acute esophageal food impaction, the possibility of EoE should be strongly considered. Particular attention on endoscopy should be made to identify features suggestive of EoE: "corrugated" or "ringed" mucosal appearance, furrowing, strictures, punctuate white exudates, smaller caliber, and edema (Figure 17.5) [45,46]. Multiple, concentric mucosal rings and longitudinal furrowing are seen in over 70% of patients. A minimum of five biopsies should be obtained from the proximal and distal esophagus [47]. Since esophageal dilation of patients with EoE may have a higher complication rate of severe chest pain and esophageal perforation, empiric dilation should be avoided [46]. Moreover, the efficacy of medical therapy often makes esophageal dilation unnecessary in many patients. Many patients will have significant edema or even mucosal tears

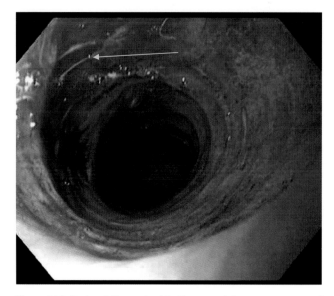

Figure 17.5 Eosinophilic esophagitis. Corrugated rings represent one of the hallmarks of eosinophilic esophagitis. The superficial tear (arrow) illustrates the friable mucosa observed in EoE patients.

immediately following disimpaction. For this reason, we typically delay endoscopic biopsies or dilation, if indicated, for at least one week after relieving a food bolus.

Conclusions

For the successful management of FB ingestions, the physician should make every effort to anticipate the potential challenges associated with endoscopic retrieval. A stepwise approach to these cases will minimize the risk of severe complications. This begins with a thorough pre-procedure assessment and concludes with an evaluation for secondary causes of esophageal obstruction when appropriate. When possible, patients with sharp or large FBs and food impactions should be referred to a high-volume center, particularly those lodged in the esophagus. Trainees who have achieved an elementary level of competence in upper endoscopy can participate in these cases and often complete the entire procedure with close supervision. Animal models provide a unique opportunity to practice using a number of retrieval instruments on a variety of FBs. By taking a stepwise approach to each patient and their endoscopy, an instructor can recognize when an experienced endoscopist should take control. Given the potential for severe complications, no case of FB retrieval should be considered routine.

Videos

Video 17.1 Sewing needle
Video 17.2 Safety pin
Video 17.3 Covered esophageal stent
Video 17.4 Retained video capsule

References

1 Webb WA: Management of foreign bodies of the upper gastrointestinal tract: update. *Gastrointest Endosc* 1995;**41**:39–51.
2 Velitchkov NG, Grigorov GI, Losanoff JE, Kjossev KT: Ingested foreign bodies of the gastrointestinal tract: retrospective analysis of 542 cases. *World J Surg* 1996;**20**:1001–1005.
3 Brady PG: Esophageal foreign bodies. *Gastroenterol Clin N Am* 1991;**20**:691–701.
4 Bloom RR, Nakano PH, Gray SW, Skandalakis JE: Foreign bodies of the gastrointestinal tract. *Am Surg* 1986;**52**:618–621.
5 Chaikhouni A, Kratz JM, Crawford FA: Foreign bodies of the esophagus. *Am Surg* 1985;**51**:173–179.
6 Li ZS, Sun ZX, Zou DW, Xu GM, Wu RP, Liao Z: Endoscopic management of foreign bodies in the upper-GI tract: experience with 1088 cases in China. *Gastrointest Endosc* 2006;**64**:485–492.
7 Little DC, Shah SR, St Peter SD, et al.: Esophageal foreign bodies in the pediatric population: our first 500 cases. *J Pediatr Surg* 2006;**41**:914–918.
8 Llompart A, Reyes J, Ginard D, et al.: [Endoscopic management of foreign bodies in the esophagus. Results of a retrospective series of 501 cases]. [Article in Spanish] *Gastroenterol Hepatol* 2002;**25**:448–451.
9 Vicari JJ, Johanson JF, Frakes JT: Outcomes of acute esophageal food impaction: success of the push technique. *Gastrointest Endosc* 2001;**53**:178–181.
10 Berggreen PJ, Harrison E, Sanowski RA, Ingebo K, Noland B, Zierer S: Techniques and complications of esophageal foreign body extraction in children and adults. *Gastrointest Endosc* 1993;**39**:626–630.
11 Blair SR, Graeber GM, Cruzzavala JL, et al.: Current management of esophageal impactions. *Chest* 1993;**104**:1205–1209.
12 Cote GA, Hirano I: Foreign bodies in the esophagus. In: Shields T, Locicero, J, Reed, CE, Feins, RH (eds), *General Thoracic Surgery*, 7th edn. York, PA: Lippincott Williams & Wilkins, 2009.
13 Hahn IH, Hoffman RS, Nelson LS: Contrast CT scan fails to detect the last heroin packet. *J Emerg Med* 2004;**27**:279–283.
14 Eng JG, Aks SE, Waldron R, Marcus C, Issleib S: False-negative abdominal CT scan in a cocaine body stuffer. *Am J Emerg Med* 1999;**17**:702–704.
15 Eisen GM, Baron TH, Dominitz JA, et al.: Guideline for the management of ingested foreign bodies. *Gastrointest Endosc* 2002;**55**:802–806.
16 Ginsberg GG: Management of ingested foreign objects and food bolus impactions. *Gastrointest Endosc* 1995;**41**:33–38.
17 Ashraf O: Foreign body in the esophagus: a review. *Sao Paulo Med J* 2006;**124**:346–349.
18 Cheng W, Tam PK: Foreign-body ingestion in children: experience with 1,265 cases. *J Pediatr Surg* 1999;**34**:1472–1476.
19 Eliashar R, Dano I, Dangoor E, Braverman I, Sichel JY: Computed tomography diagnosis of esophageal bone impaction: a prospective study. *Ann Otol Rhinol Laryngol* 1999;**108**:708–710.
20 Takada M, Kashiwagi R, Sakane M, Tabata F, Kuroda Y: 3D-CT diagnosis for ingested foreign bodies. *Am J Emerg Med* 2000;**18**:192–193.
21 Goldschmiedt M, Haber G, Kandel G, Kortan P, Marcon N: A safety maneuver for placing overtubes during endoscopic variceal ligation. *Gastrointest Endosc* 1992;**38**:399–400.
22 Bertoni G, Sassatelli R, Conigliaro R, Bedogni G: A simple latex protector hood for safe endoscopic removal of sharp-pointed gastroesophageal foreign bodies. *Gastrointest Endosc* 1996;**44**:458–461.
23 Bertoni G, Pacchione D, Sassatelli R, Ricci E, Mortilla MG, Gumina C: A new protector device for safe endoscopic removal of sharp

gastroesophageal foreign bodies in infants. *J Pediatr Gastroenterol Nutr* 1993;**16**:393–396.

24 Bertoni G, Pacchione D, Conigliaro R, Sassatelli R, Pedrazzoli C, Bedogni G: Endoscopic protector hood for safe removal of sharp-pointed gastroesophageal foreign bodies. *Surg Endosc* 1992;**6**:255–258.

25 Nelson DB, Bosco JJ, Curtis WD, et al.: ASGE technology status evaluation report. Endoscopic retrieval devices. *Gastrointest Endosc* 1999;**50**:932–934.

26 Faigel DO, Stotland BR, Kochman ML, et al.: Device choice and experience level in endoscopic foreign object retrieval: an in vivo study. *Gastrointest Endosc* 1997;**45**:490–492.

27 Katsinelos P, Kountouras J, Paroutoglou G, Zavos C, Mimidis K, Chatzimavroudis G: Endoscopic techniques and management of foreign body ingestion and food bolus impaction in the upper gastrointestinal tract: a retrospective analysis of 139 cases. *J Clin Gastroenterol* 2006;**40**:784–789.

28 Litovitz T, Schmitz BF: Ingestion of cylindrical and button batteries: an analysis of 2,382 cases. *Pediatrics* 1992;**89**:747–757.

29 Yardeni D, Yardeni H, Coran AG, Golladay ES: Severe esophageal damage due to button battery ingestion: can it be prevented? *Pediatr Surg Int* 2004;**20**:496–501.

30 Leers JM, Vivaldi C, Schafer H, et al.: Endoscopic therapy for esophageal perforation or anastomotic leak with a self-expandable metallic stent. *Surg Endosc* 2009;**23**:2258–2262.

31 Ott C, Ratiu N, Endlicher E, et al.: Self-expanding Polyflex plastic stents in esophageal disease: Various indications, complications, and outcomes. *Surg Endosc* 2007;**21**(6):889–896.

32 Gelbmann CM, Ratiu NL, Rath HC, et al.: Use of self-expandable plastic stents for the treatment of esophageal perforations and symptomatic anastomotic leaks. *Endoscopy* 2004;**36**:695–699.

33 Miehlke S, Tausche AK, Bruckner S, Aust D, Morgner A, Madisch A: Retrieval of two retained endoscopy capsules with retrograde double-balloon enteroscopy in a patient with a history of complicated small-bowel disease. *Endoscopy* 2007;**39**(Suppl 1): E157.

34 Lee BI, Choi H, Choi KY, et al.: Retrieval of a retained capsule endoscope by double-balloon enteroscopy. *Gastrointest Endosc* 2005;**62**:463–465.

35 Carey EJ, Heigh RI, Fleischer DE: Endoscopic capsule endoscope delivery for patients with dysphagia, anatomical abnormalities, or gastroparesis. *Gastrointest Endosc* 2004;**59**:423–426.

36 Longstreth GF, Longstreth KJ, Yao JF: Esophageal food impaction: epidemiology and therapy. A retrospective, observational study. *Gastrointest Endosc* 2001;**53**:193–198.

37 Mamel JJ, Weiss D, Pouagare M, Nord HJ. Endoscopic suction removal of food boluses from the upper gastrointestinal tract using Stiegmann-Goff friction-fit adaptor: an improved method for removal of food impactions. *Gastrointest Endosc* 1995;**41**:593–596.

38 Weinstock LB, Shatz BA, Thyssen SE: Esophageal food bolus obstruction: evaluation of extraction and modified push techniques in 75 cases. *Endoscopy* 1999;**31**:421–425.

39 Lacy PD, Donnelly MJ, McGrath JP, Byrne PJ, Hennessy TP, Timon CV: Acute food bolus impaction: aetiology and management. *J Laryngol Otol* 1997;**111**:1158–1161.

40 Chae HS, Lee TK, Kim YW, et al.: Two cases of steakhouse syndrome associated with nutcracker esophagus. *Dis Esophagus* 2002;**15**:330–333.

41 Breumelhof R, Van Wijk HJ, Van Es CD, Smout AJ. Food impaction in nutcracker esophagus. *Dig Dis Sci* 1990;**35**:1167–1171.

42 Waterman DC, Dalton CB, Ott DJ, et al.: Hypertensive lower esophageal sphincter: what does it mean? *J Clin Gastroenterol* 1989;**11**:139–146.

43 Yan BM, Shaffer EA: Eosinophilic esophagitis: a newly established cause of dysphagia. *World J Gastroenterol* 2006;**12**:2328–2334.

44 Croese J, Fairley SK, Masson JW, et al.: Clinical and endoscopic features of eosinophilic esophagitis in adults. *Gastrointest Endosc* 2003;**58**:516–522.

45 Gonsalves N, Kahrilas P, Hirano I: Eosinophilic esophagitis (EE) in adults: emerging entity or misdiagnosed malady. *Gastrointest Endosc* 2005;**61**:AB132.

46 Sgouros SN, Bergele C, Mantides A: Eosinophilic esophagitis in adults: a systematic review. *Eur J Gastroenterol Hepatol* 2006;**18**:211–217.

47 Gonsalves N, Policarpio-Nicolas M, Zhang Q, Rao MS, Hirano I: Histopathologic variability and endoscopic correlates in adults with eosinophilic esophagitis. *Gastrointest Endosc* 2006;**64**:313–319.

18 Endoscopic Mucosal Resection and Endoscopic Submucosal Dissection

Juergen Hochberger[1]

With the support of Elena Kruse[1], Edris Wedi[1], Karl-Friedrich Buerrig[2], SongSa Dammer[1], Peter Koehler[3], & Detlev Menke[1]

[1] St. Bernward Academic Teaching Hospital, Hildesheim, Germany
[2] Institute of Pathology, Hildesheim, Germany
[3] Federal Research Institute for Animal Health (FLI) Mariensee, Neustadt, Germany

Introduction

Endoscopic resection (ER) started with the introduction of snare polypectomy in the colon, esophagus, cardia, and stomach in Germany and in Japan at the end of the 1960s and beginning of 1970s [1]. In 1970, Deyhle, Seuberth, Jenny, and Demling performed the first colonic polypectomy [2]. In the following Classen and Demling form Erlangen, Germany, removed the first gastric polyp [3,4]. Other locations followed. In 1972, Seifert et al. removed for the first time a polyp due to neurofibromatosis from the upper esophagus [5]. Henke and Ottenjann resected an adenoma with focal cancer at the cardia in three sessions in 1973 [6]. Deyhle performed in 1974 the first "en bloc" resection of a minute early gastric cancer using a snare [7].

Polypectomy as the name says is useful for the removal of polypoid lesions. The technique frequently fails when a soft standard snare is applied to remove an only slightly elevated lesion. With the introduction of saline-assisted polypectomy in 1973 by Deyhle et al. after prior experiments in dogs, deep coagulation of the wall could be prevented and the removal of flat lesions facilitated [8]. This technique is nowadays the classic "endoscopic mucosal resection" (EMR) technique but was described in the following often also as "strip biopsy," especially in the Japanese literature and successfully applied in the removal of early gastric and colonic cancers [9–11].

There are mechanical alternatives to saline-assisted resection of mucosa. These include the use of a stiff monofilament snare to be pressed into the mucosa, the aspiration of mucosa into a tube with prograde or side opening and the aspiration of mucosa into a cap or plastic cylinder mounted onto the distal end of the endoscope [12,13]. The Makuuchi tube uses the protrusion of mucosa itself to better grab it with the snare. In a further development by Inoue, the mucosa is aspirated into a special transparent plastic cap mounted onto the distal end of the endoscope. This cylinder is preloaded with a special fine asymmetrical snare placed into a narrow inner rim at the distal end of the cylinder and closed once the mucosal "mushroom" has been aspirated [13]. The third mechanical way is to aspirate the mucosa into a transparent cylinder with externally deployable rubber bands, ligate a pseudo-mushroom after mucosal aspiration, and to consecutively snare it off underneath the rubber band [14–17].

The search for techniques to resect even large mucosal areas with early gastric cancer and to get a thorough histopathologic diagnosis led to the development of "endoscopic submucosal dissection" (ESD) in Japan at the end of the 1990s [18–20]. The concept is based on a freehand needle-knife technique as applied in needle-knife sphincterotomy for difficult access to the biliary or pancreatic duct in ERCP. A large submucosal fluid cushion serves as protective layer when the lesion is first isolated by means of a circular cut outside a safety zone marked beforehand by fine coagulation dots placed around the margins of the lesion. After this circumcision, the lesion is separated from the muscolaris propria at the level of the submucosa. This gives the technique the name of "submucosal dissection." Various knives and special tools have been developed for this scope.

In the following section, the key steps for proper acquisition of EMR and ESD techniques as well as the prerequisites are explained. There is no doubt that a theoretical explanation of the techniques even when illustrated by images, schemes, and video sequences do not replace a one-to-one supervised preclinical and clinical teaching situation. However, we hope you will find some helpful tips for you daily practice.

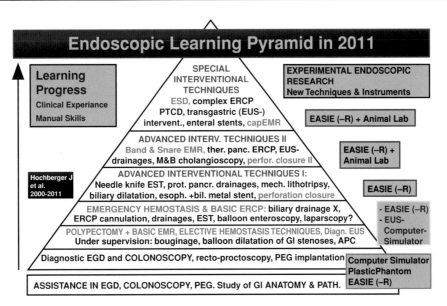

Figure 18.1 Endoscopic "learning pyramid" for stepwise clinical skills acquisition in gastrointestinal endoscopy and the possible complementary use of training simulators.

Endoscopic mucosal resection

EMR techniques to be considered

Common EMR techniques according to organs
Colon:
- Saline-assisted snare resection of flat lesions (classic "EMR")
- Resection of flat lesions using a stiff snare without prior injection

Esophagus:
- CapEMR
- Band and snare technique

Stomach:
- Cap resection for lesions up to 1 cm
- Saline-assisted snare resection of flat lesions (classic "EMR")

Small intestine:
- Saline-assisted snare resection of flat lesions (classic "EMR")

Special EMR techniques not considered
- EMR via double channel endoscope "Pull and snare"
- EMR via Machuuchi tube
- Other rarely applied techniques

Procedures to be considered
EMR is carried out in the entire gastrointestinal tract according to the same principle. Preferred localizations are colo-rectum, stomach, esophagus, and small intestine. It can be part of any primarily diagnostic intervention in these organs, for example, within preventive colonoscopy. Accordingly, it can also be part of gastroscopy, enteroscopy, and ERCP procedures.

Prerequisite level of expertise for endoscopic mucosal resection
There is a large variety in the level of expertise needed for EMR depending on the lesion itself as well as the resection technique applied. Considering our learning pyramid of training, from the base to the most sophisticated techniques, EMR is today no longer considered an expert-only technique; EMR should to be started now at the second level and be taught together with injection and clip hemostasis after trainees have gathered sufficient experience in unsupervised gastroscopy and colonoscopy [21–24] (Figure 18.1). An exact number is not known, but 50 unsupervised colonoscopies plus 100 unsupervised gastroscopies could be a good starting point for the first supervised steps in EMR. The learner should beginning with uncomplicated colo-rectal polyps of less than 2 cm, easy to reach, for example, in the rectum.

More sophisticated techniques and EMRs in difficult locations such as the duodenum, in the esophagus or stomach do require a by far higher level of expertise and a high competence in complication management.

Special considerations
The necessary skills for EMR are best obtained in an intial "hands-on" training course and subsequent clinical guidance of an experienced endoscopist. It is a prerequisite that the trainee is familiar with indications for EMR. He must know contraindications for endoscopic procedures in general and in particular for EMR. Specifically, the trainee has to be able to anticipate and to act upon procedure-related complications during and after EMR.

Specific technical and cognitive skills
EMR requires sufficient cognitive skills with regard to the
- Indication for EMR
- Ability to discriminate submucosal lesions and invasive cancers from mucosal pathologies
- Interpretation of non-invasive imaging results such as abdominal and endoscopic ultrasound (US; EUS), computed tomography (CT), or magnetic resonance imaging (MRI)

• Adequate estimation of the time needed for elective therapeutic procedures

• Knowledge of specific instrumentation or accessories that might be necessary during the procedure in order to organize logistics. Availability has to be checked best the day before the intervention

• Evaluation of clinical signs and symptoms during the procedure and following the endoscopy, for example, abdominal pain due to bloating after colonoscopy versus an "acute abdomen" due to perforation

• Available diagnostic measures and imaging techniques for the detection of procedure-related complications (e.g. CT-scan; US; plain abdominal X-ray film)

• Management of complications: endoscopic and non-endoscopic, for example, medical, minimal-invasive,or surgical

• Evaluation of the histologic result. This is true for an uneventful course but also in case of complications that may lead to the necessity of endoscopic or differenciated more or less radical surgical management

• Scheduling of endoscopic follow-up surveillance intervals according to the histologic result

• Management of late complications such as strictures or local tumor recurrences, non-surgical, or surgical

Equipment for EMR

General considerations

The equipment for EMR depends on the individual lesion and anatomical situation. Criteria to select specific equipment include size, macroscopic appearance, and location of the target lesion, and may vary considerably. Furthermore, the resection technique applied and accessories used may play a role for the overall setting.

For localizations in the lower and upper GI-tract, standard colonoscopes and gastroscopes are commonly used. However, for special localizations, for example, in the duodenum or at the gastric angulus other endoscopes such as duodenoscopes may facilitate resection. In the rectum, a therapeutic or standard gastroscope may prove favorable as it is easier to maneuver than a long routine colonoscope. A double channel gastroscope can provide an additional channel for suction and be advantageous, for example, for strongly vascularized lesions or resections over the hemorrhoidal plexus in the distal rectum. EMR in the jejunum is possible by means of a pediatric colonoscope up to 30–50 cm distal to the ligament of Treitz. Theoretically, EMR can be carried out in the entire small intestine, for example, in FAP patients by means of a special enteroscope and serve as a substitute for surgery. A large channel therapeutic enteroscope, for example, a therapeutic double-balloon enteroscope (e.g., Fujinon EN450T5) is considered best because of adequate hemostasis possibilities. ERs of tumors of the papilla of Vater (Figure 18.2) require advanced skills in ERCP and have to be discussed separately. Special locations of ERs have been described, such as the pharynx and hypopharynx or in the common bile duct on the percutaneous–transhepatic route [25,26].

Equipment independent of the procedure

Adequate monitoring and supervision during sedation

Sedation should be carried out according to national guidelines. In cases of severe comorbidity or extremely complex interventions, general anesthesia should be considered. EMR procedures in large lesions or with technically difficult anatomical access may take considerable time, for example, 1–2 hours (Figure 18.3).

Endoscopic flush pump

A separate flush pump (e.g., "Endowasher" Griessat Endotechnik, Solingen, Germany) operated by a foot switch and coupled in by means of a Y-adapter or a special "jet channel" facilitates the removal of debris, blood, or mucus and seems essential to us for ER techniques. This way, the water pump can be operated without taking an instrument out of the accessory channel during irrigation (Figure 18.4).

Organ-specific equipment

Colon

• Standard or pediatric colonoscope
• Saline-assisted EMR
   ○ Injection needle 21G (0.7 mm) with saline ± epinephrine, for example, 1:250.000 and indigocarmine blue 0.002%
   ○ different stiff snares of a size of 15–35 mm (standard snares have often a size of 20–25 mm)
   ○ Hemoclips for colonoscopic use (e.g., Olympus Optical, Tokyo, Japan; Boston Scientific, Natick, MA)
   ○ Polyp trap to be interposed into the endoscope suction at the level of the attachment to the endoscope light source
   ○ Polyp retrieval net (e.g., Roth net, US Endoscopy, Mentor, OH, USA)

Esophagus

• High-resolution standard diameter adult gastroscope
• For CapEMR
   ○ Injection needle 21G (0.7 mm) with saline ± epinephrine, for example, 1:250.000 and indigocarmine blue 0.002%
   ○ Oblique or straight transparent cap with inner rim (Olympus Optical, Tokyo, Japan) adopted to the outer diameter of the endoscope (e.g., Cap No. 3 for many standard gastroscopes)
   ○ 25 mm multifilament asymmetrical snare (which fits all types of caps; Olympus Optical, Tokyo, Japan)
   ○ Hemoclips for use in the upper (or lower) GI tract (e.g., Olympus Optical, Tokyo, Japan; Boston Scientific, Natick, MA)
• For band and snare EMR technique
   ○ Ready available kit with multiligation cylinder equipped with six rubber bands and special hexagonal snare (Cook Medical, Winston-Salem, USA; Figure 18.7)
   ○ Alternatively, a variceal band ligation set plus standard snare in case of a single lesion
   ○ Polpy retrieval net (e.g., Roth net, US Endoscopy, Mentor, OH, USA) for retrieval from the gastric fundus
   ○ Polyp trap in case of the use of a large channel gastroscope to be considered (interposed between suction tube and endoscope)

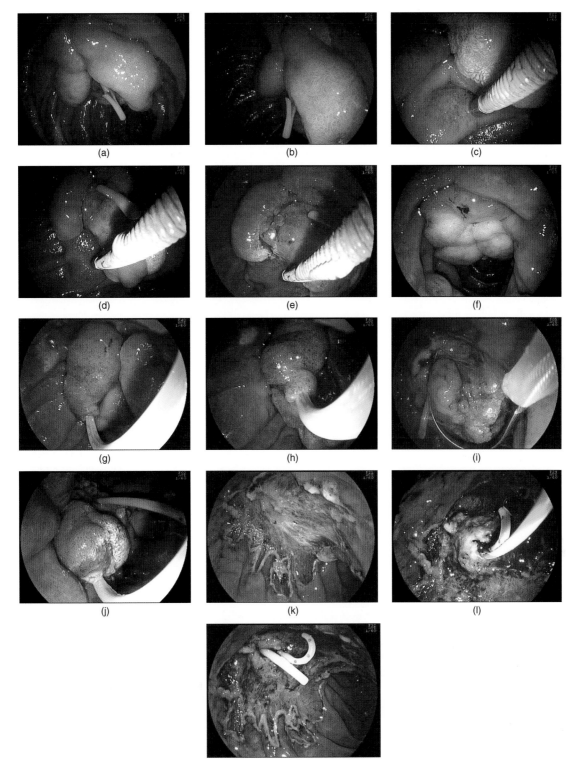

Figure 18.2 (a, b) Endoscopic snare resection of a large 2.5 cm × 3 cm ampullary tumor using a side viewing endoscope: 5 Fr polyurethane drainage still in place. EUS and ERCP with pancreatic and biliary sphincterotomy and bi-ductal stenting had been performed 2 weeks earlier to guarantee a safe ductal access even in case of complications. (c–e) Generous submucosal injection using a Carr-Locke spiral 25G injection needle (US Endoscopy, USA) and a saline/epinephrine solution (1:250.000) with 0.002% indigocarmine blue addition. (f) A complete lifting of the lesion is achieved as important diagnostic criterion for endoscopic respectability. (g–j) Piecemeal EMR is carried out using a 25 mm multifilament snare (Griessat Endotechnik Corp., Solingen, Germany). (k) Macroscopically adenoma-free resection base as final result. (l, m) As last step, a new pancreatic and biliary drainage is implanted to prevent fluid retention.

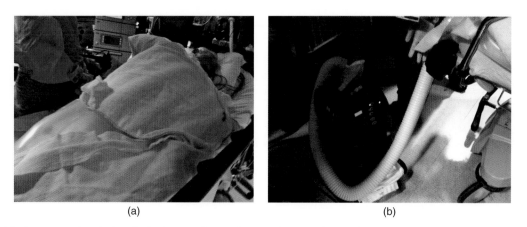

(a)   (b)

Figure 18.3 (a) Patient preparation: for long lasting interventions such as complex ESDs the use of a warming blanket may be advisable.

Stomach
- High-resolution standard diameter adult gastroscope
- Saline-assisted EMR
  - Injection needle 21G (0.7 mm) with saline ± epinephrine, for example, 1:250.000 and indigocarmine blue 0.002%
  - Different stiff snares of a size of 15–35 mm.
  - Hemoclips for use in the upper (or lower) GI tract (e.g., Olympus Optical, Tokyo, Japan; Boston Scientific, Natick, MA, USA)
  - Polyp trap to be interposed into the endoscope suction at the level of the attachment to the endoscope light source
- Polpy retrieval net (e.g., Roth net, US Endoscopy, Mentor, OH, USA)
  - Polyp trap in case of the use of a large channel gastroscope to be considered (interposed between suction tube and endoscope)

Duodenum
- High-resolution gastroscope and therapeutic side-viewing duodenoscope. In the third part of the duodenum, a pediatric colonoscope is often helpful
- Saline-assisted EMR
  - Injection needle 21–23G (0.7–0.5 mm) with saline ± epinephrine, e.g., 1:250.000 and indigocarmine blue 0.002%

- Different snares of a size of 15–20 mm
- Hemoclips for use in the upper (or lower) GI tract (e.g., Olympus Optical, Tokyo, Japan; Boston Scientific, Natick, MA, USA)
- For a sideviewing duodenoscope, disposable (yellow) Olympus clips preferred
- Polyp trap to be interposed into the endoscope suction at the level of the attachment to the endoscope light source
- Polyp retrieval net (e.g., Roth net, US Endoscopy, Mentor, OH, USA) helpful in case particles are first deposited in the gastric fundus and then removed together
- When a sideviewing duodenoscope is used. Disposable Olympus clips ("Quick Clip" and "Quick Clip long," Olympus Optical, Tokyo, Japan). The outer Teflon sheath should be shortened about 2 cm by means of a scalpel

Jejunum and deep small intestine
- Therapeutic enteroscope, for example, therapeutic double-balloon enteroscope (e.g., Fujinon EN450T5)
- Pediatric colonoscope 175 cm for the first 30–50 cm of the jejunum often feasible. For interventions using a pediatric colonoscope or enteroscope of max. 200 cm standard colonoscopy equipment often works

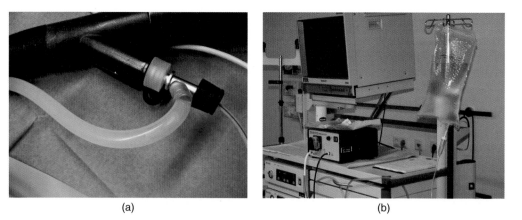

(a)   (b)

Figure 18.4 (a) The system is connected to a Y-shaped side port at the instrumentation channel inlet or a complimentary water jet channel. (b) Helpful accessory for all endoscopic resection techniques: an "endowasher" pump with 3 L bag of rinsing solution.

- Saline-assisted EMR in double-balloon enteroscopy
  - Injection needle 23G (0.5 mm) 270 cm long with saline ± epinephrine, for example, 1:250.000 and indigocarmine blue 0.002%
  - Special DBE snares of a size of 15–25 mm
  - Hemoclips DBE (Olympus Optical, Tokyo, Japan) or for the use in the lower GI tract (e.g., Boston Scientific, Natick, MA)
  - Polyp trap to be interposed into the endoscope suction at the level of the attachment to the endoscope light source
  - Polyp retrieval net (e.g., Roth net, US Endoscopy, Mentor, OH) in case of retrieval after interdisposition in the fundus of the stomach.

Salvage accessories

- "Over-the-scope-clip," "bear trap" (OTSC; e.g., Ovesco, Tuebingen, Germany).

Patient preparation

Focus on informed consent

To justify EMR within a procedure, it has to be covered within the informed consent of the patient prior to the intervention. If EMR appears to be indicated during a primarily diagnostic intervention, the physician has to decide if he needs additional information for example, a rectal ultrasound or MRI of the lesser pelvis to exclude invasive growth or if it seems justified to proceed to resection within the same session. Furthermore, it has to be cleared if alternative treatment options have been discussed sufficiently and if the patient would be ready to accept that she/he needs hospitalization after a complex procedure. Especially in the upper GI tract without the necessity of a special preparation and easy and fast access, it is rather recommended to come back in a second session than to proceed to an invasive procedure without having discussed the next steps sufficiently with the patient.

Patient condition and alternative treatment options

EMR in difficult locations or large lesions may require a longlasting procedure. Fitness of the patient for prolonged sedation during this intervention and complication management has to be checked early. For special interventions anesthesia may be required for airway management. Furthermore, the intervention has to be seen in an interdisciplinary context and alternatives be balanced. Is this the best treatment option for the patient also in the eyes of his relatives, of a general surgeon, or an outside assessor in case of a litigation? Often, it is better to postpone an elective intervention if conditions are not optimal or patient and relatives not thoroughly convinced of the procedure.

Patient preparation

The general preparation is according to the "carrier procedure," for example, gastroscopy or colonoscopy. Special medication such as anticoagulants should be discontinued according to national guidelines and individual recommendations, for example, of the attending cardiologist [27].

Key steps for proper technique in EMR (see Video 18.1)

Evaluation of the lesion

EMR is focused on the removal of epithelial lesions. The first step to an exact evaluation of the lesion is optimal visualization. One should always inspect the entire lesion, including the proximal and lateral margins. Debris or stools should completely be flushed off the lesion and its proximity. Within the last decade, new technical features such as digital chromoendoscopy (NBI, FICE, I-scan), zoom and high-resolution endoscopy (HRE) have added a significant diagnostic yield to standard video endoscopes [28]. Optical contrast such as NBI or FICE can help to better delineate the margins of the lesion and to evaluate the surface structure and the so called "pit pattern" [29,30]. Already by optical appearance, an experienced endoscopist may correctly classify a lesion as suspicious or endoscopically treatable about 80% of the time [31]. However, especially in the upper GI-tract and in the rectum, noninvasive imaging such as EUS, CT, or MRI may add significant information on local lymph node status and invasion depth. The value of submucosal (sm) injection as diagnostic tool will be discussed in the next section. In uncertain cases, clip marking 1–2 cm from the lesion, exact determination of the location, biopsies, and a second examination with more information may be a good alternative [32].

Marking

In case of suspected or proven early malignant lesions, a prior marking including a safety zone of at least 3 mm from the lesion should be performed using thermocoagulation. The by far easiest tool to use is Argon plasma coagulation (e.g., 25 W, 0.3 L gas flow "forced coag" in the VIO generator; ERBE Medizintechnik, Tuebingen, Germany). Alternatives are, for example, the tip of a snare, however, with an increased risk of deeper injury of the wall.

Submucosal injection

Submucosal injection can help in two senses as diagnostic tool. Using saline and epinephrine 1:100.000 alone for injection usually turns the mucosa pale with impaired vision, a reason some endoscopists did not like to use submucosal injection of flat polyps over the years. Adding indigocarmine blue to the injection solution (e.g., Indigo Carmin™, American Regent, Shirley, NY, 1.5–2 mL of a commercial 0.8% solution to a bag of 500 cc of saline) and epinephrine 1:250.000 turns the underground to a mid blue after submucosal injection while the lesion remains bright. This leads to wonderful images with a sharp delineation of even shallow lateral margins.

Furthermore, also the ease to separate layers at the level of the submucosa and the degree of adhesion serve as important diagnostic tools. In case of a clear "lifting" of the entire lesion, resection is almost always possible. A so-called "non-lifting sign" of the lesion with central adherence and lateral bulging, in the extreme case similar to a floating tire, always signalizes an increased perforation risk at resection. An insufficient or only moderate lifting is not always equivalent to malignant infiltration but may occur due to local scarring and prior inflammation, for example, in flat adenomata in the colon or prior incomplete attempts at resection. However, a "non lifting" even after generous fluid injection makes the lesion suspicious and should raise the question whether it is better to continue resection, send the patient to an expert, request additional information, or send the patient directly to the surgeon.

We favor submucosal injection due to the reasons mentioned. However, for single instruments/techniques namely the "ligate and snare" technique using rubber bands for tissue ligation prior to resection, it seems that a larger tissue volume of mucosa can be accomplished with less injection edema in the submucosa. Furthermore, some authors prefer to not use submucosal injection in combination with a stiff monofilament snare [33,34].

An important practical point in submucosal injection is that in contrast to ulcer hemostasis where the needle is rather pressed into the tissue to avoid leakage of fluid, in case of EMR-/ESD-injection, the target layer is the very superficial submucosa. Wall perforation of the needle leading to transmural leakage during further injection and the following resection procedure should be avoided. The needle is first advanced from the catheter and held about 1–2 mm over the mucosal surface. The assistant is asked to start injection. Only when fluid leaves the needle, it is advanced with a sharp "go" to just perforate the mucosa and then immediately pulled back 2–3 millimeters. This will lead to a typical submucosal blowing up of the mucosa. Trainees must be made aware that if the needle is deeply stuck into the tissue and nothing happens, the fluid is being injected beyond the organ wall. We use a standard 5 mm long 21G (0.7 mm) universal injection needle. However, shorter, 3 mm long needles are available for EMR purposes.

Resection techniques for EMR

In this chapter, we limit our discussion to the description in detail of the three most common EMR techniques applied. An overview on EMR and ESD techniques can be found in the current literature [27].

Lift and cut technique ("saline-assisted EMR"; "classic" snare EMR after prior submucosal injection)

Historical background and aim of this technique is to enable the resection of flat polyps in which a conventional snare would easily slip over the lesion (Figure 18.5). The technique is the most popular EMR technique applied especially for the removal of nonpedunculated colorectal polyps. Technically, submucosal saline injection provides a soft fluid cushion into which the snare can easily be pressed. A bulging of the mucosa to the interior of the snare provides a higher friction and better grip of the snare filaments when the snare is closed. This increases the tissue volume per cut. Resection proceeds often easier and faster after the first specimen has been removed. A clear step between the muscular resection base and the mucosal surface facilitates subsequent cuts. Following the first resection, the snare is placed, for example, with the left side into the mucosal defect and the right side is placed onto the lesion elevated by submucosal injection. Pressing the snare onto the ground and closing it slowly, the next piece of mucosa to the right is resected. This is repeated until the entire lesion as well as a lateral safety margin has been removed. The technique is therefore also called "piecemeal resection."

It is advisable to start at the lateral margins of the lesion, incorporating a "safety margin" of 2–3 mm in order to reduce the risk for local recurrences (Figure 18.5). The tissue removed can be pushed to the side and be collected by means of retrieval net (e.g., "Roth net," US Endoscopy, Mentor, OH). Alternatively, but more traumatic and sometimes leading to a rupture or loss of fragments is the retrieval by the snare itself or a wire basket for ERCP stone removal. The third possibility is to just suck off the fragments via the instrumentation channel and to collect them by means of a "polyp trap." Care should be taken that the particles are not smashed and that they are placed in a sufficient quantity of formalin in an appropriate recipient (e.g., for urine samples with sealed trap).

CapEMR

CapEMR is an expert technique and should be applied by advanced endoscopists. It has been developed by Inoue et al. as a further development and logical consequence of the Makuuchi tube for the removal of early esophageal cancer in the beginning of the 1990 and has been one of the major achievements in EMR [13,35]. There is a straight and oblique version of the so-called "distal attachment cap" (Figure 18.6). Caps are provided in different diameters and are in the "classic version" composed of a hard plastic part with an inner rim at the distal end and a soft silicone ring to mount the cap on the endoscope. There are different variations, including a so-called "soft-cap" with larger diameter and flexible plastic cylinder.

We usually recommend starting with a cap No. 3 and a standard HR gastroscope. For the beginner, a straight cap is easier to use. Gaining experience, many will prefer the oblique type as it provides larger resection pieces, better vision on the short side, and traumatizes less the underlying tissue. Having mounted an oblique cap onto the endoscope, one will see on the endoscopy video screen a round plastic tube with inner rim and rectangle being cut out. The purpose of this rectangle in the rim is to indicate the shortest part of the cylinder, while the oblique nose is on the opposite side. The cylinder has to be turned on the endoscope tip until the rectangle is exactly in front of the instrumentation channel (often in an 8 o'clock position). This is essential for a proper functioning of the oblique cap together with the asymmetrical snare (Figure 18.6). The cap is additionally fixed to the endoscope by means of a stripe of sterile soft adhesive (e.g., cut off from the lateral margin of an adhesive or as part of a fixation set for i.v. accesses) (Figures 18.6 and 18.8). This is necessary in order to not loosen the distal cap when retrieving the specimen after resection at the level of the mouth guard. We discourage from taking regular nonsterile "Scotch tape" used for dressings, etc., as it does not stay reliably on the neoprene end of the endoscope and is a potential carrier of hospital germs.

The cap resection technique implies the use of a special 25 mm asymmetrical multifilament snare in the form of the head of a dolphin. The working mechanism includes a stopper integrated in the distal end of the Teflon sheath, the way one side of the snare is bulging while the other one stays in place. This mechanism allows the clockwise deposition of the soft snare into the inner rim of the distal attachment cap (see Video 18.1).

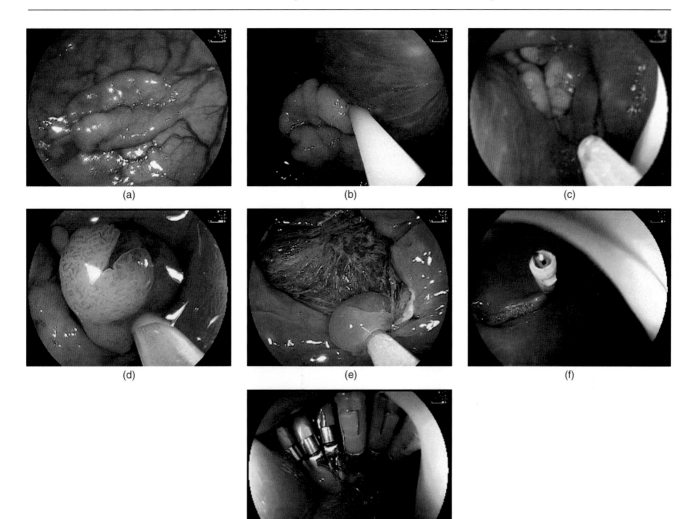

Figure 18.5 (a–e) Indigocarmine blue colorant for improved delineation of flat lesions and later resection margins. "Indigo" is added in a small quantity to the saline/epinephrine submucosal injection fluid (1:250.000; 1.5–2 mL of indigo into 500 cc of saline): flat laterally spreading colonic adenoma clearly visible for piecemeal resection of a lateral safety zone together with the lesion. (f, g) Complete clip adaptation of the margins in a patient at increased bleeding risk.

At first the endoscope is gently introduced into the upper esophagus. Pressing the rinsing and the suction button of the endoscope at the same time removes mucus from the inner side of the cylinder and leads to a clear vision. At first, a marking of the area to be resected is performed, e.g., using an argon plasma probe (25 W, "forced," 0.5 sec pulses forced coag, ERBE VIO prograde probe), including a sufficient safety zone of adjacent inconspicuous tissue (minimum 2–3, recommended 5 mm).

In the case of a circumscript Barrett's cancer, the surrounding Barrett's epithelium may be resected at the same time or just the prominent part with secondary thermal ablation [36,37]. We personally prefer a clear histology over pure ablation after endoscopic inspection and focal biopsy and try to resect 1/3 to 2/3 of the circumference in a Barretts segment containing high-grade dysplasia or early cancer. In this case, an initial marking of the resection field

is performed, extending at least 5 mm cranially and caudally of the Barrett's segment into normal squamous or gastric cylindrical epithelium.

As a second step, the mucosa is generally lifted by submucosal injection using saline/epinephrine 1:250.000 and indigocarmine blue 0.002% in relatively large quantities (e.g., 300 cc during an examination and repeat injection). One should not be afraid of "overinjection" as passing by with the endoscope from cranially to caudally after a short time the fluid will rapidly disappear.

For deposition of the snare within the cylinder, the transparent hood is gently pushed against normal mucosa, for example, in the proximal esophagus, in order to not disturb the lesion itself until the snare is properly seated along the rim of the cylinder. The snare catheter with the snare closed is then advanced until it can be seen within the cylinder. The assistant has then to slowly open the snare

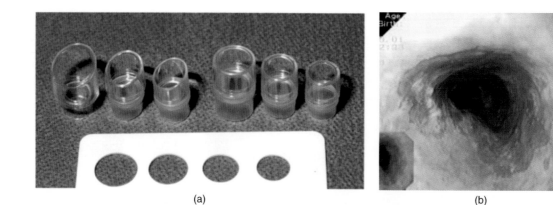

(a)

(b)

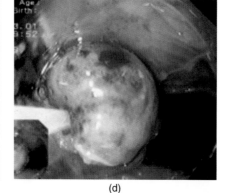

(c)

(d)

(e)

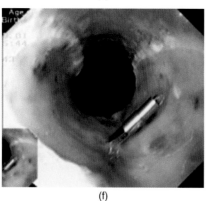

(f)

(g)

(h)

Figure 18.6 (a) Cap resection (EMRc) for flat esophageal lesions: "distal attachment" caps (Olympus Optical, Tokyo, Japan) of various sizes with straight or oblique distal ends according to H. Innoe, Japan. (b) Clinical application in a patient with long-segment Barrett's esophagus and multifocal HG-IEN. (c) After marking of the proximal and distal ends of the Barrett's segment and generous submucosal injection (not shown), a transparent cap is mounted onto the distal end of the endoscope. We use size number 3 oblique with inner rim in combination with an HR standard endoscope, here applied in the proximal esophagus. The rectangle indicates the shortest point of the cylinder and should be aligned with the instrumentation channel. A snare catheter can be seen in the 8'o clock position. The 25 mm asymmetrical snare consists of a special soft wire of 20 multifilaments and is placed into the inner rim of the cylinder, best in a clockwise direction. (d) Resection is started at the proximal end of the lesion including a 2–5 mm safety margin. The endoscope is rotated until the snare catheter directs towards the lesion.

The end of the cylinder is then gently pressed tangentially against the mucosal surface and aspiration is activated. This way only mucosa distally to the cylinder is aspirated and the resection area better defined. When there is a "red out" and the cylinder completely filled the snare, the inner rim of the cylinder is closed and a mushroom-like area of mucosa is captured. After releasing the suction and gently pulling back the endoscope, the mucosa mushroom is released with the snare still closed and resection performed. (e) This can be repeated several times from cranially to caudally over the total length of the long Barrett's segment. (f) Resection of more than two-third of the circumference should be avoided at a time to prevent structuring. Fibrin-covered clean resection base is performed after 5 days. (g) Resection is continued in this case 2 weeks after the first resection but should preferably be carried out after complete healing; usually, 2–3 months after the first resection session. (h) Final result after 3 months with complete removal of the dysplastic area and all Barrett's mucosa. (*continued*)

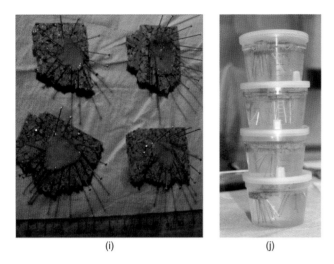

(i) (j)

Figure 18.6 (*Cont.*) (i) capEMR specimen up 3 cm, pinned on cork. (j) Specimen upside down in transport recipients filled with formalin. A second layer of cork is used to securely keep the specimen in the fluid and avoid insufficient fixation or drying.

the way it is deployed in a clockwise fashion onto the inner rim of the distal cylinder. This just as much that the snare surrounds completely the cylinder but does not protrude over the rim into the lumen. The snare catheter is then fixed with the little finger of the left hand at the endoscope in order to avoid dislocation from the inner rim while the endoscopist is moving.

Resection itself is usually started at the cranial end of the Barrett's epithelium or the respective lesion if not Barrett's. The endo-

scope is rotated within the longitudinal axis in order to bring the instrumentation channel with the snare catheter close to the esophageal wall. Again resection is carried out by including in the first resection at least 2–3 mm if not more of normal appearing mucosa in order to be radical enough. The transparent cylinder is therefore placed in an oblique way onto the cranial end to be resected the way the snare catheter is close to the esophageal wall as possible. Aspiration is performed and the mucosa will stepwise creep into the transparent cylinder until there is a "red out" like in variceal band ligation. At this point, the endoscopist stays with his left index on the suction and has his right hand at the snare catheter above the instrumentation channel valve. The assistant now slowly closes the snare while the endoscopist advances the snare catheter into the instrumentation channel just as much as necessary to compensate shrinking of the Teflon tube by compression of the tissue under traction. The assistant has to close the snare to the maximum with the snare handle. A round to oblique area of mucosa is now caught like a mushroom in the snare. At this point, it is important to release the suction with the index of the left hand and to push the closed snare catheter about 2 cm forward out of the cylinder and shake it gently. This helps release possibly entrapped muscularis propria and avoids perforation. Now the entrapped piece of mucosa is cut through with blended current (e.g., "Endocut Q," setting 2, ERBE VIO, or 60W setting 3 ERBE ICC 200). The created little "meat ball" of resected mucosa is then aspirated into the cylinder and the endoscope is withdrawn. With a standard gastroscope and 2.8 mm channel, a polyp trap at the level of the suction is usually not needed. Outside the patient, suction is released best over a sterile metal recipient filled with saline

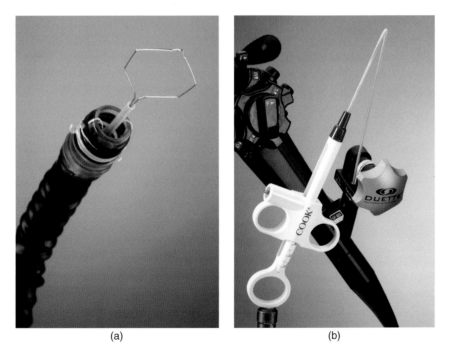

(a) (b)

Figure 18.7 Commercial "Band and Snare" mucosal resection kit ("Douette", Cook Medical, Winston-Salem, USA). A hexagonal monofilic snare (a) is used in combination with a special multiligation system (b) for repeated mucosal aspiration, rubber band ligation, and snare resection under the rubber band.

and the specimen flushed out or if necessary caught by a pair of forceps without damaging it (see Video 18.1).

Time should not be wasted to take of the specimen at this point but rather to go back to the esophagus again and see if there is any bleeding or wall defect. Both should be fixed immediately in the case that either of this has occurred.

Multiple resections can be accomplished this way in the same session. The second resection should adjoin the first one caudally the way the transparent cylinder with the snare is placed precisely at the transition of prior resection base and mucosa to be resected. Again, the cylinder touches at the side of the snare catheter the muscularis propria and suction is applied. The snare should then slip exactly under the mucosal edge between muscular resection abase and mucosa in order to allow a seamless transition and enlargement of the resection. Even more than 10 particles can be taken out going from cranially to caudally, for example, in a Barrett's esophagus and the resection street can be enlarged by a second or third directly adjacent track.

After resection, care should be given to hemostasis of small vessels using, for example, APC at a low gas flow or hemoclips.

Ligate and cut EMR-technique

A technically simple method to resect Barrett's mucosa with HG-IEN in piecemeal fashion is the so-called "ligate and cut" technique [16,34]. Recent advances in refining the technique include the development of the "Duette" system (Cook Medical Bloomington, Indiana) [17,38]. A transparent cylinder with six rubber bands similar to the "sixshooter" variceal band ligation device is mounted on the distal end of the endoscope. In contrast to the variceal band ligator set, the EMR set has a different handle and contains a hexagonal snare that can be introduced into the instrumentation channel via an additional access port in the handle (Figure 18.7).

The technique is applied without prior injection. The mucosa is sucked into the cylinder and the band is fired. The snare is introduced and resection of the created ligation mushroom underneath the band is carried out. Immediately after the next band is placed adjacent to the previous resection site in order to avoid tissue bridges. Tang et al. from Dallas reported a successful removal of a 14 cm Barrett's esophagus with HG-EIN in two sessions. However, in the second resection session alone, they applied 64 bands and 11 EMR/ligation kits, a considerable medical but also economic effort [38]. Wall perforations using the ligate and cut technique are rare [17,39].

Endoscopic submucosal dissection

ESD is composed of a sequence of different steps:
1 Identification and marking of the lesion with a sufficient lateral safety margin
2 Submucosal injection and tissue elevation
3 Circumcision of the lesion
4 Submucosal dissection, "en bloc" removal and subsequent retrieval of the lesion
5 Careful hemostasis and prophylactic occlusion of vessels at the resection base

6 Preparation of the specimen for histopathologic evaluation.
In the following, we will go through personal and technical prerequisites as well as the different steps of ESD

Procedures to be considered for ESD

Procedures to be considered for ESD in the upper and lower GI tract are comparable to those of EMR, with the exception of the small intestine beyond the ligament of Treitz where ESD has not been described so far.

Skills for ESD and who should do it

Prerequisite level of expertise and skill for learning ESD

ESD is currently a technique for the "high-end" endoscopist requiring a long practice in interventional endoscopy and complication management. ESD originated in Japan and is a relatively new procedure in the Western world. The prerequisites and the learning curve to perform a "safe" and sufficiently fast ESD still have to be defined. ESD is a "freehand" needle-knife technique similar to needle-knife sphincterotomy when gaining access to the common bile duct in difficult ERCP situations. In the beginning, ESD is time-consuming and carries an increased complication risk, especially for perforation.

Special considerations for ESD

Initial steps in learning ESD should be accompanied by a training program and expert teaching. Early training steps include a progressive approach to the technique in "*ex vivo*" pig stomachs. Training in live pigs is a useful next step to acquire ESD hemostasis skills and to train the technique in an environment with natural GI motility. For clinical practice, a close student–teacher relationship and sufficient phases of watching the procedure seem important before a student goes to unsupervised clinical ESD. Japanese say that at least 100 ESD procedures are required before the trainee reaches a sufficient speed and safety for standard "en bloc" resections. Systematic training programs will help to avoid pitfalls and lead to a successful spread of this undoubtedly fascinating technique.

Specific technical and cognitive skills for ESD

All statements given for EMR in section are also valid for ESD. Beside these points, the trainee should have the following personal prerequisites:
• Extensive experience in complication management in the upper and lower GI tract especially in adequate treatment of perforations and bleedings
• Several years of experience in interventional endoscopy including different EMR techniques for benign and early malignant lesions.

Equipment for ESD

General considerations on ESD equipment

The equipment for ESD depends much on the individual preferences and resection technique used [40]. For lesions located in the lower and upper GI-tract standard gastroscopes and colonoscopes may be used. However, our personal preference is a slim therapeutic HR double channel gastroscope (Fujinon EG 530D Fujifilm Medical, Tokyo, Japan; Table 18.1) with the advantage of a large suction channel reserved exclusively for aspiration while the smaller channel takes the accessory, for example, the resection knife and is equipped with a Y-side-port for additional coaxial rinsing using a flush pump. We like the double channel instrument as it gives an optimal orientation and overview even in difficult situations. Especially, in a strongly vascularized environment as in the distal rectum, two different channels for rinsing and suction are a major advantage.

Essential equipment for ESD
Upper GI tract, recto-sigmoid, left-sided colon
- Respectively preferred instruments: double-channel gastroscope, standard gastroscope, standard, or pediatric colonoscope.

Colo-rectum
- Standard or pediatric colonoscope.

Special equipment for ESD
- R-scope or M-scope [Olympus Optical, Tokyo, Japan] as experimental articulating endoscopes with two elevators in order to allow up and down and left and right movements of instruments.

Equipment independent of the procedure

Adequate monitoring and supervision during sedation
See section "EMR."

Endoscopic flush pump
See section "EMR."

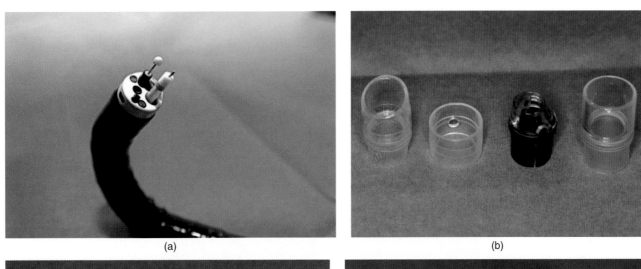

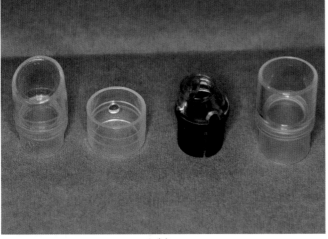

Figure 18.8 (a) Helpful accessories for endoscopic submucosal dissection (ESD): a high resolution double channel gastroscope (EG530D; Fujifilm, Tokyo, Japan) offers optimal suction and overview even in bleeding situations and can be used in the upper GI tract as well as in the recto-sigmoid. Two resection knifes are inserted for demonstration only. (b–d) Transparent caps of different shapes and sizes significantly improve vision during ESD and offer a safe working space for resection knifes. Furthermore, they mechanically help to separate mucosal layer and muscolaris propria in analogy to surgical triangulation. (*continued*)

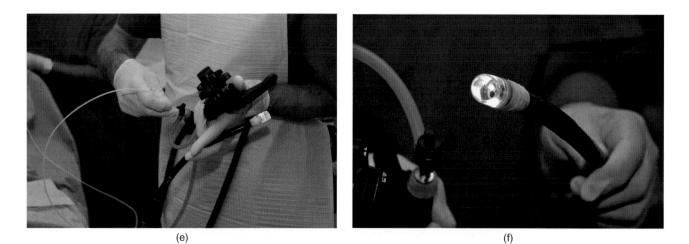

(e)

(f)

(g)

Figure 18.8 (*Cont.*) (e–g) The cylinders should be fixed on the distal end using a sterile tape, for example, as used in dressing kits for IV accesses. This prevents a loss or displacement of the cap during the procedure.

Table 18.1 Typical technical features of different endoscopes (Fujinon EG 590 WR gastroscope, EC 590 ZW colonoscope, EG 530 D therapeutic double channel gastroscope) The EG 530 D (Figure 18.8 e,k) is the preferred standard endoscope for ESD with optimal rinsing and suction capabilities especially in the strongly vascularized distal rectum [40].

Endoscope denomination	Endoscope type	Distal end	Channel Ø	Bending
EG 590 WR	Gastroscope	9.6 mm	2.8 mm	UD 210°/90° LR 100°
EC 590 ZW	Colonoscope	12.8 mm	3.8 mm	UD 180° LR 160°
EG 530 D	Therapeutic double-channel gastroscope	11.5 mm	2.8 mm 3.8 mm	UD 180° LR 160°

UD, up/down; LR, leftright.

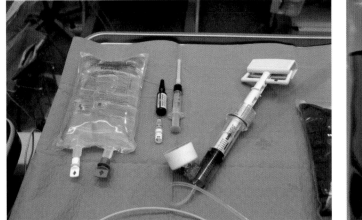

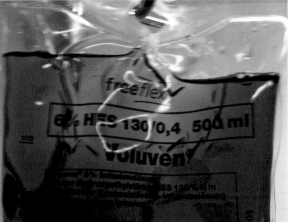

(a)   (b)

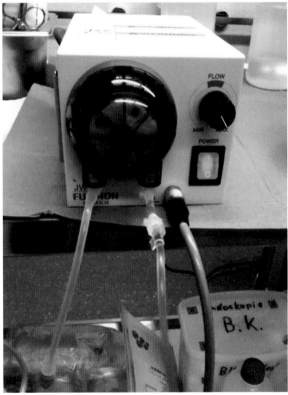

(c)

Figure 18.9 Viscous substances are preferably used in ESD for creation of a longer persisting fluid cushion compared to submucosal saline alone. As using syringes alone for application is cumbersome, the viscous fluid, for example, hydroxy ethylic starch (HAES 6%) is applied by means of commercial 30 cc balloon insufflation pressure manometer (a, b). An electric pump with a foot switch can be a helpful accessory alternative for submucosal fluid injection (c).

Positioning of the patient for ESD

ESD procedures can be prepared like other interventional upper and lower GI interventions. However, they can be long-standing procedures and take hours in large lesions or in case of unexpected events. At least in Germany, ESD is so far not yet an established outpatient procedure. We like to carry out ESD procedures in a left lateral position in a modern hospital bed after adequate

hygienic coverage. This seems a good prevention against any kind of compression damage under deep and long sedation and is not a hygienic problem. In single, very long-standing cases even a warming cover can be helpful (Figure 18.3). After the procedure, the patient recovers in this bed, which may be exchanged then in the ward. We found it helpful to cover the part of the bed close to the assistant with a sterile drape. This provides a good place for a short deposit of instruments when rapid exchanges of instruments are necessary, for example, in case of hemostasis. The other accessories are better stored on a separate height-adjustable table for the assistant.

Antibiotics and PPI
See section "EMR".

Pre-interventional endosonography (EUS)
For ERs of suspicious or early malignant lesions in the upper GI tract and rectum EUS is still the gold standard in order to have a status quo concerning regional lymph nodes and depth infiltration of the lesion [41–45].

See also "Evaluation of the lesion."

Transparent distal endoscope cap for ESD
A special cap at the distal endoscope end serves as transparent "cage" and provides a safe workspace in front of the endoscope. Tissue is kept at distance by means of this atraumatic plastic cylinder, and instruments can be pulled back into this "safety zone" without damaging the working channel. When "diving" with the endoscope underneath the lesion during resection at ESD, the cap serves as important window for local orientation. During initial circumcision, the cap helps to keep a constant distance to the tissue surface and to prevent slipping of the needle-knife into the depth of the cutting rim. There are different caps according to the preferences of the endoscopist (Figure 18.8). The most universal cap is in our experience a short 4 mm soft cylinder cap (Olympus Optical, Tokyo, Japan) as used for zoom endoscopy. It provides a broad field of vision and does not substantially prolong the bending section of the endoscope. Alternatively, a longer oblique distal attachment cap can be used as described for capEMR (endoscope dependent No. 3 or 4 oblique, Olympus Tokyo; Figure 18.8). The advantage lies in the rounded distal end of the cap on the outside, enabling an atraumatic work at the resection base without mechanical irritation. Unfortunately, the inner rim of the cap has to be removed by a scalpel to prevent instruments from getting caught on the rim. The third option is a funnel-like cap that eases tunneling under the lesion during ESD (Fujifilm Medical, Tokyo, Japan). However, this needs some experience with the technique as the field of vision is restricted. As mentioned above, all caps should be fixed to the tip of the endoscope by means of sterile tape.

Injection substances for ESD
In contrast to EMR, ESD requires a stable at least 3–5 mm fluid cushion to safely perform "freehand" needle dissection in the submucosa without injuring the muscularis propria and/or damaging the mucosal lesion for histopathologic evaluation. Furthermore, a sufficiently broad fluid cushion facilitates detection of submucosal vessels. This gives the chance to adequately obturate them, avoiding hemorrhage.

Pure saline rapidly diffuses into tissue. Within the last few years, a wide variety of viscous or osmotically active substances have been evaluated in order to achieve a stable cushion. In order to find a biocompatible, easy to apply, and not too expensive substance, for example, hyaluronic acid, sugars such as dextrose and

fructose, glycerole, or hydroxyethylic starch as well as different mixtures have been evaluated. New substances are in preclinical testing [46]. In Japan, often a mixture of 1% 1900 kD hyaluric acid (Suvenyl™, Chugai Pharmaccutical Co., Tokyo, Japan) and saline 1:3 to 1:7 is used (Mucoup™, Johnson & Johnson, KK, Tokyo, Japan). Also a mixture of 10% glycerin, 5% fructose, and saline (Gyceol™, Chugai Pharmaceutical Co., Tokyo, Japan) is often used [47]. Other substances that have been used are, for example, hydroxyprpyl methylcellulose as used in artificial eye drops [48]. However, these substances are often not available or not officially approved for this indication [49–57].

More than three years ago, we switched successfully to 6% hydroxyethyl starch (e.g., Voluven®, Fresenius Kabi, Germany) as used over years as parenteral volume substitute in emergency and intensive care medicine. To a bag of 500 mL of the solution, we add 2 mL of 1:1000 epinephrine solution, leading to a dilution of 1:250.000. As colorant, 1.5 mL of sterile indicarmin blue solution 0.8% (e.g., Indigo Carmin™, American Reagents, Shirley, NY) is added (Figure 18.9). Other substances in use in Germany are Glycerosteril 10% (a mixture of glucose 1-water 13.75 g, 50 g glycerol, and 2.25 g of sodium chloride per 500 mL) [58]. However, availability and approval for submucosal injection should be individually checked.

Needle injection for tissue elevation
Different modes of tissue elevation can be applied. Aspects of needle injection and the correct technique are described above, A constant cushion formation with just a few injection sites is desirable in order to avoid a leakage of fluid through mucosal needle perforations ("shower head effect"). Furthermore, a deep penetration of the needle into the muscle with transmural (e.g., peritoneal) spillage should to be avoided.

Submucosal injection is usually performed using a sufficiently large sclerotherapy injection needle (21 G = 0.7 mm diameter, 3–5 mm long; Figure 18.10). Contrary to a smaller 23G standard needle, rapid injection of even large quantities of fluid becomes possible for the deposit of a sufficiently high local cushion, preventing escape of the fluid to the periphery. There is little experience with the use of a 19G (1 mm) needle. Although feasible in our experience, a leakage of fluid from needle perforation sites in the mucosa is disadvantageous. Furthermore, it is unclear whether initial excessive local pressure in the submucosa may lead to a transmural escape of fluid through muscle gaps.

Resection knifes

Conventional resection knifes (Figure 18.11)
First ESDs had been performed with standard needle-knives often attached with tape on the distal end of the endoscope, leaving the instrumentation channel free [59,60]. A big step ahead was the development of the so-called "isolated tip knife" (IT knife) at the end of the 1990s (Olympus Optical, Tokyo, Japan) [19]. The advantage over a standard needle-knife was the protection of the muscle layer from the needle tip during dissection. A further development is the IT2-knife. The "IT2-knife" is equipped with an only hemi-spherical isolated white tip with

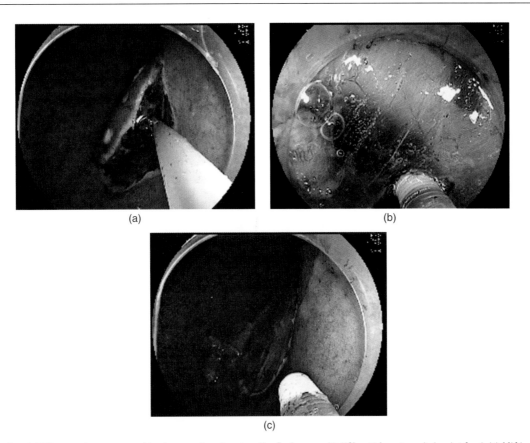

(a)   (b)

(c)

Figure 18.10 Gastric ESD procedure supported by the use of an electric roller flush pump (Fujifilm, Tokyo, Japan). (a–c) After initial lifting of the lesion using a 21G standard needle connected to the pump, the fluid cushion can be re-established during the procedure by pressing the flush-knife catheter into the submucosa and subsequent pump activation.

"Mercedes"-star-like metal base with better lateral resection capabilities (Olympus Optical, Tokyo, Japan) [61,62]. The "hook-knife" is a miniature version of laparoscopic surgical hook-knife and can be rotated by the assistant. Resection of the mucosa as well as dissection of the submucosa is achieved by first "hooking" the tissue and then transection it by electrocautery. The assistant can steer the direction of the hook at the handle. This resection technique is considered the safest, for example, for resections in the colon and esophagus but probably also the most time consuming [63]. The flex-knife, developed by Yahagi, consists in a miniature monofilament snare resembling a broad nose at the tip of the Teflon catheter [18,64,65]. The triangular knife tries to combine hooking capabilities and enforced by means of a small triangular anchor at the tip of the knife [66]. To be mentioned also is the "'dual-knife" (Olympus Optical, Tokyo, Japan) developed as along with the flex-knife by Naoisha Yahagi, one of the pioneers in the field of ESD. The knife has a drop-like distal end, which allows easier coagulation of vessels and reduces the risk of a sharp damage to the muscle layer.

There is a little truth in the sentence "every expert has his own resection knife" as efficiency using a resection tool is closely related to personal experience. To that end, it is reasonable for trainees to gain exposure to a variety of available instruments during the early animal tissue work phases of training.

Resection knifes with integrated fluid injection capability

Water jet technology and "hybrid-knife" (Figure 18.11)

In open surgery, a so-called "water-jet" technology is known over years but plays only a minor role today in surgical organ resection [67–72].

Within the last few years, this technique has been rediscovered for flexible endoscopy by many due to work by Kähler, Yahagi, Neuhaus, and Enderle [64,73,74]. Via an only 0.9-mm wide polyamide catheter (the "capillary"), creation of a submucosal fluid cushion is possible. The capillary does not even have to penetrate the submucosa. It is rather sufficient to just gently place it on the mucosal surface. By activation via a foot pedal, a pressure-controlled electronic pump drives the fluid through the catheter at a pressure of up to 100 bars. The just 60 µm wide flow penetrates the mucosa but is captured at the level of the submucosa as disruption of the muscularis propria would require much higher pressures than penetration of mucosal or submucosal tissue [75]. The system is integrated in a central bore of a needle-knife catheter and the device is called "hybrid-knife" (Erbe Elektromedizin, Tuebingen, Germany) [73]. This allows to elegantly first create a submucosal fluid cushion at a defined pressure and to then use the needle-knife as an electrosurgical tool for circumcision and dissection. Intermittent submucosal

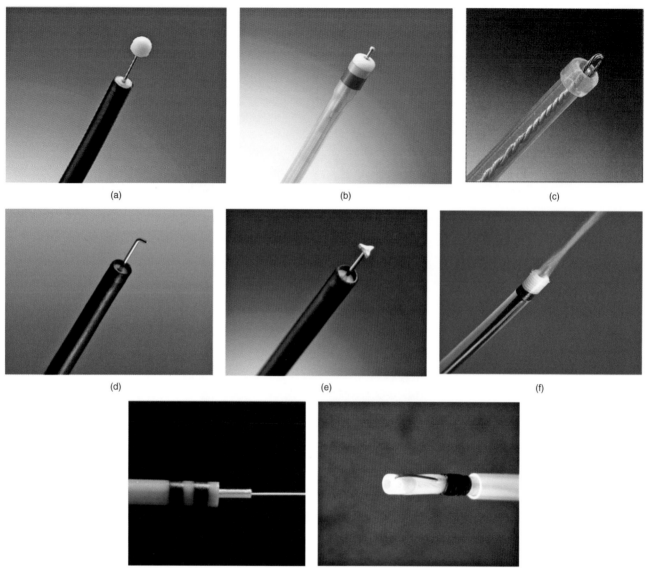

Figure 18.11 8 different ESD cutting knifes are shown. The IT Knife (a), Dual Knife (b) and Flex Knife (c) show an isolated respectively broadened tip to reduce the risk of inadvertent penetration of the knife. The Hook Knife (d) and Triangular Tip Knife (e) are used for 'fishing' and traction of submucosal fibres towards the knife before cutting them through which is considered a safety factor. The same is true for the Flush Knife (f) and the Hybrid Knife (g) which allows intermittent fluid injection for flushing of debris and re-establishment of the necessary submucosal fluid cushion during resection. The Mucosetome (h) somewhat resembles a mini-papillotome.

reinjection is simple. Disadvantages of the system are so far costs and the fact that this is a bit stiffer catheter compared to standard instruments. First preclinical and clinical results are promising [64,74,76,77].

Flush-knife

The so-called "flush-knife" (Fujifilm, Tokyo, Japan) is an interesting alternative to the hybrid-knife and consists of two components. The needle-knife itself exists in different lengths from 1 to 4 mm available in 0.5 mm graduations. We use exclusively the 1 and 1.5 mm knives. The chrome-plated needle is contrary to the hybrid-knife rounded at its tip and has a supple Teflon catheter

with a broad base of 2.7 mm compared to the short nose of the knife. This gives a nice guideway during circumcision, reducing the risk of deeper penetration of the knife during circumcision like a jigsaw [78]. For rectum, esophagus, and colon, we use mostly the 1 mm knife, and for the stomach, we use the 1.5 mm knife [78]. The short length and rounded tip of the knife is responsible for the high safety and precise dissection of the knife. The flush-knife comes together with a roller pump activated by a foot switch and variable in rotation speed (Figure 18.10). A side connection at the level of the handle allows to couple-in fluid that is directed to the catheter tip. Pressing the catheter intermittently into the submucosa and activating the pump rebuilds effectively a decreasing fluid cushion (Figure 18.10). However, initial conventional needle injection is advisable in our experience. Activating the pump intermittently also helps to better identify bleeding sources at the resection base with only limited flushing volume compared to flushing with the endowasher through the endoscope itself. An advantage of the flush-knife/pump combination is the reasonable price. A direct comparison of flush-knife and hybrid-knife does not exist yet.

The "ball-tip flush-knife" (Fujifilm, Tokyo, Japan) is needle-knife similar to the flush-knife with a broad catheter and short knife that is enlarged at the tip to a ball for better coagulation and questionably a reduced perforation risk. However, this may be at the cost of the very fine and clean resection capabilities of the original straight knife.

Electrosurgical settings

Concerning electrosurgery, there are big variations as well in the literature in regard to the settings used. While circumcision is mostly performed with a pure or blended cutting, current dissection is, at least in Japan, often carried out with pure coagulation current. Electrosurgical settings vary for different accessories and may not be comparable for generators of different companies. We use a "VIO 300" generator (Erbe Elektromedizin, Tuebingen, Germany) in combination with a 1 mm flush-knife (Fujifilm, Tokyo, Japan) for the circumcision with the following settings: "Endocut Q," pulse duration 1, pulse length 1, effect 2 or 1. For coagulation with this knife, "Swift Coag" 30 W. For dissection under a strongly vascularized lesion, for example, in the distal rectum, "Forced Coag" 50 W setting 2 is often well suited. By changing

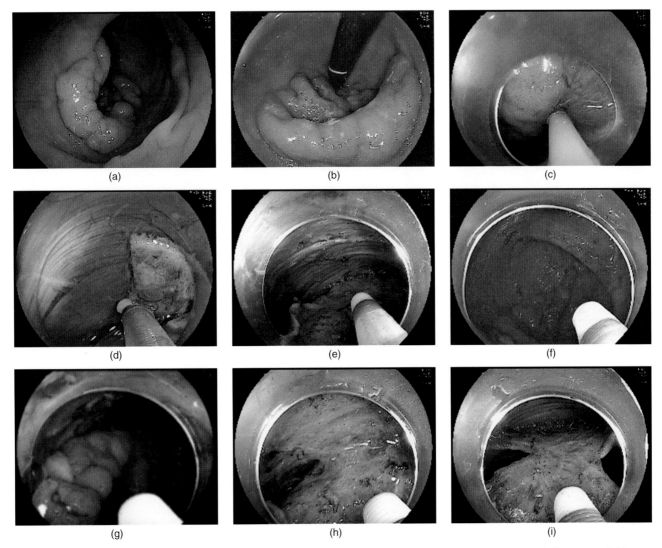

(a) (b) (c)

(d) (e) (f)

(g) (h) (i)

Figure 18.12 Steps of endoscopic en bloc resection using submucosal dissection technique (ESD). (a, b) A large, 8 cm × 6 cm, laterally spreading tumor in the mid and upper rectum is shown from a prograde and retroflexed position (LST-NG type; Paris IIa+c, tubulovillous adenoma with multifocal HG-IEN). (c) After circular marking of the lesion with small coagulation dots, injection of a large 300 cc fluid cushion helps to establish a more than 1 cm submucosal fluid cushion as safe dissection plane. Figures (d)–(i) show the stepwise ESD resection process preserving a single specimen until reaching the upper end of the subtotal circumcision of the lesion. (*continued*)

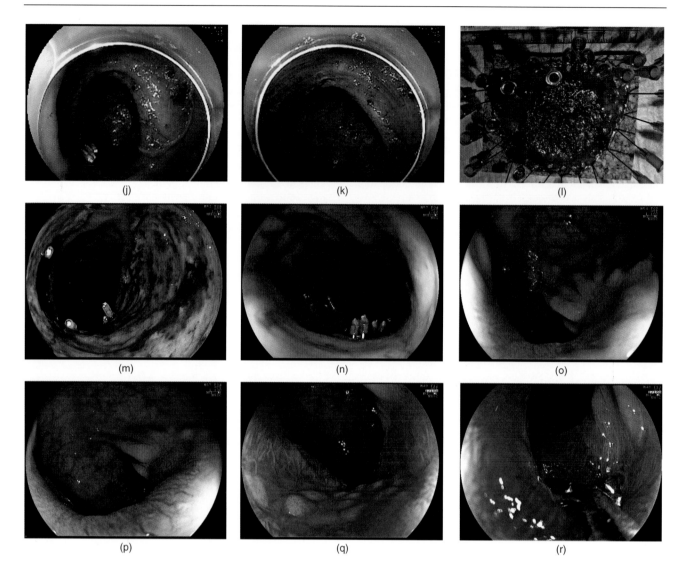

(j) (k) (l)

(m) (n) (o)

(p) (q) (r)

Figure 18.12 (*Cont.*) Figures (j) and (k) show the final dissection result with a clean base of the large resection area leading over rectal Kohlrausch folds. Resection steps as well as the coagulation of all vessels had been performed using an only 1.5 mm short flush-knife (Fujifilm, Tokyo, Japan) in combination with HAES 6% as submucosal fluid cushion and an electric flush pump. (l) 10 cm × 12 cm resection specimen pinned on cork before being placed upside-down in formalin for histopathologic evaluation. Fibrinoid resection bed after 1 week. (m) Single prophylactic hemoclips had additionally been placed on larger coagulated vessel stalks at the end and on day 1 after the procedure. Still fibrinoid wound bed after 6 weeks (n), and progressive shrinking with purely red scar after 4 months (o–r).

between cutting and coagulation current, a smooth resection is possible with effective coagulation of vessels up to 1 mm and rapid dissection using just one knife. Using a "coagulation forceps" (e.g., "Coag Grasper," Olympus Optical, Tokyo, Japan) with a larger contact area, a higher power setting may be necessary (e.g., "Soft Coag," effect 5, 30–60 W). It is important to keep always in mind that excessive coagulation may lead to late necroses even after 24–72 hours with secondary perforation. Basically, a stepwise testing of the coagulation capabilities of one's own generator seems essential, and it is always helpful to take some time to compare coagulation depth of different instruments at various settings on a piece of meat, for example, beef or pig liver, even though this cannot be directly transferred to "*in vivo* settings." The trainee needs to understand the general principles of electrosurgical generators, a topic covered in detail in another chapter in this book and become well versed in the specific settings required for dissection and coagulation of bleeding vessels.

Using the 1–1.5 mm flush-knife at the abovementioned settings, we do not use any coagulation forceps anymore. In case of big vessels, we carefully start fulgurization at a distance of 1 mm from the vessel and close to the overlaying lesion as the vessel will shrink. If after shrinkage of the vessel this has to be performed at a distance too close to the muscular layer, and if one has to continue to coagulate due to ongoing bleeding, then retraction of the vessel into the muscular layer or creation of a coagulation defect in the muscle layer may occur. To avoid this, a short-arm (green or yellow) hemoclip should be applied at the penetration site of the vessel at the muscular layer.

Novel dissection tools are in preclinical and first clinical testing, such as flexible "Maryland Dissector," which applies gentle mechanical lateral force by opening its long jaws similar to the same named surgical tool. It may as well be used for the application of the electrocautery of vessels [79]. Other instruments and devices tested are, for example, submucosal balloon dissection or an automatic submucosal circumcisor ("Circular Cutter," Apollo Endosurgery, Austin, TX, USA). These developments, which introduce traditional surgical techniques and principles into the realm of luminal ER, may be an indicator of trends leading in the not too distant future to the entity of the *Endoscopic Interventionelist*, a new hybrid endoscopic specialist who encompasses the skill sets of today's tradtional gastroenterologists and minimally invasive surgeons [80–82].

Procedural steps of endoscopic submucosal dissection (Figures 18.10; 18.12–18.15)

There is a big variety of ESD techniques depending often on the individual preferences of the physician and personal level of expertise. There are common features of the technique such as marking of the lesion, creating a preferably stable submucosal fluid cushion, circumcision of the lesion outside the safety zone, and markings and separation of the mucosal layer from the muscularis propria at the level of the submucosa in a single piece.

ESD is therefore composed of a sequence of different steps:
1 Identification and marking of the lesion with a sufficient lateral safety margin
2 Submucosal injection and tissue elevation
3 Circumcision of the lesion

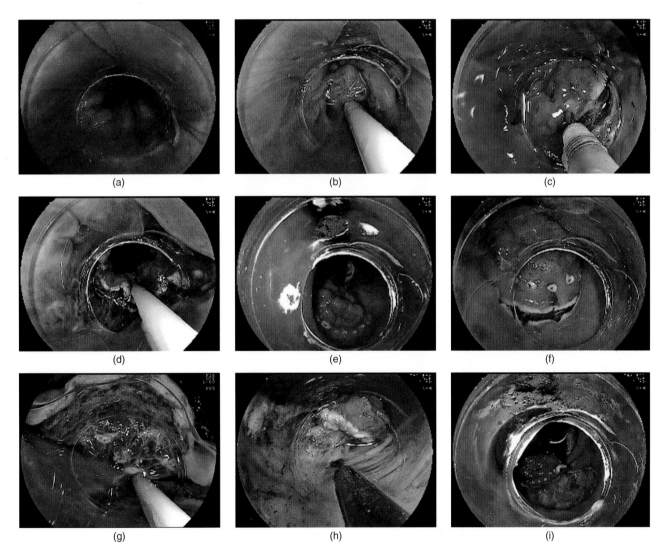

(a)   (b)   (c)

(d)   (e)   (f)

(g)   (h)   (i)

Figure 18.13 Endoscopic "en bloc" resection in submucosal dissection technique (ESD) of a wide spread flat polyp in the distal rectum reaching down the anal channel to the dentate line (a). Injection of lidocain 1% at the dentate line as well as repeat large-volume submucosal needle injection of an HAES 6%/epinephrine/indigocarmine blue solution (b–g) under the proximal lesion is effected before and during the resection process in combination with an IT2 knife (Olympus Optical, Tokyo, Japan) (h). (*continued*)

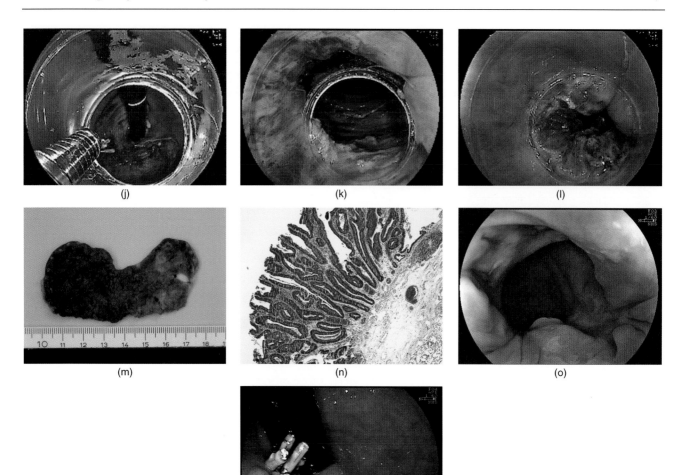

(j) (k) (l)

(m) (n) (o)

(p)

Figure 18.13 (*Cont.*) Resection site with about 60–85% of the circumference resected in the distal rectum and anal channel over the hemorrhoidal plexus (j, k, l). Macropathologic and histopathologic aspects of the 7.7 cm × 3.6 cm specimen showing a tubulovillous adenoma with LGD (m, n). Resection site 6 months after resection with a white scar (o, p). Massive shrinkage of the formerly large resection area

to about 1.5 cm × 1.5 cm with clips in situ can be seen with compensatory extension of the remaining healthy mucosa due a continuous dilatation effect with the storage function of the rectal ampulla. This would not have taken place with a 100% circular resection without retaining healthy mucosa.

4 Submucosal dissection, "en bloc" removal and subsequent retrieval of the lesion
5 Careful hemostasis and prophylactic occlusion of vessels at the resection base
6 Preparation of the specimen for histopathologic evaluation.

Submucosal injection
See p. 218 section 'Needle injection for tissue elevation'

Circumcision
Care should be given that even distant parts of the lesion are sufficiently lifted by submucosal injection before proceeding to circumcision. One can imagine that with point-shaped needle injection, the fluid distributes in a circular or oval shape. To sufficiently reach and elevate the center of the lesion from an

injection at the level of the peripheral markings, the same area will be lifted in a centripedal direction. Japanese carefully avoid central needle perforation of the tumor in order not to potentially seed tumor cells into the depth, therefore, to the submucosa or even to the muscularis propria.

After complete elevation of the lesion, one should uninterruptedly proceed to circumcision. It is advisable to start circumcision always at the most difficult part of the lesion, which is often the most distant one. In the ano-rectum, it is often the cranial and left-lateral side of the lesion. The importance of the markings is usually realized when it comes to circumcision. The cut is performed about 1–2 mm outside the markings. Placing the endoscope gently on top of the elevated mucosa with the transparent cap, the field of vision is often that close to the mucosa one will only see the next marking point as pathfinder for the right direction and to avoid to get lost toward the periphery or worse toward the lesion. Circumcision should be in every case be completed before one proceeds to submucosal dissection, even if there is often a nice bulging of the isolated central mucosal island, having performed only part of the circumcision. Otherwise, one risks to undermine the lateral margins under-tunneling the specimen with incomplete circumcision, or one has difficulties to free the specimen at the end due to a lack of submucosal fluid cushion at the end of the dissection. Often, it is necessary to circle a second time around the circumcision in order to completely transect tissue bridges.

A lateral submucosal dissection of the "normal" surrounding peripheral mucosa for about 5 mm helps to nicely form a broad rim at the circumcision as the freed mucosa tends to retract due to contraction of the muscularis mucosa after liberation from the submucosa. Care should further be given that the fluid cushion is not too much depressed by the cap and force of the endoscope. This may result in a superficial cut into the muscle layer. The shorter the knife is and the broader the catheter, the less is the risk of damage when using a needle-knife. We usually perform circumcision with the 1 mm flush-knife in the distal stomach with the 1.5 mm flush-knife at the EC settings described above. An alternative concerning safety is the use of a hook-knife.

Submucosal dissection

Before switching from circumcision to submucosal dissection, it is often considerable to first reinject in order to have an optimal

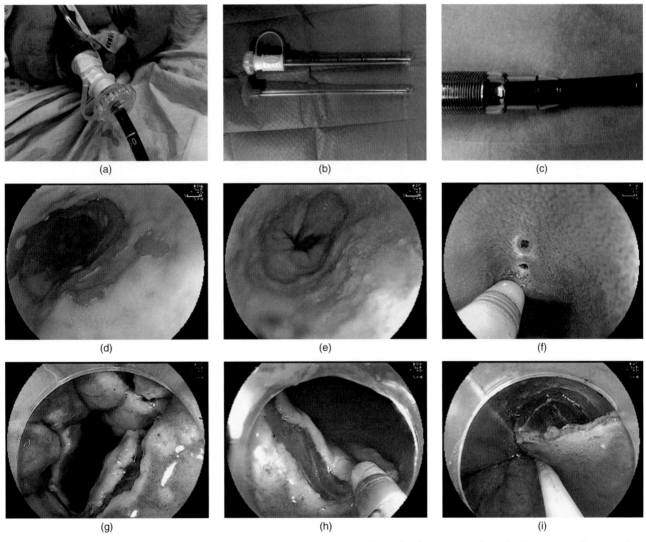

(a)　　　　　　　　　　　(b)　　　　　　　　　　　(c)

(d)　　　　　　　　　　　(e)　　　　　　　　　　　(f)

(g)　　　　　　　　　　　(h)　　　　　　　　　　　(i)

Figure 18.14 Widespread "en bloc" resection using ESD in the esophagus. (a–c) An overtube can be used as an alternative to endotracheal intubation for airway protection avoiding aspiration due to flushing or bleeding for lesions in the mid and distal esophagus. (d, e) Steps of the ESD procedure itself for "en bloc" resection of a long segment Barrett's esophagus with multifocal HG-IEN. A 75–80% circumferential resection was performed using a 1.5 mm short resection knife (Flush Knife, Fujifilm, Tokyo, Japan). (f–j) After marking and repeat submucosal injection, a U-shaped circumcision was performed including a 1 cm safety zone at the proximal and distal ends of the Barrett's segment. (*continued*)

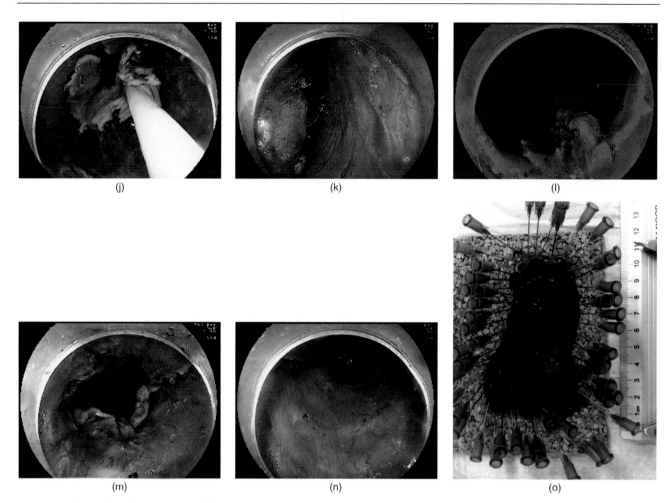

Figure 18.14 (*Cont.*) (k–n) Step submucosal dissection from cranium to caudal with a clean resection base at the end. (o) Esophageal resection specimen pinned on cork histopathologically confirmed the initial diagnosis (multifocal HG-IEN; R0 within specimen). Local status after 3 months with a circumscript residual Barrett's area (p), and after 6 months with complete removal (q).

fluid cushion. Submucosal dissection is carried out in parallel to the mucosal layer often in a semilunar fashion. Vessels have to be respected and are better first coagulated than cut through with secondary coagulation. Depending on the diameter of the vessel, this is best be achieved by

- Switching the foot pedal from "cut" to "coag" current
- Withdrawing the knife and switching to a coagulation grasper
- Placing a short-arm clip close to or at the exit of the vessel from the muscular layer.

The latter is usually avoided because of a possible accidental mechanical removal of the clip by the endoscope. Furthermore, the metal of the clip is conductant and the clip impairs vision and free maneuverability of the endoscope. Last but not least, the clip has later to be removed in order to get a "clean" scar for further follow-up inspection and biopsies.

After a short course of 7–10 mm, the lesion can be lifted and tunneled by the cap. This helps to stretch the submucosal tissue and eases resection. The function simulates traction forces applied during "triangulation" in laparoscopic surgical dissection.

Retrieval of the specimen

Attention should be paid especially in large resections not to destroy the specimen during retrieval. This is especially the case for large specimen in the stomach or rectum. In the rectum, this can be facilitated by first removing the flexible endoscope and introducing a rigid proctoscope for adults (e.g., 16–18 mm). After removal of the obturator, the proctoscope is held by an assistant and the flexible endoscope is reintroduced via the proctoscope. The specimen can now be pulled into the proctoscope and can be easily removed. For retrieval, a large braided snare or a stone extraction basket can be using moderate force at the handle when closing.

In the stomach, retrieval of big specimen can be facilitated by first introducing a flexible overtube (US Endoscopy, Mentor, OH; Figure 18.14) The specimen is first stretched and about 1/3rd grabbed by a snare. Removal of the specimen is then performed with slow and constant traction, fixing the catheter at the level of the instrumentation channel cap. The specimen is then first put temporarily in a recipient with sufficient saline (e.g., a metal basin accommodating 250–500 cc of saline).

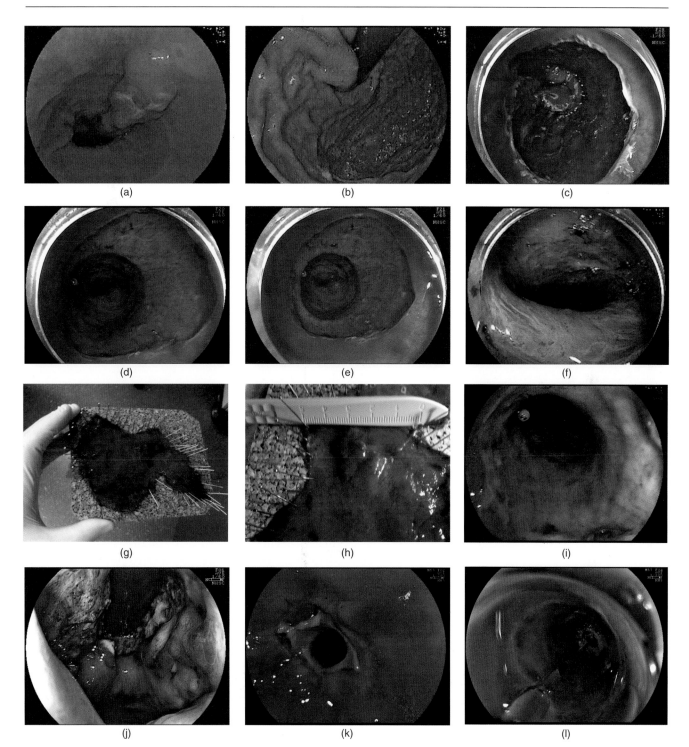

Figure 18.15 Limits of endoscopic resection at the gastroesophageal junction. (a) Widespread "en bloc" resection using ESD of a 3 cm early cancer Siewert Type II extending to the distal esophagus and proximal stomach in a patient repeatedly refusing surgery. In analogy to the case in Figure (a), a 16.5 cm × 10 cm specimen is resected including 7 cm of the tubular esophagus, the cardia and proximal stomach (c–i). (*continued*)

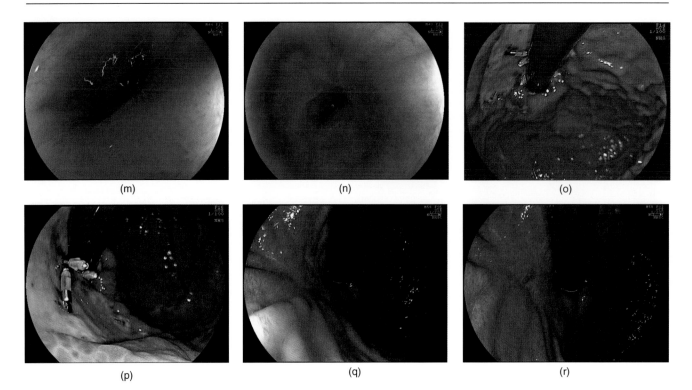

(m)　　　　　　　　　　(n)　　　　　　　　　　(o)

(p)　　　　　　　　　　(q)　　　　　　　　　　(r)

Figure 18.15 (*Cont.*) (i–r) Different states of wound healing with stricture formation and repeat bouginage and balloon dilatation.

Inspection of the resection base and occlusion of vessels

Careful inspection of the resection base should be performed directly after temporary deposit of the specimen in saline. Protruding resected vessels, sometimes still pulsating, should be checked for sufficient occlusion. In doubtful cases, coagulation with a coag grasper or clip application in vessels of more than 1.5 mm is advisable.

Preparation of the specimen for histopathologic evaluation

After a short immersion in saline, the specimen is pinned on cork. A pair of splinter tweezers as used in hand surgery and conventional fixing pins are well suited for this purpose, if not available usual 21 G cannulas (Figure 18.16). Cork as used in pin boards does a good job for this purpose. A rectangular piece of cork about $1^{1}/_{2}$ to 2-folds, the size of the estimated ER area, is cut from the board and placed on a disposable underlay. At first, the specimen is orientated with the epithelial surface upward. Pinning is performed about 1–1.5 mm from the margin, holding the specimen at the border with the tip of the forceps and avoiding damage by excessive compression. After the first pin is placed, the specimen is not (!) stretched out, placing the next pin at the opposite side, as this would lead to a disruption of the margins and impaired histopathologic evaluation. The margin of the specimen is instead caught about 5 mm away from the first needle and pulled laterally. The second fixation pin is placed 2–3 mm at the side of the first one. This way the whole specimen is stretched out like a tambourine (Figure 18.16.d). As the next step, the size of the specimen, if possible also of the lesion should be determined

and documented. We found it the most hygienic way to use a pair of stainless steel compasses with locking possibility and to first determine the greatest longitudinal diameter. This distance is then transferred from the compasses to a metal ruler as used for engineering drawings and the size read off. The same is done for the largest perpendicular diameter. We usually perform then a photo documentation of the specimen with a ruler at the side. For fixation and transportation, the specimen is then placed upside-down in a recipient filled with usual buffered formalin 4%, the way it swims on the surface. Excessive cork material can be shortened before if necessary by a pair of scissors or a scalpel, avoiding getting injured by the needles. The piece of cork with the pinned specimen is slightly kept under water, charging it with a second cork plate or cork surpluses on top. The recipient is then covered at least by a stretched latex glove in case the lab is next door or safely sealed for further transportation (Figure 18.16.e).

In addition to standard histopathological documentation, the pathologist should be asked for macropathologic documentation, and in the case of submucosal infiltration of a tumor, the pathologist needs to report the precise vertical infiltration depth in microns.

Post-EMR and post-ESD management

Control endoscopy

We routinely inspect resection bases the next day after upper GI ESDs even in asymptomatic patients, for the purpose of detecting bleeding or other complications. However, first analyses indicate that this practice might be unnecessary [83].

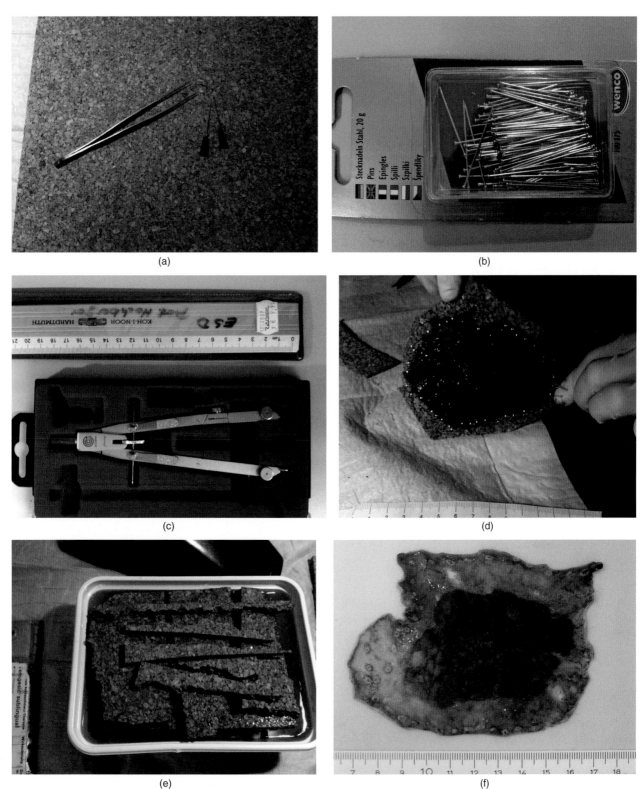

(a)

(b)

(c)

(d)

(e)

(f)

Figure 18.16 Tools for adequate preparation of a mucosal specimen for histopathology: the specimen should be spread out and pinned on cork in order to facilitate lateral evaluation of the resection margins. A pair of splinter tweezers (a) is used in hand surgery and conventional fixing pins (b) are well suited for fixation of the specimen on a piece of cork. The pins are applied one-by-one in a circular fashion to avoid laceration of the specimen (see text) (d). A pair of compasses (c) is well suited to transfer the size of the lesion to a metal spacer (e). The lesion is then placed upside-down into a robust recipient with formalin for transfer to the pathologist. The fixed specimen shows a broad lateral safety zone important for histopathological evaluation (f).

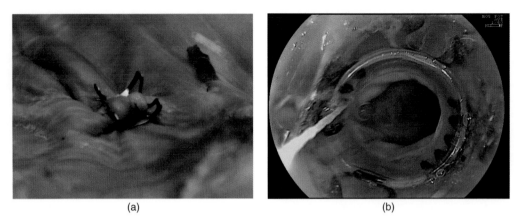

(a)   (b)

Figure 18.17 (a) An over-the-scope clip (OTSC; Ovesco, Tüebingen, Germany) can be helpful salvage tool in ESD.

Risk of secondary bleeding

In case of a clinically uneventful procedure and postinterventional course, a second-look endoscopy is usually not necessary after EMR in colonic lesions. For EMR in the esophagus and stomach, it may clearly depend on the complexity of the procedure. However, as in ulcer hemostasis, a second look endoscopy might be unnecessary [83]. A recent retrospective analysis after ER of 454 gastric epithelial neoplasms (386 early gastric cancers and 68 gastric adenomas) showed an overall postinterventional bleeding rate of 5.7%. However, 2.8% and 2.5% occurred before or after a scheduled second day gastroscopy. All cases occurred within 14 days after the procedure.

Peri-interventional antibiotics and PPIs

Peri-interventional antibiotics are not routinely administered or supported by any data [84–86]. However, in complex procedures and in case of suspected intercurrent perforation or microperforation, an antibiotic prophylaxis should be given [85,87]. Established substances are a second- or third-generation cephalosporine (e.g., ceftriaxone 2 g/1 × die i.v.) plus metronidazole (3 × 500 mg i.v.) or ampicillin plus sulbactam (e.g., 1g plus 0.5 g, 3×/die i.v.). The duration has to be decided on the clinical course and ranges from 1 to 5 days. We routinely place patients undergoing upper GI ESD on PPI medication to prevent delayed bleeding. Data supporting the role of PPI is limited.

Management of complications

Acute procedure-related complications

Procedure-related complications are defined as being clinically evident within 1 week after the procedure. Complications in total are rare but are more frequent in ESD than in EMR. The most common ones are bleeding, perforation, and sequelae associated with perforation. Sequelae of open or covered perforation may be air leakage and infection. Gastric perforation is often associated with pneumoperitoneum and peritonitis, esophageal perforation with mediastinal and subcutaneous emphysema, pneumothorax, and mediastinitis. Large colonic perforations are associated

with pneumoperitoneum and peritonitis, duodenal perforations often with retroperitoneal emphysema, and secondary peritonitis. Biliary leakages due to perforations in the second or third part of the duodenum are feared by surgeons. Other intrainterventional complications may involve cardiorespiratory depression (hypotension, arrythmia, hypoxemia) and may be procedure- or sedation-induced.

Perforation

The incidence of intrainterventional gastric perforation ranges from 1–6% in gastric ESD and is described in a much lower percentage in gastric EMR (0.2%), maybe due to smaller lesions resected endoscopically at the time of EMR compared to nowadays.

Minami et al. from the National Cancer Center Hospital in Tokyo, Japan, followed 121 of 2460 patients (4.9%) who underwent gastric EMR between 1987 to 2004 with perforation during the procedure [88]. The initial four patients were treated with emergency surgery, the subsequent 117 patients with endoclips. Endoscopic closure with endoclips was successful in 115 patients (98.3%), only two patients had to undergo emergency surgery. Patients with perforation during gastric EMR treated with endoscopic closure had a recovery rate similar to that of the nonperforation cases. The authors conclude that gastric perforation during ER can be conservatively treated by complete endoscopic closure with endoclips in the hands of experienced endoscopists [88].

A new promising tool is the so-called "Over-the-scope-clip" (OTSC; "Bear-Trap"; Ovesco Tuebingen, Germany; Figure 18.17) [89,90–93]. The nitinol macroclip comes already mounted on a transparent plastic cylinder and is fired similar to a variceal band ligator. However, the perforation site is actively pulled into the cylinder by means of grasper forceps as aspiration alone would be inefficient due to the air leak within the defect. First clinical applications for perforation closure, severe bleedings, and chronic fistulae are promising [94–96].

Hemorrhage- and procedure-related mortality

With the development of more aggressive interventional techniques in between traditional GI endoscopy and minimally invasive surgery such as ESD and NOTES® hemorrhage needs a

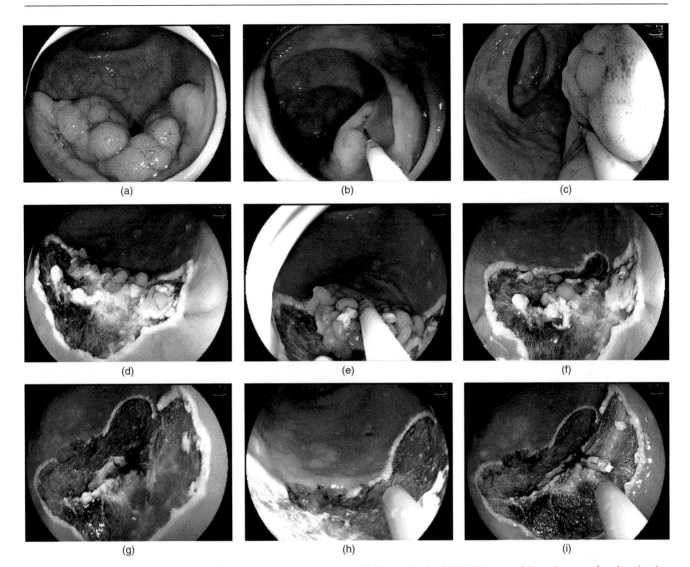

Figure 18.18 (a–i) WHAT NOT TO DO: Difficult piecemeal snare resection of a flat rectal polyp (LST-GT) as one of the main causes for a later local recurrence into or aside a scar. This situation should be avoided especially in lesions at elevated risk for HG-IEN or mucosal cancer such as rectal polyps larger than 3 cm.

new definition. Acute bleeding during ESD cutting through a vessel due to insufficient coagulation cannot primarily be regarded as complication unless it cannot be treated endoscopically comparable to a surgical ligature during an operation. Only bleedings that cannot be stopped or hemorrhages with a consequent drop of hemoglobin more than 2 g/dL in addition to patients with relevant clinical signs of acute hemorrhage (shock, hemotochezie, etc.) should be considered to be a complication. Data from large multicenter studies from Japan or South Korea including over 1000 patients are unfortunately all of retrospective nature [97–101]. Acute and delayed bleeding rates given are between 0.5% and 15.6% for acute bleeding during the first 48 hours and the same for delayed bleedings occurring at the most within the first 14 days after the procedure. In three large trials, cited procedure-related mortality was 0% [99,101,102].

Late and secondary complications

Stricture formation

When more than 75% of the circumference is resected in a tubular GI structure, especially in the esophagus, pylorus, sigmoid, or anus, secondary stricture formation may occur (Figure 18.14.m) [103]. Stricture formation often initiates between 10 and 20 days after resection. However, at least in our opinion, an individual's tendency to stricture formation plays a relevant role. Treatment consists of balloon dilation or bouginage and should be started early as soon as tissue retraction starts to become symptomatic. A sufficient diameter of 18–20 mm should be sought. In the case of esophageal strictures placement of a temporary self expanding covered metal stent after the first bouginage sessions is a possible treatment alternative [47,104,105].

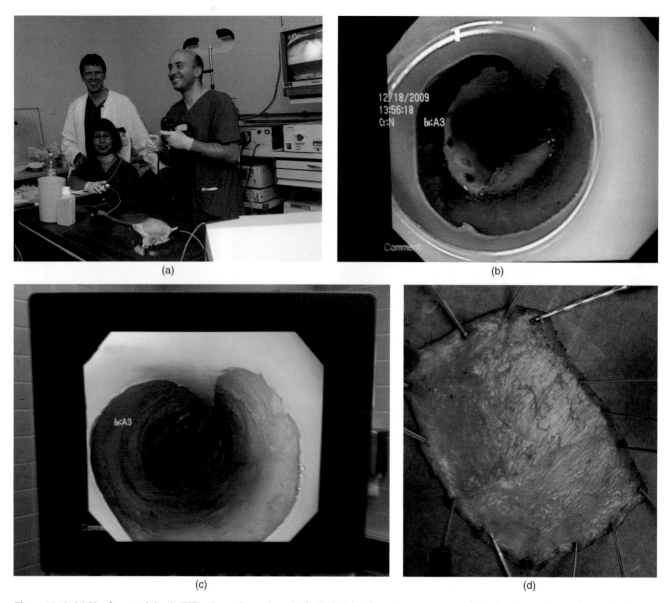

Figure 18.19 (a) Hands-on training in ESD using a pig specimen in the EASIE simulator. A one-to-one teaching situation and more than 50 in vitro training sessions are desirable. (b–d) New ESD locations, for example, in the esophagus should first be trained in the model, even for the experienced.

When to use EMR and when ESD?

This question has to be answered individually and no general rule is applicable. In case of a known or suspected malignant lesion, transection of the tumor should be avoided and "en bloc" resection for adequate histological evaluation should clearly be favored. Furthermore, a clearly lower local recurrence rate favors ESD over EMR even in benign lesions. However, ESD is still a new technique in the "Western Word" and not yet a standard. We will have to learn it step by step and will have to take care that proper training is provided [106] (Figure 18.18).

Training and first steps in ESD

At present, endoscopic skills are mostly acquired under supervision by an experienced colleague while examining a patient.

The usual method of teaching is similar to that of a craft apprenticeship. The trainees start gradually, at first only observing the examination and the handling of the equipment by the endoscopist and assistance. More complex procedures follow simple ones starting, for example, with gastroscopy, recto-proctoscopy, and colonoscopy. First interventional procedures include, for example, PEG implantation, then polypectomy. This kind of clinical learning we described in the past as a "learning pyramid" (Figure 18.1) [21–24,82].

Learning certain new techniques in the course of clinical practice as opposed to during formal fellowship training may be possible. However, it requires a very slow approach in multiple little steps under close clinical surveillance. Under the pressure of maximized efficiency in today's clinical medicine, this way of learning is often not very realistic anymore. This may induce several consequences. Or, there is no real change in skills acquisition over years and an endoscopist, for example, working in private practice will just continue to perform procedures as he learned them during his clinical training at the hospital for the rest of his professional career. The second extreme is that one sees a new technique in advertisement or heard from a colleague about it and just orders the kit and tries it for the first time in the next more or less suitable case. The slightly nicer version is to see it during a live video transmission and to do it for the first time with assistance of the local sales representative. The best practical setting is to visit a department with a high frequency in the specific procedure and see it performed in the morning and train it in an EASIE simulator in the afternoon under the guidance of an experienced endoscopist for several days (Figure 18.19). Any therapeutic intervention a learner may approach in endoscopy should at the same time be accompanied by a training program on how to manage unintended outcomes and complications. Main complications in any ER technique are bleeding and perforation. Training in EMR and ESD will therefore always has to include hemostasis training. The degree of skill and expertise and amount of time required to gain necessary proficiency for such complicated and high-risk procedures as ESD make it extremely difficult to pick up in the course of a busy practice without a concerted effort and devotion of considerable time to the endeavor.

Systematic training studies for ESD do not exist so far up to our knowledge. We are currently registering the learning curves in ESD for ESD-novices of different prior levels of experience. We think that training in ESD includes obviously building up a sufficient theoretical background of the procedure and starting with the resection of a defined area of tissue in a pig stomach "in vitro" in the EASIE simulator. The next step is "in vivo" resection in the stomach of live pigs. Parallel first clinical steps are made beginning with marking the surrounding of the lesion carefully with APC dots at a distance of 2–3 mm from each other and from the lesion plus submucosal injection. The next step after at least 10 successful ESDs in the simulator without perforation is to perform short sections of circumcision under supervision. Training in the pig stomach and animal model should continue while first sections of dissection and complete circumcision in the patient are performed under supervision. This means that an experienced colleague is in the room and sits, for example, on the computer with intermittent following of the procedure and immediate intervention in case of problems. Japanese say that it takes about 100 ESDs before the endoscopist has gathered sufficient experience and has reached a satisfying speed for most standard situations. ESD is performed probably with the lowest risk in the gastric antrum to the greater curvature or anterior/posterior wall. Also, the distal rectum is a good location to start with. However, the distal rectum below the peritoneal fold is just theoretically without risk. We find that it requires most attention to not damage the wall and to occlude even small defects immediately in order to not risk free air in

the surroundings and pain or fever of the patient. It should be emphasized that the width of the fluid cushion and the shortness of the needle-knife are important safety factors. The less experience one has, the shorter the knife should be, in our eyes preferably a 1 mm "flush-knife" and a large cushion of hydroxyethylic starch should be used.

As emphasized above, for the future structured training courses at expert centers including a clinical demonstration of the technique in the morning and lectures and "hands-on" training in pig stomach models and finally animal training as step 2 should become mandatory for a safe introduction of this fascinating technique in the Western world.

Conclusions and perspectives

EMR has developed to a standard technique for the removal of laterally spreading premalignant polyps in the Western world and has changed from an experts-only technique to one of the essential techniques to train after diagnostic gastroscopy/colonoscopy and parallel to or right after hemostasis techniques. ESD is currently the experts-only technique and will probably remain for the next years as it requires a high level of manual dexterity and experience in complication management as well as the oncologically correct treatment of early malignant GI lesions. The learning curve of ESD in the Western world is not known yet. However, growing experience in the West as well as in its locus of origin Japan and recently Korea will lead to far steeper learning curves. New developments as short-knife allowing injection and resection at the same time will further reduce resection times and complication risk. Special cases and locations of ERs have been described, such as ESD in the pharynx and hypopharynx or in the common bile duct on the percutaneous transhepatic route with special instrumentation [25,26].

ESD is a fascinating technique as is its concept of "en bloc resection" as oncologically correct treatment for high-risk or early malignant lesions is with no doubt convincing. Proper training will be one of the key issues for a successful spread of this promising technique.

Nonstandard Abbreviations

APC	Argon plasma coagulation
CT	Computed tomography
DBE	Double-balloon enteroscopy/enteroscope
EC	Electrocoagulation
EGD	Esophagogastroduodenoscopy
EMR	Endoscopic mucosal resection
ESD	Endoscopic submucosal dissection
EUS	Endoscopic ultrasound
FAP	Familiar adenomatous polyposis
GI	Gastrointestinal
GIT	Gastrointestinal tract
HG-IEN	High-grade intraepithelial neoplasia (synonymous to "high-grade dysplasia")
HR	High resolution
LG-IEN	Low-grade intraepithelial neoplasia (synonymous to "low-grade dysplasia")

MRI   Magnetic resonance imaging
NOTES   Natural orifice translumenal endoscopic surgery
PEG   Percutaneous endoscopically controlled/assisted
              gastrostomy implantation
PPI   Proton pump inhibitor
sm   Submucosal

Videos

Video 18.1 Key principles of successful cap EMR technique
Video 18.2 Endoscopic submucosal dissection
Video 1.3 Use of simulator to teach what not to do: improper submucosal lift in EMR leads to perforation on purpose
Video 23.4 Closure of gastrointestinal perforations
Video 30.1 Ampulectomy
Video 30.4 Management of immediate bleeding during cap EMR
Video 30.5 Detection and endoscopic management of mucosal tear complicating upper endoscopy

References

1 Niwa H: New challenges in gastrointestinal endoscopy. In: Niwa H, Tajiri H, Nakajima M, Yasuda K (eds), *The History of Digestive Endoscopy*. Tokyo: Springer, 2008: 3–28.

2 Deyhle P, Seuberth K, Jenny S, Demling L: Endoscopic polypectomy in the proximal colon. *Endoscopy* 1971;**2**:103–105.

3 Classen M, Demling L: [Surgical gastroscopy: Removal of gastric polyps using a fiber-optic gastroscope]. [Article in German] *Dtsch Med Wochenschr* 1971;**96**:1466–1467.

4 Deyhle P: Results of endoscopic polypectomy in the gastrointestinal tract. *Endoscopy* 1980: 35–46.

5 Seifert E, Huchzermeyer H, Otto P, Wagner H: Therapeutic polypectomy of the esophagus. *Endoscopy* 1972;**4**:228.

6 Henke M, Ottenjann R: Therapeutic snare-ectomy of an early carcinoma in the cardia. *Endoscopy* 1973;**5**:225–228.

7 Deyhle P, Sulser H, Säuberli H: Endoscopic snare ectomy of an early gastric cancer—A therapeutical method? *Endoscopy* 1974;**6**:195–198.

8 Deyhle P, Largiadér F, Jenny S, Fumagalli I: A Method for endoscopic electroresection of sessile colonic polyps. *Endoscopy* 1973;**5**:38–40.

9 Tada M, Karita M, Yanai H, Takemoto T: [Endoscopic therapy of early gastric cancer by strip biopsy]. *Gan To Kagaku Ryoho* 1988;**15**:1460–1465.

10 Karita M, Tada M, Okita K, Kodama T: Endoscopic therapy for early colon cancer: The strip biopsy resection technique. *Gastrointest Endosc* 1991;**37**:128–132.

11 Waye JD: Endoscopic mucosal resection of colon polyps. *Gastrointest Endosc Clin N Am* 2001;**11**:537–548, vii.

12 Makuuchi H, Yoshida T, Ell C: Four-step endoscopic esophageal mucosal resection (EEMR) tube method of resection for early esophageal cancer. *Endoscopy* 2004;**36**:1013–1018.

13 Inoue H, Endo M, Takeshita K, Yoshino K, Muraoka Y, Yoneshima H: A new simplified technique of endoscopic esophageal mucosal resection using a cap-fitted panendoscope (EMRC). *Surg Endosc* 1992;**6**:264–265.

14 Ell C, May A, Wurster H: The first reusable multiple-band ligator for endoscopic hemostasis of variceal bleeding, nonvariceal bleeding and mucosal resection. *Endoscopy* 1999;**31**:738–740.

15 Ell C, May A, Gossner L, et al.: Endoscopic mucosal resection of early cancer and high-grade dysplasia in Barrett's esophagus. *Gastroenterology* 2000;**118**:670–677.

16 Soehendra N, Seewald S, Groth S, et al.: Use of modified multiband ligator facilitates circumferential EMR in Barrett's esophagus (with video). *Gastrointest Endosc* 2006;**63**:847–852.

17 Seewald S, Ang TL, Omar S, et al.: Endoscopic mucosal resection of early esophageal squamous cell cancer using the Duette mucosectomy kit. *Endoscopy* 2006;**38**:1029–1031.

18 Yamamoto H, Yahagi N, Oyama T: Mucosectomy in the colon with endoscopic submucosal dissection. *Endoscopy* 2005;**37**:764–768.

19 Ono H, Kondo H, Gotoda T, et al.: Endoscopic mucosal resection for treatment of early gastric cancer. *Gut* 2001;**48**:225–229.

20 Gotoda T: Endoscopic resection of early gastric cancer: The Japanese perspective. *Curr Opin Gastroenterol* 2006;**22**:561–569.

21 Hochberger J, Maiss J: Currently available simulators: Ex vivo models. *Gastrointest Endosc Clin N Am* 2006;**16**:435–449.

22 Hochberger J, Maiss J, Hahn EG: The use of simulators for training in GI endoscopy. *Endoscopy* 2002;**34**:727–729.

23 Cohen J, Cohen SA, Vora KC, et al.: Multicenter, randomized, controlled trial of virtual-reality simulator training in acquisition of competency in colonoscopy. *Gastrointest Endosc* 2006;**64**:361–368.

24 Hochberger J, Maiss J, Cass O, Roesch T, Hahn EG: Training and Education in Gastrointestinal Endoscopy. In Classen M, Tytgat GNJ, Lightdale CJ (eds), *Gastroenterological Endoscopy*. Stuttgart, New York, Georg Thieme Verlag 2002:102–9.

25 Suzuki H, Saito Y, Oda I, Nonaka S, Nakanishi Y: Feasibility of endoscopic mucosal resection for superficial pharyngeal cancer: A minimally invasive treatment. *Endoscopy* 2010;**42**:1–7.

26 Hochberger J, d'Addazio G: Endoscopic tumor treatment in the bile duct. *Gastrointest Endosc Clin N Am* 2009;**19**:597–600.

27 Kantsevoy SV, Adler DG, Conway JD, et al.: Endoscopic mucosal resection and endoscopic submucosal dissection. *Gastrointest Endosc* 2008;**68**:11–18.

28 Cohen J: *Advanced Digestive Endoscopy—Comprehensive Atlas of High Resolution Endoscopy and Narrow Band Imaging*. Hoboken, NJ: Blackwell Publishing, 2007.

29 Kudo S, Kashida H, Tamura T, et al.: Colonoscopic diagnosis and management of nonpolypoid early colorectal cancer. *World J Surg* 2000;**24**:1081–1090.

30 Kudo S, Kashida H, Nakajima T, Tamura S, Nakajo K: Endoscopic diagnosis and treatment of early colorectal cancer. *World J Surg* 1997;**21**:694–701.

31 May A, Gunter E, Roth F, et al.: Accuracy of staging in early oesophageal cancer using high resolution endoscopy and high resolution endosonography: A comparative, prospective, and blinded trial. *Gut* 2004;**53**:634–640.

32 Cohen J: The impact of tissue sampling on endoscopy efficiency. *Gastrointest Endosc Clin N Am* 2004;**14**:725–734, x.

33 Soehendra N, Binmoeller KF, Bohnacker S, et al.: Endoscopic snare mucosectomy in the esophagus without any additional equipment: A simple technique for resection of flat early cancer. *Endoscopy* 1997;**29**:380–383.

34 Seewald S, Akaraviputh T, Seitz U, et al.: Circumferential EMR and complete removal of Barrett's epithelium: A new approach to management of Barrett's esophagus containing high-grade intraepithelial neoplasia and intramucosal carcinoma. *Gastrointest Endosc* 2003;**57**:854–859.

35 Inoue H, Takeshita K, Hori H, Muraoka Y, Yoneshima H, Endo M: Endoscopic mucosal resection with a cap-fitted panendoscope for esophagus, stomach, and colon mucosal lesions. *Gastrointest Endosc* 1993;**39**:58–62.

36 Pouw RE, Wirths K, Eisendrath P, et al.: Efficacy of radiofrequency ablation combined with endoscopic resection for barrett's esophagus with early neoplasia. *Clin Gastroenterol Hepatol* 2010;**8**:23–29.

37 van Vilsteren FG, Bergman JJ: Endoscopic therapy using radiofrequency ablation for esophageal dysplasia and carcinoma in Barrett's esophagus. *Gastrointest Endosc Clin N Am* 2010;**20**:55–74, vi.

38 Tang SJ, Tang L, Jazrawi SF: Circumferential endoscopic mucosal resection of a 14-cm Barrett's dysplasia with the Duette mucosectomy device (with videos). *Gastrointest Endosc* 2008;**68**:786–789.

39 Gerke H, Siddiqui J, Parekh KR, Vanderheyden AD, Mitros FA: Esophageal perforation complicating band ligator-assisted mucosal resection. *Gastrointest Endosc* 2009;**69**:153–154.

40 Hochberger J, Dammer S, Kruse E, et al.: Endoskopische Submukosa-Dissektion—Technische Voraussetzungen. *Verdauungskrankheiten* 2009;**27**:260–268.

41 Tanabe S, Koizumi W, Higuchi K, et al.: Clinical outcomes of endoscopic oblique aspiration mucosectomy for superficial esophageal cancer. *Gastrointest Endosc* 2008;**67**:814–820.

42 Rampado S, Bocus P, Battaglia G, Ruol A, Portale G, Ancona E: Endoscopic ultrasound: Accuracy in staging superficial carcinomas of the esophagus. *Ann Thorac Surg* 2008;**85**:251–256.

43 Waxman I: EUS and EMR/ESD: Is EUS in patients with Barrett's esophagus with high-grade dysplasia or intramucosal adenocarcinoma necessary prior to endoscopic mucosal resection? *Endoscopy* 2006;**38**(Suppl 1):S2–S4.

44 Akashi K, Yanai H, Nishikawa J, et al.: Ulcerous change decreases the accuracy of endoscopic ultrasonography diagnosis for the invasive depth of early gastric cancer. *Int J Gastrointest Cancer* 2006;**37**:133–138.

45 Larghi A, Lightdale CJ, Memeo L, Bhagat G, Okpara N, Rotterdam H: EUS followed by EMR for staging of high-grade dysplasia and early cancer in Barrett's esophagus. *Gastrointest Endosc* 2005;**62**:16–23.

46 Fernandez-Esparrach G, Shaikh SN, Cohen A, Ryan MB, Thompson CC: Efficacy of a reverse-phase polymer as a submucosal injection solution for EMR: A comparative study (with video). *Gastrointest Endosc* 2009;**69**:1135–1139.

47 Ono S, Fujishiro M, Niimi K, et al.: Long-term outcomes of endoscopic submucosal dissection for superficial esophageal squamous cell neoplasms. *Gastrointest Endosc* 2009;**70**:860–866.

48 Arantes V, Albuquerque W, Benfica E, et al.: Submucosal injection of 0.4% hydroxypropyl methylcellulose facilitates endoscopic mucosal resection of early gastrointestinal tumors. *J Clin Gastroenterol* 2010;**44**:615–619

49 Fujishiro M, Yahagi N, Nakamura M, et al.: Successful outcomes of a novel endoscopic treatment for GI tumors: Endoscopic submucosal dissection with a mixture of high-molecular-weight hyaluronic acid, glycerin, and sugar. *Gastrointest Endosc* 2006;**63**:243–249.

50 Sakai Y, Eto R, Kasanuki J, et al.: Chromoendoscopy with indigo carmine dye added to acetic acid in the diagnosis of gastric neoplasia: a prospective comparative study. *Gastrointest Endosc* 2008;**68**:635–641.

51 Sohn DK, Chang HJ, Choi HS, et al.: Does hyaluronic acid stimulate tumor growth after endoscopic mucosal resection? *J Gastroenterol Hepatol* 2008;**23**:1204–1207.

52 Iizuka T, Kikuchi D, Hoteya S, Yahagi N: The acetic acid + indigocarmine method in the delineation of gastric cancer. *J Gastroenterol Hepatol* 2008;**23**:1358–1361.

53 Lee SH, Cho WY, Kim HJ, et al.: A new method of EMR: Submucosal injection of a fibrinogen mixture. *Gastrointest Endosc* 2004;**59**:220–224.

54 Yamamoto H: Endoscopic submucosal dissection of early cancers and large flat adenomas. *Clin Gastroenterol Hepatol* 2005;**3**:S74–S76.

55 Yamasaki M, Kume K, Kanda K, Yoshikawa I, Otsuki M: A new method of endoscopic submucosal dissection using submucosal injection of jelly. *Endoscopy* 2005;**37**:1156–1157.

56 Yamasaki M, Kume K, Yoshikawa I, Otsuki M: A novel method of endoscopic submucosal dissection with blunt abrasion by submucosal injection of sodium carboxymethylcellulose: An animal preliminary study. *Gastrointest Endosc* 2006;**64**:958–965.

57 Sato T: A novel method of endoscopic mucosal resection assisted by submucosal injection of autologous blood (blood patch EMR). *Dis Colon Rectum* 2006;**49**:1636–1641.

58 Probst A, Golger D, Arnholdt H, Messmann H: Endoscopic submucosal dissection of early cancers, flat adenomas, and submucosal tumors in the gastrointestinal tract. *Clin Gastroenterol Hepatol* 2009;**7**:149–155.

59 Hoteya S, Yahagi N, Iizuka T, et al.: [Endoscopic resection for early gastric cancers by EMR/ESD]. *Gan To Kagaku Ryoho* 2007;**34**:16–20.

60 Tsuruta O, Tsuji Y, Kawano H, et al.: Indication for endoscopic resection of submucosal colorectal carcinoma: Special reference to lymph node metastasis. *Diagn Ther Endosc* 2000;**6**:101–109.

61 Ono H, Hasuike N, Inui T, et al. Usefulness of a novel electrosurgical knife, the insulation-tipped diathermic knife-2, for endoscopic submucosal dissection of early gastric cancer. *Gastric Cancer* 2008;**11**:47–52.

62 Con SA, Oda I, Suzuki H, Kusano C, Kiriyama S, Gotoda T: Risk of perforation during endoscopic submucosal dissection using latest insulation-tipped diathermic knife (IT knife-2). *Endoscopy* 2009;**41**(Suppl 2):E69–E70.

63 Oyama T, Tomori A, Hotta K, et al.: Endoscopic submucosal dissection of early esophageal cancer. *Clin Gastroenterol Hepatol* 2005;**3**:S67–S70.

64 Yahagi N, Neuhaus H, Schumacher B, et al.: Comparison of standard endoscopic submucosal dissection (ESD) versus an optimized ESD technique for the colon: An animal study. *Endoscopy* 2009;**41**:340–345.

65 Kodashima S, Fujishiro M, Yahagi N, Kakushima N, Omata M: Endoscopic submucosal dissection using flexknife. *J Clin Gastroenterol* 2006;**40**:378–384.

66 Chiu PW, Chan KF, Lee YT, Sung JJ, Lau JY, Ng EK: Endoscopic submucosal dissection used for treating early neoplasia of the foregut using a combination of knives. *Surg Endosc* 2008;**22**:777–783.

67 Toth S, Vajda J, Pasztor E, Toth Z: Separation of the tumor and brain surface by "water jet" in cases of meningiomas. *J Neurooncol* 1987;**5**:117–124.

68 Terzis AJ, Nowak G, Rentzsch O, Arnold H, Diebold J, Baretton G: A new system for cutting brain tissue preserving vessels: Water jet cutting. *Br J Neurosurg* 1989;**3**:361–366.

69 Une Y, Uchino J, Horie T, et al.: Liver resection using a water jet. *Cancer Chemother Pharmacol* 1989;**23**(Suppl:S74–S77.

70 Schmidbauer S, Hallfeldt KK, Sitzmann G, Kantelhardt T, Trupka A: Experience with ultrasound scissors and blades (UltraCision) in open and laparoscopic liver resection. *Ann Surg* 2002;**235**:27–30.

71 Schurr MO, Wehrmann M, Kunert W, et al.: Histologic effects of different technologies for dissection in endoscopic surgery: Nd:YAG laser, high frequency and water-jet. *Endosc Surg Allied Technol* 1994;**2**:195–201.

72 Baer HU, Stain SC, Guastella T, Maddern GJ, Blumgart LH: Hepatic resection using a water jet dissector. *HPB Surg* 1993;**6**:189–196; discussion 196–198.

73 Kaehler GF, Sold MG, Fischer K, Post S, Enderle M: Selective fluid cushion in the submucosal layer by water jet: Advantage for endoscopic mucosal resection. *Eur Surg Res* 2007;**39**:93–97.

74 Neuhaus H, Wirths K, Schenk M, Enderle MD, Schumacher B: Randomized controlled study of EMR versus endoscopic submucosal dissection with a water-jet hybrid-knife of esophageal lesions in a porcine model. *Gastrointest Endosc* 2009;**70**:112–120.

75 Kroh M, Hall R, Udomsawaengsup S, Smith A, Yerian L, Chand B: Endoscopic water jets used to ablate Barrett's esophagus: Preliminary results of a new technique. *Surg Endosc* 2008;**22**:2498–2502.

76 Lingenfelder T, Fischer K, Sold MG, Post S, Enderle MD, Kaehler GF: Combination of water-jet dissection and needle-knife as a hybrid knife simplifies endoscopic submucosal dissection. *Surg Endosc* 2009;**23**:1531–1535.

77 Fernandez-Esparrach G, Matthes EL, Maurice D, Enderle M, Thompson CC, Carr-Locke DL. A novel device for endoscopic submucosal dissection that combines water-jet submucosal hydrodissection and elevation with electrocautery: Initial experience in a porcine model. *Gastrointest Endosc* 2010;**71**:615–618.

78 Toyanaga T, Man IM, Ivanov D, et al.: The results and limitations of endoscopic submucosal dissection for colorectal tumors. *Acta Chir Iugosl* 2008;**55**:17–23.

79 von Renteln D, Pohl H, Vassiliou MC, Walton MM, Rothstein RI: Endoscopic submucosal dissection by using a flexible Maryland dissector: A randomized, controlled, porcine study (with videos). *Gastrointest Endosc* 2010;**71**:1056–1062.

80 Hochberger J, Lamade W, Matthes K, Menke D, Köhler P: Wer macht in Zukunft NOTES? Gastroenterologe, Chirurg, endoskopischer Interventionalist? *Endoskopie heute* 2008;**21**:217–221.

81 Hochberger J, Lamade W, Matthes K, Menke D, Köhler P: Transluminale Interventionen (NOTES)—Aktueller Stand. *Deutsch Med Wschr* 2009;**134**:467–472.

82 Hochberger J, Maiss J, Matthes K, Costamagna G, Hawes R: Training and education in endoscopy. In: Classen M, Tytgat GNJ, Lightdale C (eds), *Gastroenterological Endoscopy*. Stuttgart, New York: Georg Thieme Verlag, 2010: 92–105

83 Goto O, Fujishiro M, Kodashima S, et al.: A second-look endoscopy after endoscopic submucosal dissection for gastric epithelial neoplasm may be unnecessary: A retrospective analysis of postendoscopic submucosal dissection bleeding. *Gastrointest Endosc* 2010;**71**:241–248.

84 Min BH, Chang DK, Kim DU, et al.: Low frequency of bacteremia after an endoscopic resection for large colorectal tumors in spite of extensive submucosal exposure. *Gastrointest Endosc* 2008;**68**:105–110.

85 Jeon SW, Jung MK, Kim SK, et al.: Clinical outcomes for perforations during endoscopic submucosal dissection in patients with gastric lesions. *Surg Endosc* 2010;**24**:911–916.

86 Banerjee S, Shen B, Baron TH, et al.: Antibiotic prophylaxis for GI endoscopy. *Gastrointest Endosc* 2008;**67**:791–798.

87 Onogi F, Araki H, Ibuka T, et al.: "Transmural air leak": A computed tomographic finding following endoscopic submucosal dissection of gastric tumors. *Endoscopy* 2010;**42**:441–447.

88 Minami S, Gotoda T, Ono H, Oda I, Hamanaka H: Complete endoscopic closure of gastric perforation induced by endoscopic resection of early gastric cancer using endoclips can prevent surgery (with video). *Gastrointest Endosc* 2006;**63**:596–601.

89 Kirschniak A, Kratt T, Stuker D, Braun A, Schurr MO, Konigsrainer A: A new endoscopic over-the-scope clip system for treatment of lesions and bleeding in the GI tract: First clinical experiences. *Gastrointest Endosc* 2007;**66**:162–167.

90 Schurr MO, Hartmann C, Ho CN, Fleisch C, Kirschniak A: An over-the-scope clip (OTSC) system for closure of iatrogenic colon perforations: Results of an experimental survival study in pigs. *Endoscopy* 2008;**40**:584–588.

91 von Renteln D, Vassiliou MC, Rothstein RI: Randomized controlled trial comparing endoscopic clips and over-the-scope clips for closure of natural orifice transluminal endoscopic surgery gastrotomies. *Endoscopy* 2009;**41**:1056–1061.

92 von Renteln D, Schmidt A, Vassiliou MC, Rudolph HU, Gieselmann M, Caca K: Endoscopic closure of large colonic perforations using an over-the-scope clip: A randomized controlled porcine study. *Endoscopy* 2009;**41**:481–486.

93 Kratt T, Kuper M, Traub F, et al.: Feasibility study for secure closure of natural orifice transluminal endoscopic surgery gastrotomies by using over-the-scope clips. *Gastrointest Endosc* 2008;**68**:993–996.

94 Repici A, Arezzo A, De Caro G, et al.: Clinical experience with a new endoscopic over-the-scope clip system for use in the GI tract. *Dig Liver Dis* 2009;**41**:406–410.

95 Iacopini F, Di Lorenzo N, Altorio F, Schurr MO, Scozzarro A: Over-the-scope clip closure of two chronic fistulas after gastric band penetration. *World J Gastroenterol* 2010;**16**:1665–1669.

96 Kirschniak A, Traub F, Kueper MA, Stuker D, Konigsrainer A, Kratt T: Endoscopic treatment of gastric perforation caused by acute necrotizing pancreatitis using over-the-scope clips: A case report. *Endoscopy* 2007;**39**:1100–1102.

97 Hotta K, Oyama T, Akamatsu T, et al.: A comparison of outcomes of endoscopic submucosal dissection (ESD) for early gastric neoplasms between high-volume and low-volume centers: Multi-center retrospective questionnaire study conducted by the Nagano ESD Study Group. *Intern Med* 2010;**49**:253–259.

98 Kurokawa Y, Hasuike N, Ono H, Boku N, Fukuda H. A phase II trial of endoscopic submucosal dissection for mucosal gastric cancer: Japan Clinical Oncology Group Study JCOG0607. *Jpn J Clin Oncol* 2009;**39**:464–466.

99 Isomoto H, Shikuwa S, Yamaguchi N, et al.: Endoscopic submucosal dissection for early gastric cancer: A large-scale feasibility study. *Gut* 2009;**58**:331–336.

100 Chung IK, Lee JH, Lee SH, et al.: Therapeutic outcomes in 1000 cases of endoscopic submucosal dissection for early gastric neoplasms: Korean ESD Study Group multicenter study. *Gastrointest Endosc* 2009;**69**:1228–1235.

101 Oda I, Saito D, Tada M, et al.: A multicenter retrospective study of endoscopic resection for early gastric cancer. *Gastric Cancer* 2006;**9**:262–270.

102 Kim JJ, Lee JH, Jung HY, et al.: EMR for early gastric cancer in Korea: A multicenter retrospective study. *Gastrointest Endosc* 2007;**66**:693–700.

103 Ono S, Fujishiro M, Niimi K, et al.: Predictors of postoperative stricture after esophageal endoscopic submucosal dissection for superficial squamous cell neoplasms. *Endoscopy* 2009;**41**: 661–665.

104 Wong VW, Teoh AY, Fujishiro M, Chiu PW, Ng EK: Preemptive dilatation gives good outcome to early esophageal stricture after circumferential endoscopic submucosal dissection. *Surg Laparosc Endosc Percutan Tech* 2010;**20**:e25–e27.

105 Ishii N, Horiki N, Itoh T, et al.: Endoscopic submucosal dissection with a combination of small-caliber-tip transparent hood and flex knife is a safe and effective treatment for superficial esophageal neoplasias. *Surg Endosc* 2010;**24**:335–342.

106 Yahagi N: Is esophageal endoscopic submucosal dissection an extreme treatment modality, or can it be a standard treatment modality? *Gastrointest Endosc* 2008;**68**:1073–1075.

19 Mucosal Ablation Techniques

John A. Dumot[1], Bruce D. Greenwald[2], & Virender K. Sharma[3]

[1]Digestive Health Institute, University Hospitals, Cleveland, OH, USA
[2]University of Maryland, School of Medicine and Greenebaum Cancer Center, Baltimore, MD, USA
[3]Arizona Center for Digestive Health, Gilbert, AZ, USA

Introduction

Ablation literally means to remove abnormal growths or harmful substances by mechanical means. Endoscopic mucosal ablation can be achieved through traditional thermal energy devices (multipolar electrocautery (MPEC), argon plasma coagulator (APC), heater probe, Nd:YAG laser), biochemical means with sclerotherapy, photochemical injury with photodynamic therapy (PDT), and by newer thermal methods—radiofrequency ablation (RFA) and cryotherapy. Training in endoscopic ablation involves developing an understanding of the mechanism of injury, risks, benefits, and alternatives to each therapy. Practical considerations include experience with simple cases such as APC ablation of small mucosal lesions initially followed by more complex lesions once the endoscopist and assistants are familiar with the patient preparation and operation of the devices. Endoscopic ablation requires a treatment plan that considers several clinical characteristics such as the size, stage, location, and topography of lesion(s). Physicians must consider the patient's overall medical condition when dealing with advanced lesions, such as intramucosal cancer, because treatment failures or recurrences can be fatal.

The unifying principal of endoscopic ablative therapy is that the mucosa tends to heal with normal native epithelium. In Barrett's esophagus (BE) patients, "neo-squamous" epithelium forms after ablation in an acid-free environment [1]. The origin of the new squamous epithelium is debated. All patients are treated with acid suppression, typically with twice-daily proton pump inhibitors. Some patients receive antireflux procedures such as Nissen fundoplication before or after ablation for control of acid reflux. In some trials, 24 hour pH monitoring was performed to confirm acid suppression. The duration of acid suppression after treatment is variable, although experts generally recommend lifelong acid suppression to minimize the risk of developing new intestinal metaplasia in the esophagus. The risk of buried dysplastic epithelium or malignancy after ablation cannot be taken lightly. The term total Barrett's eradication refers to the tenet that once ablation has been pursued, attempts to remove all intestinal metaplasia from the esophagus and esophagogastric junction is the goal. Guidelines for follow-up of patients after ablation have not been established.

This chapter considers the specific information about technique that trainees need to master and discusses the optimal means by which they can develop the knowledge and skills needed to perform these procedures well.

Procedures and equipment involved in mucosal ablation

Endoscopic mucosal ablation is typically performed in the upper gastrointestinal tract via upper endoscopy. Close follow-up is needed after ablation, and this is best performed with high-resolution endoscopes with narrow-band imaging or the equivalent. If this is not available, chromoendoscopy with Lugol iodine staining can be used in the esophagus. There are specific specialized sets of tools for the particular ablative techniques and these will be described below.

Prerequisite cognitive and technical skills for trainees prior to learning mucosal ablation

Endoscopists should have expertise in identifying and treating early neoplastic lesions in the GI tract. An understanding of the advantages and disadvantages of different ablative treatment modalities is essential, as well as appreciation of the importance of close follow-up to detect ablation failures and treat them appropriately. Technical skills required include solid basic skills in upper endoscopy, proper biopsy technique for surveillance, identification of early neoplastic lesions using chromoendoscopy or optical contrast imaging (narrow-band imaging, FICE®, I-Scan®), endoscopic mucosal resection, and familiarity with the devices used to perform ablation (discussed below). (The acquisition of skill in chromoendoscopy and interpretation of advanced imaging

Successful Training in Gastrointestinal Endoscopy, First Edition. Edited by Jonathan Cohen.
© 2011 Blackwell Publishing Ltd. Published 2011 by Blackwell Publishing Ltd.

modalities is addressed in detail in a separate chapter in this volume.) The trainee in mucosal ablation should be trained to take full advantage of these image enhancements both to find the areas to ablate and to delineate the margins of these lesions accurately.

Setting of training

Mucosal ablation skills are best acquired in a high-volume center where patients are seen in a multidisciplinary setting by experts in surgery, medical oncology, and radiation therapy. A working relationship with colleagues in surgery and oncology is essential. Use of monitored anesthesia care should be strongly considered for these procedures, since they may be prolonged and uncomfortable to the patient.

Specific knowledge trainees must acquire during training to perform esophageal mucosal ablation

Patient selection

Patient selection for mucosal ablation requires a thorough understanding of the limitations of mucosal ablation techniques—endoscopic or surgical resection may be the preferred method of treating some lesions. Training in a variety of ablation methods affords the endoscopist the option to use alternative techniques to manage difficult locations and topography. Trainees must develop a solid knowledge of indications and know whom it is best not to treat at all and advise only ongoing surveillance. Understanding the pros and cons of such alternative options is needed for both optimal management decisions and providing thorough informed consent.

Selection of particular ablation method

In order to learn how to make appropriate decisions about which specific ablative technique to use, trainees must consider existing literature and expert opinion about current options. No study has compared mucosal ablation techniques in a prospective fashion. The choice of ablation technique is typically based on endoscopist and patient preference. APC and MPEC/bipolar probe have not been well studied in treatment of dysplastic Barrett's epithelium and should not be used as the primary treatment modality. They are useful for treating small focal areas of residual intestinal metaplasia after primary treatment. RFA and spray cryotherapy with liquid nitrogen have demonstrated efficacy in treatment of BE with high-grade dysplasia. RFA should not be used if the mucosa to be treated is not flat due to limited depth of injury with this modality. Endoscopic resection of these areas or use of cryotherapy is appropriate in this setting. Endoscopic resection of more than one-half the circumference of the esophagus is a contraindication to circumferential RFA due to risk of mucosal laceration during balloon expansion. Cryotherapy should not be used in patients who have undergone procedures to reduce or restrict gastric volume (such as gastric bypass or partial gastrectomy with gastrojejunostomy) or in those with diseases that significantly reduce elasticity of the

gastrointestinal tract (such as Marfan's syndrome and eosinophilic esophagitis).

Anticoagulation considerations

Recent American Society of Gastrointestinal Endoscopy and British Society of Gastroenterology guidelines discuss general management of antithrombotic agents for endoscopic procedures [2,3]. The risk of bleeding after mucosal ablation is low; however, this risk may be increased with the use of antithrombotic agents. Many procedures with planned mucosal ablation may be combined with other high-risk procedures, such as esophageal dilation and mucosal resection. Decisions on whether to continue these therapies during ablation must be individualized based on the patient's risk of a thromboembolic event and the procedural risk of bleeding. Endoscopists may consider using the following approach.

Warfarin

In patients with low risk of thromboembolic event, warfarin may be stopped 3–5 days before the procedure and resumed the day following the procedure. In high-risk individuals, the use of intravenous or low molecular weight subcutaneous heparin may be used as bridge therapy while the INR is below the target level.

Heparin

Heparin should not be given on the day of the procedure.

Aspirin

Aspirin can probably be safely continued in patients undergoing endoscopic mucosal ablation.

Clopidogrel

In patients with low risk of thromboembolic event, clopidogrel may be stopped at least 5 days before the procedure and resumed in 1–3 days following the procedure. In high-risk patients, it may be continued. If clopidogrel is stopped, continuing or starting aspirin should be considered.

Acid suppression

Adequate acid suppression is critical for effective ablation of Barrett's epithelium and is an important consideration in assessing possible causes of ineffective treatment. Proper acid-suppressant therapy is important, not only to minimize patient discomfort, but also to allow the esophagus to heal optimally and regenerate with squamous epithelium. All patients should be prescribed a high-dose proton-pump inhibitor twice a day (omeprazole 40 mg BID, esomeprazole 40 mg BID, lansoprazole 30 mg BID, pantoprazole 40 mg BID, or equivalent) beginning 1 week before ablation and continuing for at least one month after ablation is complete. H2-receptor antagonists and sucralfate were prescribed in some trials, but there is no scientific evidence that these improve healing. All patients should be queried for persistent heartburn symptoms on high-dose therapy, with consideration given to increasing PPI dosage if symptoms persist. The cause of incomplete regression to squamous mucosa after ablation is not clear, but consideration should be given to inadequate acid suppression. Ambulatory

24-hour pH monitoring on therapy can be helpful in confirming adequacy of acid suppression in problematic patients.

Postablation analgesia

Frequently, patients undergoing mucosal ablation require post-treatment medications to control pain, nausea, and dysphagia. After ablation, patients are advised to adhere to a liquid or soft diet overnight. A soft diet is continued if dysphagia or pain persists and can be increased as symptoms dissipate. Citrus- and tomato-based products may also cause symptoms and may be avoided. Patients may experience symptoms of chest discomfort, sore throat, difficulty or pain with swallowing, and nausea, which usually improve each day. Lidocaine oral solution (sometimes mixed with liquid antacid and/or diphenhydramine solution), liquid acetaminophen with or without codeine or hydrocodone, and antiemetic medication are often helpful to palliate symptoms. Use of nonsteroidal anti-inflammatory medications is not advisable. Patients are advised to avoid alcoholic beverages during the healing process, which typically takes at least 2 weeks. Some patients may present with severe chest pain and fever. Inpatient observation and conservative management with an intravenous proton pump inhibitor, analgesic regimen, and hydration usually suffices in these cases. Trainees must also be mindful to prepare patients for these specific postablation symptoms and their management during the consent process.

Pacemakers and implantable cardiac defibrillators (ICDs)

In general, pacemakers are not affected by RFA techniques, which involve the use of bipolar current. (Training in electrosurgical principles is covered in a separate chapter in this volume, but is important knowledge for individuals who perform RFA.) ICDs may be affected by monopolar coagulation such as APC. All patients should undergo standard cardiac monitoring during the procedure. The grounding pad for APC should not be placed near a pacemaker or ICD. Cardiology consult is recommended before performing APC in a patient with an ICD to determine proper ICD management during the procedure. Typically, the ICD is temporarily deactivated by appropriately trained personnel before performing APC, and external defibrillation may be necessary in the event of a life-threatening arrhythmia during treatment.

Postablation surveillance

No study has validated the appropriate surveillance interval or proper technique after successful ablation. For BE with high-grade dysplasia, surveillance intervals after successful ablation are typically every 3 months for one year, every 6 months for 2 more years, then annually up to year 5. At each endoscopy, optical contrast, such as narrow-band imaging or Lugol iodine staining should be used to identify subtle areas of residual intestinal metaplasia in the treated area of esophagus. Any nodules within the treated area are generally removed by endoscopic mucosal resection. Surveillance biopsies should be taken at each endoscopy with large capacity or jumbo biopsy forceps. Biopsies should be taken of any abnormal appearing areas and in four quadrants every 1 cm

within the treated segment in what is now normal-appearing squamous mucosa. Biopsies should also be taken in four quadrants below the squamocolumnar junction to assess for residual intestinal metaplasia in the esophagogastric junction and cardia.

Equipment and technical steps

Argon plasma coagulation

Argon plasma coagulation (APC) is a noncontact thermal technique using ionized argon gas to deliver a monopolar high-frequency current, which effectively coagulates tissue. The APC device and endoscopic catheter most commonly used are manufactured by ERBE Elektromedizin GmbH (Tübingen, Germany). The depth of tissue destruction is thought to be limited due to increased resistance and diminished current flow through coagulated tissue, although perforation has occurred with this device. The second-generation device (VIO/APC2) incorporates several improvements over the first-generation device. The overall efficiency of the device is improved by 30–50%, so lower power settings can be used to produce the same thermal effects and conversely, the same power settings may cause deeper and more extensive tissue injury than expected. Three different modes are now available on the device—forced, pulsed, and precise. Forced APC provides continuous output and corresponds to settings on the earlier system. Pulsed APC provides intermittent current with two options. Effect one setting pulses approximately once per second, with increasing energy output with each successive pulse. Effect two pulses approximately 16 times per second with lower energy output per pulse. This may be preferred when superficial treatment of large surface areas is desired. Trainees must acquire detailed knowledge of the settings for the generator in their unit and are well advised to have written charts of settings used for specific procedures readily available in the unit. Successful trainees should not need to rely upon knowledgeable endoscopy nurses and technicians for specific information regarding electrosurgical generators, accessories, and how to use them.

Equipment

APC device

Both 7 Fr and 10 Fr catheter sizes are available for use in endoscopic procedures. The 7 Fr catheter is favored due to its ability to pass through the working channel of a standard upper endoscope with minimal resistance and provide enough power to treat most all lesions. Straight-fire catheters are preferred by the authors due to overall ease of use compared to sidefire catheters. Porcelain tip round fire catheters are not used for ablation in this setting.

Key steps

1 *Patient preparation.* Bowel preparation with a purgative is required prior to APC use in the colon to reduce the incidence of explosion of combustible gases (hydrogen and methane). An electrosurgical skin ground is placed across the flank or hip avoiding

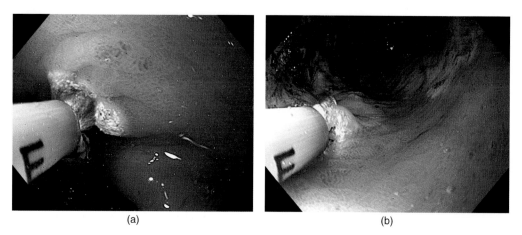

(a)   (b)

Figure 19.1 ERBE argon plasma coagulator being applied to a focal area of Barrett's mucosa (a) and over a wide area of the esophagus (b).

prior surgical sites that may contain implants. As stated above, patients with indwelling electronic devices (pacemakers and especially ICDs) will require special attention by the cardiology unit. Detailed information about any implanted device should be obtained in advance of the actual procedure.

2 *Treatment.* APC is applied to tissue until a white coagulum appears, and then the catheter and endoscope are manipulated in a vertical or circumferential linear pattern to coagulate additional tissue (Figure 19.1). Controlling the insufflated argon gas with judicious use of suction is important to prevent over distention in the lumen and subsequent thinning of the wall as well as patient discomfort. Care should be taken to not touch the target lesion because inadvertent impaction of the APC probe into the mucosa can result in injection of the gas into the submucosal layer or through the bowel wall, resulting in a possible pneumomediastinum or pneumoperitoneum. In the esophagus, pain is more likely with treatment of longer segments of esophagus, and stricture is more likely with circumferential treatment.

A variety of reports have evaluated APC for ablation of BE [4]. Energy settings of 40–90 watts have been used. In some studies, circumferential ablation of all metaplastic tissue was attempted, while in others noncircumferential ablation was performed or the length of tissue treated was limited. Considerable variation exists between studies in terms of energy used, endpoints, duration of follow-up, and use of chromoendoscopy to identify recurrent or persistent intestinal metaplasia. Most experts do not recommend routine ablation of nondysplastic BE by APC. The relatively high incidence of complications, low rate of progression to cancer, and lack of long-term data on effectiveness of eradication in preventing cancer progression confines ablation of nondysplastic BE to the research setting in most cases. Ablation of high-grade dysplasia (HGD) in BE has been studied, but the limited data available in this patient group makes it difficult to recommend APC for routine care. However, the availability of APC in most endoscopy units, ease of use, and endoscopists' familiarity with the device make it useful as a "touch-up" therapy to ablate small residual areas of intestinal metaplasia after treatment with other ablative techniques.

Bipolar or multipolar electrocoagulation

Bipolar electrocautery or multipolar electrocoagulation (MPEC) was one of the earliest technologies applied to ablation in endoscopic procedures. No data exists to suggest noncontact methods, such as APC or thermal laser, function any better than this widely available device. Bipolar electrocautery is favored by experts when the patient has implantable devices (pacemaker, defibrillators, etc.) because the electrical current does not travel beyond the depth of thermal injury, compared to monopolar technology with a grounding device, which can disrupt the programming of these devices.

Equipment

Electrosurgical generator

Both 10 Fr and 7 Fr endoscopic catheters are available. The 10 Fr catheters provide slightly larger surface area for larger lesions or bleeding vessels but must be used with a colonoscope or therapeutic upper endoscope.

Key steps

1 *Patient preparation:* Bowel preparation with a purgative to reduce the incidence of explosion of combustible gases (hydrogen and methane) in the colon is generally not required prior to use MPEC, which makes it a preferred method of hemostasis in acute lower gastrointestinal bleeding. Patients with indwelling electronic devices (pacemakers, ICDs, etc.) do not require special attention.

2 *Treatment:* The catheter is applied to the target mucosa and electrical current administered until a white coagulum is noted in a similar fashion to APC.

Radiofrequency ablation

The RFA system (BARRX Medical, Sunnyvale, CA) comprises two distinct ablation systems: the HALO[360] system for primary circumferential RFA and the HALO[90] system for secondary focal RFA of BE or primarily as treatment for short segment BE [5,6]. Treating longer segments of esophageal mucosa generally increases patient symptoms including pain and nausea. Typically, 9 cm

(3 balloon segments) is the maximal treatment length using the circumferential ablation catheter.

Ablation should be repeat every 2–3 months until all BE has been eradicated visually, and then histological response is confirmed. Most patients will need one circumferential ablation session and 1–2 focal ablation sessions to eradicate all dysplasia and intestinal metaplasia [7].

Equipment

Circumferential and focal ablation energy generators
- Balloon-based ablation catheters (18 mm, 22 mm, 25 mm, 28 mm, and 31 mm. All sizes should be available at the time of procedure) (single use only)
- Focal ablation catheters (single use only)
- Sizing balloon (single use only)
- 0.038″ guide wire
- Soft endoscopic friction-fit cap (single use only)
- Acetylcysteine diluted to 1%, 30–60 mL in syringe capable of injecting through the working channel of endoscope.

Key steps

Circumferential ablation (Figure 19.2, Video 19.1)

1 *Patient preparation:* Since there is no significant risk of bleeding with the RFA procedure, antiplatelet/anticoagulant drugs can be continued from a safety standpoint. However, even minimal amounts of blood can interfere with adequate delivery of RF energy and can compromise the efficacy of RFA procedure. Hence, if possible, minimizing or stopping antiplatelet/anticoagulant drugs is desirable. Unlike standard bipolar or multipolar coagulation probes, delivery of RF energy may interfere with the proper functioning of electromedical devices such as pacemakers and implantable devices. Standard electrosurgical precautions for electronic medical devices should be taken while performing RFA in these patients. Patients should be consented for possible empiric dilation prior to the procedure as passage of the balloon RFA catheter may be impeded by anatomical abnormalities such as cricopharyngeus hypertrophy or cervical osteophytes. In these patients, empiric dilation with a 14–16 mm dilator may facilitate the passage of the catheter.

2 *Recording esophageal landmarks:* Lubrication jelly should not be used on the endoscope to ensure effective delivery of the RF energy to the target mucosa. The scope is lubricated with water only. A routine upper endoscopy is performed, preferably using optical contrast endoscopy, to assess for location of BE and evaluate for other abnormalities. After performance of routine upper endoscopy, wash the esophageal wall with acetylcysteine (1%) followed by water to remove excessive mucus. The following distances from the incisors are measured and recorded: top of the gastric folds, maximum proximal extent of circumferential and noncircumferential BE, and maximum extent of Barrett's islands.

3 *Guide wire placement:* With the scope in the gastric antrum, insert the guide wire and remove the endoscope, leaving the guide wire in place.

4 *Sizing esophageal inner diameter:* Connect the sizing balloon to the circumferential RFA generator. Calibrate by pressing the calibration button, which will inflate and deflate the balloon. After deflation, disconnect the balloon from the generator. Lubricate the balloon with water only (lubricants may decrease effectiveness of ablation) and introduce the catheter into the esophagus over the guide wire. The sizing procedure can be performed under endoscopic visualization or as a "blind" procedure using the 1-cm scale on the catheter shaft for reference. Endoscopic visualization can assess the response of the esophagus to balloon inflation. In special cases (e.g., localized narrowing), endoscopic visual control may assure that the sizing is performed at the required level. For the first measurement, the catheter is placed 5 cm above the maximum proximal extent of the BE or 12 cm above the gastric folds. The distal end of the balloon is then located 1 cm above the most proximal extent of any Barrett mucosa. The measurement cycle is initiated by activating the inflation footswitch, the sizing balloon inflates, and the esophageal inner diameter and recommended ablation balloon catheter size are automatically calculated and reported by the generator. Record this information. This action is repeated for every centimeter of the targeted portion of the esophagus,

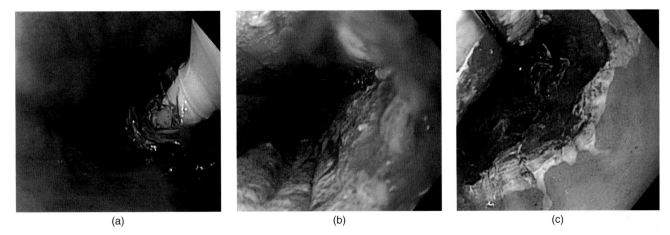

(a) (b) (c)

Figure 19.2 Circumferential radiofrequency ablation in long segment Barrett's esophagus before ablation (a), after the first treatment passes before debridement of coagulated mucosa (b), and after debridement of coagulum (c).

advancing the balloon distally in 1 cm linear increments, until an increase in measured diameter indicates the transition to the hiatal hernia or stomach. Disconnect and remove the sizing balloon, leaving the guide wire in place in the stomach for passage of the ablation catheter.

5 *Selecting the appropriate circumferential RFA catheter:* On the basis of the esophageal inner diameter measurements, an appropriate circumferential RFA ablation catheter is selected to ensure good contact of the inflated balloon with the mucosal surface. The diameter of the ablation balloon is the smallest diameter recommended during sizing. Selecting a larger size balloon may result in mucosal tearing, especially if a mucosal tear or oozing is noted after the esophageal sizing or in patients who have scarring in the esophagus due to a previous stricture or prior endoscopic mucosal resection.

6 *First circumferential ablation pass:* Connect the ablation catheter to the generator to confirm proper function, but do not inflate the balloon. Disconnect the catheter, lubricate the balloon with water, and introduce over the guide wire. Reconnect the catheter and insert the endoscope alongside the ablation catheter, positioning the tip just proximal to the inflation balloon. Confirm appropriate energy settings on the generator. In general, the energy density setting is 12 J/cm^2 and power density setting is 40 W/cm^2. Position the proximal margin of the electrode 1 cm above the maximum proximal extent of the BE using endoscopic visualization and the centimeter markings on the catheter. The balloon is inflated via the left foot pedal, the esophagus is deflated to optimize tissue contact using endoscopic suction, and the right footswitch is activated to deliver the RF energy to the electrode and the Barrett epithelium when the appropriate tone is sounded by the generator. Energy delivery typically lasts <1.5 seconds after which the balloon is automatically deflated by the generator. Moving from proximally to distally, the balloon is repositioned, allowing a minimal overlap with the previous ablation zone of <5 mm. Ablation is repeated in a sequential fashion until the entire targeted BE has received one application of RF energy or three segments have been treated.

7 *Cleaning procedure between ablation cycles:* After the first ablation pass, disconnect the catheter from the generator. The endoscope, guide wire, and ablation catheter are removed. Outside the patient, the catheter is inflated to clean the electrode surface of

coagulum with wet gauze or a soft brush until all coagulum is removed. A soft distal attachment cap is fitted on the tip of the endoscope to assist with cleaning of the ablation zone. The endoscope is reinserted, and the tip of the endoscope with the cap in place is used to gently remove the coagulum from the esophageal wall in the ablation zone. After most of the coagulum has been removed with the cap, forceful spraying of water through a spraying catheter using a high-pressure pistol or a pump can be used to remove residual coagulum. Although the extensive cleaning procedure requires extra procedure time, it has been proven to increase the efficacy of ablation.

8 *Second ablation pass:* After the cleaning procedure, the guide wire is reinserted in the gastric antrum and left in place while the scope is removed. The clean ablation catheter is reinserted over the guide wire, and then the scope is reinserted. The entire treated area is again ablated using the same energy settings and technique described in step 6, resulting in double treatment of the entire targeted segment.

9 *Follow-up treatments:* Endoscopy is repeated after a minimum of 8–12 weeks to allow healing. In cases of residual circumferential BE > 2 cm, patients are treated with a second circumferential ablation. In case of an irregular Z-line, small tongues, circumferential extent < 2 cm, or diffuse islands of residual Barrett's epithelium, patients are treated with focal ablation (described below).

Focal ablation (Figure 19.3, Video 19.2)

1 *Patient preparation:* See comments above concerning use of antiplatelet and anticoagulants and use of acid suppression prior to ablation. Patients should be consented for possible empiric dilation prior to the procedure as passage of the focal RFA catheter may be impeded by anatomical abnormalities such as cricopharyngeus hypertrophy or cervical osteophytes. In these patients, empiric dilation with a 17–18 mm dilator may facilitate the passage of the catheter.

2 *Esophageal preparation:* Lubrication jelly should not be used on the endoscope to ensure effective delivery of the RF energy to the target mucosa. The scope is lubricated with water only. A routine upper endoscopy is performed, preferably using optical contrast endoscopy, to assess for location of BE and evaluate for other abnormalities. After performance of routine upper endoscopy,

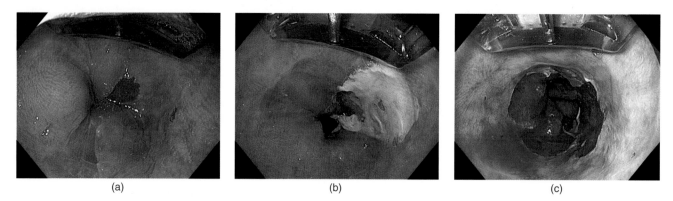

(a)	(b)	(c)

Figure 19.3 Focal radiofrequency ablation of a small residual island of Barrett's mucosa before treatment (a), after the first treatment with coagulum (b), and circumferential application at the esophagogastric junction (c).

wash the esophageal wall with acetylcysteine (1%) followed by water to remove excessive mucus. The following distances from the incisors are measured and recorded: top of the gastric folds, maximum proximal extent of circumferential and noncircumferential BE, and maximum extent of Barrett's islands.

3 *Introduction of the focal RFA catheter:* The focal RFA catheter is fitted on the tip of the endoscope and positioned at the 12 o'clock position in the endoscopic video image (Figure 19.3). Connect the catheter to the generator to confirm proper function. Disconnect the catheter, lubricate the electrode with water, and introduce under visual control. When the laryngeal cavity is visualized the tip of the endoscope is deflected slightly downward, allowing the leading edge of the catheter to be passed behind the arytenoids. The patient is asked to swallow and the endoscope is gently advanced. In <10% of cases introducing the focal RFA catheter may prove difficult due to cricopharyngeus hypertrophy, cervical osteophytes, or other anatomical deformities at the pharyngeal–esophageal junction. In such instances, use of a biopsy forceps or a soft tip guide wire or the spraying catheter as a guide may facilitate passage into the proximal esophagus. In difficult cases, proximal esophageal dilation by balloon or a wire-guided dilator may be used to open the upper esophageal sphincter.

4 *First ablation pass:* Barrett epithelium targeted for ablation is positioned at the 12 o'clock position in the endoscopic video image. The electrode is brought into contact with the mucosa and the tip of the endoscope is deflected upward with pressure against the Barrett's mucosa. The esophagus is deflated to get good contact with the mucosa using endoscopic suction, and the generator is activated via the footswitch. Once the generator tone is heard, the footswitch is activated a second time, while keeping the electrode in position against the esophageal mucosa, resulting in a double application of energy to the same area. All areas of residual Barrett's mucosa are treated in the same manner. If this is the first focal ablation treatment session, ablation of the entire Z-line circumferentially generally is recommended, even if no clear tongues are observed, to ensure eradication of any residual IM at the gastroesophageal junction.

5 *Cleaning procedure:* After all Barrett's mucosa has been ablated, the coagulum is carefully pushed off the esophageal wall with the leading edge of the focal RFA electrode. The catheter is disconnected from the generator, and the endoscope is removed. The electrode is cleaned using water and gauze if needed. The ablation zone may be cleaned with a spraying catheter and pressure pistol or water pump as described above under circumferential ablation.

6 *Second ablation pass:* Using the ablation zones from the first ablation pass for orientation, all ablated areas are treated with a double application of energy using the same energy settings and technique described in step 4, resulting in four total ablations of the entire targeted segment. Note that each Halo 90 catheter will deliver a maximum of 80 pulses.

Cryotherapy

Two endoscopic catheter devices have been developed by independent investigators. The carbon dioxide system (Polar Wand, GI Supply, Camp Hill, PA) uses the Joule–Thompson effect of rapid cooling during expansion of gas and appears to be a safe and effective treatment for vascular lesions of the gastrointestinal tract [8,9]. Preliminary results of the high pressure carbon dioxide system in BE in abstract form show promise [10]. The liquid nitrogen system (CryoSpray Ablation, CSA Medical, Baltimore, MD) applies the much colder cryogen at low pressure to the target tissue in order to achieve the treatment effect. The majority of available human data pertaining to ablation of Barrett's dysplasia and neoplasia are with the liquid nitrogen system [11–14]. Spray cryotherapy has been studied in both BE with high-grade dysplasia, squamous dysplasia, and esophageal carcinoma. It may be more useful than other ablation techniques for nodular mucosa because of the ability to achieve a greater depth of injury.

Spray cryotherapy presents a unique challenge in the GI tract. The expansion of gas within a closed system presents a risk of over distension and perforation. Careful monitoring of the patient during cryotherapy is necessary to prevent these complications. This requires specific training of ancillary personnel in addition to the endoscopist for proper performance of this procedure. Contraindications to this procedure include conditions that alter or limit compliance of the esophagus or stomach (such as Marfan's syndrome, severe eosinophilic esophagitis, intrathoracic stomach, and partial or total gastrectomy) and the presence of food in the stomach, which may impair proper decompression tube function.

Equipment

• CryoSpray ablation™ system console filled with liquid nitrogen (LN2)
• Cryotherapy spray catheters
• Kit (supplied by the device manufacturer) containing 20 Fr dual-lumen cryotherapy decompression tube (CDT) and suction tubing for connecting tube to system console
• Suction trap for console (supplied by the device manufacturer)
• Portable or wall suction
• Soft friction-fit cap (Olympus D-201-11804—12.1 mm × 4 mm or dedicated size per endoscope) to help with visualization (use optional)
• 0.038″ stainless steel guide wire
• Glycopyrrolate (Robinul), an antimuscarinic agent, to reduce salivary, tracheobronchial, and pharyngeal secretions intravenous (use optional)

Key steps (Figure 19.4, Video 19.3)

1 *Patient preparation:* Patients with indwelling electronic devices (pacemakers, defibrillators, etc.) do not require special attention. A prolonged fast may be necessary if the patient has delayed gastric emptying because food particles can occlude the CDT. In some patients, excessive secretions may impair visibility during treatment. Intravenous glycopyrrolate 0.1–0.2 mg can be given in these circumstances, ideally at least 20 minutes before the procedure. Care must be taken to assure proper fitting of the endoscopic bite block even in edentulous patients because the extreme cold from the endoscope can cause thermal injury to the lips.

2 *Esophageal preparation:* Routine upper endoscopy is performed, and all secretions are suctioned from the stomach. Small amounts

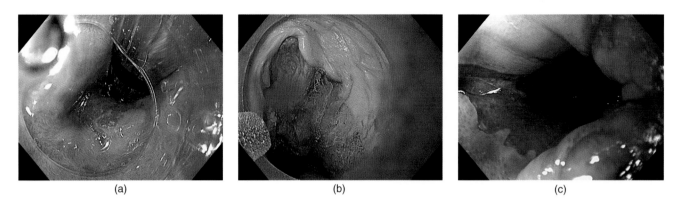

(a)	(b)	(c)

Figure 19.4 Soft cap adjacent to the liquid nitrogen cryotherapy decompression tube at the esophagogastric junction (a), cryotherapy freeze spray after 20 seconds (b), and cryotherapy posttreatment hyperemia (c).

of residual food should be removed. If removal of all retained food is not possible, the procedure must be aborted. The following distances from the incisors are measured and recorded: top of the gastric folds, maximum proximal extent of circumferential and noncircumferential BE, and maximum extent of Barrett's islands.

3 *Decompression tube placement:* With the endoscope in the gastric antrum, a guide wire is passed through the scope into the stomach. The guide wire is left in place as the scope is withdrawn and removed. Water-soluble lubricant is applied to the CDT which is inserted into the stomach over the guide wire. The optional soft cap is applied to the tip of the endoscope, and the scope is reinserted alongside the CDT. The CDT is adjusted so that the double black band is located at the gastroesophageal junction. The wire is removed taking care to maintain position of the CDT. The CDT is connected to the suction canister tubing on the console. Some users secure the CDT to the bite block with tape to prevent movement, while others attach a small piece of tape to the CDT to note possible migration as the scope is maneuvered. The suction control pedal should be activated to clear any gastric fluids that have accumulated.

4 *Spray cryotherapy:* The cryotherapy spray catheter is connected to the console and an audible beep will sound confirming proper connection. Hold the catheter with gauze to protect from the extreme cold ($-196°C$) when LN2 begins to flow. The catheter and console are cooled by continuously pressing the spray control pedal (blue) until a steady stream of liquid (not gaseous) nitrogen is observed flowing from the end of catheter. Release the pedal and stop the flow of LN2. A small spring-wire is available for use in the accessory channel cap to prevent kinking of the spray catheter. The spray catheter is passed through the working channel of the scope and extended to the distal edge of the cap or approximately 4–6 mm beyond the tip.

An assistant must palpate the upper abdomen to obtain a baseline measurement for potential abdominal distention. The suction pedal is depressed, activating suction, and the assistant monitors for distension with their hand on the patient's upper abdomen. Throughout the procedure, this assistant is applying gentle intermittent pressure to the left upper quadrant to monitor for distension and assist in decompression. The scope is maneuvered

to the treatment area, and the spray pedal is depressed, spraying liquid nitrogen onto the mucosa. The catheter is kept in place until a white frost is seen. The endoscope is manipulated to move the catheter tip back and forth, freezing adjacent tissue. When the entire target area is frozen, the timer is started. Current freeze time for most treatments is 20 seconds. After 20 seconds, the spray pedal is released. Suction may be left on or turned off, and the tissue is allowed to thaw. Thawing is complete when no ice crystals are seen and should take at least 30–60 seconds. Shorter thaw times suggest incomplete freezing. After thawing, the target area is treated again in the same manner. Most tissues are treated for two to three freeze–thaw cycles. The catheter is then moved to an adjacent treatment area and the freeze–thaw cycles are repeated.

Typically, one-fourth to one-third of the circumference of the esophagus can be kept frozen at one time over a length of 2–3 cm. Overlap of treatment sites is common to assure a uniform treatment effect. After treating several sites, the tissue may be cool enough to allow freezing of the entire circumference of the esophagus. Endoscope suction and air/water function are not available during the treatment because the channels freeze. No deterioration of endoscope function has been reported to date. Columnar epithelium appears hyperemic and friable after treatment, which serves as a guide to identify areas completely treated.

5 *Equipment removal:* The endoscope and CDT are removed at the end of the procedure. It is not necessary to wait for tissue to thaw before removing the scope and CDT. If the catheter is removed while the scope is still inserted, the heat function on the console can be activated. Suction must remain on and the abdomen monitored for distension during heating of the catheter when the scope is inserted. Several heat cycles may be necessary to thaw the catheter during prolonged cases. The scope channel may be flushed with warm water to restore function of the air/water nozzle.

Photodynamic therapy

There is ample literature on the use of PDT to achieve mucosal ablation. However, because of the side effects of skin sensitization, cost, and higher rate of complications such as stricturing, this technique is seldom performed and accordingly not covered in detail.

Opportunities and methods for training in mucosal ablation

Mucosal ablation skills are taught in a variety of ways. Professional society-sponsored courses and sessions during national or regional meetings allow endoscopists to become familiar with the techniques and equipment available through hands-on demonstration and use (Video 33.1). Tissue explants of the esophagus and stomach or live animal training may be available as well. The amount of training to gain technical proficiency in each procedure is unknown, although the authors believe that at least ten procedures are required to gain basic technical proficiency. Proficiency is best maintained if procedures are performed on a regular basis.

Defining competency

No data exist on the definition or assessment of competency for mucosal ablation. Any competency determination must assess the ability to identify appropriate patients for mucosal ablation, perform appropriate assessment of those patients prior to treatment, choose an appropriate ablation modality and perform this modality proficiently, and manage the patient after ablation, including assessment and treatment of complications and appropriate surveillance for recurrent disease. Published high success rates in achieving eradication of Barrett's epithelium and dysplasia for RFA may be used as benchmarks for recent trainees to try to reproduce as they track their own success rates in practice. In recent studies, complete eradication of low-grade dysplasia was 90.5% and high-grade dysplasia was 81%, with 77.4% success rate at eradicating all intestinal metaplasia at 12-month follow-up [7]. Complete eradication of nondysplastic Barrett's mucosa was seen in 97% of patients with 30-month follow-up in another study [5]. Careful recording of outcomes including both success rates and adverse events will allow trainees to rate their progress during training and provide them with the confidence once they are on their own that they have been successfully trained.

Maintaining skill level

It is unknown how frequently ablation techniques must be performed to maintain an adequate skill level. Those performing these techniques less frequently can refamiliarize themselves with appropriate technique through the review of peer-reviewed publications, device manufacturer supplied physician education materials, and computer-based or Internet-based instructional videos.

Videos

Video 19.1 RFA circumferential
Video 19.2 RFA focal
Video 19.3 Circumferential radiofrequency ablation
Video 33.1 Endofest 2010

References

1 Berenson MM, Johnson TD, Markowitz NR, Buchi KN, Samowitz WS: Restoration of squamous mucosa after ablation of Barrett's esophageal epithelium. *Gastroenterology* 1993;**104**:1686–1691.

2 Anderson MA, Ben-Menachem T, Gan SI, et al.: Standards of Practice Committee of the American Society for Gastrointestinal Endoscopy. ASGE guideline: management of antithrombotic agents for endoscopic procedures. *Gastrointest Endosc* 2009;**70**:1053–1059.

3 Veitch AM, Baglin TP, Gershlick AH, Harnden SM, Tighe R, Cairns S: Guidelines for the management of anticoagulant and antiplatelet therapy in patients undergoing endoscopic procedures. *Gut* 2008;**57**:1322–1329.

4 Dumot JA, Greenwald BD: Argon plasma coagulation, bipolar cautery and cryotherapy: ABC's of ablative techniques. *Endoscopy* 2008;**40**: 1026–1032.

5 Fleischer DE, Overholt BF, Sharma VK, et al.: Endoscopic ablation of Barrett's esophagus: a multicenter study with 2.5 year follow up. *Gastrointest Endosc* 2008;**68**:867–876.

6 Pouw RE, Sharma VK, Bergman JJ, Fleischer DE: Radiofrequency ablation for total Barrett's eradication: a description of the endoscopic technique, its clinical results and future prospects. *Endoscopy* 2008; **40**:1033–1040.

7 Shaheen NJ, Sharma P, Overholt BF, et al.: Radiofrequency ablation in Barrett's esophagus with dysplasia. *N Engl J Med* 2009;**360**:2277–2288.

8 Cho S, Zanati S, Young E, et al.: Endoscopic cryotherapy for the management of gastric antral vascular ectasia. *Gastrointest Endosc* 2008;**68**:895–902.

9 Pasricha PJ, Hill S, Wadwa KS, et al.: Endoscopic cryotherapy: experimental results and first clinical use. *Gastrointest Endosc* 1999;**49**: 627–631.

10 Canto MI, Dunbar KB, Okolo P, Jagannath SB, Kantsevoy SV: Low flow CO2-cryotherapy for high risk Barrett's esophagus (BE) patients with high grade dysplasia and early adenocarcinoma: a pilot trial of feasibility and safety. *Gastrointest Endosc* 2008;**67**:AB179.

11 Dumot JA, Vargo JJ, Falk GW, Frey L, Lopez R, Rice TW: An open-label, prospective trial of cryospray ablation of Barrett's esophagus high-grade dysplasia and early esophageal cancer in high-risk patients. *Gastrointest Endosc* 2009;**70**:635–644.

12 Greenwald BD, Dumot JA, Horwhat JD, Abrams JA, Lightdale CJ: Safety, tolerability, and efficacy of endoscopic low-pressure liquid nitrogen spray cryotherapy in the esophagus. *Dis Esophagus* 2009;**23**: 13–19.

13 Shaheen NJ, Greenwald BD, Peery AF, et al.: Safety and efficacy of endoscopic spray cryotherapy for Barrett's esophagus with high-grade dysplasia. *Gastrointest Endosc* 2010;**71**:680–685.

14 Greenwald BD, Dumot JA, Abrams JA, et al.: Endoscopic spray therapy for esophageal cancer: safety and efficacy. *Gastrointest Endosc* 2010;**71**:686–693.

20   Complicated Polypectomy

Jerome D. Waye[1] & Yasushi Sano[2]

[1] Mt. Sinai Hospital, New York, NY, USA
[2] Sano Hospital, Tarumi-ku, Kobe, Hyogo, Japan

One of the major advances in medicine during the last 50 years has been the colonoscopic removal of colon polyps, which has decreased the incidence, morbidity, and mortality of colorectal cancer. Most polyps in the large bowel are less than 1 cm in diameter, a size that has enabled successful treatment of polyps and has permitted the relatively easy removal of polyps throughout the world. Only 20% of polyps are over 1 cm in size, with most large polyps (over 20 mm) being adenomas.

The removal of colon polyps requires the ability to transect a polyp, while simultaneously preventing bleeding and maintaining the integrity of the colon wall during use of electrothermal current. The successful removal of colon polyps by the snare and cautery technique involves a balance between the act of transection and the hemostasis that is required. During removal of large polyps, the two forces that must be balanced are the shearing force from closing the wire loop and the thermal energy, which results in cauterization of blood vessels providing hemostasis. Both the shearing force and hemostasis must be achieved simultaneously to permit removal of polyps without bleeding and with the safe application of thermal energy to the thin colon wall without a deep zone of thermal destruction. The closure of the snare can result in cutting through a polyp but guillotine of a polyp can often be associated with bleeding; the application of thermal energy alone through the wire loop without a shearing force will cause deep thermal injury without the ability to sever a polyp. It is important that both forces, shearing and application of heat, must be used simultaneously. Small polyps, up to 5 mm in diameter, have small nutrient blood vessels and are often successfully removed by "cold" snare transection (without the application of thermal energy) with no significant bleeding. Most polypectomies are performed without any blood loss because hemostasis during polypectomy is very similar to hemostasis in any type of bleeding: pressure on a blood vessel to stop the flow of blood. In polypectomy, that principle is achieved by squeezing a blood vessel with the snare to occlude the vascular channel prior to heat sealing it with thermal energy. By tightly closing the snare around a polyp, the blood vessel walls are coapted in a similar fashion to that employed for cessation of hemorrhage from an ulcer in the upper intestinal tract. In a bleeding gastric ulcer, for example, hemostasis is usually achieved by pushing on a vessel with a probe (BICAP or heater probe) and then applying heat which obliterates the vascular channel. During polypectomy, once the blood vessel walls have been coapted by squeezing the snare, permanent hemostasis is achieved by employing thermal energy, which seals the coapted blood vessel through which blood is no longer flowing. This is effective for pedunculated polyps that have a single arterial supply as well as for sessile polyps where several smaller vascular channels exist.

The electrosurgical unit

It is important for the successful achievement of polypectomy to be aware of the electrosurgical unit that is employed for polypectomy. There are no generally accepted criteria for the type of current that is used for polypectomy, nor for the amount of energy delivered during polypectomy. Most doctors that perform polypectomy use pure coagulation current for snare polypectomy, others use a blended current, and some use the endocut capability whereby a burst of cutting current is followed by coagulation current on an alternate basis. Pure cutting current is not used for polypectomy since this type of energy explodes cells, including vascular structures, and delivers no hemostasis.

Coagulation current on the other hand tends to heat tissue and will seal a coapted blood vessel squeezed tightly by the snare. Experience has shown that there is no need to strangulate a polyp and see it turn purple before current application: once closed tightly around a polyp, a burst of coagulation current may be given and then current application maintained along with slide bar retraction until severance is achieved. Blended current, a combination of cutting current and coagulation current is used by some, but does have the propensity to explode cells and may result in immediate postpolypectomy bleeding. New electrocoagulators may provide a range of settings that include a combination of cutting and coagulation current in alternating fashion called endocut. This may not be the optimal current setting for polypectomy, since during a portion of the active cycle, pure cutting current is introduced. which destroys cells with high frequency current even though the next portion of the cycle delivers coagulation current. In general, a low setting for coagulation current can be successfully used for polypectomy in the colon, without the need to vary the current setting for polypectomy on the left or right side of the colon.

Successful Training in Gastrointestinal Endoscopy, First Edition. Edited by Jonathan Cohen.
© 2011 Blackwell Publishing Ltd. Published 2011 by Blackwell Publishing Ltd.

The heat produced by snare activation is localized to the area around the wire loop, but the thermal effect also spreads toward the colon wall and may travel through the mucosa to the muscularis propria and the serosa. The distended colon wall is quite thin, measuring about 1.4–2.3 mm on EUS reports [1,2]. These studies by EUS have demonstrated that there is no "thick area" in the sigmoid colon where the endoscopist can feel complacent in snare application because of the perceived notion that the sigmoid is much thicker than the right colon.

An adenoma actually replaces the mucosal surface and removal of the polyp leaves only a portion of the submucosa with the muscularis propria and serosa, with a total thickness of less than 1.5 mm of tissue. The larger the polyp, the greater will be the volume of tissue within the snare loop and more thermal energy will be required to sever the polyp. The increase in energy required to sever a large polyp or a large portion of a polyp may result in a full thickness burn of the colon wall, which can ultimately result in a perforation.

Snares for polypectomy

Any type of snare may be used whether reusable or disposable, oval or hex shaped, but the size should correspond to the diameter of the polyp. After several applications of a snare, the wire loop often becomes distorted, primarily because of the pulling force on the snare wire exerted during snare closure. As the slide bar on the snare handle is retracted during polypectomy, there is considerable pressure on the pointed tip of the snare as the polyp is squeezed between the tip of the wire and the tip of the snare sheath. As the loop is being retracted into the sheath, the wires at the tip are squeezed tightly together with captured tissue at the retraction site so that the next opening of the wire loop may not result in as wide an aperture as exists in a virgin snare. This happens with repeated use of a reusable snare or during resection of multiple polyps in the same patient with a disposable snare. The distortion of the wire loop may be reversed by withdrawal of the snare from the colonoscope, and with the wire loop opened, spreading the wires apart with force reconstituting the normal shape of the loop. This stretching can make the loop wider to fit around a larger polyp if necessary. One aspect of wire distortion that is difficult to overcome is the bending of the loop that distorts it from opening in a flat plane. When the wire loop can no longer be applied in a flat manner, further use is often not possible.

During snare application of any polyp, it is important to place the tip of the snare sheath at the point at which closure is desired. With a pedunculated polyp, the desired location is usually considered to be at the midpoint of the stalk. Since the tip of the snare sheath is the fixed point in the snare closure system, the tip of the wire always retracts toward the tip of the sheath. In the case of a pedunculated polyp, once the wire loop is placed around the stalk, closure of the snare will be toward the tip of the sheath, which should be placed on the pedicle where transection is to occur, either at the midpoint of the stalk or close to the colon wall if there is a concern about malignancy. If, however, the wire loop catches on the interstices of the frond-like head of a polyp, it is possible to draw a portion of the polyp head into the closing loop and have part of the polyp head caught into the loop along with capture of the pedicle. The application of electrocurrent to the closed snare will therefore cut across part of the head of the polyp as well as the stalk.

Small polyps, less than 5 mm may be transected readily with a cold snare [3], but polyps with a base attachment less than 1.5 cm can be ensnared and transected with the wire snare and cautery application. Sessile polyps may be removed with one application of the snare if the base of attachment is 1.5 cm or less. Polyps larger than 1.5 cm in diameter should be taken off in piecemeal fashion. The intention of snare closure around a wide-based sessile polyp is to bunch the adenomatous tissue up into the snare so that transection can take place with the mucosa and submucosa bunched up into the snare loop. However, because the colon wall is thin [1,2] (the thickness of the distended colon wall varies from 1.4 to 2.3 mm in diameter as noted in several reports) and the muscularis propria is not a strong or thick muscle, it is possible that closing the snare around a large sessile polyp may invert not only the submucosa into the closed snare, but also the muscularis propria and serosa so transection will completely cut through the entire thickness of the colon wall, resulting in a perforation when the polyp is severed. In order to prevent this complication, fluid can be injected into the submucosa to elevate the polyp away from the deeper tissues greatly expanding the submucosal layer. This fluid injection will separate the mucosa from the muscularis propria and serosa, resulting in the ability to close the snare around an adenoma and averting the possibility of catching deeper tissue into the snare loop during closure.

The snare handle as an information center

Safety in snare polypectomy can be enhanced by using the snare handle as an information system [4].

All snares are made with a thumbhole on the end of the handle and a two-ring slide bar that moves along the handle shaft. The slide bar opens and closes the snare in a direct 1:1 ratio. A mark can be made on the handle shaft that will transmit information to the person who closes the snare. This mark is made by the assistant prior to the endoscopic polypectomy. The technique to partially close the slide bar; watch the tip of the wire loop as it retracts into the sheath and stop slide bar movement when the tip of the wire meets the tip of the sheath. Any further closure of the slide bar will move the tip of the wire into the sheath. At the closure point where both tips are at the same location (the tip of the wire is at the tip of the sheath), a mark should be made on the handle shaft where the slide bar has been stopped. This is called the "closure point" or "the line." This mark should be made toward the thumbhole side of the slide bar. After this, with the assistant not looking at the tip of the sheath, the slide bar can always be closed to the mark without retracting the tip of the wire into the snare sheath. This can also be accomplished by looking at the handle shaft and stopping slide bar motion at the line that has been inscribed by the assistant on the handle shaft (the closure point). This is an extremely useful tool when dealing with small polyps, since the trained assistant always stops at "the line," which will prevent guillotining small polyps or soft polyps which do not have any "closure sensation" as the slide bar is retracted. Oftentimes, it will be desired to "cold cut" or "cheese wire" a small polyp to guillotine it without electrocautery current; however, this should be at the discretion of the endoscopist and not inadvertently severed by the gastrointestinal assistant as the snare is closed. The mark (line) on the handle shaft will always signal the assistant to use that as a stop mark before further slide bar closure.

This same mark can very effectively be used during removal of larger polyps in order to promote safety during polypectomy. There is a 1:1 correlation with the amount of wire loop that extends beyond the tip of the snare sheath and the slide bar. Often, as the slide bar is retracted around a large polyp, there is a "closure sensation" to the assistant as the volume of the polyp resists further slide bar movement. This resistance to further closure is usually felt as a "spongy" or "rubbery" sensation. For relatively small polyps or very soft polyps, the "closure sensation" may not be reached until the slide bar has reached "the line" and indeed, there may be no "closure sensation." However, the assistant should stop at the line to prevent slicing the polyp off the wall. If the closure sensation is reached when the slide bar is at the "line," it means that the polyp base has been compressed to a small size. Although the diameter of the base may be 1–2 cm, it frequently is compressed during snare closure so that the "closure sensation" is perceived when the slide bar is at or just a few millimeters from "the line." On the other hand, if a polyp whose base is 2 cm in diameter is captured, and the assistant perceives the closure sensation when the slide bar is several centimeters from the line, that information should be transmitted to the endoscopist, since that is an indication that a significant amount of snare wire is outside the sheath, and the wire loop may have engaged a large portion of mucosa, submucosa, and perhaps serosa within the tightened loop. Cutting through the polyp at this point may cause deep injury to the wall of the bowel proximal to the polyp itself. Given the information that closure sensation is felt when the slide bar is several centimeters from the line, the endoscopist must consider various scenarios: that the polyp is large and the distance from the line to the slide bar is consistent with the size of the polyp and the application of cautery current should commence; the wire loop bar is tangentially placed across the polyp, has closed around a large section of the polyp, and was not applied parallel to the colon wall or the snare has caught a large piece of tissue behind the polyp that has been drawn into the closed loop. If this has occurred, the loop should be repositioned in order to avoid transecting a portion of the normal colon wall. In order to assure that the snare will not become incarcerated (stuck) around a polyp during polypectomy, it is necessary that the tip of the snare wire must retract into the sheath at least 1.5 cm before the snare is used for polypectomy. During polypectomy, the plastic sheath tends to buckle inside the colonoscope as the wire is retracted and the loop is being tightened around a polyp. The 1.5 cm retraction of the tip of the wire loop ensures that even with shortening of the sheath, the guillotine force exerted by the closing wire loop against the sheath tip will result in severance of the polyp. Before each snare is used, this should be tested by retracting the snare handle completely since this maneuver will prevent the snare from being stuck around a polyp and not being able to transect it.

Safety in snare handling

When an assistant is requested to open the snare, the tip of the sheath should be pointed toward the lumen and not directly toward the colon wall. The pointed tip of the wire loop can easily penetrate the colon wall if opened rapidly when it is close to the mucosal surface. Conversely, the fully opened wire is quite flexible and can be pushed against the wall either to anchor its tip during entrapment of a polyp or can be pushed on the wall to widen the loop to place it over a large polyp. A safety measure to permit the endoscopist to have full control over the snare is to have the endoscopist advance the snare sheath until the tip is visible in the visual field. The endoscopist then withdraws the sheath into the instrument channel while the snare wire is still extended. The endoscopist needs to keep only the distal few millimeters of the wire loop in view as the sheath and the loop are withdrawn into the instrument channel. The assistant should open the loop fully as the sheath is being withdrawn by the endoscopist. In this manner, the opened wire loop is almost completely within the instrument channel. When snare capture of the polyp is desired, the sheath can be pushed out and the wire loop will open as it exits from the tip of the scope. The operator then has complete control over the length and width of the loop as it opens by pushing or pulling on the sheath and no longer requires the assistant to open and close the snare to position it around a polyp because it has been fully opened and is lying within the instrument channel.

Techniques for successful removal of sessile polyps

In order to successfully perform polypectomy, the endoscopist must have excellent control of the instrument at all times during the procedure, and especially during the snare capture of a polyp and when applying electrical current. The skill and knowledge of colonoscopy techniques can only be acquired through performance of multiple colonoscopic examinations prior to attempting colonoscopic polypectomy. The endoscopist should start polypectomy with small polyps and once familiar with the technique of placing the snare over a polyp, closing the snare, and application of electrocautery current while keeping the polyp properly in view with the instrument in a stable position, the endoscopist can move on to larger polyps. There is no literature on the learning curve concerning removal of large polyps, but since the same techniques required for colonoscopic polypectomy of small- and medium-sized polyps are used in removing large polyps, once basic skills are learned, it would seem sufficient to watch several being performed and then do a few under tutelage (minimum of 5) before embarking on the task of removing large sessile polyps. Since most colon polyps are sessile, the approach to smaller lesions can readily be applied to those that require more expertise.

It is important to fully assess a polyp before beginning polypectomy. The surface must be inspected for irregularity, for ulceration, and scanned for blood vessel abnormalities. The edges can be more clearly defined by use of chromoendoscopy or narrow-band imaging. Most endoscopists do not employ endoscopic ultrasound to delineate the depth of invasion, but narrow-band imaging and magnification endoscopy may provide useful information in this regard.

The techniques that must be learned for polypectomy are as follows:

1 Use an appropriate size snare that is optimal for the polyp size. Most polyps are 1 cm or less, and it is easier to capture these with a small snare (3 cm long × 1 cm wide). It is often difficult to capture a small polyp with a standard snare (6 cm long × 3 cm wide), which must be almost fully extended before the arms of the wire loop expand sufficiently to capture a polyp. Having to extend the wire to its full extent of 6 cm to capture a polyp can often be problematic because of the folds and bends of the colon may prevent the ability to fully open the snare.

2 It is important that the polyp to be removed is placed in the 5–6 o'clock position in the visual field in order to permit snare capture [5] (Figure 20.1, Video 20.1). The instrument channel is oriented toward the 5 o'clock position and a polyp in that position is considerably easier to entrap with the snare. It is extremely difficult to have the snare encircle a polyp located in the 12 o'clock or 9 o'clock position in the visual field.

3 Place the snare over the polyp with the wire in the plane of the surrounding mucosa so that it lies flat on the mucosal surface. This maneuver ensures that the snare will close at the junction of the polyp and mucosal surface. Since the tip of the sheath is the stationary portion of the snare complex, the open wire always retracts to the position of the tip of the sheath. If the sheath is advanced to the edge of the polyp at any angle over 10° from the plane of the mucosal surface and is then pushed on the junction of the adenoma with mucosa, oftentimes the tip of snare will rise up and no longer remain flat on the colon wall. If closure occurs with the snare in this position, the snare will capture a tangential part of the polyp, leaving a portion on the proximal edge, which then has to be further resected. One of the important aspects of polypectomy is to keep the snare wire flat on the wall during closure.

4 Aspirate air once the snare is in place. The aspiration of air causes the entire circumference of the colon to become smaller and its diameter to decrease. The decrease in circumference causes the polyp to actually rise up within the snare that has been placed over the polyp. The elevation of the polyp into the snare occurs because when the circumference decreases, the footprint of the polyp also decreases. Since the polyp volume does not change in size as its base gets smaller, the polyp actually elevates into the snare. Frequently, air aspiration results in loss of visual contact with the closing snare since folds may collapse over the polyp.

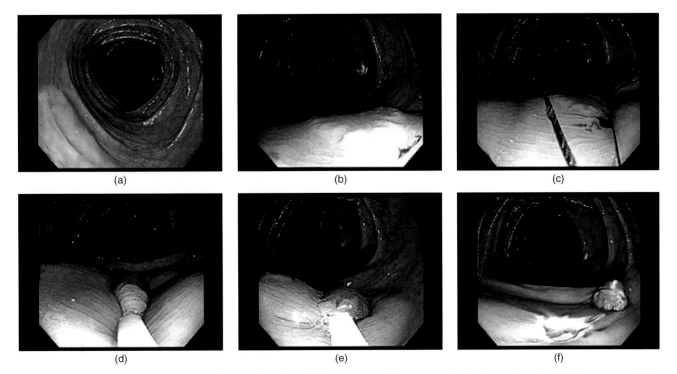

(a)   (b)   (c)

(d)   (e)   (f)

Figure 20.1 Endoscopic mucosal resection. A flat polyp is at the 7 o'clock position (a). Although the polyp can be injected in that position, it must be brought to the 5–6 o'clock position in order to perform polypectomy (b). The injection fluid contains a small amount of methylene blue to provide a contrast between the fluid-filled submucosa and the pink polyp on top. The open snare is placed over the polyp (c). The snare is pushed down on the polyp as air is aspirated, having placed the sheath on the point of desired separation (d). The snare is closed and tightened on the polyp (e) and severed using coagulation current without bleeding (f).

Even if the snare capturing the polyp cannot be readily seen, the assistant is asked to close the snare to the mark or until there is a closure sensation. Air is then reinsufflated and an assessment is made with full vision as to the relationship of the snare to the polyp. If only part of the polyp has been captured, the snare can be opened and repositioned.

5 The closed snare should be jiggled back and forth by holding the sheath near the biopsy port and moving it in and out. This maneuver will ensure that a large piece of the colon wall has not been captured within the snare loop behind the polyp (and out of sight). Entrapped proximal mucosa will result in the colon wall behind the polyp also moving back and forth as the snare is jiggled.

6 Once the snare is closed snugly onto the polyp, electrocautery is applied with a foot switch. The assistant (or the person who closes the snare) should not begin snare closure until requested by the endoscopist. In training circumstances, it is not unusual for the trainee, deeply involved in snare position, air aspiration, and then reinsufflation, maintaining the polyp in sight, and application of electrocautery current with the foot switch, to forget to ask the endoscopy assistant to close the snare. Often the nurse/assistant will have considerably more experience in polyp removal than the trainee and the result is that the nurse/assistant will close the snare without waiting for the request from the trainee endoscopist. However, once becoming familiar with the techniques of polypectomy, it is better to have the assistant wait until requested by the endoscopist to begin snare closure. This request for snare closure should be made after having briefly activated electrosurgical energy. With small polyps, snare closure will be relatively rapid and as soon as the foot switch is pressed, the request may be given to close the snare. However, if a polyp is relatively large, has a wide sessile base, or a thick pedicle, usually a few seconds of electrosurgical current should be given prior to a request for snare closure.

Once foot switch application has started the flow of current, the foot switch should be pressed continuously until the polyp has been severed. There is no advantage in pumping the foot switch up and down in an on-off-on-off sequence during polypectomy.

For all sessile polyps over 1 cm in diameter, the technique is the same. These include placing the open loop directly over the polyp, keeping the snare flat on the wall, aspiration of air, requesting slow snare closure, moving the sheath as necessary during snare closure, and having the assistant close to the line before beginning the application of electrosurgical power.

Pedunculated polyps

Pedunculated polyps are relatively easy to remove, since the snare wire only needs to be placed on the pedicle and tightened prior to the application of electrocautery current. If the pedunculated polyp is large, the pedicle is often thick and may be of variable length. When a large pedunculated polyp is seen, it should be moved around with the closed snare sheath in an attempt to ascertain the location, width, and length of the stalk and its relationship to the colon wall. Once this has been established, the colonoscope should be passed proximal to the polyp into an open area of the lumen. The scope is then rotated so that the polyp attachment is at the 5 o'clock position. With the standard snare fully opened, and the sheath tip near the tip of the colonoscope, the colonoscope and snare should be withdrawn slowly until the leading edge of the polyp is visualized or the attachment of the polyp is seen if the head is pointed toward the anus. Upon withdrawal of the colonoscope, the open wire loop is dragged along the colon wall over the polyp when the head is in a proximal position. As the scope with wire loop extended is withdrawn while holding the shaft with the right hand, the scope can be torqued to the right or to the left in order to place the loop over the polyp. If the snare cannot fully capture the polyp, rapid left/right rotation of the shaft can help to engage other portions of the polyp as withdrawal continues. After the shaft of the colonoscope with its wire has been withdrawn to the point where the pedicle is identified, slow closure of the snare handle should be accomplished as the endoscopist steadies the scope and moves the right hand from the shaft of the instrument to the snare sheath advancing it as closure is accomplished. In this fashion, the wire loop that passed underneath the polyp will always close toward the tip of the sheath that the endoscopist places on the pedicle at the point where closure is desired. If the wire snare becomes enmeshed within nodular portions of the polyp head, it is possible that they will be dragged down to the area of the pedicle and be captured within the closed wire loop. If a large portion has been captured, it will be evident by the assistant who will inform you that the slide bar is not close to "the mark" previously placed on the snare handle. If a large portion of the polyp head is caught, it may be necessary to have the assistant slowly open the snare while the endoscopist pulls the sheath back into the instrument channel. If the assistant opens the snare slowly as the endoscopist retracts the snare into the instrument channel, this will allow the endoscopist to manipulate the snare by jiggling it and dislodging a portion of polyp that may be caught in the snare. If this is not possible, the snare should be jiggled back and forth with the intention of seeing if the back wall moves along with the polyp when it is jiggled. If the back wall moves with the polyp, there is a strong possibility that the wall may be captured within the snare loop giving rise to the possibility of injuring the colon wall during polypectomy. If the back wall moves with the jiggling maneuver, the endoscopist must consider that it is caught within the snare loop, and further attempts should be made to dislodge it.

Fluid injection for polypectomy

Injection of fluid under a polyp is a useful tool to elevate the polyp away from deeper layers of the colon wall and make polypectomy safer [6]. The injection is made using a 23-gauge needle on a long flexible catheter. For successful elevation of any polyp, the injection must be placed into the submucosal space under the lesion, and the needle is usually inserted into an area of normal mucosa adjacent to the sessile polyp. If the needle is not inserted into the right plane, fluid may leak out into the lumen if too superficial or may be injected into the peritoneal cavity if too deep. A trick to get the insertion into the submucosal plane is to start the injection as the needle approaches the mucosa and as the

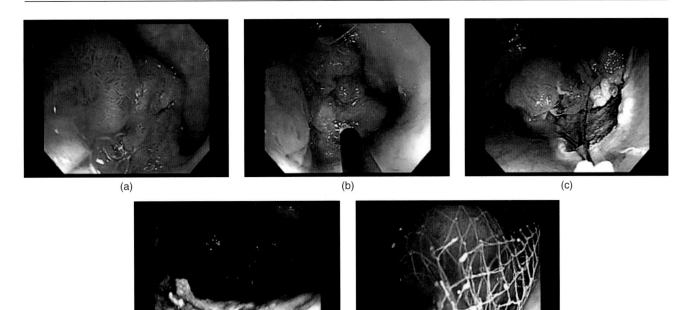

(a) (b) (c)

(d) (e)

Figure 20.2 Endoscopic mucosal resection. A large sessile polyp in the rectosigmoid (a) is injected with fluid. Because the polyp was located at a bend of the colon, the fluid injection could not be performed proximal to the polyp base (b). The polyp was resected in piecemeal fashion (c), with the submucosal injection fluid with added methylene blue seen at the base of the polypectomy site. After resection is complete, the base and edges are viewed with the assistance of narrow band imaging to observe if any fragments of adenomatous tissue remain (d). The fragments are recovered with the Roth net basket (e).

fluid flowing out of the needle reaches the submucosal space, it will balloon out the submucosa, causing the polyp to become visibly elevated. Occasionally, the fluid will create an intramucosal bleb that rapidly fills with blood but that does not cause a problem for subsequent polypectomy. A new injection device has been introduced, which uses a high-pressure fluid jet though an open tip catheter sans needle that drives the injection solution through the mucosa into the submucosa, creating a fluid cushion similar to that produced by a needle injector. This has been combined with an integral cutting tip (through which the stream is directed) to provide one device that can provide more than a single function [7–9]. Fluid that may be injected for polypectomy is often saline, and some endoscopists add a few drops of methylene blue to the injection solution to add color, which may assist in visualization of the edges of the adenoma, which will appear as pink tissue on a bed of blue fluid, rendering easier visualization of the polyp edge. As the polyp rises up on the fluid-filled submucosa, the peripheral margins of the polyp can be readily determined (Figure 20.2, Video 20.2).

Various substances other than those mentioned above have been used to create the submucosal cushion when resecting sessile polyps: these include 0.5% sodium hyaluronate [10] (via a 21-guage needle), glycerol, sugars, and 0.83% hydroxypropyl methylcellulose [11]. The former is quite expensive, but the latter is relatively cheap, an ingredient of "artificial tears," a component that is universally available. The high viscosity fluid remains at the injection site longer than saline, which makes piecemeal polypectomy less time-dependent. Endoscopic submucosal dissection (ESD) requires more time to complete a polypectomy and large volumes of a long-lasting solution are used. Epinephrine may be added to the injection solution to decrease bleeding and retain the injected fluid for a longer time [12].

Sometimes, very large headed polyps require piecemeal resection to sever portions of the polyp so that the site of attachment can be ensnared. Since most of these large thick-stalk pedunculated polyps will be in the sigmoid colon, the twists and bends of the sigmoid colon may prevent the standard snare (6 cm long by 3 cm wide) to be fully extended when approaching the polyp from its distal aspect. However, once the instrument tip has been passed beyond the polyp into the proximal lumen and is being withdrawn, it is easy to open the snare to its full 6 cm length, providing a 3-cm wide loop to maneuver over the polyp as the scope and fully extended snare are withdrawn. Most endoscopists do not inject the stalk of a pedunculated polyp with epinephrine, but this has been reported [4].

Sessile polyps less than 1.5 cm can be resected with one snare application [13], but larger polyps require piecemeal resection. Shrinking large polyps with an intralesional injection of epinephrine has been reported but not been widely used [14]. For larger polyps, one edge of the wire should be placed on the margin between the adenoma and normal tissue, with the other limb of the wire placed over a substantial portion of the polyp.

The sheath is then advanced to the desired point of separation. The plane of the wire loop should be positioned flat on the colon wall and air is then aspirated to result in capture of a portion of the polyp. The pieces that are removed should be less than 2 cm in diameter. Fragments are removed usually from one edge of the polyp the other, placing one limb of the wire into the divot caused by the removal of the preceding portion. Sometimes, it is easier to take one or two snare applications from the one side of the polyp and then move to the other side for further resection.

When most of a polyp is hidden from view behind a fold or wrapped around a fold in clamshell fashion, injection of the part nearest to the colonoscope may elevate that portion, but result in the inability to see the rest of the polyp because the mound of fluid injected into the submucosal space will block vision. When confronted by this type of polyp, an attempt should be made to pass the scope to the far edge of the polyp and deflect the tip toward the polyp. Fluid should be injected into the normal mucosa just at or near the proximal edge of the polyp (the part farthest from the colonoscope tip). After the back portion (proximal part) has been removed, then additional fluid may be injected into the residual polyp closest to the scope for its removal.

The nonlifting sign

In general, malignant tumors should not be removed using the submucosal fluid injection method. If a polyp fails to elevate (the "nonlifting sign"), it may be an indication of infiltration by cancer into deeper tissues, limiting the expansion of the submucosal layer [15,16]. Although deep or superficial needle placement may be the cause for failure to raise a bleb under a polyp, a submucosal bulging or bleb on one side of a polyp in response to injection without any visible elevation of the tumor itself (or only minimal elevation of one portion) is a clue that there is fixation into the submucosa. This phenomenon may also be caused by a prior attempt at polypectomy with healing and scarring of the mucosa and submucosa, preventing their separation by fluid injection.

Any tumor that can be elevated with submucosal injection of fluid may be totally removed by endoscopic resection, even if invasive cancer is found on tissue examination. The ability to elevate a tumor indicates that there is no deep fixation, or only a limited degree of fixation to the submucosal layer, with the probability of complete removal.

Retroversion

A technique for removal of a polyp located on the far side of a fold is to perform a U-turn maneuver. With standard instruments, this can only be accomplished in the cecum, ascending colon, and sometimes in the transverse colon, although it is somewhat easier with pediatric colonoscopes. The method for making a retroversion in the colon is to get to the cecum and visualize the appendiceal orifice. Turn the large dial maximally up and the small dial maximally to the right, and lock it in place. Hold the scope shaft and withdraw it with a clockwise rotation until the U-turn is seen. In the rectum and lower sigmoid, the use of a gastroscope can be considered. It is difficult but not impossible to resect a polyp in a U-turn mode because the tip deflection responses are opposite to those usually expected. Using special scopes with marked tip angulation, it is often possible to achieve total polypectomy in instances where the straightforward approach is not feasible.

Large right colon polyps with a clamshell configuration may present with only the most distal portion being visible to the endoscopist. In fact, even though the most distal portion of polyp may be removed endoscopically, there often is a portion of the polyp on the proximal aspect of the fold that may not be visible. This area can be seen by performing a retroversion maneuver in the right colon (Video 20.3). This maneuver is best accomplished using a pediatric colonoscope, with a short "nose," and a shorter bending radius than the standard colonoscope. With the instrument straightened, and the tip in the cecum, retroversion is performed by markedly deflecting the up/down control and advancing the instrument to push the angulated tip bending section into the caput, increasing the angle of deflection similar to rectal retroversion. Once the turn has been made, it is usually necessary to markedly adjust the right/left control to permit visualization of the colonoscope shaft in the U-turn mode. Often, pulling back the endoscope shaft will complete the turning maneuver. Polyps can be removed in the retroversion mode, but all the intraluminal events are upside down and backward from the usual control functions, since the instrument is now in a 180° opposite view than on straightforward colonoscopy. However, saline may be injected, the snare may be utilized, and the argon plasma coagulator can all be passed through the accessory channel in the retroverted scope.

A gastroscope can also be used for removal of polyps in a tortuous sigmoid colon, laden with diverticuli. The short nose and acute angulation capability usually permits accurate positioning of the scope and snare to perform polypectomy when the standard adult colonoscope is unable to get the polyp and snare into the proper configuration.

EMRC

To assist in removal of flat sessile polyps, a plastic cap may be attached to the colonoscope tip, with a preloaded snare placed at the mouth of the cap [17]. The cap is similar to that used for esophageal variceal banding. Once the polyp elevated with saline injection has been aspirated into the cap, a sizable portion of the mucosa can be removed using coagulation current. This technique has received the acronym "EMRC," for endoscopic mucosal resection with cap. Caution is urged for using this technique above the peritoneal reflection because of the risk of full-thickness resection when the entire wall of the colon is aspirated into the cap. Full suction cannot be applied, nor should the aspirated tissue fill the cap before transection. A large volume submucosal fluid cushion is necessary for safety.

Endoscopic submucosal dissection (Videos 20.4 and 20.5)

A recent extension of EMR is ESD developed in Japan. Large flat-elevated/sessile lesions in the colorectum tend to have a relatively benign nature despite their large size. These lesions need to be completely resected; however, on follow-up, after piecemeal EMR, local residual or recurrent lesions are occasionally detected, which tends to be more frequent in larger lesions after piecemeal EMR. The margins of lesions need to be accurately determined prior to resection by EMR or ESD. Although visual identification is often sufficient to provide this information, the edges of a polyp can be enhanced by augmentation with chromoendoscopy (Video 20.6) or with the use of narrow-band imaging (Video 20.7). To reduce the incidence of residual or recurrent tumors, en bloc resection of the neoplasm can be performed using ESD. This collection of techniques aims to remove a large sessile lesion in one piece by injecting fluid deep to the lesion, as for EMR, then incising the mucosa just near the tumor margin that has been elevated by the submucosal fluid injection. The initial mucosal incision usually involves approximately 30–60% of the perimeter of the polyp with a small margin of normal mucosa. This is followed by careful dissection underneath the polyp, staying in the fluid-filled superficial submucosal plane undermining the entire polyp until the resection is complete [18–20]. Although originally intended for removing early gastric cancer, ESD has been successfully applied to the colon, and several accessories are available [21,22]. Among these ESD accessories are a variety of cutting tools of various sizes and shapes, some with insulated tips and others that have the appearance of a snare device with only the tip of the cutting electrode protruding from the catheter sheath. Since repeated fluid injections are necessary to maintain the infiltration of the submucosa, several types of devices are available, some of which combine the cutting tool and the injector in the same catheter.

There is growing evidence that lesions with submucosal invasion limited to less than 1,000 µm without lymphovascular involvement or a poorly differentiated component do not have lymph node metastases [23]. The Paris endoscopic classification [24,25] of superficial neoplastic lesions states that the "depth of cancer invasion into the submucosa is a critical factor in predicting the risk of nodal metastases in superficial tumors of the digestive tract." This classification also states that the micrometric measure cut-off value between the superficial and deep layers of the submucosa is 1,000 µm. In this regard, it is important to determine the vertical depth of invasion of submucosal colorectal cancers. At the present, ESD is indicated for large, flat sessile lesions (especially more than 20 mm in size, called lateral spreading tumors), very large pedunculated polyps, or a lesion with submucosal fibrosis such as in residual or recurrent adenoma after polypectomy or EMR (Figures 20.3–20.5). The learning curve to develop the collection of techniques required for safe and effective ESD is quite steep as meticulous tool manipulation is necessary during this prolonged procedure. The procedure should be reserved for those who have been able to develop familiarity with this procedure under tutelage by experts in the field.

Where EMR provides a safety factor at the deep margin of resection by virtue of the submucosal fluid injection, ESD actually dissects in that fluid-filled submucosal plane just above the muscularis propria.

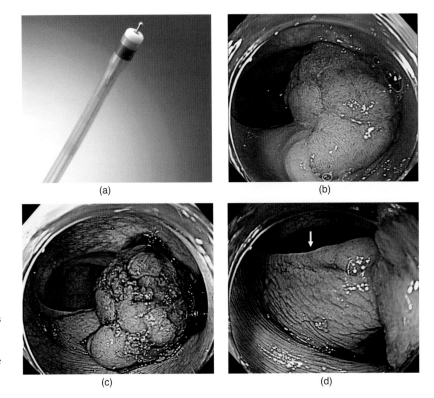

(a)

(b)

(c)

(d)

Figure 20.3 Large pedunculated polyp and ESD knife. (a) Electrosurgical knife for endoscopic submucosal dissection (ESD). Dual knife (KD-650; Olympus Company, Tokyo, Japan). The needle is 1.5 mm in diameter with a small insulated disc at its tip. (b) Colonoscopy revealed a large pedunculated sigmoid polyp. (c) A lobular surface without ulceration can be visualized after indigocarmine dye spraying. (d) Lateral extension can be seen on the stalk (white arrow).

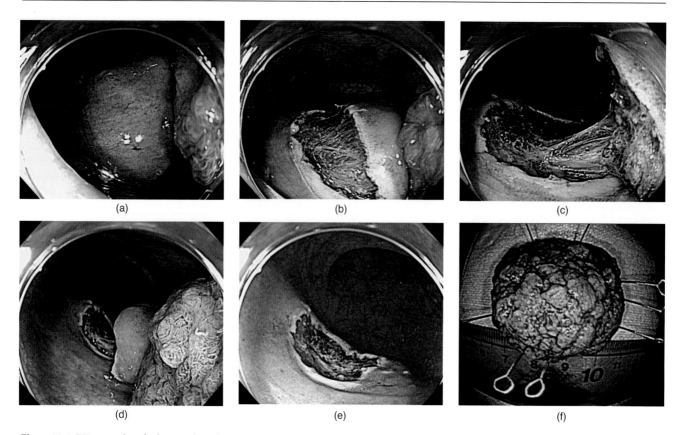

Figure 20.4 ESD procedure for large pedunculated polyp. (a) The lesion shows a prominent lifting after adequate submucosal injection of glycerol. (b–d) ESD using electrosurgical knife (Dual knife). Normal but infiltrated mucosa at the edge of the polyp was incised. Submucosal dissection was started beginning at the incision site. Further mucosal incisions and submucosal dissections were repeated under direct vision until completion. (e) The lesion was completely resected without complications. (f) Resected material, 35 mm in size. Histologically, the resected material had the features of tubulovillous adenoma with low grade to focal high grade dysplasia without lymphatic or venous invasion and the cut margin was clear.

The argon plasma coagulator

After piecemeal resection of sessile polyps, there are often small fragments of tissue left at the intersections of snare loop application and at the edges of the polypectomy site. Narrow band imaging may enhance the ability to visualize whether residual adenomatous tissue is present. These bits of adenoma usually will, with healing, reform as viable but small polyps. Immediately following snare polypectomy, these can be destroyed by using a thermal energy source, such as a Bicap electrode, heater probe, or argon plasma coagulator. There are no series that have reported on the first two, but articles on the APC have shown that its use on the polyp base to ablate residual tissue will decrease the recurrence rate [26–28]. Occasionally, some lesions cannot be completely removed during one or more sessions of polypectomy but may be amenable to ablation by a combination of repeated snare and cautery application and the use of APC (Video 20.8). Some expert endoscopists [29] have the opinion that the entire polyp and a surrounding portion of normal adjacent mucosa should be included in the piecemeal resection to avoid postpolypectomy recurrence and eschew the use of APC postpolypectomy.

Three different kinds of probes are available with the argon coagulator: a straightforward probe, a side fire probe, and a 360° probe tip. Of all of the probe tips, the straight end-on probe is preferred for most polypectomy completions. The straight end-on probe affords the ability to precisely pinpoint the area where electron beams will be transmitted. A side fire probe and the 360° probe have ceramic tips at the end of the probe and will prevent burning through the mucosal surface (or through the entire thickness of the colon wall) even if the probe tip is touched to tissue. However, in both these probes, when the tip is close to tissue, the electrons jump through the argon gas (producing the argon "plasma," which is the term used for any ionized gas), and the site of electron transfer cannot be precisely predicted because the electrons beams are not in the long axis of the probe but flow around the probe to the closest conductive tissue.

The delivery of energy depends on electrically activated plasma. The monopolar circuit is completed as a spark is produced, which contacts the bowel wall. If the tip of the catheter is pointed into the lumen or is several centimeters from the target tissue, no spark occurs, and inactivated and inert argon gas escapes harmlessly into the colon lumen. It is necessary to monitor the patient's abdominal distention by having an assistant gently palpate the

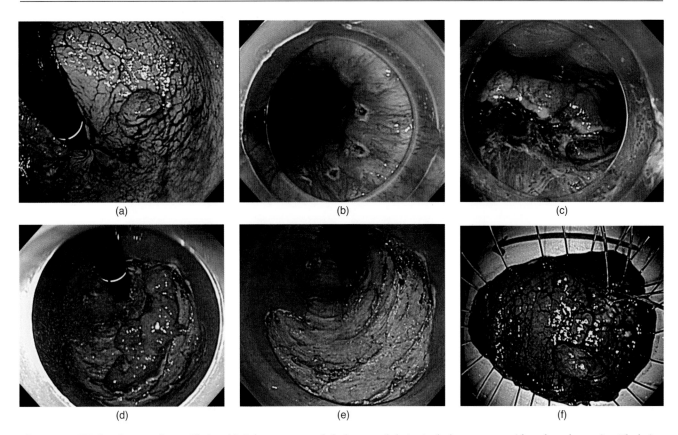

Figure 20.5 ESD for a large sessile rectal lesion. (a) Colonoscopy revealed a large sessile lesion in the lower rectum with anal canal extension. The lesion was hemicircumferential in its upper extent. (b) ESD using electrosurgical knife (Dual knife). Part of the normal mucosa was incised on the anal side of the tumor after a large volume of sodium hyaluronate was injected. Marking with APC or a snare tip is intended to delineate the edge of the tumor as these marks will persist even when the area becomes edematous from the injection solution. (c) Submucosal dissection was started from the incision in the anal canal using a transparent hood. (d and e) Mucosal incision and submucosal dissection under direct vision was repeated until completion. (f) Resected material, 60 mm in size. Histologically, the resected material had the features of tubular adenoma with low grade to focal high grade dysplasia. There was no lymphatic or vascular invasion and the deep margin was negative.

abdomen during each activation of the APC. Since this modality is not a laser, it requires no special protection for personnel during its use.

The depth of coagulum is variable, and can, to a large extent, be controlled by the duration of application and the total energy delivered. During use of the heat-producing argon plasma coagulator, the generated spark desiccates tissue. With the low power output settings used in the colon (40 watts with the original model or 25 watts with the ERBE VIO), the spark will only jump a few millimeters from the tip of the probe to the bowel wall with a burn depth of approximately 1 mm. The argon plasma coagulator can safely treat the base of a polypectomy site to ensure total ablation of adenoma, once piecemeal polypectomy has been performed (Figure 20.6, Video 20.9). The longer that the transfer of energy is directed to one area of the colon wall, the deeper will be the thermal damage. To prevent a deep burn, the tip of the probe should be kept in motion during activation. Because of the ability to maintain a superficial depth of thermal injury, the argon plasma coagulator can be successfully used to "paint" a large area of flat adenoma or residual tissue at the base of a

polypectomy site without damage to deep layers of the colon wall.

Hemostasis

In general, when coagulation current is used, bleeding during polypectomy is unusual. If bleeding does occur from the cut margins, it may be controlled by application of the wire loop to another adjacent portion of the polyp, where its removal results in cautery of the bleeding site with hemostasis. If this is not possible, there are several ways of stopping immediate polypectomy bleeding. One is to use the tip of the almost closed snare to act as a cautery device depositing point cautery at a specific location at the polypectomy site. This can readily be accomplished by closing the snare almost to the sheath with only approximately 1 mm of wire extended. Placing it directly on the bleeding site with application of cautery (at the same setting as for polypectomy) often results in hemostasis. Hemostasis can also be achieved with a clip (Figure 20.7, Video 20.10), although clips may interfere with further attempts

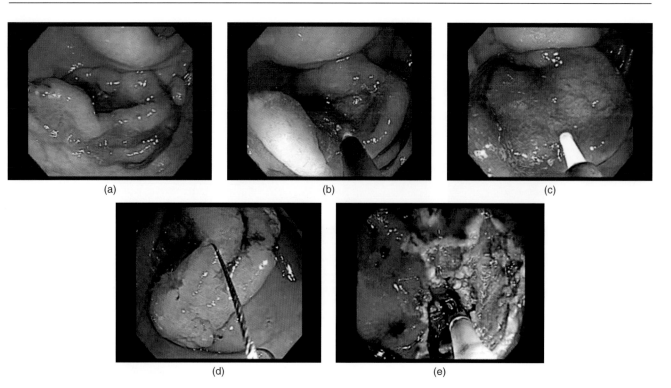

Figure 20.6 Endoscopic mucosal resection. A sessile polyp with an indented, but not ulcerated center (a) is injected with fluid with the needle directly into the depressed center (b) to elevate the central portion so that it can be removed (c). The polyp was removed in piecemeal fashion (d). The blue tinged submucosal fluid injection is visualized in contrast to the pink polyp. One portion could not be removed in spite of further injection. Therefore it was biopsied (e) before being ablated with the argon plasma coagulator.

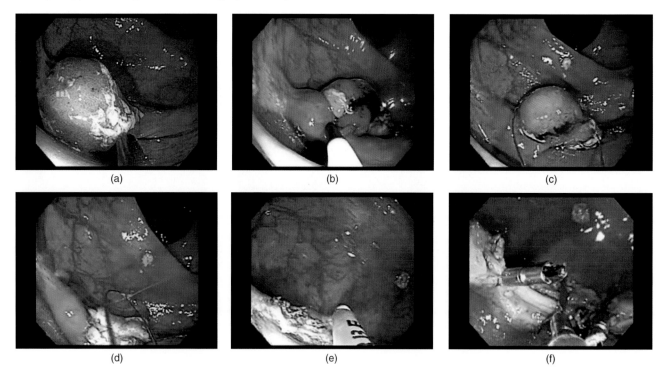

Figure 20.7 Endoscopic mucosal resection. A needle injector is shown about to place fluid into the submucosa. The needle was placed proximal to the polyp and then withdrawn bringing the polyp toward the endoscope (a). The injection is being made on the side and proximal to the polyp. Another injection is given at the base of the polyp (b). The snare is placed over the polyp for resection (c). A small amount of residual adenomatous tissue on the proximal edge of the polypectomy site is being removed with the snare (d). The base and edges are fulgurated with the argon plasma coagulator to ensure its total removal (e). The patient is on anticoagulation therapy and clips are used (f) to close the defect to ensure hemostasis, although clips are not usually deployed for routine colonoscopic polypectomy sites.

at completion of polypectomy. Any bleeding that occurs during polypectomy should be actively controlled although it has little hemodynamic significance but is a nuisance since it often interferes with vision. The argon plasma coagulator can also be used effectively to control bleeding, but that is rarely necessary during polypectomy. Once controlled, the remainder of the polyp procedure can continue. The topic of training in hemostasis skills is explored in greater detail in a separate chapter in this volume.

Endoscopic closure using hemoclips

Clips are not usually needed to close the mucosal defect after polypectomy following EMR or ESD (Video 20.11). An endoscopic closure using hemoclips can be performed as the first management for immediate therapeutic perforation regardless of the location (Figure 20.8). Taku et al. [30] reported that a successful closure using hemoclips was possible in nearly 70% of patients with mini-perforation (usually less than 10 mm in diameter) that can happen just after endoscopic resection. Most patients with successful closure can be managed conservatively without peritonitis

or diffuse peritoneal symptoms [30]. Training in techniques of closure of mucosal defects is also covered in more depth in a separate chapter.

Recent studies have suggested the usefulness of endoscopic clipping for the prevention of leakage of intestinal contents in patients with perforations associated with endoscopic treatment, such as EMR and ESD in the upper gastrointestinal tract [31,32]. The usefulness of clipping in patients with perforation in the lower gastrointestinal tract has also been reported [33]. Moreover, Raju et al. [34] recently reported that endoscopic closure of small iatrogenic colon perforations with clips results in mucosal and submucosal healing and prevented fecal soiling of the peritoneal cavity in a porcine model. After an iatrogenic perforation, an endoscopic closure using hemoclips can be performed as the first management for this complication regardless of the location. Many of the patients will do well without surgery if the patient's vital signs are stable and there are no peritoneal signs.

To facilitate treatment of a perforation after ESD, endoscopists should focus on (1) obtaining a good bowel preparation, (2) adequate washing of the area around the lesion and adequate aspiration of fecal fluid at the time of resection, (3) changing the patient's

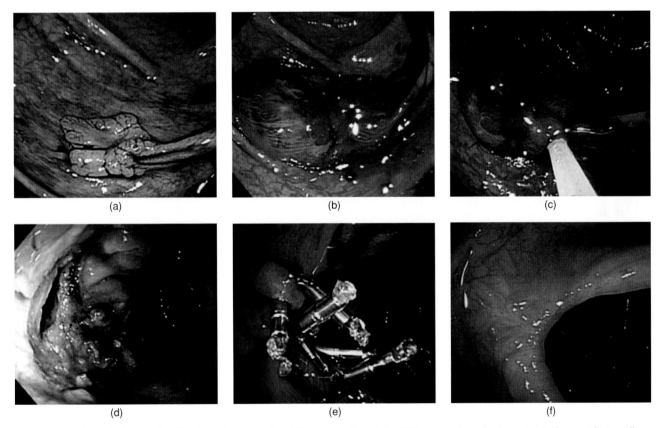

(a)   (b)   (c)

(d)   (e)   (f)

Figure 20.8 Endoscopic closure of perforation using hemoclips. A bite biopsy specimen was taken from center of the lesion by biopsy forceps and the patient was referred to our hospital for further evaluation and treatment. (a) Colonoscopy revealed a flat 15 mm lesion in the ascending colon. The lesion shows fold convergence after indigo carmine dye spraying. The fold convergence is judged to have been created by the earlier biopsy. (b) The lesion shows a nonlifting-sign, especially at the point of fold convergence, after adequate submucosal injection of glycerol. (c) EMR was performed using a standard snare. (d) A small longitudinal perforation was seen immediately after resection. (e) Six endoclips were applied for complete closure of the miniperforation. (f) Two months after EMR, the perforation site shows a scar without residual neoplasm. Histologically, the resected material had the features of tubular adenoma with moderate atypia containing part of the muscularis propria. Submucosal fibrosis was also recognized at the point of fold convergence.

position to place the perforation site in a superior position (in relation to gravity), and (4) use of CO_2 to facilitate absorption of gas, a transparent cylindrical hood to enhance the effect of suction to draw the edges together, and special injection liquids (glycerol, sodium hyaluronate) to maintain the base of submucosal fluid at the site. For the trainee, immediate recognition of a complication is a paramount skill. With the advent of animal tissue simulators, individuals along with their staff assistants learning to perform EMR and ESD of very large polyps can take advantage of safe, controlled opportunities to practice closing intentionally made perforations in order to gain proficiency when these skills are needed.

Precolonoscopic laboratory testing

A query should be made to every patient as to their tendency to bleed excessively if cut, injured, or having a tooth extraction. This is sufficient to identify most patients that may have a bleeding diathesis. There is no indication for ordering a blood count prior to colonoscopy or colonoscopic polypectomy in the usual patient who presents for polypectomy. A guideline from the ASGE [35] states that aspirin may be continued without an adverse effect on safety during polypectomy. There is some controversy as to whether clopidogrel therapy must be discontinued prior to colonoscopic polypectomy [36]. If warfarin anticoagulation is discontinued 4 days prior to the procedure, there is no mandate to perform a blood test to determine the prothrombin time or INR prior to the polypectomy procedure [37,38].

Intraoperative colonoscopy

It is possible to localize the site of a tumor, or a resected polypectomy site, by performing intraoperative colonoscopy This technique has been avoided by most endoscopists because of the need to perform an endoscopic examination in the operating room with all the constraints of positioning the patient, handling the scope, and trying to use maneuvers such as torque and straightening techniques with the abdomen open. The amount of air insufflated for colonoscopy can create problems with surgical techniques once the endoscopist has completed the necessary localization. Because the base of a polypectomy may heal within a few weeks, there is a possibility that the site may not be seen during an intraoperative endoscopy. Lesion identification can also be accomplished by colonoscopy and submucosal injection of radioactive-labeled albumin microaggregates just prior to surgery. The surgeon can then localize the precise area with detection by a gamma probe during laparotomy or laparoscopy.

Follow-up after polypectomy

When teaching complex colonoscopy, it is important that the trainee realize that their responsibility to the patient does not end once a polyp is removed. In order to ensure total removal of large polyps (over 2 cm), it is necessary to perform an interval colonoscopic reevaluation of the polypectomy site in 3–6 months after polypectomy has been performed [39]. A 1-month follow-up is rarely required since complete healing without an ulcer will permit removal of residual adenomas. The larger the initial polyp, the greater the chance of recurrence. Usually, after the major portion of the polyp has been removed via an initial colonoscopy, the residual polyp is much smaller than the original lesion and can readily be either removed with the snare or treated with the argon plasma coagulator.

If a large sessile polyp has been removed and the polypectomy appears to have been complete, the patient may have repeat polypectomy in 2–3 years because there is a tendency for other polyps to grow in the colon, and these patients need to be followed up for the rest of their lives. On the other hand, if the polyp is large, or if there is any residual fragments of polyp that remain or that were fulgurated with the argon plasma coagulator, the site of polyp removal must be identified since polyps tend to recur at the same site of polypectomy, especially if there is any visible residual tissue left at the polypectomy site.

A permanent mark can be placed anywhere in the colon to allow the endoscopist to find the site of polypectomy in the future at follow-up or to alert the surgeon as to the site of polypectomy so that surgical resection can be readily and safely performed knowing the exact location [17]. The technique is to inject through a standard injection needle, carbon particles in solution. This permanent stain can be seen by the endoscopist during follow-up or by the surgeon since it actually stains the serosal surface where it has been deposited into the submucosal tissues during injection. The injection solution for tattooing the colon was India ink when tattooing was first begun by Ponsky in 1972, and now can be performed with a suspension of pure carbon particles in a premeasured, prediluted, and sterilized form (SPOT). The important part of injection of a surgical marker (tattoo) is that the carbon particles be deposited directly into the submucosa. Oftentimes, as the injector needle is inserted into the colon wall after polypectomy, the tip of the needle is not placed directly into the submucosa, and this may result in fluid running out of the site of injection and not being deposited into the submucosal space. Indeed, if a visible bluish black bleb is not seen to elevate in the area of the needle injection, there is a high likelihood that no injection has been made, and that the site will not be able to be identified by either the endoscopist or the surgeon on subsequent endoscopic examinations.

Summary

Submucosal injection polypectomy is a safe and effective method for removal of sessile polyps. By paying attention to detail, raising a sufficient submucosal bleb of fluid, aspiration of air, keeping the snare loop parallel to the mucosal surface, and following accepted piecemeal polypectomy techniques, removal of large polyps throughout the colon is possible in a high percentage of patients. The technique of EMR is within the capability of any person who has learned how to remove polyps since the method for removal of large sessile neoplasms is only an extension of the skills required to resect smaller polyps, applied repeatedly to larger lesions. ESD is a new and exciting development in the field of colon polypectomy where developments and tools and techniques are progressing rapidly.

The welfare of the patient is the most important factor in the approach to the difficult polyp. If the impending polypectomy has a high risk of complication, or the endoscopist is concerned that the lesion is too large or cannot be approached in a safe manner, polypectomy should not be performed. The risks and benefits to the patient must be evaluated in any polypectomy, and especially when dealing with the difficult polyp.

Videos

Video 20.1 Endoscopic mucosal resection

Video 20.2 Endoscopic mucosal resection

Video 20.3 A retroversion for polypectomy

Video 20.4 Endoscopic submucosal dissection for a flat sigmoid lesion

Video 20.5 Endoscopic submucosal dissection for a large sessile lesion

Video 20.6 Chromoendoscopy

Video 20.7 Narrow band imaging for delineation of margins: the iceberg effect

Video 20.8 Multiple session polypectomy

Video 20.9 Endoscopic mucosal resection

Video 20.10 Endoscopic mucosal resection

Video 20.11 Giant lipoma resection with clip application

References

1 Gast P, Belaiche J: Rectal endosonography in inflammatory bowel disease: Differential diagnosis and prediction of remission. *Endoscopy* 1999;31:158–166.

2 Tsuga K, Haruma K, Fujimura J, et al.: Evaluation of the colorectal wall in normal subjects and patients with ulcerative colitis using an ultrasonic catheter probe. *Gastrointest Endosc* 1998;48: 477–484.

3 Tappero G, Gaia E, DeFiuli P, Martini S, Gubetta L, Emmnuelli G: Cold snare excision of small colorectal polyps. *Gastrointest Endosc* 1992;38:310–313.

4 Waye JD: Polypectomy: Basic principles. In: Waye JD, Rex DK, Williams CB (eds), *Colonoscopy: Principles and Practice*. London: Wiley-Blackwell, 2009, Chapter 42.

5 Tanaka S, Oka S, Chayama K, Kawashima K: Knack and practical technique of colonoscopic treatment focused on endoscopic mucosal resection using snare. *Dig Endosc* 2009;21(Suppl 1):S38–S42.

6 Repici A, Pellicano R, Strangio G, Danese S, Fagoonee S, Malesci A: Endoscopic mucosal resection for early colorectal neoplasia: Pathologic basis, procedures, and outcomes. *Dis Colon Rectum* 2009;52:1502–1515.

7 Yahagi N, Neuhaus H, Schumacher B,: Comparison of standard endoscopic submucosal dissection (ESD) versus an optimized ESD technique for the colon: an animal study. *Endoscopy* 2009;41: 340–345.

8 Neuhaus H, Wirths K, Schenk M, Enderle MD, Schumacher B: Randomized controlled study of EMR versus endoscopic submucosal dis-

section with a water-jet hybrid-knife of esophageal lesions in a porcine model. *Gastrointest Endosc* 2009;70:112–120.

9 Lingenfelder T, Fischer K, Sold MG, Post S, Enderle MD, Kaehler GF: Combination of water-jet dissection and needle-knife as a hybrid knife simplifies endoscopic submucosal dissection. *Surg Endosc* 2009;23:1531–1535.

10 Fujishiro M, Yahagi N, Kashimura K, et al.: Comparison of various submucosal injection solutions for maintaining mucosal elevation during endoscopic mucosal resection. *Endoscopy* 2004;36:579–583.

11 Feitoza AB, Gostout CJ, Burgart LJ, Burkert A, Herman LJ, Rajan E: Hydroxypropyl methylcellulose: A better submucosal fluid cushion for endoscopic mucosal resection. *Gastrointest Endosc* 2003;57: 41–47.

12 Lee SH, Lee KS, Park YS, et al.: Submucosal saline-epinephrine injection in colon polypectomy: Appropriate indication. *Hepatogastroenterology* 2008;55:1589–1593.

13 Waye JD: How big is too big? *Gastrointest Endosc* 1996;43:256–257.

14 Hogan RB, Hogan RB 3rd: Epinephrine volume reduction of giant colon polyps facilitates endoscopic assessment and removal. *Gastrointest Endosc* 2007;66:1018–1022.

15 Uno Y, Munakata A: The non-lifting sign of invasive colon cancer. *Gastrointest Endosc* 1994;40:485–489.

16 Ishiguro A, Uno Y, Ishiguro Y, Munakata A, Morita T: Correlation of lifting versus non-lifting and microscopic depth of invasion in early colorectal cancer. *Gastrointest Endosc* 1999;50:329–333.

17 Conio M, Repici A, Demarquay JF, Blanchi S, Dumas R, Filiberti R: EMR of large sessile colorectal polyps. *Gastrointest Endosc* 2004;60:234–241.

18 Ono H, Kondo H, Gotoda T, et al.: Endoscopic mucosal resection for treatment of early gastric cancer. *Gut* 2001;48(2):225–229.

19 Soetikno R, Kaltenbach T, Yeh R, Gotoda T: Endoscopic mucosal resection for early cancers of the upper gastrointestinal tract. *J Clin Oncol* 2005;23(20):4490–4498.

20 Yamamoto H, Sekine Y, Higashizawa T, et al.: Successful en bloc resection of a large superficial gastric cancer by using sodium hyaluronate and electrocautery incision forceps. *Gastrointest Endosc* 2001;54(5):629–632.

21 Saito Y, Uraoka T, Matsuda T, et al.: Endoscopic treatment of large superficial colorectal tumors: A case series of 200 endoscopic submucosal dissections (with video). *Gastrointest Endosc* 2007;66(5):966–973.

22 Fujishiro M, Yahagi N, Kakushima N, et al.: Outcomes of endoscopic submucosal dissection for colorectal epithelial neoplasms in 200 consecutive cases. *Clin Gastroenterol Hepatol* 2007;5(6):678–683.

23 Kitajima K, Fujimori T, Fujii S, et al.: Correlations between lymph node metastasis and depth of submucosal invasion in submucosal invasive colorectal carcinoma: A Japanese collaborative study. *J Gastroenterol* 2004;39:534–543.

24 Participants in the Paris Workshop: The Paris endoscopic classification of superficial neoplastic lesions: Esophagus, stomach, and colon. November 30 to December 1, 2002. *Gastrointest Endosc* 2003;58:S3–S43.

25 Lambert R, Kudo SE, Vieth M, et al.: Pragmatic classification of superficial neoplastic colorectal lesions. *Gastrointest Endosc* 2009;70:1182–1199.

26 Brooker JC, Saunders BP, Shah SG, Thapar CJ, Suzuki N, Williams CB. Treatment with argon plasma coagulation reduces recurrence after piecemeal resection of large sessile colonic polyps: A randomized trial and recommendations. *Gastrointest Endosc* 2002;55:371–375.

27 Norton ID, Wang L, Levine SA, et al.: In vivo characterization of colonic thermal injury caused by argon plasma coagulation. *Gastrointest Endosc* 2002;55:631–636.

28 Regula J, Wronska E, Polkawski M, et al.: Argon plasma coagulation after piecemeal polypectomy of sessile colorectal adenomas: Long-term follow-up study. *Endoscopy* 2003;**35**:212–218.

29 Bourke M: Current status of colonic endoscopic mucosal resection in the west and the interface with endoscopic submucosal dissection. *Dig Endosc* 2009;**21**(Suppl 1):S22–S27.

30 Taku K, Sano Y, Fu KI, et al.: Iatrogenic perforation associated with therapeutic colonoscopy: A multicenter study in Japan. *J Gastroenterol Hepatol* 2007;**22**(9):1409–1414.

31 Tsunada S, Ogata S, Ohyama T, et al.: Endoscopic closure of perforations caused by EMR in the stomach by application of metallic clips. *Gastrointest Endosc* 2003;**57**:948–951.

32 Yoshikane H, Hidano H, Sakakibara A, Niwa Y, Goto H: Feasibility study on endoscopic suture with the combination of a distal attachment and a rotatable clip for complications of endoscopic resection in the large intestine. *Endoscopy* 2000;**32**:477–480.

33 Fu KI, Sano Y, Kato S, et al.: Hazards of endoscopic biopsy for flat adenoma before endoscopic mucosal resection: A case report. *Dig Dis Sci* 2005;**50**(7):1324–1327.

34 Raju GS, Pham B, Xiao SY, et al.: A pilot study of endoscopic closure of colonic perforations with endoclips in a swine model. *Gastrointest Endosc* 2005;**62**(5):791–795.

35 Zuckerman MJ, Hirota WK, Adler DG, et al.; Standards of Practice Committee of the American Society for Gastrointestinal Endoscopy: ASGE guideline: The management of low-molecular-weight heparin and nonaspirin antiplatelet agents for endoscopic procedures. *Gastrointest Endosc* 2005;**61**:189–194.

36 Singh M, Mehta N, Murthy UK, Kaul V, Arif A, Newman N: Postpolypectomy bleeding in patients undergoing colonoscopy on uninterrupted clopidogrel therapy. *Gastrointest Endosc* 2010;**71**:998–1005.

37 Kwok A, Faigel DO: Management of anticoagulation before and after gastrointestinal endoscopy. *Am J Gastroenterol* 2009;104: 3085–3097.

38 Veitch AM, Baglin TP, Gershlick AH, Harnden SM, Tighe R, Cairns S; British Society of Gastroenterology; British Committee for Standards in Haematology; British Cardiovascular Intervention Society: Guidelines for the management of anticoagulant and antiplatelet therapy in patients undergoing endoscopic procedures. *Gut* 2008;**57**: 1322–1329.

39 Caputi Iambrenghi O, Ugenti I, Martines G, Marino F, Francesco Altomare D, Memeo V: Endoscopic management of large colorectal polyps. *Int J Colorectal Dis* 2009;**24**:749–753.

21 Natural Orifice Translumenal Endoscopic Surgery (NOTES®)

Kai Matthes[1], Mark A. Gromski[2], & Robert Hawes[3]

[1] Beth Israel Deaconess Medical Center, Harvard Medical School, Boston, MA, USA
[2] Beth Israel Deaconess Medical Center, Harvard Medical School, Boston, MA, USA
[3] Medical University of South Carolina, Charleston, SC, USA

Introduction

Natural orifice translumenal endoscopic surgery (NOTES®) is an emerging experimental alternative to open or laparoscopic surgery that eliminates abdominal incisions and incision-related complications by combining endoscopic and laparoscopic techniques to diagnose and treat abdomino–pelvic pathology. The advantages of this "scarless" approach are improved cosmesis, avoidance of the risk of abdominal wall herniation and infection, potentially less perioperative analgesic requirement, and potentially fewer perioperative complications.

The term "pure NOTES®" or "total NOTES®" implies performing a surgical procedure without any incisions of the abdomen, instead gaining access to the region of interest by traversing a natural orifice (e.g., vagina, anus, mouth), and thereby making a translumenal incision (i.e., in the vaginal wall, colon or stomach). NOTES® is a recent concept and early in its development, having been first described in an animal model in 2004 [1]. The experimental NOTES® technique is being studied largely in animal studies. There are, however, a number of human case reports and a handful of human case series presently [2–4]. The vast majority of human case reports are hybrid-NOTES® procedures, with laparoscopic ports utilized for visualization, retraction and technical assistance. Some NOTES® procedures involve the use of rigid laparoscopic instruments, while others use flexible endoscopic instruments. Procedures in the upper abdomen may be performed using rigid instruments through a transvaginal or transcolonic approach. The use of a peroral transgastric approach requires the use of flexible endoscopes with flexible equipment (Video 21.1).

Clinical Interest in NOTES®

There has been growing interest among surgeons, gastroenterologists and industry regarding the development of NOTES® as a surgical alternative. For example, in a recent survey carried out among general surgeons, 72% of responding surgeons would be interested in becoming trained in NOTES®, representing a great degree of interest in the field [5]. As may be expected, respondents with minimally invasive surgery (MIS) specialization and surgeons less than 60 years old had increased interest in training in NOTES® [5]. Of responding surgeons, 44% revealed that they would perform NOTES® rather than laparoscopic cholecystectomy if NOTES® was feasible, that NOTES® was an available modality in their hospital and they were trained effectively. Of the surgeons who responded that they would not prefer NOTES® cholecystectomy over laparoscopic cholecystectomy, the vast majority (88%) noted that they would change to a NOTES® procedure if there were sufficient data to demonstrate improved outcomes compared to the standard of care [5].

Words of Caution

With the onset of any new technique, caution must be exercised in the adoption of techniques that have little human experience or long-term follow-up. In the case of NOTES®, there are certain unique aspects that require perhaps even more caution, such as the nexpertise in multiple skill groups (MIS and flexible endoscopy). Some have argued that the laparoscopic cholecystectomy was introduced by surgeons in a less than orderly fashion that did not optimize patient safety and proper surgical training. There must be caution in the adoption of NOTES® technology in humans without adequate training and experience in animal models and simulations. Surgeons and/or teams that attempt to perform NOTES® procedures without adequate training are more likely to have poor results, which may result in patient harm and may hinder the development and adoption of this new technology [6].

With an eye towards this, the Natural Orifice Surgery Consortium for Assessment and Research (NOSCAR) was created by a joint initiative of the leaders of the Society of American

Successful Training in Gastrointestinal Endoscopy, First Edition. Edited by Jonathan Cohen.
© 2011 Blackwell Publishing Ltd. Published 2011 by Blackwell Publishing Ltd.

Gastrointestinal and Endoscopic Surgeons (SAGES) and the American Society of Gastrointestinal Endoscopy (ASGE). In 2006, NOSCAR published a White Paper addressing important considerations for conducting NOTES® research and provided recommendations for the clinical development and implementation of NOTES® [7]. One of the areas singled out as a priority is the area of training. While the entire process of setting out guiding principles for development of a field at the inception is novel and admirable, the fact that NOSCAR recognized that training considerations must be considered at the inception represents a major advance in the whole field of medical technology advancement. To coordinate research efforts, the consortium also directs funding and has established an international registry for human NOTES® procedures.

Knowledge and Skills Sets of NOTES® Training

Translumenal Access

Using a translumenal approach, the abdominal cavity is accessed with flexible endoscopes or rigid laparoscopic instruments through an incision in the stomach, colon or vagina, which may be created with various endoscopic, laparoscopic or surgical techniques. Translumenal access is associated with a risk of injury to adjacent organs, particularly in a nonhybrid procedure, with lack of visualization internal to the access location.

Transgastric Access

Knowledge

A transgastric approach to the abdominal cavity is commonly performed using a flexible endoscope and flexible endoscopic instruments operated through the working channel of the endoscope. The advantage of choosing the stomach as an entry point is that organs in the lower abdomen such as the appendix or the fallopian tubes may be accessed in a direct fashion. Surgical sites in the upper abdomen are more difficult to access with this approach since certain locations distant from the access port (e.g., the gallbladder) are difficult to reach without the ability to fix the endoscope in space. Retroversion of the endoscope allows areas to be accessed if they are located adjacent to the gastric incision. Some multiplatforms with endoscope fixation technology or additional bending sections may help to overcome this limitation.

Skills

For transgastric NOTES®, trainees should be proficient in flexible endoscopy, with pre-experience using guide wires, controlled radial expansion balloons, sphincterotomes and needle knives. Of utmost importance is avoidance of injury to adjacent organs, such as liver, spleen, pancreas, colon, or small bowel, with the gastric incision. These injuries may be undetected and can lead to infection or hemorrhage resulting in high morbidity and mortality. The transillumination technique will help the trainee to verify that no adjacent organs are on the other side of the stomach wall at the incision site. The PEG technique described by Kantsevoy and colleagues is considered to be a safe transgastric NOTES®

access technique [8]. It involves the combination of transillumination, percutaneous insertion of an angiocatheter into the stomach under visualization by the endoscope, grasping of the guide wire using a forceps and retrieving the guide wire through the working channel of the endoscope, insertion of a sphincterotome over the guide wire to incise the stomach wall, dilatation of the stomach incision with a dilation balloon, which is then used to direct the endoscope thorough the stomach wall into the abdomen by pushing the endoscope forward led by the guide wire and the dilation balloon [8]. Some institutions may prefer to obviate some of the steps described above and limit the access to the use of the needle knife alone or a combination of guide wire and sphincterotome. Some investigators use endoscopic ultrasound to avoid injury to adjacent organs. Using linear ultrasound, a guide wire may be introduced safely into the abdominal cavity using this technique and then combined with a sphincterotome incision and/or balloon dilatation.

Transvaginal Access

Knowledge

Currently, the transvaginal access is most frequently used in human studies, based on consideration that the closure of a vaginal incision has been proven to be safe for gynecological procedures in the past. Of course, transvaginal access is only possible in female patients. A manual closure of the incision site may be performed by a gynecologist skilled in this approach.

Skills

Rigid instruments may be used to operate in the upper abdomen (e.g., cholecystectomy or nephrectomy). If rigid instruments are used, the trainee should be familiar with the standard laparoscopic approach before attempting NOTES®. If flexible instruments are used, the trainee should become familiar with advanced interventional endoscopy before using these instruments for abdominal surgery.

Transcolonic or Transanal/TEM Access

Knowledge

Wilhelm, Meining and colleagues demonstrated an innovative method for creating transcolonic access by using a specially designed guide tube, which is inserted via a transcolonic approach into the abdominal cavity after intraperitoneal instillation of a decontamination solution through a Veress needle in the umbilicus [9]. The solution provides an artificial fluid level in the abdomen, allowing the bowel loops to float on top of the fluid that collects in the pelvis by positioning the patient in 30° reverse Trendelenburg. After verifying a clear space on the opposite side of the colon by using an endoluminal ultrasound probe (10 MHz) inserted transanally, abdominal access is obtained with a transanal endoscopic microsurgery device (TEM; Storz, Tuttlingen, Germany) by advancing a trocar through the colon. Following the procedure, the access site is closed with a purse string suture that is placed before entering the abdominal cavity in addition to 1–2 applications of a linear stapler [9]. Other investigators use a needle knife in addition to the TEM or simply a double-channel colonoscope to enter the abdomen. Bacterial contamination of the abdomen with colonic bacteria is certainly the biggest concern of this NOTES® approach and requires special considerations and further clinical testing.

Skills

The trainee should be made familiar with the use of the TEM device and how to operate a double-channel colonoscope. Alternatively, rigid laparoscopic instruments may be used to access the right or left upper quadrants of the abdomen. Here, laparoscopic pre-experience with the standard approach is required before attempting NOTES®.

Transvesical Access

Knowledge

Lima and colleagues demonstrated the feasibility of using the bladder as a translumenal access point [10–12]. Use of this technique is limited by the small size of the endoscope that can fit through the urethra. However, advantages of this technique are the applicability to both genders, the avoidance of the colon with more harmful bacterial flora and the sterile conditions of the bladder, with presumably smaller risk of abdominal infection in the setting of closure insufficiency.

Skills

The creation of transvesical access requires urological experience regarding the performance of advanced vesicoscopy.

Surgical Procedures

Visualization

Knowledge

Proper visualization of anatomical structures is of utmost importance to safely perform NOTES®. The light source of flexible endoscopes provides limited illumination of the abdominal cavity compared to standard surgical laparoscopes, since they are designed to illuminate smaller lumens such as the stomach or the colon. The light source can be adjusted manually, but with a change of scope orientation the illumination may then be too strong if the scope is operated closer to the organ wall, leading to reflection of light and glaring of the optical lens.

Skills

Meticulousness is required to examine all structures and to verify that the correct structures are identified and dissected. This requires certain expertise of the trainee and some training to manually adjust the light source as needed. Simulator training may be sufficient to obtain this level of expertise before proceeding with live animals.

Tissue Dissection

Knowledge

As mentioned above, the identification of correct anatomical structures is absolutely necessary to perform NOTES® safely.

Tissue dissection can be achieved with flexible endoscopic instruments such as forceps, graspers, endoscopic scissors and the needle knife. The needle knife must be used with caution because the depth of dissection may be difficult to perceive since the trajectory of the instrument and the optical camera are parallel in current endoscopes. The further development of new endoscopes which provide triangulation may help to overcome this problem.

Skills

Blunt dissection with a flexible endoscope is different from laparoscopic instruments and requires excellent endoscopic skills, which should be acquired in a simulator or in live animals before proceeding to humans. Particularly, the use of endoscopic scissors or needle knives requires advanced endoscopic experience. If a needle knife is used to dissect large vessels such as the renal artery or the splenic vein, minor unintentional movements of the tip of the endoscope (from releasing one of the wheels of the endoscope, for example) may move the needle knife a few millimeters laterally, potentially resulting in laceration of the vessel being focused on.

Rigid versus Flexible Operation

Knowledge

Depending on the background of the "digestivist" performing NOTES®, either flexible or rigid instruments may be chosen depending on the preference and clinical background of the surgeon or gastroenterologist. Flexible instruments are required for the transgastric access route, but transcolonic or transvaginal procedures are amendable to rigid instrumentation.

Skills

Using rigid instruments requires little adaptation of the surgeon to perform NOTES®. If flexible endoscopes are required and the physician is not performing flexible endoscopy on a daily or weekly basis, additional skills need to be acquired to gain proficiency in this technique before advancing to humans. Flexible endoscopic skills can be enhanced with the aid of virtual reality, plastic or tissue simulators. However, there are no clear guidelines or data as to how much simulator training or real endoscopic procedures are needed to be sufficiently trained to perform flexible NOTES® on patients.

Retraction

Knowledge

Retraction of organs and structures is important to perform surgical procedures, but is more challenging if the procedure is performed using a NOTES® approach. The lack of triangulation provides a challenge since retracting instruments exit the endoscope parallel to the imaging source and the dissecting device. Additional anchor points can be created with abdominal ports using a hybrid approach, with magnetic anchoring systems or retracting sutures placed in the peritoneum endoscopically.

Skills

The NOTES® approach, with limited retraction possibilities, provides a challenge to both gastroenterologists as well as minimally invasive surgeons. To overcome poor retraction and visualization, trainees may undergo simulation in *ex vivo* models followed by live animals to get adjusted to the different circumstances in comparison to standard laparoscopy.

Ligation

Knowledge

Ligation of vessels and other structures can be achieved endoscopically with Endoloops (Olympus America Inc., Center Valley, PA, USA). However, the ligating force of these endoscopic devices is likely not comparable to a surgical suture or a laparoscopically placed ligation clip. If rigid instruments are chosen, standard laparoscopic conditions apply, overcoming the limitations of endoscopic devices.

Skills

Interventional endoscopy skills are required for the trainee to learn how to efficiently ligate structures with flexible endoscopic devices. The ligation of the appendix using a NOTES® approach is not much different from the ligation of a large pedunculated colonic polyp. Here, a background in advanced endoscopy appears to be helpful.

Clip Application

Knowledge

Endoscopic clips may not provide the safety of laparoscopically applied surgical clips, as the strength of the smaller nitinol clips is not comparable to surgical clips. Current endoscopic clips will need to be redesigned because when closed, a gap exists between the two arms of the clip that does not assure adequate sealing. This underscores the importance of ongoing training as new devices are developed to improve on many of the above mentioned components of the NOTES® operations.

Skills

The trainee should understand the limitation of using commercially available clips for flexible endoscopy and use them with caution for hemostasis or the clipping of ducts. Insufficiency of clip application on the cystic duct after cholecystectomy may result in dangerous yet avoidable consequences.

Organ or Specimen Retrieval

Knowledge

The retrieval of organs following NOTES® resection (e.g., the appendix, gallbladder, or kidney) can provide challenges depending on the size of the organ. Retrieving the appendix is not challenging, but a transvaginal retrieval of the gallbladder, for example, could lead to rupture of the gallbladder with spillage of bile or may lead to a laceration of the access organ, complicated by hemorrhage or postoperative infection.

Skills

The retrieval of organs through a natural orifice should be practiced in *ex vivo* models or live animals before it is performed in humans. Observing the exit of the organ through the access organ with laparoscopy may provide additional safety in human procedures.

Closure of Access Site (Video 23.4)

Knowledge

One important concern regarding NOTES® is the safety of closure of the translumenal access point. The closure of a transvaginal access port may be less critical since the bacterial flora of the vagina is rather benign and may be less likely to lead to a significant infection of the abdomen. However, with transgastric or transcolonic access, the efficiency of closure is of utmost importance, due to the increased potential of an intra-abdominal infection in the setting of closure insufficiency. When providing perioperative care for patients undergoing NOTES® procedures, significant abdominal discomfort, tenderness or clinical signs of infection may point towards a complication in relation to the translumenal closure. The closure of the access site may be performed with endoclips applied laparoscopically in a hybrid approach, or endoscopically using clips used for endoscopic hemostasis. The latter technique does not appear to be safe to close a stomach incision as the strength of adaptation of the incision wall is questionable and cannot be considered safe [13]. Recently, clips using an over-the-scope technique appear to be more promising since they provide a stronger adaptation force. Devices such as the Ovesco OTSC clip (Ovesco Inc., Tübingen, Germany) (Video 21.2) or the Aponos clip (Aponos Inc., Kingston, NH, USA) have recently been developed for such applications. Special closure devices using suction are available and under investigation. Ultimately, the safest closure may be by using surgical staplers or hand-sewn closure of the access site in the rectum or the vagina.

Maintenance of Sterility

Knowledge

If flexible endoscopy is chosen for a NOTES® approach, the increased length of the endoscopic instruments is associated with an increased risk of infection as the instruments may touch unsterile areas in the OR. This may go unrecognized, especially as this is a new technique and the operating team may be too focused on the procedure, which may lead to an oversight of break of sterility.

Skills

Care should be taken by the surgical team to avoid contamination of the instruments. Sterile overtubes for the endoscopes are increasingly available to provide a sterile tunnel between the orifice and the translumenal incision. Sterility of flexible instruments can be maintained by using dedicated operating room space (e.g., a table with sterile covers where instruments are placed when not used for the surgery). The operating room team should maintain OR hygiene standards by routinely wearing hats, face masks, sterile gowns and gloves. The anesthesiologist may be helpful by alerting the surgical team regarding a potential source of infection.

Management of Intraoperative Complications

Hemodynamic Changes

Knowledge

Preliminary data suggest that, in the porcine model, NOTES® peritoneoscopy is associated with higher peak inspiratory pressures and marked increases in median intra-abdominal pressure with wide variation compared to laparoscopic peritoneoscopy [14]. This increase in intra-abdominal pressure leads to a decreased cardiac output based on decreased cardiac return, or preload [14]. Increases in peak inspiratory pressure correlate with increases in intra-abdominal pressure [14]. If the pneumoperitoneum is maintained with on-demand insufflation using a standard endoscopic insufflator, higher intra-abdominal pressures are detected than with controlled insufflation through a Veress needle using carbon dioxide [14]. While NOTES® is currently being studied extensively in animal models, there is still insufficient evidence of the impact of intraoperative cardiopulmonary effects during NOTES® procedures.

Skills

The trainee should be made aware of potential increases in intra-abdominal pressure if the abdomen is insufflated through the working channel of the endoscope and without a pressure regulation device. The tension of the abdomen should be reassessed on occasion throughout the case and the blood pressure and heart rate monitored by the anesthesiologist, who should be aware of this potential side effect.

Intra-abdominal Hemorrhage

Knowledge

One of the challenges of providing anesthesia for NOTES® procedures is the limited knowledge or experience with unexpected complications. A pure NOTES® approach implicates minimally invasive surgery (MIS) with flexible endoscopic devices that are generally not designed for this particular purpose. Due to the accelerated development of this disruptive minimally invasive approach and early clinical application of prototypes or use of devices other than for their intended purposes, the development of advanced equipment specifically for NOTES® is lagging behind. Some devices used for intra-abdominal surgery during NOTES® were designed for the endolumenal use of interventional gastrointestinal endoscopy. In the setting of vascular injury during a nonhybrid NOTES® procedure, the ability to achieve hemostasis is limited by lack of access and functionality of flexible endoscopic devices. This may result in an unexpected blood loss and a potential conversion to laparotomy if hemostasis cannot be achieved endoscopically. Even in NOTES® centers with research experience, surgeons still operate at the steep part of the learning curve. The management of unexpected complications may challenge even experienced surgeons. A limited visualization of the abdominal cavity with flexible endoscopes could lead to minor bleeding being unrecognized, as the source may be hidden behind other structures.

Skills

With the current standard of endoscopic devices used for NOTES®, there is limited ability to treat a major vascular injury. In the setting of a significant intra-abdominal hemorrhage, transabdominal laparoscopic ports may need to be inserted or a laparotomy performed. Due to the lack of sufficient expertise with this emerging surgical technique, anesthesiologists must be prepared for a major blood loss, even with minor procedures such as a transvaginal cholecystectomy or appendectomy. This is primarily based on the fact that surgeons operate on the steep part of the learning curve when performing NOTES®. NOSCAR strongly discourages surgeons interested in NOTES® from advancing to human application too quickly. The establishment of translumenal access, especially, is different from current laparoscopic procedures. With the access of the abdominal cavity, adjacent organ structures may be injured. There may be a time delay until sufficient visualization of the peritoneal cavity is accomplished, and there may be a lack of visualization of the entire abdominal cavity, which may lead to significant hemorrhage being detected late or not at all. Proper surgical ligation of major vessels may take longer than expected in comparison to standard laparoscopic or open procedures. Complications can be realistically simulated in live animal or *ex vivo* models and should be an important consideration during the training process prior to human work.

Air Embolism and Pneumothorax

Knowledge

Possible complications of NOTES® procedures include air embolism and pneumothorax. Sumiyama and colleagues described a procedure of submucosal tunneling using carbon dioxide injection [15]. Two out of four animals died intraoperatively, with at least one sustaining a venous CO_2 air embolism, resulting in death [15]. Even without the use of CO_2, venous air embolism must be taken into consideration since the intra-abdominal pressure may be higher than during laparoscopy if the abdomen is insufflated through the working channel of the endoscope and without the use of a pressure control mechanism. Willingham and colleagues experienced a fatal pneumothorax in the NOTES® animal group in comparison to laparoscopic distal pancreatectomy [16]. In particular, transesophageal procedures can lead to pneumothorax or pneumomediastinum with possible fatal consequences.

Skills

A similar vigilance and meticulousness is required by surgeons and anesthesiologists to carefully select patients for NOTES®, to observe for any possible complications and to be prepared for complications like venous air embolism and pneumothorax, even during standard surgical procedures.

Anesthesia Considerations

Due to the potentially less invasive character of NOTES® procedures, patients may require less perioperative analgesics. Due to the less stimulating character of the surgery, it may be discovered through studies that some interventions may be carried out under monitored anesthesia care instead of general anesthesia. It is unclear, however, if this different management would be associated with decreased morbidity and mortality.

Guidelines

As of now, there are no formal clinical guidelines for training or education in NOTES®, as there is not sufficient human experience to acknowledge the most appropriate procedures to attempt NOTES® [6]. At the 4th International NOSCAR Conference in Boston in 2009, the training and credentialing committee debated critical points to be included in guidelines suggested for implementation by the ASGE and SAGES. These suggested guidelines for establishment and safe introduction of NOTES® include that NOTES® procedures should only be performed under IRB-approved protocols. Physicians engaging in NOTES® procedures should demonstrate competency in the requisite skills set, such as therapeutic flexible endoscopy, laparoscopy, knowledge of gross and endoscopic anatomy, and colpotomy if a transvaginal access point is chosen. During initial phases of adoption of the technique, team training is recommended to be multidisciplinary to complete and demonstrate adequate skills sets. This team training should include surgeons, gastroenterologists, physician assistants, operating room nurses and possibly anesthesiologists. Use of the NOSCAR registry is mandatory to publish the results of human studies. As of now, credentialing is left to individual institutions and the use of proctors as part of the credentialing process is recommended.

Assessment of Competency

There are not, as of yet, generally agreed upon competencies for NOTES®. As procedures mature and more experience is achieved, a specific set of competencies will emerge. Through existing animal and human experience, however, it is clear that competencies from general surgery, MIS and flexible endoscopy are required in a NOTES® team. Frequently, for the establishment of transvaginal access procedures, gynecologists are consulted to assist with the incision and closure. At present, it is prudent to insist that a multidisciplinary NOTES® team consist of members that fulfill competencies and principles present in guidelines for general surgery, MIS and flexible endoscopy, as described by respective authorities (i.e., ACGME, SAGES and ASGE, respectively) [17–20]. Procedure-specific benchmarking will clearly influence future definitions of competency in NOTES® with an emerging availability of published outcome data on human experience.

The development of a NOTES® assessment tool is considered a prerequisite for the credentialing process. Recently, the FITNESS (Formative Intraoperative Tool for NOTES® Evaluation of Surgical Skills) tool has been demonstrated by Vassiliou and colleagues as a method of assessing competency in NOTES® [21]. This assessment tool consists of six items scored on a Likert scale from 1 to 5: access (A), navigation and orientation (NO), visualization and stabilization (VS), instrument manipulation and targeting (IMT), closure (C), and application of surgical principles (SP) [21]. However, there is limited data regarding the validity of this tool since the preliminary study involved only eight participants (4 novice and 4 experienced). Multicenter trials are currently warranted to establish inter-rater reliability and construct validity of FITNESS. It is currently not clear whether a team versus individual assessment is mandatory.

The experimental Fundamentals of NOTES® Surgery (FNS) is based on Fundamentals of Laparoscopic Surgery (FLS) and Fundamentals of Endoscopic Surgery (FES) training tools, which are supported by the SAGES/ASGE Task Force. Prerequisites for FNS would be FLS and FES certification. FNS aims to assess cognitive and manual skills components specific to NOTES® procedures and challenges related to different accesses and platforms. FNS may develop into modules that are access and procedure specific.

Team Development

Those interested in learning and training in the novel NOTES® technique should assemble a multidisciplinary team devoted to NOTES® training and procedures, composed of members who are proficient and experienced in general surgery, MIS, flexible endoscopy, anesthesiology, nursing and technological support. The creation of a dedicated team that undergoes a thorough training, initially with simulation models followed by a transition to animal models, ensures that the team learns the premise of the procedures and mastery of the necessary interdisciplinary communication skills that are imperative to NOTES®.

Furthermore, NOSCAR has created the following guidelines for team development:
- Multidisciplinary team, possessing skills in advanced therapeutic endoscopy and advanced laparoscopy
- Should include members of SAGES and/or ASGE
- Access to animal laboratory facilities for research and training
- Lab results should be shared at semiannual NOSCAR group meetings
- Any and all human procedures performed after IRB approval
- Human cases should be submitted to NOSCAR registry

Simulation

Prior to attempting NOTES® procedures in the animal lab with large live animals, it is beneficial for the multidisciplinary NOTES® team to gain facility with the procedures, techniques and communication through simulated procedures. Existing computer trainers for laparoscopic surgery and gastrointestinal endoscopy are valuable for developing the basic skills necessary for NOTES®. These trainers are especially valuable for cross-training, such as allowing a surgeon to develop or refine advanced endoscopy skills with a virtual reality endoscopy trainer and vice versa. There are no existing virtual reality simulation trainers, however, specific to NOTES® procedures.

The ELITE trainer (Endoscopic–Laparoscopic Interdisciplinary Training Entity) is a plastic phantom developed by the Technical

University of Munich. The group demonstrated the construct validity of the model in a study involving 15 novices and 15 experts [22]. Significant differences were observed for the total time required to perform the respective procedures between these two different groups (first pass: 394.3 ± 176.6 s for experts vs. 531.9 ± 166.7 s for beginners, p = 0.040) [22]. All participants passed a significant learning curve during the assessment (total time needed: 473.1 ± 178.5 s for first pass vs. 321.9 ± 182.0 s for fifth pass; p = 0.02) [22]. In regards to laparoscopic skills, the group consisted of 9 experts and 21 novices. There was no statistically significant difference between these two groups with respect to total time required [22]. The limitation of the plastic model is the limited realism in terms of simulating haptics.

The EASIE-R™ simulator (Endosim, LLC, Berlin, MA, USA) uses *ex vivo* porcine specimens harvested from the meat production industry that are thoroughly cleaned, sterilized and surgically altered to resemble human anatomy (Figure 21.1). This model is currently the only real-tissue NOTES® simulator available and provides the opportunity to use commercially available surgical and endoscopic devices and prototypes. Participants of the learning center of the SAGES Annual Meeting in 2008 performed a NOTES® hands-on station utilizing both the ELITE and EASIE-R™ simulators (Figure 21.2). The participants rated the realism of the EASIE-R™ higher than the ELITE plastic phantom (Abstract, SAGES 2010 Annual Meeting).

Also, after the multidisciplinary NOTES® team has progressed to procedures with live animals in the lab or with humans in the operating room, it is useful to hone the unique skills required in NOTES® in a simulated environment. Some procedures may be undertaken in human cadavers. The advantage is the adequacy of human anatomy with proper dimensions. The disadvantages are the limited availability of cadavers and ethical concerns involved with this training modality. In comparison to plastic models and *ex vivo* models, there is a concern of infection from human blood borne viruses.

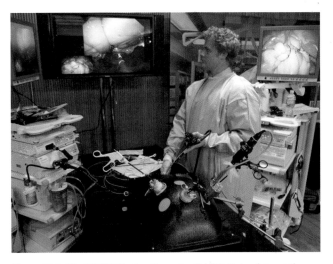

Figure 21.2 Live NOTES instruction using EASIE-R simulator at the 2009 CIMIT Exploratorium in Boston, MA, USA (Endosim, LLC, Berlin, MA, USA)

Training with simulation provides a safe environment to attempt new procedures or refine new ones, and also saves time and money that would have been spent in the animal laboratory.

Animal Lab Experience

It is difficult to overemphasize the necessity of ample experience in the animal laboratory before any attempt is made to perform human NOTES® procedures. Large animals, particularly pigs, but also sheep and dogs, have been utilized in the majority of the research that has been produced regarding the development of NOTES® as a surgical technique. Performing NOTES® procedures on large animals allows the multidisciplinary team to develop acceptable techniques while monitoring effects on physiology. It also allows the team to become facile with the available technology and tools, as well as the management of complications as they arise, such as intraperitoneal bleeding. Importantly, animal lab studies allow NOTES® procedures to be analyzed for efficacy, complications and physiologic sequelae.

Although similar in many regards to humans, large animals will never be able to reproduce perfectly the effect of a certain procedure or technique on humans. Thus, after multidisciplinary groups have spent a great amount of time in the animal and simulation laboratories, and are comfortable in the safety and efficacy of the procedure(s), well-controlled and well-designed human studies should be undertaken.

Preceptorship/Training Centers

Since NOTES® is a new technique in minimally invasive surgical intervention, with a unique set of skills necessary, very few teams exist in the world that are approaching competency to regularly apply the technique to human subjects. The initial few teams that

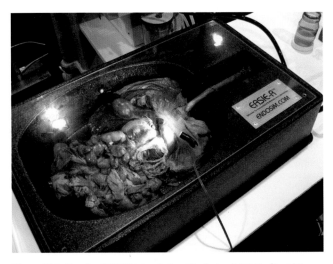

Figure 21.1 Ex-vivo NOTES simulation (Endosim, LLC, Berlin, MA, USA)

are leading the development of NOTES® techniques and technology will need to train and share results with each other, as has been occurring through professional meetings and site visitations [6]. As the number of practitioners interested in NOTES® increases and more practitioners and medical centers invest in the resources necessary to develop a qualified multidisciplinary team (technology, animal lab access, simulators), a centralized preceptorship system, with oversight from the professional societies (ASGE/SAGES), should be organized around "centers of excellence". The "centers of excellence" should be established with the support of the current leaders and innovators in the field.

This preceptorship system should follow the design of acquisition of a "major skill", as defined by the ASGE [23]. The ASGE defines a major skill as "a new technique or procedure which by its nature involves a high level of complexity, interpretative ability, and/or new type of technology" [23]. For major skills, a vehicle of formal instruction, such as a preceptorship, is the appropriate mode of instruction and acquisition of skills. Actively participating in a workshop or brief course is not sufficient to acquire the skills for a major skill [23].

The preceptors will be the principal members of groups currently leading NOTES® research and clinical application. It is likely that they will be selected either through NOSCAR or ASGE/SAGES, based on their extensive experience with the development and application of NOTES®. The preceptor, as an extension of the authority of the professional societies, will be responsible for developing a curriculum, teaching select NOTES® procedures, demonstrating NOTES® techniques, supervising and evaluating the preceptee and documenting competency of certain NOTES® techniques [23]. The preceptee will develop an understanding of the history of NOTES®, its indications and alternatives, a proficiency in certain NOTES® procedures, an ability to develop care plans based upon initial findings and the ability to avoid, recognize and manage complications encountered [23]. These should start as preceptorships in large animal NOTES® (i.e., pigs) to allow new multidisciplinary groups to gain proficiency with certain NOTES® procedures in the animal laboratory. Eventually, with more widespread application of NOTES® procedures to humans, these preceptorships will expand to include human preceptorships for more experienced NOTES® teams.

Privileging and Credentialing

Currently, there are no formal avenues for credentialing or awarding privileges in NOTES®. As the technology and techniques develop, guidelines for credentialing will likely be created by the professional societies, either the ASGE or SAGES or both, with credentials determined after completion of a recognized preceptorship and documentation of competency. Due to the multidisciplinary nature of NOTES®, it is possible that there may be discussion and conflict over which specialties will be credentialed to perform NOTES® procedures [6].

Credentialing today is institution-based and not uniform. As suggested by the members of the training and credentialing committee at the NOSCAR conference in 2009, to maximize safety and to ensure competency in each critical aspect, the following should be present for an individual or a team performing NOTES® procedures:

- Baseline credentialing in the procedure (operative privileges)
- Endoscopic credentialing
- Platform training
- Credentialing in the organ of access
- Currently by teams only

Postgraduate and Residency Training

Due to NOTES® being in an early stage of development, there is currently little role for postgraduate and residency training, except for perhaps a few pioneering academic centers of the world. However, this may change as certain NOTES® procedures become clinically acknowledged. Today, training for NOTES® occurs currently in the form of ad hoc fellowships, proctoring, case observations and hands-on courses at various centers and the annual NOSCAR conference. In the short term, development of accredited fellowship programs including both GI and surgical trainees may develop. A few academic institutes recently introduced "NOTES® fellowships" for surgeons and gastroenterolgists after completing a residency in general surgery or a fellowship in gastroenterology. These, so far nonaccredited programs, involve research projects and participation in human NOTES® procedures, which vary in content and actual exposure to clinical cases from institution to institution. As the number of NOTES® cases increase nationally, some fellowships may become endorsed by the ASGE and/or SAGES. In the medium term, the basic NOTES® skills set may be increasingly integrated into surgical and gastroenterology training. Providing exposure to animal laboratory NOTES® procedures is an effective way to demonstrate the experimental frontiers of MIS and flexible endoscopy, which may be an encouraging and thought-provoking experience for postgraduate and resident trainees [24]. With the maturation of NOTES® as a surgical technique, it can be expected that postgraduate and residency training programs will evolve to include components of NOTES® exposure and training, complete with curricula containing objectives and learning strategies. In the long run, with further establishment of NOTES® as an accepted discipline, the societies may consider creating the dedicated education of a "digestivist" as a combined training in general surgery and gastroenterology with emphasis in laparoscopy and flexible endoscopy during residency. The creation of a hybrid training program if accessed through gastroenterology might be facilitated by eliminating or shortening the internal medicine section. In surgery, sections of nongastrointestinal surgery such as vascular surgery, breast, and head and neck surgery similarly may be streamlined or even omitted. This form of education would require the boards of internal medicine, gastroenterology and surgery to participate and reach a consensus.

A specific NOTES® fellowship may be accessed after a general surgery, MIS fellowship or advanced GI training. It is currently unclear whether it should be area or technique specific. The educational paradigm should be competency-based and not time-based.

The assessment of cognitive competency specific to area of interest in addition to preoperative and postoperative care and assessment of patients is paramount.

Continuing Education

As new procedures and technical equipment are developed to support NOTES®, there will need to be a reliable way for those proficient in NOTES® to become familiar with the latest products and procedures. This will likely take place through independent NOTES® courses directed by experts of recognized academic centers or through NOTES® courses as part of national and/or regional meetings. A well conducted hands-on training program with a low faculty-to-student ratio will allow existing NOTES® practitioners to gain proficiency in new techniques, with the opportunity to use novel equipment and devices.

Videos

Video 21.1   Ex vivo simulator for the simulation of Natural Orifice Translumenal Endoscopic Surgery (NOTES®)

Video 21.2   NOTES® gastrojejunostomy for treatment of duodenal obstruction

Video 23.4   Closure of gastrointestinal perforations

References

1 Kalloo AN, Singh VK, Jagannath SB, et al.: Flexible transgastric peritoneoscopy: a novel approach to diagnostic and therapeutic interventions in the peritoneal cavity. *Gastrointest Endosc* 2004;**60**(1):114–117.

2 Decarli LA, Zorron R, Branco A, et al.: New Hybrid Approach for NOTES transvaginal cholecystectomy: preliminary clinical experience. *Surg Innov* 2009;**16**(2):181–186.

3 Horgan S, Cullen JP, Talamini MA, et al.: Natural orifice surgery: initial clinical experience. *Surg Endosc* 2009;**23**(7):1512–1518.

4 Zornig C, Mofid H, Siemssen L, et al.: Transvaginal NOTES hybrid cholecystectomy: feasibility results in 68 cases with mid-term follow-up. *Endoscopy* 2009;**41**(5):391–394.

5 Volckmann ET, Hungness ES, Soper NJ, et al.: Surgeon perceptions of Natural Orifice Translumenal Endoscopic Surgery (NOTES). *J Gastrointest Surg* 2009;**13**(8):1401–1410.

6 Rattner D, Kalloo A: ASGE/SAGES working group on natural orifice translumenal endoscopic surgery. October 2005. *Surg Endosc* 2006;**20**(2):329–333.

7 Rattner D: Introduction to NOTES white paper. *Surg Endosc* 2006;**20**(2):185.

8 Kantsevoy SV, Jagannath SB, Niiyama H, et al.: A novel safe approach to the peritoneal cavity for per-oral transgastric endoscopic procedures. *Gastrointest Endosc* 2007;**65**(3):497–500.

9 Wilhelm D, Meining A, von Delius S, et al.: An innovative, safe and sterile sigmoid access (ISSA) for NOTES. *Endoscopy* 2007;**39**(5):401–406.

10 Lima E, Henriques-Coelho T, Rolanda C, et al.: Transvesical thoracoscopy: a natural orifice translumenal endoscopic approach for thoracic surgery. *Surg Endosc* 2007;**21**(6):854–858.

11 Lima E, Rolanda C, Correia-Pinto J: Transvesical endoscopic peritoneoscopy: intra-abdominal scarless surgery for urologic applications. *Curr Urol Rep* 2008;**9**(1):50–54.

12 Lima E, Rolanda C, Pego JM, et al.: Transvesical endoscopic peritoneoscopy: a novel 5 mm port for intra-abdominal scarless surgery. *J Urol* 2006;**176**(2):802–805.

13 Arezzo A, Morino M: Endoscopic closure of gastric access in perspective NOTES: an update on techniques and technologies. *Surg Endosc* 2010 Feb;**24**(2):298–303. Epub June 30, 2009.

14 von Delius S, Huber W, Feussner H, et al.: Effect of pneumoperitoneum on hemodynamics and inspiratory pressures during natural orifice transluminal endoscopic surgery (NOTES): an experimental, controlled study in an acute porcine model. *Endoscopy* 2007;**39**(10):854–861.

15 Sumiyama K, Gostout CJ, Rajan E, et al.: Transgastric cholecystectomy: transgastric accessibility to the gallbladder improved with the SEMF method and a novel multibending therapeutic endoscope. *Gastrointest Endosc* 2007;**65**(7):1028–1034.

16 Willingham FF, Gee DW, Sylla P, et al.: Natural orifice versus conventional laparoscopic distal pancreatectomy in a porcine model: a randomized, controlled trial. *Gastrointest Endosc* 2009;**70**(4):740–747.

17 American Society for Gastrointestinal Endoscopy. Principles of training in gastrointestinal endoscopy. *Gastrointest Endosc* 1999;**49**(6):845–853.

18 Greenberg JA, Irani JL, Greenberg CC, et al.: The ACGME competencies in the operating room. *Surgery* 2007;**142**(2):180–184.

19 Peters JH, Fried GM, Swanstrom LL, et al.: Development and validation of a comprehensive program of education and assessment of the basic fundamentals of laparoscopic surgery. *Surgery* 2004;**135**(1):21–27.

20 Levy LC, Adrales G, Rothstein RI: Training for NOTES. *Gastrointest Endosc Clin N Am* 2008;**18**(2):343–360.

21 Vassiliou M MD, Kaneva P, Park P, et al.: Development of an assessment tool to measure technical skills for NOTES®. *Gastrointestinal Endoscopy* 2009;**69**(5):AB306.

22 Gillen S SA, Fioka A, Von Delius S, et al.: The "ELITE": construct validation of a new training system for NOTES. *Gastrointestinal Endoscopy* 2008;**67**(5):AB117.

23 American Society for Gastrointestinal Endoscopy. ASGE Guidelines for clinical application. Methods of privileging for new technology in gastrointestinal endoscopy. *Gastrointest Endosc* 1999;**50**(6):899–900.

24 Kavic MS, Mirza B, Horne W, et al.: NOTES: issues and technical details with introduction of NOTES into a small general surgery residency program. *Jsls* 2008;**12**(1):37–45.

22 Bariatric Endoscopy

Sohail N. Shaikh[1,2], Marvin Ryou[1,2], & Christopher C. Thompson[1,2]

[1]Brigham and Women's Hospital, Boston, MA, USA
[2]Harvard Medical School, Boston, MA, USA

The procedure(s) to be considered

Bariatric endoscopy encompasses (1) endoscopic management of surgical complications, (2) revisional procedures for failed gastric bypass, and (3) primary weight loss procedures (Table 22.1). Endoscopic therapy provides minimally-invasive treatment of common postsurgical complications such as fistulae, leaks, stenoses, marginal ulcers, and erosion of foreign material. Revisional weight loss procedures focus on reduction of the dilated gastrojejunal anastomosis and/or the dilated gastric pouch, which are considered potential mechanical etiologies of weight regain. Primary endoscopic weight loss procedures seek to create a "first-option" transoral bariatric procedure with current strategies focusing on gastric volume alteration and luminal prosthetics that target metabolic mechanisms. This chapter delineates basic therapeutic techniques relevant to each aforementioned category of bariatric endoscopy.

Endoscopic management of postbariatric surgery complications

A variety of postsurgical complications may be addressed endoscopically. These include leaks or fistulae, stomal stenosis, small bowel obstruction, ulcers, and erosion of bands and foreign material. Although their incidence varies for various bariatric interventions, they are all germane to the most common procedure—Roux-en-Y gastric bypass. Currently, the standard approach to many of these complications is surgical revision; however, with increasing skills and tools an endoscopic approach may be preferable. Incidences of the major complications are:

- Postsurgical leaks in 2–5% of cases [1,2,3]
- Stenosis in 1–20% [4,5,6]
- Ulcers reported as high as 16–20% [7,8]
- Band erosion in 0.3–11% [9,10]

Endoscopic management of complications may provide a means of avoiding the increased complication rates and mortality associated with surgical revision [1]. The skill level required for procedures that address these complications range from moderate to high (which may be more readily accomplished by operators trained in advanced intraluminal therapeutics).

Revisional endoscopic procedures for failed gastric bypass

Postsurgical weight loss failure is often of great concern to patients. Most weight is lost over the first 2 years following gastric bypass, with a wide range of 20–70% subsequently regaining weight from their nadir [11,12,13,14]. Surgical revision is the standard of care for those patients with significant regain or recurrent comorbid disease; however, this carries significant risk of morbidity and up to 2% mortality. The exact mechanisms for regain are not clear; however, mechanical complications of the pouch are thought to play a role. A dilated gastrojejunal (GJ) anastomosis, dilated pouch, or large fistula may all lead to decreased satiety and subsequent increased caloric intake. Endoscopic suturing can be used to reduce the size of the pouch or anastomosis, thus improving satiety, or may be used as a tool to retrain proper eating habits [15,16]. Additionally, clinical investigations have shown utility in outlet reduction using sclerosing agents [17]. Prior to any endoscopic intervention, dietary indiscretion must be evaluated and properly addressed. Skill levels for these maneuvers range from simple submucosal injection to endoscopic suturing that requires considerable technical ability.

Primary endoscopic obesity procedures

These currently fall into the following three major device categories, although application of each device may vary according to its particular attributes:

1 *Space occupying devices*: Gastric balloons have been studied as early as 1958 as a research tool in the pathophysiology of duodenal ulcers, with weight loss investigations as early as 1982 [18,19]. To date, intragastric balloons have been the most frequently employed endoscopic procedure for weight loss; however, most data is retrospective and of fair quality. Long-term durability is also questionable; nevertheless, balloons may find a niche as a bridge to decrease operative risk for various surgical interventions. Several complications including mucosal damage, spontaneous deflation, and small bowel obstruction have been encountered, and are important considerations for any training program [20]. Many devices have been placed over the years with recent publications from European and Far East countries [21,22,23]. Precise steps in balloon deployment are specific to each manufacturer and require moderate

Successful Training in Gastrointestinal Endoscopy, First Edition. Edited by Jonathan Cohen.
© 2011 Blackwell Publishing Ltd. Published 2011 by Blackwell Publishing Ltd.

Table 22.1 Summary of bariatric endoscopy—categories, specific procedures, and skill sets.

Categories	Specific procedures/devices	Optimal skill sets
1. Management of postsurgical complications	Fistulae/leak closure Stenosis dilation Foreign body removal Hemostasis of marginal ulcers	Stents, glue delivery Endoscopic suturing Balloon dilation Foreign body removal, Endoscopic shears Endoscopic hemostasis
2. Revision of failed gastric bypass	Sclerotherapy Endocinch* IOP* StomaphyX*	Endoscopic injection Endoscopic suturing
3. Primary weight loss procedures	Intragastric balloons EndoCinch* TOGA* Endo Barrier* ValenTx* Endo Stitch* OverStitch* Other emerging technologies (injectables, neuromodulation, etc.)	Endoscopic suturing Implant placement

*Manufacturer information in text

endoscopic skill. Additionally, with a large number of balloons currently in use familiarity with removal techniques is requisite for bariatric endoscopists.

2 *Endoluminal gastric volume reduction*: Suturing is the primary tool that enables endoscopists to emulate surgical tasks and has been a major stepping stone for transoral bariatric surgery. This method was first used for endoluminal bariatric surgical revision, in patients with weight regain or gastro-gastric fistulae, due to the high rate of morbidity and mortality associated with traditional surgical revision [24,15]. The objective of these primary obesity procedures is to reduce functional gastric volume by a variety of stitch patterns, with the goal of achieving earlier satiety. Currently it is unknown what exact neurohormonal mechanisms may also play a role. There have been many abstract presentations on suturing technologies with limited peer-reviewed publications to date [25,26,27,28,29,30]. These procedures may find a role in early intervention for those patients who do not yet qualify for traditional bariatric surgery, or as an alternative to traditional bariatric surgery. This will ultimately depend on their safety profile and long-term efficacy. Endoluminal staplers have also been used to achieve similar gastric volume reduction and are currently under clinical investigation. Endoscopic volume reduction strategies require a high level of endoscopic skill and will demand a robust therapeutic background with subsequent device specific training.

3 *Endoluminal metabolic prosthetics*: Other endoscopic endeavors have utilized a sleeve-like barrier to bypass the stomach, and/or proximal segments of the small bowel, to trigger a metabolic mechanism leading to weight loss and improvement in comorbid illness. Direct calorie malabsorption is not thought to be a major component to this procedure. Initial porcine studies have shown technical feasibility and preliminary human studies have demonstrated a 19–23% excess weight loss (EWL) at 3 months [31,32,33]. Results from long-term studies have not yet been reported. These prosthetics may prove useful as a treatment for comorbid illnesses (such as type 2 diabetes), as an adjunct therapy for weight loss, or as a bridge to various surgical procedures. Complications known thus far include nausea, vomiting and bleeding. Although placement currently requires a modest amount of skill, management of complications may necessitate a high degree of endoscopic competence, specifically with hemostasis.

Prerequisite level of expertise and technical ability

Mentee

Bariatric endoscopy is technically challenging. No guidelines have yet been established regarding training or level of expertise necessary to perform specific bariatric procedures. Ideally candidates should have basic training through an ACGME approved gastroenterology fellowship or surgical program, and should be proficient with advanced endoscopic procedures, as would be acquired through supplementary training in advanced intraluminal therapeutics.

Mentor

Desired attributes for a mentor include intricate anatomical knowledge of postbariatric surgical anatomy, expertise in advanced intraluminal techniques, and experience in endoscopic suturing or other endoscopic weight loss modalities. At this early stage, an experienced mentor will likely have been involved in device and procedure development, preclinical large animal studies, and clinical trials. A mentor may be further qualified by their case load, and publication history.

Special considerations/setting

Training in bariatric endoscopy may best be pursued within a certified Bariatric Center of Excellence. Such centers are multidisciplinary and provide a well-rounded experience, including nutritional, metabolic, psychosocial, and other medical elements that are critical to proper bariatric care. They also have experienced surgeons to provide further mentorship and procedural backup in the case of endoscopic complications. Such centers also have adequate procedure volumes to permit proper training. Additional special considerations include a dedicated advanced nursing team specifically familiar with bariatric patients and the custom endoscopic devices used in their care. This is critical as bariatric hardware requires an intricate interplay between assisting staff and the primary operator.

Essential cognitive and technical skill sets

Bariatric endoscopy requires cognitive skills in patient assessment, and interpretation of clinical data, including evaluation of small bowel series, chest and abdominal computer tomography or magnetic resonance imaging, and fistula-grams in real time. Clinically, it is important to understand the natural history of the postsurgical bariatric patient and which complications may be amenable to endoscopic therapy. Additionally, physicians should be well versed in nonsurgical options for weight loss as these play an important role pre- and postoperatively and should be emphasized prior to any surgical intervention.

A range of technical expertise is needed for bariatric endoscopy. These include basic hemostatic techniques, stricture dilation, foreign body removal, stent placement, small bowel enteroscopy, and endoluminal suturing or similar techniques.

Procedural complications and postbariatric surgery complications

Many postsurgical bariatric complications fall under the purview of bariatric endoscopy. Such patients present with a variety of clinical problems including ulceration, erosion of prosthetics, pain syndromes, strictures, retained suture, small bowel obstruction, staple-line dehiscence, and leaks. Skill sets required to address these situations include basic endoscopy for diagnostic evaluation, and advanced therapeutics, including hemostasis, mucosal ablation, use of endoscopic sealants, and enteral stent placement. Performance of these techniques often differs in the postsurgical patient and attention must be paid to specific methodological details.

Revisional endoscopic procedures for failed gastric bypass

RYGB is the most commonly performed bariatric surgery. Some RYGB patients experience weight regain that may be due to outlet or pouch dilation. Many of the technical aspects are similar to primary bariatric procedures; however, difficulty may be significantly greater in some revision procedures, as the total working space is reduced and anatomical reference points may shift or be completely absent. Various methods of outlet reduction have been investigated including suturing, tissue anchors, and submucosal injection of sclerosants. Technical and cognitive skills needed are scope proprioception, specific device knowledge, and device haptics. It is also critical to understand methods of device failure and possible complications, so that these can be avoided or the effects minimized.

Primary endoscopic obesity procedures

Endoscopic Suturing

Primary endoscopic bariatric procedures currently invoke two principles: gastric volume reduction and small bowel barrier/exclusion. At present, it is unclear if either imparts a neurohumoral response that may contribute to weight loss such as ghrelin inhibition or PYY alterations. Current suturing type platforms are relatively complex and require a team approach. Technical skill sets involve adept upper endoscope maneuvering, scope proprioception and technical dexterity in scope and device management. Another important aspect is the coordination of primary operator and secondary operator tasks. Assisting staff are critical to a successful procedure as these devices may be complicated and necessitate concise and frequent communication between the endoscopist and the assistant. The assistant's education and training is also invaluable to improve efficiency and minimize complications.

Endoscopic metabolic prosthetics

Initial prosthetics utilized were intragastric space occupying balloons. Although relatively straightforward in placement, they may prove challenging to remove. Other devices employ a sleeve that anchors in the gastric cardia or the pylorus/duodenal bulb. Initial sizing and deployment utilize many tenants required for enteral stenting. Some devices in clinical trials may also require suturing or placement of tissue anchors. Technical and cognitive skills needed are similar to enteral stenting, with advanced techniques needed for certain devices.

Essential equipment

Procedures for endoluminal bariatrics require an array of different devices and equipment. In addition to forward viewing endoscopes, these procedures often utilize CO_2 insufflation with or without distal instillation of simethicone. The following list outlines additional equipment:

1 *Postbariatric surgery complication management*:
   - Balloon dilators
   - Endoscopic scissors
   - Endoscopic clips
   - Rat-tooth forceps
   - Nitinol wires—biliary
   - Mechanical lithotripter
   - Range of esophageal stents—metal (preferably fully covered) or plastic
   - Mucosal ablative therapies including argon plasma coagulation (APC)
   - Endoscopic sealants such as fibrin glue (requires a warmer)
   - Steroids and/or saline for injection
   - Needle-knife cautery
   - Methylene blue/contrast

2 *Endoscopic revisional procedures*:
   - Suturing or tissue anchoring device (EndoCinch*, StomaphyX*, IOP*)
   - Sodium morrhuate
   - Small caliber scope (4 mm) in addition to a forward viewing endoscope
   - Measuring devices
   - Suture cutting scissors

- Overtube/bougie system
- Standard hemostasis equipment (epinephrine, injection needle, clips)
- Extra suture material and associated knot tying device/materials

3 *Primary endoscopic weight loss procedures*: Different equipment will be required depending on which system is employed. Typical equipment needs are listed below:

- Small caliber scope (4 mm) in addition to a standard forward viewing endoscope
- Suture cutting scissors
- Measuring devices
- Overtube/bougie system
- Standard hemostasis equipment (epinephrine, injection needle, clips, cautery equipment)

4 *Various custom devices (currently in trials)*:

- Balloon systems (BIB*, Heliosphere Bag*)
- Suturing device (EndoCinch*, IOP*, Endo Stitch*, Over-Stitch*)
- Stapling system (TOGA*)
- TERIS (Barosense Inc., Redwood City, CA, USA)
- Custom Barrier device and anchoring systems (EndoBarrier*, ValenTx*)
- Extra suturing material and associated knot tying device/materials

*See text for manufacturer information

Key steps of proper technique

Multiple specific endoscopic procedures will be addressed as well as keys to proper technique. Key elements of proper technique are specific to each unique device and method. Endoscopic interventions for the bariatric patient include management of postbariatric surgical complications, revisional procedures, and primary weight loss therapies. Endoscopic treatments of post-surgical complications typically require advanced skills with subtle modification in standard methods. Revisional procedures typically require advanced skill sets with novel equipment and methods. Primary therapies are similar to revisional procedures in skill demand and methodology. General skill sets and specific patient-population knowledge must be provided by medical societies and fellowship training programs. Evolving device specific elements are best addressed by ongoing corporate training programs. It is critical that these programs concentrate on potential failure mechanisms and complications, and ways of mitigating or addressing such issues. This portion of the chapter concentrates on some unique elements of the various devices in development and some differentiating features. The focus is on elements of use that are less likely to be covered in a standard industry-sponsored training program.

Initial evaluation of patients that may be eligible for an endoscopic obesity procedure includes psychological and nutritional assesment. After meeting clinical criteria necessary for primary endoscopic intervention (not yet established), upper endoscopy is performed to evaluate the native anatomy and assess any pathology that may preclude endoscopic surgery. Currently, these procedures are performed under general anesthesia; as tools improve and procedure times shorten conscious sedation may prove adequate. We first concentrate on endoscopic solutions for surgical complications and revision, and then focus on primary bariatric interventions.

Endoscopic management of postbariatric surgery complications

After bariatric surgery there are a variety of complications that may be addressed endoscopically. These include leaks and fistulae, stomal stenosis, foreign body erosion, band erosion, small bowel obstruction, and ulceration.

Leaks/fistulae

Up to 2–5% of bariatric surgeries may result in postoperative leaks manifesting as constitutional symptoms, abscess, or fistulae [1,2,3,33,35]. Surgical remedies are technically difficult due to minimal residual gastric tissue, and carry significant mortality risk. Endoscopic therapy allows for a noninvasive alternative to surgical revision.

An upper endoscopy is performed and suspected sites of leak are carefully evaluated. These are typically located high in the gastric pouch at the staple-line, or at the gastrojejunal anastamosis. Leak sites are confirmed with Methylene blue injection through an existing drain and/or by fluoroscopy using water-soluble contrast. Once identified, the mucosa surrounding the outflow tract is typically ablated with APC. A sealant is also often applied. Our group has used fibrin glue to help address the 20% leak rate that occurs around stents when used alone. Fibrin glue is injected through a double-lumen cannula, with the two components mixing at the tip of the cannula becoming activated. Once the fistula is filled, endoscopic clips may be used as an adjunct for aperture/mucosal apposition. Alternatively, a fully covered esophageal stent may be placed bridging the leak site and effectively isolating it from ingested food. The stent is removed after approximately 6 weeks. It is recommended to obtain a chest radiograph to confirm optimal stent positioning 2 days after original stent placement. Stent migration is a concern and may be partially mitigated by early removal (in under 6 weeks) and placement of longer stents, or a stent within a stent.

Outlet stenosis

Outlet stenosis following bariatric surgery has been reported as high as 20% [4,5,6]. Although careful measures are taken intraoperatively to ensure adequate outlet size, some patients may experience symptoms due to a narrow outlet. Obstructive symptoms may be attributed to outlet stenosis if the diameter is < 10 mm [34,36].

Endosocpically this can be managed by balloon dilation, injection therapy or cautery incision. Therapy should not be performed in the setting of active ulceration. Balloon dilation is the standard approach and is successful in over 93% of cases, often requiring 2–3 sessions [6,36]. Safety has been shown dilating to 15 mm; however, overdilation of the outlet must be cautioned against as this may lead to a loss of restriction and ultimately weight regain. Outlets refractory to balloon dilation should be examined for adjacent suture material that may prevent balloons from achieving their maximal radial force. If suture material is present, endoscopic shears and forceps may be used for removal. If no extrinsic barriers are present, inflammatory, fibrotic, and postsurgical tissue changes should be considered and potentially addressed using injection therapy with saline or steroids. This potentially breaks up scar tissue and may aid in subsequent dilations. A more invasive approach for stenosis refractory to dilation therapy involves the use of a needle-knife. This is an advanced technique and is performed by creating short perpendicular linear incisions around the outlet with subsequent dilation [37,38].

Key concepts for the management of outlet stenosis include avoidance of overdilation as this carries an increased risk of perforation and weight regain, and careful inspection of the surrounding mucosa for suture material.

Foreign body reaction/pain syndromes

Some RYGB patients complain of abdominal pain despite trials of proton pump inhibitors and normal radiographic studies. Although there are a variety of etiologies that may be responsible from ischemia to ulceration, our group has discovered some cases that improve with foreign body (FB) removal [39]. Under direct visualization suture material or staples may be appreciated within the gastric pouch or at the gastrojejunal anastamosis. Frequently, they are associated with an inflammatory FB reaction. We perform these procedures under light sedation in order to intra-operatively affirm reproducibility of symptoms by placing tension on the FB [40]. FB removal can be achieved using rattooth forceps and endoscopic scissors through a double-channel endoscope. Loop cutters may be used for prolene suture removal; however, they should not be used for silk suture as this may become lodged in the loop cutter making removal difficult. Key to success is elimination of other possible etiologies of abdominal pain prior to endoscopic intervention. Multiple sessions may be required to achieve complete FB removal.

Band erosion

Gastric band erosion is reported in up to 11% of adjustable gastric band patients, and may occur at any time after initial surgery [9,10,39,41,42]. These patients may present with nausea, vomiting and abdominal pain. Before endoscopic removal the abdominal port must be surgically removed. Subsequently, under direct visualization the band is transected to allow removal through the esophagus. This is not possible with endoscopic scissors, but common endoscopic equipment may be used to cut and remove the band. For example, a nitinol biliary wire may be looped through the band and externally threading the free ends through a mechanical lithotripter that is advanced over the wires abutting the metal catheter tip against the gastric band. The nitinol wire is cinched until it transects the gastric band, which can then be removed transorally by forceps, graspers, or a snare [43]. The key to success includes being able to identify the band buckle before attempting the procedure. If the buckle is not visualized the band will be very difficult, if not impossible, to remove endoscopically. The

reservoir must also be surgically removed before band removal. This may be done under local injection or in the endoscopy suite during the procedure.

Ulceration

Ulcers have been found in up to 20% of postsurgical patients [7,8]. Common ulcer etiologies must be considered including bacterial infection, NSAID use and hyperacidity states. Unique to the postsurgical patient, however, is ischemia [44] and FBs. In our center, we have observed some ulcers improve after FB (i.e., suture or staple) removal from the ulcer base [45]. A pearl for assessment includes checking *H. pylori* fecal antigen as pouch biopsies and breath test may result in false negative results. Smoking cessation is also critical for ulcer healing.

Revisional endoscopic procedures for failed gastric bypass

Despite the multifactorial nature of obesity, mechanical changes to the postbariatric anatomy are thought to contribute to weight regain. Examples of mechanical etiologies include dilation of the gastrojejunal anastomosis and dilation of the gastric pouch—both of which are thought to cause loss of satiety. Ideal pouch length is approximately 4 cm and ideal stoma diameter is less than 12 mm. Several endoscopic revisional procedures are potential solutions.

Sclerotherapy

Using traditional endoscopic techniques with an injection needle, sodium morrhuate is injected around the gastric outlet. This is repeated at 12-week intervals and often requires a total of 2–3 sessions to achieve the desired outlet size of less than 12 mm. Approximately 2 cc per injection for a total of up to 20 cc per session is best. The proper technique is to create a submucosal bleb in the area and to avoid overinjection as this may lead to bleeding. On repeat procedures, blebs may be difficult to create due to tissue sclerosis. Of note, if dark maroon or black discoloration is noted while creating a bleb, injection in that site should be halted immediately as this is a harbinger of bleeding. Initial studies reported on 45 patients showed 75% of patients achieved weight loss/stabilization over 6 months compared to 50% of matched controls [46].

EndoCinch

The EndoCinch (BARD Endoscopic Technologies, Billerica, MA, USA) consists of a small rounded metal cap that is placed on the end of an upper endoscope with an externally connected suction port. Within this cap is a channel (in the same axis of the endoscope) that allows vacuum-assisted tissue acquisition and needle puncture for stitch placement. Care must be taken to ensure proper loading of the needle and suture line. The proximal user interface is a plunger-like handle that attachs to the endoscopic working channel. Pushing this handle inward guides a needle through acquired tissue within the metal cap, thereby placing a stitch. To ensure safe passage of the endoscope an overtube is used for the procedure (Video 22.1). The original iteration of this device allowed for single suture placement and was used for fistula repair and gastric pouch reductions. The first reported endoscopic post-bypass pouch reduction on eight patients with 5-months weight follow-up reported 23.4% EWL; however, varying interpatient results spurred additional studies [16]. Stoma reduction using the EndoCinch was evaluated by a randomized sham control trial with 6 month crossover. This technique, with an average of four sutures per patient, yielded 4.7% weight loss compared to 1.9% in the sham arm with weight loss/stabilization in 96% of patients compared to 78% of sham procedures [47]. Important technical steps include assessing adequate tissue acquisition by looking for agitation in suction lines and applying gentle tip pressure. Prior to handle activation, the control knobs must be released to a neutral position to assure full needle stroke and stitch placement. If stitches are left to cinch at the end of suture placement, care must be taken to avoid knotting.

StomaphyX

The StomaphyX (EndoGastric Solutions, Redmond, WA, USA) device is a specialized clear overtube that is placed transorally after initial measurements of the existing pouch. The distal end of the device contains an opening through which pouch tissue is secured by vacuum-acquisition and a polypropylene fastener is delivered to create a plication. A recently published study of 39 patients at 3–12 months follow-up showed 7.4–19.5% EWL [48]. A key concept for this procedure is to maintain careful positioning in regard to pouch position as visualization may be limited during deployment of the polypropylene fasteners.

Incisionless operating platform (IOP)

The IOP (USGI Medical, San Capistrano, CA, USA) has the appearance of a large endoscope. In function it is a modified steerable overtube with four lumens designed to house specialized equipment (Figure 22.1). The additional channels are used for a 4 mm endoscope, corkscrew tissue acquisition device (g-lix) and specialized 2.5 cm grasping jaws (g-prox) (Figure 22.2) [49]. This system performs serosal tissue plications under direct visualization to adjust dilated pouches and gastric outlets. Plications are made with specialized jaws that pass a curved hollow needle through which nitinol tissue anchors are deployed (Figure 22.3) (Video 22.2). This is repeated until the desired pouch and/or outlet size is achieved. Key steps include careful site selection for tissue plication and watchful deployment of the tissue anchors through the needle as gentle pressure is needed to ensure individual basket deployment and prevent premature release. This system requires

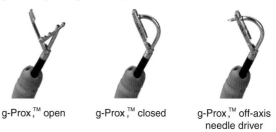

g-Prox™ grasping/tissue approximation device

g-Prox,™ open   g-Prox,™ closed   g-Prox,™ off-axis needle driver

US**ǵi** medical®

Figure 22.2 Incisionless Operating Platform (IOP) tissue approximation device with needle driver and exiting tissue anchor (Reproduced by permission of USGI)

short purposeful movements as several devices are in a small field of operation and bimanual coordination requiring effective communication with assistant operators. Initial feasibility studies in 17 patients have shown 8.8 kg EWL at 3-months follow-up [50,51].

Primary endoscopic obesity procedures

Gastric balloons

Intragastric balloons historically have been used as space occupying devices for weight loss since the early 1980s [19,52]. Placement requires balloon positioning in the stomach under direct visualization with subsequent air/saline insufflation. The Bioenterics Balloon (BIB; Allergan Inc., Irvine, CA, USA) and Heliosphere Bag ® (Helioscopie Medical Implants, UK Surgical, UK) are two currently available models recently used in a prospective randomized study in 33 patients with 27–30% EWL at 6 months [53]. Although there have been several studies showing short-term benefit, long-term studies are lacking and these devices have several complications including esophagitis, nausea, vomiting, abdominal pain, and rupture [54]. Key steps in placement involve proper positioning and adequate insufflation (physician choice dictates amount of solution used).

g-Cath™ tissue anchor delivery catheter with expandable tissue anchors™

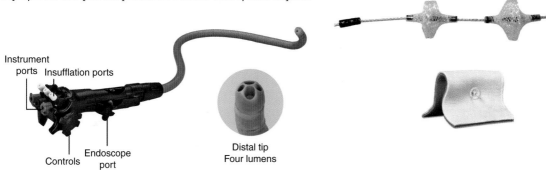

US**ǵi** medical®

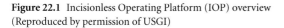

Figure 22.1 Incisionless Operating Platform (IOP) overview (Reproduced by permission of USGI)

Instrument ports Insufflation ports

Controls Endoscope port

Distal tip Four lumens

Figure 22.3 Incisionless Operating Platform (IOP) tissue anchors (Reproduced by permission of USGI)

Intragastric balloon insertion is relatively straightforward with slight variations according to manufacturer. Data published by Genco et al. reviewed 2,515 patients over 6 months revealing a 33.9% EWL [55]. Knowledge for proper removal is important as intragastric balloons have been the most frequent endoscopically-placed weight loss device to date. Removal kits are not yet available in the US and are not completely reliable when available. Using a double-channel endoscope the balloon shell must first be penetrated. Rat-tooth forceps are used to firmly grasp the outer shell while endoscopic scissors create a hole. Scissors or an endoscopic needle may be used to puncture the inner bladder and aspirate the liquid. All fluid should be completely removed from both bladders. This is important as reducing balloon size will minimize risk of esophageal perforation during removal. Once fully deflated the rat-tooth forceps are placed through a snare which is then lowered over the balloon. The snare is tightened and the endoscope is removed as one unit with the snare and balloon.

Endoscopic Suturing Platforms

There are several types of volume reduction devices under investigation in various stages of development. Some attach to the scope tip and others are designed as guide tubes that accept an endoscope. Many platform types accommodate both primary and revisional therapeutic strategies. Suturing devices currently achieve volume reduction by anterior and posterior gastric wall approximation (EndoCinch). Alternatively, the TOGA® system (Satiety Inc., Palo Alto, CA, USA) uses staples to create a gastric sleeve similar to an unsupported vertical banded gastroplasty.

Other suturing devices in preclinical stages that have shown encouraging results include the Endo Stitch (Covidien AG, Mansfield, MA, USA) and OverStitch (Apollo Endosurgery Inc., Austin, TX, USA), both of which allow for transoral suturing.

EndoCinch

The EndoCinch is attached to the endoscope and has a specialized distal suturing tip. Initial versions of this device required removal of the endoscope for individual sutures. Current stitch patterns employ individual or complex running sutures [26,27]. For example, in Fogel's study, suturing sites were identified starting in the proximal body with one running suture engaging anterior and posterior walls (seven sites) in a zigzag pattern moving up the stomach from the antrum to the cardia [25] (Figure 22.4). Recent follow-up of 233 patients demonstrated 45 patients achieving 49% EWL at 2 years [56]. Our group similarly has favored placing the first stitch in the cardia/fundus with ensuing sutures then proceeding cephalad from the antral/body junction towards the initial suture.

Approximately five sets of suture are placed depending on the stomach's anatomical measurements. These procedures are still

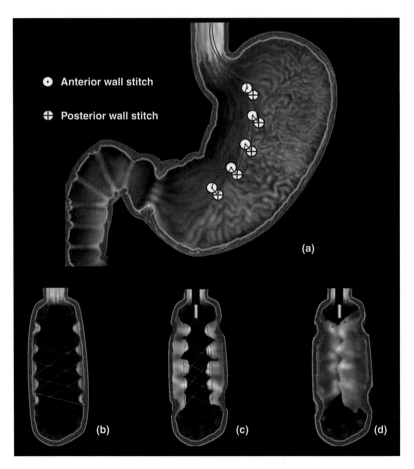

Figure 22.4 EndoCinch suturing pattern illustration as used by Fogel et al. (a) Anticipated suture sites, (b) After suture placement prior to closure (lateral view), (c) and (d) Suture tension with closure (lateral views) (Reproduced by permission of GIE)

evolving, and device features and methodology will continue to change.

TOGA

This device currently under clinical investigation uses staples to create a sleeve restriction of the stomach. The device is passed over a wire into the stomach. An endoscope is then passed through the device and retroflexed for visualization. A sail is deployed towards the greater curvature ensuring anterior and posterior wall apposition when suction is applied. Once tissue is acquired, the sail is displaced and a vertical row of staples deployed, thereby creating a gastric tissue sleeve extension from the LES. This procedure may be repeated to allow for a longer sleeve along the lesser curvature. Initial studies in 21 and 11 patients showed 24.4% EWL and mean weight loss of 24 kg, respectively, at 6 months [57,58]. Ongoing clinical trails are underway to assess weight loss, durability and metabolic effects with initial results on nine subjects showing an improvement in insulin sensitivity and reduction in BMI from 42.49 to 35.65 at 3 months [59].

Endo Stitch

The flexible Endo Stitch is a preclinical suturing device that is placed into the stomach along side the endoscope. The Endo Stitch's proximal interface has a pull handle similar to a laparoscopic tool and navigation wheels similar to those of an endoscope that allow four degrees of freedom. The distal end of the device has opposable jaws that pass a detachable short needle. Both sides of the needle are sharpened with suture anchored at the center allowing it to pierce tissue in both directions. The suture material has a unique one-way barb that prevents retrograde tissue movement when acquired.

Once the device and endoscope are in place, a series of suture tasks are performed retracting the fundus and creating three horizontal runs in the gastric body (proximal, mid, and distal). Starting from the greater curvature these horizontal stitches engage the anterior and posterior walls extending medially leaving a 2 cm column free at the lesser curvature. This procedure requires adept maneuvering of the endoscope in tandem with the suturing device to supervise suture placement and aid tissue manipulation. Initial investigations have shown 72% gastric volume reduction in an *ex vivo* porcine model [30]. Key to this procedure is maintaining adequate visualization while applying suture tension. This may prove challenging in the confines of a reduced stomach as the needle and suture line are divorced from the endoscope.

OverStitch

An additional device under investigation, the OverStitch has been used to reduce gastric volume. Used with a double-channel endoscope and overtube its proximal control is similar to a laparoscopic handle permitting single operator deployment (Figure 22.5). The suturing assembly is mounted on the distal tip secured through the working channel by a retention wire. Needle, suture and anchor elements are passed down this channel into the suture arm (Figure 22.6). Having undergone several iterations, recent in vivo experiments demonstrated technical feasibility in four porcine models creating 30 mL pouches [60]. Key to this procedure is safeguarding

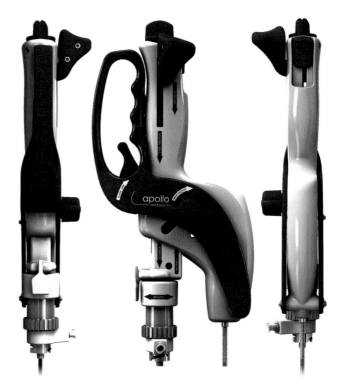

Figure 22.5 OverStitch proximal user interface (Reproduced by permission of Apollo Endosurgery)

adequate space for suture-arm movement and ensuring sufficient slack in the suture line when placing multiple stitches.

All of the aforementioned bariatric devices require a high degree of coordination between primary endoscopist and assistant. Overall success is determined by calculated suture/anchor placement following a predetermined suture plan, careful patient selection, maintaining adequate visualization, and effective communication with assistant operators.

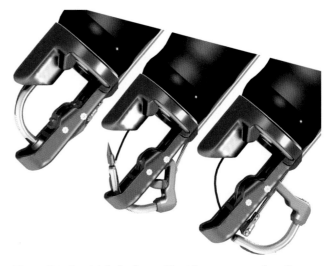

Figure 22.6 OverStitch distal assembly with suture arm and needle (Reproduced by permission of Apollo Endosurgery)

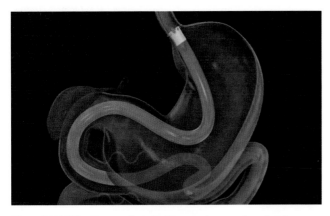

Figure 22.7 ValenTx gastrointestinal bypass sleeve anchored at the esophagus extending into the small bowel (Reproduced by permission of ValenTx Inc.)

Primary endoscopic metabolic prosthetics

Surgical weight loss procedures, such as RYGB, change anatomy to bypass the proximal small bowel. Similar intestinal bypass may be accomplished endoscopically by placement of a barrier in the small bowel. Currently, two models exist: sleeves that engage the distal esophagus (ValenTx, Inc., Hopkins, Minnesota, USA) and the duodenum (EndoBarrier; GI Dynamics Inc., Lexington, MA, USA).

ValenTx

The ValenTx device consists of a cuff with a distally deployed sleeve. Anchored into the esophago–gastric junction by a specialized device the sleeve extends 120 cm through the stomach into the midjejunum (Figure 22.7). The sleeve is impermeable thereby bypassing proximal bowel nutrient absorption. Metabolic effects occur when undigested material is presented to the distal small bowel although the mechanism is not clearly understood. An initial study utilizing laparoscopic assistance reported 12-week (nine patients) and 8- week (12 patients) follow-up with 39.9 and 40.5% EWL, respectively, and an improvement in diabetic parameters [61]. Key to this procedure is careful site selection and positioning of the cuff.

EndoBarrier

The EndoBarrier (GI Dynamics Inc., Watertown, MA, USA) is similar in concept to ValenTx; however, anchors in the duodenal bulb using a nitinol self-expanding cuff, and extends a polyethylene sleeve 60 cm into the small bowel (Figures 22.8, 22.9). It does not require additional equipment for anchoring as the proximal portion is similar to a self-expanding stent and is easily removable by a proximal removal loop. Recent publications with 41 patients (26 of whom received the device) over 3 months have shown a 19% EWL with an improvement in hemoglobin A1C and glucose control medications [62]. Key to placing this device is adequate assessment of the duodenal bulb to ensure appropriate seating of the cuff.

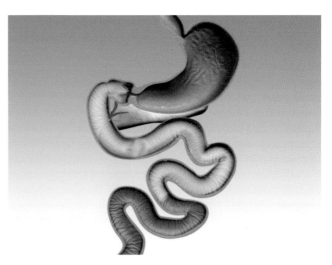

Figure 22.8 Illustration of Endobarrier's duodenal cuff with distally extending sleeve (Reproduced by permission of GI Dynamics)

Setting and tools for training

These procedures should be conducted in a hospital setting with a strong referral for obesity. Ancillary services should include bariatric surgical expertise, anesthesia, psychological evaluation, and nutritional and radiological services. Currently, with limited training models available, these skills are taught in *ex vivo* and in vivo animal models. Advanced fellows (4th year of training) may have some exposure; however, the range of procedures covered by bariatric endoscopy may necessitate additional training time. Training would likely be most effective if conducted in the manner advanced procedures are currently taught: initial observation progressing to assistance and then primary participation. Currently, no data exists on how to measure proficiency in these procedures; however, as with all new techniques, a basic barometer should be patient outcomes including weight loss and adverse events.

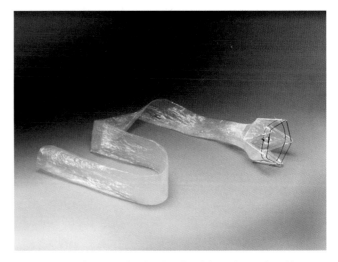

Figure 22.9 EndoBarrier duodenal cuff and sleeve (Reproduced by permission of GI Dynamics)

Defining competency for this particular skill

Competency evaluation can be separated into procedural technique and clinical application. Both require adequate exposure. No standards currently exist for the number of patients that may confer competency in bariatric endoscopy. Exposure to all aspects of bariatric endoscopy may be difficult as pathology may vary by region, population, surgical expertise, and equipment availability. Skill sets that should be mastered include suture placement for volume reduction, deployment of metabolic prosthetics, postsurgical revisional components including tissue anchors and sutures, and the management of postbariatric complications.

Clinical competency is acquired by exposure and management under a mentor's guidance. Imperative to the clinical experience is to also learn when a procedure is not indicated. No definitive case load has been established to determine the learning curve.

Maintaining skill level

Currently, these procedures are performed in advanced centers with specialized equipment. As these procedures evolve, less technically demanding tools may become available. However, it is unclear what procedure volume is needed to maintain skill level.

Conclusion

Obesity is reaching epidemic proportions, now present in over 30% of Americans according to the World Health Organization and National Health and Nutrition Examination Survey [63]. Many endoscopic bariatric procedures will require considerable technical expertise that will likely necessitate additional training outside of traditional fellowship. Training will involve clinical as well as technical components covering the gamut from primary bariatrics to revisional endoscopy and complication management. Industry's role will also be augmented as education and careful application of these tools will be paramount to ensure viability in this new arena. As future studies prove efficacy of techniques and utility of equipment, better teaching models and guidelines can be established. Bariatric endoscopy opens new frontiers to manage obesity and will give bariatric patients more options for care.

Videos

Video 22.1 Teaching new methods: Endocinch endoscopic suturing

Video 22.2 The ROSE procedure—an endolumenal suturing platform for managing weight regain after bariatric surgery

References

1 Cariani S, Nottola D, Grani S, et al.: Complications after gastroplasty and gastric bypass as a primary operation and as a reoperation. *Obes Surg* 2001 Aug;**11**(4):487–490.

2 Mondeturo F, Cappello I, Mazzoni G, et al.: Radiological contrast studies after vertical banded gastroplasty (VBG) and Roux-en-Y gastric bypass (RYGBP) in patients with morbid obesity. Study of the complications. *Radiol Med* 2004 Jun;**107**(5–6):515–523.

3 Lee S, Carmody B, Wolfe L, et al.: Effect of location and speed of diagnosis on anastomotic leak outcomes in 3828 gastric bypass cases. *J Gastrointest Surg* 2007 Jun;**11**(6):708–713.

4 Fobi MAL: Surgical treatment of obesity: a review. *J Natl Med Assoc* 2004 Jan;**96**(1):61–75.

5 Kellum JM, DeMaria EJ, Sugerman HJ: The surgical treatment of morbid obesity. *Curr Probl Surg* 1998 Sep;**35**(9):791–858.

6 Alasfar F, Sabnis AA, Liu RC, et al.: Stricture rate after laparoscopic Roux-en-Y gastric bypass with a 21-mm circular stapler: the Cleveland Clinic experience. *Med Princ Pract* 2009;**18**(5):364–367.

7 Pope GD, Goodney PP, Burchard KW, et al.: Peptic ulcer/stricture after gastric bypass: a comparison of technique and acid suppression variables. *Obes Surg* 2002 Feb;**12**(1):30–33.

8 Sapala JA, Wood MH, Sapala MA, et al.: Marginal ulcer after gastric bypass: a prospective 3-year study of 173 patients. *Obes Surg* 1998 Oct;**8**(5):505–516.

9 Lunde OC: Endoscopic laser therapy for band penetration of the gastric wall after gastric banding for morbid obesity. *Endoscopy* 1991 Mar;**23**(2):100–101.

10 Mittermair RP, Weiss H, Nehoda H, et al.: Uncommon intragastric migration of the Swedish adjustable gastric band. *Obes Surg* 2002 Jun;**12**(3):372–375.

11 Alger-Mayer S, Polimeni JM, Malone M: Preoperative weight loss as a predictor of long-term success following Roux-en-Y gastric bypass. *Obes Surg* 2008 Jul;**18**(7):772–775.

12 Powers PS, Rosemurgy A, Boyd F, et al.: Outcome of gastric restriction procedures: weight, psychiatric diagnoses, and satisfaction. *Obes Surg* 1997 Dec;**7**(6):471–477.

13 McCormick JT, Papasavas PK, Caushaj PF, et al.: Laparoscopic revision of failed open bariatric procedures. *Surg Endosc* 2003 Mar;**17**(3):413–415.

14 Karlsson J, Taft C, Rydén A, et al.: Ten-year trends in health-related quality of life after surgical and conventional treatment for severe obesity: the SOS intervention study. *Int J Obes (Lond)* 2007 Aug;**31**(8):1248–1261.

15 Thompson CC, Slattery J, Bundga ME, et al.: Peroral endoscopic reduction of dilated gastrojejunal anastomosis after Roux-en-Y gastric bypass: a possible new option for patients with weight regain. *Surg Endosc* 2006 Nov;**20**(11):1744–1748.

16 Borao F, Gorcey S, Capuano A: Prospective single-site case series utilizing an endolumenal tissue anchoring system for revision of post-RYGB stomal and pouch dilatation. *Surg Endosc* 2010 Sept;**24**(9):2308–2313. (Epub March 4, 2010).

17 Madan AK, Martinez JM, Khan KA, et al.: Endoscopic sclerotherapy for dilated gastrojejunostomy after gastric bypass. *J Laparoendosc Adv Surg Technol A* 2010 Apr;**20**(3):235–237.

18 Cooper P, Harrower HW, Stein HL, et al.: The effect of cigarette smoking on intragastric balloon pressure and temperature of patients with duodenal ulcer. *Gastroenterology* 1958 Aug;**35**(2):176–182.

19 Nieben OG, Harboe H: Intragastric balloon as an artificial bezoar for treatment of obesity. *Lancet* 1982 Jan 23;**1**(8265):198–199.

20 Tsesmeli N, Coumaros D: Review of endoscopic devices for weight reduction: old and new balloons and implantable prostheses. *Endoscopy* 2009 Dec;**41**(12):1082–1089.

21 Forlano R, Ippolito AM, Iacobellis A, et al.: Effect of the BioEnterics intragastric balloon on weight, insulin resistance, and liver steatosis in obese patients. *Gastrointest Endosc* 2010 May;**71**(6):927–933.

22 Donadio F, Sburlati LF, Masserini B, et al.: Metabolic parameters after BioEnterics intragastric balloon placement in obese patients. 2009 Feb;**32**(2):165–168.

23 Mui WL, Ng EK, Tsung BY, et al.: Impact on obesity-related illnesses and quality of life following intragastric balloon. *Obes Surg* 2010 Aug;**20**(8):1128–1132. (Epub November 18, 2008.)

24 Thompson CC, Carr-Locke DL: Endoscopy in Roux-en-Y gastric bypass patients: novel techniques for common problems DDW. *Gastrointest Endosc* 2004 Apr;**59**(5):SP221.

25 Fogel R, De Fogel J, Bonilla Y, et al.: Clinical experience of transoral suturing for an endoluminal vertical gastroplasty: 1-year follow-up in 64 patients. *Gastrointest Endosc* 2008 Jul;**68**(1):51–58.

26 Brethauer SA, Chand B, Schauer P, et al.: V-04: transoral gastric volume reduction as an intervention for weight management (TRIM trial). *Surgery for Obesity and Related Diseases* 2009 May;**5**(3 Suppl 1):S59.

27 Thompson CC, Brethauer SA, Chand B, et al.: M1259 transoral gastric volume reduction as an intervention for weight management (TRIM) multicenter feasibility study: a report of early outcomes. *Gastroenterology* 2009 5;**136**(5):A-384.

28 Moreno C, Closset J, Dugardeyn S, et al.: Transoral gastroplasty is safe, feasible, and induces significant weight loss in morbidly obese patients: results of the second human pilot study. *Endoscopy* 2008 May;**40**(5):406–413.

29 Devière J, Ojeda Valdes G, Cuevas Herrera L, et al.: Safety, feasibility and weight loss after transoral gastroplasty: first human multicenter study. *Surg Endosc* 2008 Mar;**22**(3):589–598.

30 Shaikh SN, Azagury DE, Ryou MK, et al.: M1500: quantitative comparison of endoscopic primary gastric volume reduction strategies. *Gastrointestinal Endoscopy* 2010 4;**71**(5):AB238.

31 Tarnoff M, Shikora S, Lembo A, et al.: Chronic in-vivo experience with an endoscopically delivered and retrieved duodenal-jejunal bypass sleeve in a porcine model. *Surg Endosc* 2008 Apr;**22**(4):1023–1028.

32 Tarnoff M, Shikora S, Lembo A: Acute technical feasibility of an endoscopic duodenal-jejunal bypass sleeve in a porcine model: a potentially novel treatment for obesity and type 2 diabetes. *Surg Endosc* 2008 Mar;**22**(3):772–776.

33 Rodriguez-Grunert L, Galvao Neto MP, Alamo M, et al.: First human experience with endoscopically delivered and retrieved duodenal-jejunal bypass sleeve. *Surg Obes Relat Dis* 2008 Feb;**4**(1):55–59.

34 Msika S: Surgery for morbid obesity: complications. Results of a technologic evaluation by the ANAES. *J Chir (Paris)* 2003 Feb;**140**(1):4–21.

35 Fullum TM, Aluka KJ, Turner PL: Decreasing anastomotic and staple line leaks after laparoscopic Roux-en-Y gastric bypass. *Surg Endosc* 2009 Jun;**23**(6):1403–1408.

36 Ukleja A, Afonso BB, Pimentel R, et al.: Outcome of endoscopic balloon dilation of strictures after laparoscopic gastric bypass. *Surg Endosc* 2008 Aug;**22**(8):1746–1750.

37 Hagiwara A, Sonoyama Y, Togawa T, et al.: Combined use of electrosurgical incisions and balloon dilatation for the treatment of refractory postoperative pyloric stenosis. *Gastrointest Endosc* 2001 Apr;**53**(4):504–508.

38 Catalano MF, Chua TY, Rudic G: Endoscopic balloon dilation of stomal stenosis following gastric bypass. *Obes Surg* 2007 Mar;**17**(3):298–303.

39 Yu S, Jastrow K, Clapp B, et al.: Foreign material erosion after laparoscopic Roux-en-Y gastric bypass: findings and treatment. *Surg Endosc* 2007 Jul;**21**(7):1216–1220.

40 Ryou M, Mogabgab O, Lautz DB, et al.: Endoscopic foreign body removal for treatment of chronic abdominal pain in patients after

41 Suter M, Giusti V, Héraief E, et al.: Band erosion after laparoscopic gastric banding: occurrence and results after conversion to Roux-en-Y gastric bypass. *Obes Surg* 2004 Mar;**14**(3):381–386.

42 Karmali S, Snyder B, Wilson EB, et al.: Endoscopic management of eroded prosthesis in vertical banded gastroplasty patients. *Surg Endosc* 2010 Jan;**24**(1):98–102.

43 Offodile AC, Okafor P, Shaikh SN, et al.: Duodenal obstruction due to erosion and migration of an adjustable gastric band: a novel endoscopic approach to management. *Surg Obes Relat Dis* 2010 Mar 4;**6**(2):206–208.

44 Ruutiainen AT, Levine MS, Williams NN: Giant jejunal ulcers after Roux-en-Y gastric bypass. *Abdom Imaging* 2008 Oct;**33**(5):575–578.

45 Azagury DE, Dayyeh BKA, Greenwalt IT, et al.: T1055 marginal ulcers after Roux-en-Y gastric bypass surgery: risk factors, treatment and outcomes. *Gastroenterology.* 2010 5;**138**(5):S-478.

46 Ryou MK, Dayyeh BKA, Yu S, et al.: M1356 endoscopic revision of dilated gastrojejunostomy in gastric bypass patients experiencing weight regain: a matched cohort comparison of transoral sutured revision versus sclerotherapy versus controls. *Gastroenterology* 2010 5;**138**(5):S-387.

47 Thompson CC, Roslin MS, Chand B, et al.: M1359 restore: randomized evaluation of endoscopic suturing transorally for anastomotic outlet reduction: a double-blind, sham-controlled multicenter study for treatment of inadequate weight loss or weight regain following Roux-en-Y gastric bypass. *Gastroenterology* 2010 5;**138**(5):S-388.

48 Mikami D, Needleman B, Narula V, et al.: Natural orifice surgery: initial US experience utilizing the StomaphyX device to reduce gastric pouches after Roux-en-Y gastric bypass. *Surg Endosc* 2010 Jan;**24**(1):223–228.

49 Swanstrom LL, Whiteford M, Khajanchee Y: Developing essential tools to enable transgastric surgery. *Surg Endosc* 2008 Mar;**22**(3):600–604.

50 Mullady DK, Lautz DB, Thompson CC: Treatment of weight regain after gastric bypass surgery when using a new endoscopic platform: initial experience and early outcomes (with video). *Gastrointest Endosc* 2009 Sep;**70**(3):440–444.

51 Ryou M, Mullady DK, Lautz DB, et al.: Pilot study evaluating technical feasibility and early outcomes of second-generation endosurgical platform for treatment of weight regain after gastric bypass surgery. *Surg Obes Relat Dis* 2009 Aug;**5**(4):450–454.

52 Garren M, Garren LR, Giordano F: The Garren gastric bubble for the morbidly obese. *Endoscopic Rev'* 1984;**2**:57–60.

53 De Castro ML, Morales MJ, Del Campo V, et al.: Efficacy, safety, and tolerance of two types of intragastric balloons placed in obese subjects: a double-blind comparative study. *Obes Surg* 2010 Dec;**20**(12):1642–1646.

54 Mathus-Vliegen EMH: Intragastric balloon treatment for obesity: what does it really offer? *Dig Dis* 2008;**26**(1):40–44.

55 Genco A, Bruni T, Doldi SB, et al.: BioEnterics intragastric balloon: the Italian experience with 2,515 patients. *Obes Surg* 2005 Sep;**15**(8):1161–1164.

56 Fogel R, De Fogel JF: S1578: endoluminal vertical gastroplasty for weight reduction – a study of 233 patients with up to 24 months follow-up. *Gastrointestinal Endoscopy* 2010 4;**71**(5):AB199.

57 Devière J, Ojeda Valdes G, Cuevas Herrera L, et al.: Safety, feasibility and weight loss after transoral gastroplasty: first human multicenter study. *Surg Endosc* 2008 Mar;**22**(3):589–598.

58 Moreno C, Closset J, Dugardeyn S, et al.: Transoral gastroplasty is safe, feasible, and induces significant weight loss in morbidly obese patients:

results of the second human pilot study. *Endoscopy* 2008 May;**40**(5): 406–413.

59 Chiellini C, Iaconelli A, Familiari P, et al.: Study of the effects of transoral gastroplasty on insulin sensitivity and secretion in obese subjects. *Nutr Metab Cardiovasc Dis* 2010 Mar;**20**(3):202–207.

60 Kantsevoy S, Hu B, Jagannath S, et al.: Technical feasibility of endoscopic gastric reduction: a pilot study in a porcine model. *Gastrointestinal Endoscopy* 2007 3;**65**(3):510–513.

61 Scientific Session of the Society of American Gastrointestinal and Endoscopic Surgeons (SAGES) National Harbor, Maryland, USA, 14–17 April 2010. *Surgical Endoscopy* 2010 Apr 1;**24**(1):192–269.

62 Schouten R, Rijs CS, Bouvy ND, et al.: A multicenter, randomized efficacy study of the EndoBarrier gastrointestinal liner for presurgical weight loss prior to bariatric surgery. *Ann Surg* 2010 Feb;**251**(2): 236–243.

63 Flegal KM, Carroll MD, Ogden CL, et al.: Prevalence and trends in obesity among US adults, 1999–2008. *JAMA* 2010 Jan 20;**303**(3):235–241.

23 Repair of Mucosal Defects: A Primer on Endoscopic Closure of Gastrointestinal Perforations

Gottumukkala S. Raju

University of Texas, MD Anderson Cancer Center, Houston, TX, USA

Introduction

We have witnessed rapid development of various endoscopic techniques for closure of intentional or iatrogenic gastrointestinal perforations during the last two decades. Learning how to close perforations will help us serve our patients better by avoiding the need for surgery. The goal of this chapter is to review the closing devices currently available in the market and provide a manual on how to take care of patients with gastrointestinal perforations including the techniques of closure.

Learning to close perforations

Two important issues involved in learning how to close perforations include learning about the device and its operation, and learning how to use it in various clinical circumstances. In order to help trainers and trainees make it easy to understand the learning process, I have taken the liberty of summarizing step by step my own learning process that lasted a decade.

Perspectives on learning endoscopic closure

Reflecting on my learning process, one could divide the process into the following steps: (1) Learn from an expert; (2) Practice of the art; (3) Read to expand the horizons; (4) Write to share the knowledge; (5) Experiment to refine and define the process; and (6) Teach the art to get better.

1 *Learn from an expert:* About a decade ago, I spent a half-day at the exhibitor booths during the Digestive Diseases Week (DDW) learning from a couple of engineers how to assemble an Olympus reusable clip device, load the device with a clip, and deploy it. At that time not much was available in the literature on endoscopic closure of perforations, except for a couple of reports on this subject.

2 *Practice the art:* Immediately after return to my medical center, we bought three reusable clip delivery devices and a box of 100 clips. Reusable clip devices are cheaper than currently available single use clip devices and are preferable for some one who wants to learn how to deploy the clips and perfect the technique without much cost. I trained my nurses and technicians in the use of the device and started using clips routinely to control bleeding, prevent postpolypectomy bleeding, and close mucosal defects after endoscopic mucosal resection. This has helped me develop confidence in the use of clip devices.

3 *Reading:* Exciting work on the endoscopic use of clips for hemostasis and closure started appearing in the premier endoscopy journals, *Gastrointestinal Endoscopy* and *Endoscopy*. Reading extensively on this subject provided me an opportunity to learn how other experts in the world used clips and expand my understanding of their role in endoscopy.

4 *Writing:* Based on my preliminary experience with the use of clips and review of all the print media and multimedia (videos) on this subject presented by the American Society of Gastrointestinal Endoscopy (ASGE) Learning Library, I submitted a broad-based review on this subject to *Gastrointestinal Endoscopy* journal followed by a series of case reports on this subject [1,2–5]. Appreciating the benefits of endoscopic closure of esophageal perforations from my reading of the case reports and case series, I decided to write a review on this topic in collaboration with an expert thoracic surgeon and an expert therapeutic endoscopist [6].

5 *Experimenting:* Both extensive reading and writing have helped me focus my research on endoscopic closure of colon perforations in the animal laboratory [7–13]. Eventually, knowledge gained from extensive reading and skills developed during experimental studies on closure helped in the endoscopic closure of gastrointestinal leaks in patients who were at high risk for surgery [14,15].

6 *Teaching:* Conducting the hands-on-course on endoscopic closure of gastrointestinal defects in collaboration with Roy Soetikno, MD and other experts in the world during the last three DDW meetings has helped me learn what is required to train and help others learn endoscopic closure of gastrointestinal defects.

Successful Training in Gastrointestinal Endoscopy, First Edition. Edited by Jonathan Cohen.
© 2011 Blackwell Publishing Ltd. Published 2011 by Blackwell Publishing Ltd.

Although any trailblazer will have to go through the various steps as outlined above to learn and become an expert in the field, the learning process could be hastened for the next in line by sharing what to do and what not to do.

I will focus my attention on the use of clips based on my experience with the use of these devices.

Endoscopic closure devices

In the United States, the following clip devices are available in the market:

1 QuickClip2™ (Olympus Corp., Melville, NY, USA)
2 TriClip™ (Cook Medical Inc., Winston-Salem, NC, USA)
3 Resolution Clip™ (Boston Scientific, Natick, MA, USA)

InScope Multiclip Applier™ (Ethicon Endosurgical Inc., Cincinnati, OH, USA) and over-the-scope clip (OSTC) (Ovesco Endoscopy, Tüebingen, Germany) are not available in the United States at the time of submission of this manuscript. All the currently available clip devices are ready to use immediately after taking them out of the packet without the need for reloading and are single-use products.

Clips result in inverted closure of perforation compared to parallel closure created by surgical suture closure and everted T-tag closure (Figure 23.1).

1 *QuickClip2™ (Olympus Corp., Melville, NY, USA):* This is a rotatable clip device that permits adjustment of the clip angle with rotation of the handle.

2 *TriClip™ (Cook Medical Inc., Winston-Salem, NC, USA):* This is a tri-pronged single-use clip device designed to orient on the target site without the need for rotation of the prongs.

3 *Resolution Clip™ (Boston Scientific, Natick, MA, USA):* This has the ability to reopen up to five times prior to final deployment, thus offering a second chance for better tissue approximation if necessary.

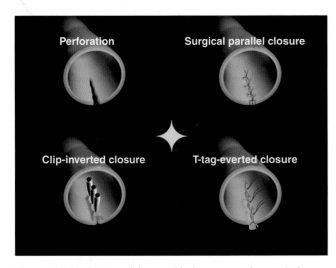

Figure 23.1 Mechanism of closure with clips compared to surgical suture closure and T-tag closure. Reproduced with permission from American Society of Gastrointestinal Endoscopy

Key steps in endoscopic management of gastrointestinal perforations

First and foremost is to avoid accidental perforation during endoscopy so as to prevent the morbidity and mortality associated with such a complication. Second is to identify the perforation immediately and manage it successfully. Third is attention to details on postoperative care for a successful outcome.

Prevent perforation

One could avoid or limit the risk of instrumental perforation by being cautious and gentle with an endoscope. Adherence to the following principles during diagnostic and therapeutic endoscopy may be helpful in the prevention of perforation under various circumstances:

1 *Esophageal perforation:*
- Excessive force should be avoided during esophageal intubation in patients with cervical spondylosis.
- Perforations from balloon dilation of an esophageal stricture could be limited by gradually increasing the size of dilation after starting with the smallest dilator and avoiding the use of excessive force during bougie dilation.

2 *Rectal perforation:*
- Evaluate the size of the rectum during slow withdrawal of the endoscope before retroflexion of the endoscope. Patients with a small rectum are at risk for perforation during retroflexion of the endoscope. In patients with a small rectum, consider examining the rectum by slow deflation of rectum or by using a thinner caliber upper endoscope if retroflexion is absolutely necessary to examine the rectum.

3 *Colon perforation:*
- Avoid the use of excessive force during the insertion of an endoscope through a sigmoid colon that is either fixed by adhesions or is redundant; instead, use a smaller caliber endoscope, use a variable stiffness colonoscope, insertion of a stiffening wire or a forceps through the biopsy channel, use of an overtube or a double balloon endoscope.
- Dry up the colon segment to prevent escape of luminal contents through the perforation, if it were to happen during excision of polyps.
- Applying a snare on the stalk of a pedunculated polyp away from the wall and tenting it up prior to cautery could limit transmural burn and perforation.
- Injection of ample amount of submucosal fluid and separating the lesion from the muscularis propria is critical to prevent thermal injury to the muscle.
- Piece-meal resection of large polyps may limit deeper injury to the muscle compared to the large en bloc resections.
- Consider surgery if the risk of perforation is high during endoscopic removal of large lesions.
- Spillage of luminal microbial soup through a perforation can precipitate septic shock; hence, *it is critical and preferable to avoid elective endoscopy, especially any therapy with a risk of perforation, in a patient with debris in the lumen until it is cleared and cleaned out.* For example, poorly prepared colon can lead to fecal contamination of peritoneal cavity, if perforation were to occur; hence, a clean colon is critical. (Similarly, a clean

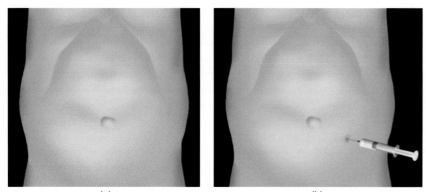

(a)   (b)

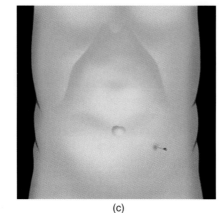

(c)

Figure 23.2 Technique of l decompression of tension pneumoperitoneum. (a) Tension pneumoperitoneum. (b) Needle insertion to release the air from the peritoneal cavity. (c) Decompression of the abdomen. Reproduced with permission from American Society of Gastrointestinal Endoscopy

esophagus is critical prior to dilation, especially in patients with achalasia.)

• Because carbon dioxide gets absorbed quickly by the body compared to air [16,17], use of carbon dioxide instead of air for endoscopy may be beneficial in patients undergoing endoscopic procedures at high risk for perforation.

Diagnosis of perforation

Perforations from mechanical trauma are clinically obvious either during or immediately after the procedure, while those from cautery damage may take a few hours or days to develop. Act immediately if a patient complains of pain by examining the patient and do not brush off the complaint as trivial due to gas. Delay in the diagnosis is associated with a poor outcome. Since perforations of the gastrointestinal tract are rare, it is hard for novices to recognize it on endoscopy. This could be improved by encouraging trainees to watch videos on endoscopic submucosal dissection to identify small perforations. Such videos are readily available from the ASGE Learning Center and for free viewing on the DAVE project [http://daveproject.org/].

In addition, development of abdominal pain, abdominal distension that cannot be decompressed and cardiopulmonary deterioration (as evidenced by tachycardia, hypotension, and drop in pulse oximetry of vital signs) due to tension pneumoperitoneum or pneumothorax should raise an alarm about a gastrointestinal perforation. Immediately after the recognition of tension pneumoperitoneum or tension pneumothorax, consider emergency decompression of the abdomen or chest with a wide bore needle puncture (Figure 23.2).

Contrary to traditional teaching, endoscopy is safe to diagnose esophageal perforations and should be undertaken if necessary after negative CT scan or esophogram to exclude the diagnosis.

Immediate endoscopic management

Currently, endoscopic clips are the only devices available in the market for closure of perforations, while suturing and stapling devices are not available for clinical use. Clips can be used to close perforations of less than 2 cm size. There is no data in the literature on endoscopic closure of iatrogenic perforations in patients that return to the emergency room after discharge from the endoscopy unit. Endoscopic management of such patients should be considered as part of an investigational protocol in close collaboration with surgeons.

Endoscopic clip closure of perforation involves a technique that is quite different from the one that is used for mechanical hemostasis, as described below. One could learn this art by attempting to close mucosal defects after endoscopic mucosal resection in clinical practice, by attending hands-on-courses on this technique, or during the investigation of the endoscopic closure of colon perforations in the animal laboratory (as I have done). Clip closure of perforations is not for the novice with no prior experience in the use of clips. It is critical for both the endoscopist and his assistant to be conversant with the use of clips before undertaking endoscopic closure of perforations.

Attention to the details as outlined below is critical for successful clip closure of perforations:

1 *Technique of clip closure of perforations (personal reflections; see Video 23.1):*
- Keep the clip close to the end of the endoscope with the clip–endoscope acting as a single unit.
- Positioning the wide-open clip across the defect at 90° to the defect.
- Gently push the clip–endoscope unit as one unit while applying gentle suction to collapse the lumen so that as much tissue away from the edge of perforation as possible could be grasped while slowly closing the clip.
- Confirm satisfactory clip closure of the perforation with approximation of the edges before deployment of the clip.
- Be patient while applying a clip because a misplaced clip to one edge of the perforation could lead to difficulty in applying additional clips for satisfactory closure.
- Application of the clip just above the upper end of a linear perforation may pucker the edges below for easier application of the second clip below the first one.
- Place additional clips from top-to-down in linear perforations or left-to-right in circular perforations after satisfactory application of the first clip, which is the most critical component of closure (Figures 23.3 and 23.4).
- Suction and decompress the lumen before withdrawal of the endoscope.

2 *Technique of clip closure—what should be avoided:*
- Avoid panic. Be calm and steady for proper use of the equipment by you and your assistant.
- Keep the endoscope close to the site of perforation. Avoid long shots as these will interfere with proper control of the device and delivery of the clip.
- Avoid air insufflation and stretching of the wall as this leads to increase of the pneumoperitoneum or pneumothorax and worsening of the cardiopulmonary status of the patient.
- Avoid stretching the tissue by pushing the clip against the wall as this limits successful approximation of the edges together.
- Avoid hasty deployment of the first clip without checking whether both the edges were successfully approximated as this will result in a wasted deployment to one edge of the perforation without complete tissue apposition of both edges of perforation.

3 *Consider alternatives to clips in special circumstances:*
- Stents may be a better option in perforations or fistulas larger than 2 cm and defects with everted edges because current clips (with wingspan less than 2 cm) fail to close such defects and in patients with a leak occurring in the setting of a malignant lesion because clips tend to tear through cancerous tissue and fail to keep the edges of perforation approximated.
- Drainage of infection before closing the defect is critical because clips may tear through edematous tissue, resulting in failure of closure.
- Use of rotatable clips or cap-fitted endoscope may be useful in closing defects in the esophagus, especially if *en face* approach to the defect is unsuccessful [18].

Postendoscopic perforation closure management
It is critical to involve surgeons right from the beginning in the management of the patients after endoscopic closure of

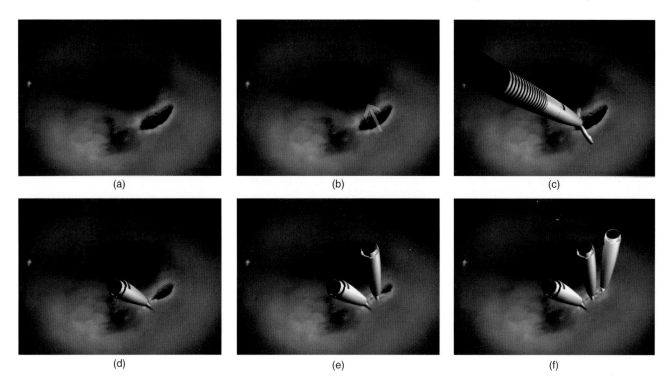

(a) (b) (c)

(d) (e) (f)

Figure 23.3 Technique of circular perforation closure. Sequential steps in the clip closure of a circular perforation (a) starting to approximate the lower edge to the upper edge (b) starting at one end of the perforation and moving along to the other end (c–f). Reproduced with permission from American Society of Gastrointestinal Endoscopy

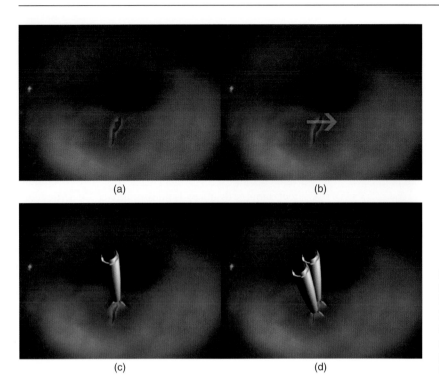

Figure 23.4 Technique of linear perforation closure. Sequential steps in the clip closure of a linear perforation (a) starting to approximate the left edge to the right edge (b) starting at the top end of the perforation and moving along to the lower end of perforation (c–d). Reproduced with permission from American Society of Gastrointestinal Endoscopy

perforations because of their extensive experience in the management in this area. Both bowel rest and broad-spectrum intravenous antibiotics are critical for healing of the perforation after endoluminal closure. Patients with esophageal perforation may benefit from minimizing gastroesophageal reflux by elevating the head end of the bed. Intermittent tube suction of luminal secretions keeps the lumen collapsed and limits escape of luminal contents through any smaller defects after clip closure. Parenteral nutrition should be considered in patients with leaks that take more than a few days to heal. All patients should be closely monitored for signs of peritoneal irritation in close collaboration with the surgeons. Oral intake could be resumed as soon as the pain and fever resolve, appetite and bowel function return, and laboratory signs of inflammation such as leukocytosis and elevated C-reactive peptide return to normal. In patients with an esophageal perforation, an esophogram is undertaken prior to the resumption of oral intake.

Setting and tools for training

Currently, endoscopic closure of gastrointestinal perforations are currently taught by expert endoscopists at the ASGE during hands-on-courses at the Institute for Training and Technology (IT&T) Center in Oakbrook, IL, and during the DDW. These sessions provide an opportunity to learn the basics of operating the clip device and deploy clips in a thawed porcine stomach model. Although live pig models provide better training opportunities to learn clip application as the tissue behaves similar to the one encountered in clinical practice, they have not become popular because of the high cost of learning in such models. There are several educational videos available at the ASGE Learning Library to help in the learn-

ing process. It is critical for the endoscopic assistants to be familiar with the use of clips, which could be accomplished by preliminary training on how to use the device followed by maintenance of the skills by regular use of the devices. Endoscopists who have majority of their practice in ambulatory surgical centers may not have the opportunity to use clips because of the low complexity of the cases managed there. Use of clips for control of bleeding, prevention of postpolypectomy bleeding and tissue approximation after endoscopic mucosal resection may help them learn the skills involved in handling the device.

Information on competency on the use of clips for endoscopic closure of perforations is lacking. Literature reveals only case reports and small case series on the use of clips for closure of perforations. As knowledge evolves one could define what is required to be competent in closure of perforations and what is required to maintain such a skill.

In summary, data on endoluminal closure of gastrointestinal perforations are encouraging. With proper training in endoluminal closure of perforations and endoscopists working in close collaboration with surgeons, patients with gastrointestinal perforations and leaks could be managed better.

Conclusion

- Endoscopic closure of gastrointestinal perforations, fistulas and anastomotic leaks is possible.
- Reports of endoscopic clip closure of esophageal, gastric, intestinal, and colonic perforations are encouraging.

- Endoscopic closure is comparable to surgery in the closure of esophageal, gastric, and colon perforations in animal studies.
- Training in endoscopic closure of perforations is needed for this technique to be used to manage patients with iatrogenic gastrointestinal perforations as an alternative to surgery.
- Close collaboration with surgeons is critical in the management of patients after endoscopic closure of perforations.

Videos

Video 23.1 Graphic demonstration of closure of a linear and circular perforation. Reproduced with permission from American Society of Gastrointestinal Endoscopy

Video 23.2 Closure of defect. Reproduced with permission from American Society of Gastrointestinal Endoscopy

Video 23.3 Use of clips to close esophageal perforation. Reproduced with permission from American Society of Gastrointestinal Endoscopy

Video 23.4 Closure of gastrointestinal perforations.

References

1 Raju GS, Gajula L: Endoclips for GI endoscopy. *Gastrointest Endosc* 2004;**59**:267–279.

2 Raju GS, Faruqi S, Bhutani MS, et al.: Catheter probe EUS-assisted treatment with hemoclips of a colonic Dieulafoy's lesion with recurrent bleeding. *Gastrointest Endosc* 2004;**60**:851–854.

3 Raju GS, Kaltenbach T, Soetikno R: Endoscopic mechanical hemostasis of GI arterial bleeding (with videos). *Gastrointest Endosc* 2007;**66**:774–785.

4 Raju GS, Nath S, Zhao X, et al.: Duodenal diverticular hemostasis with hemoclip placement on the bleeding and feeder vessels: a case report. *Gastrointest Endosc* 2003;**57**:116–117.

5 Warneke RM, Walser E, Faruqi S, et al.: Cap-assisted endoclip placement for recurrent ulcer hemorrhage after repeatedly unsuccessful endoscopic treatment and angiographic embolization: case report. *Gastrointest Endosc* 2004;**60**:309–312.

6 Raju GS, Thompson C, Zwischenberger JB: Emerging endoscopic options in the management of esophageal leaks (videos). *Gastrointest Endosc* 2005;**62**:278–286.

7 Raju GS, Pham B, Xiao SY, et al.: A pilot study of endoscopic closure of colonic perforations with endoclips in a swine model. *Gastrointest Endosc* 2005;**62**:791–795.

8 Pham BV, Raju GS, Ahmed I, et al.: Immediate endoscopic closure of colon perforation by using a prototype endoscopic suturing device: feasibility and outcome in a porcine model (with video). *Gastrointest Endosc* 2006;**64**:113–119.

9 Raju GS, Ahmed I, Brining D, et al.: Endoluminal closure of large perforations of colon with clips in a porcine model (with video). *Gastrointest Endosc* 2006;**64**:640–646.

10 Raju GS, Ahmed I, Xiao SY, et al.: Controlled trial of immediate endoluminal closure of colon perforations in a porcine model by use of a novel clip device (with videos). *Gastrointest Endosc* 2006;**64**:989–997.

11 Raju GS, Ahmed I, Shibukawa G, et al.: Endoluminal clip closure of a circular full-thickness colon resection in a porcine model (with videos). *Gastrointest Endosc* 2007;**65**:503–509.

12 Raju GS, Shibukawa G, Ahmed I, et al.: Endoluminal suturing may overcome the limitations of clip closure of a gaping wide colon perforation (with videos). *Gastrointest Endosc* 2007;**65**:906–911.

13 Raju GS, Fritscher-Ravens A, Rothstein RI, et al.: Endoscopic closure of colon perforation compared to surgery in a porcine model: a randomized controlled trial (with videos). *Gastrointest Endosc* 2008;**68**:324–332.

14 Groce JR, Raju GS, Hewlett A, et al.: Endoscopic clip closure of a gastric staple-line dehiscence (with video). *Gastrointest Endosc* 2007;**65**:321–2;Discussion 322.

15 Mummadi RR, Groce JR, Raju GS, et al.: Endoscopic management of colocutaneous fistula in a morbidly obese woman (with video). *Gastrointest Endosc* 2008;**67**:1207–1208.

16 Hussein AM, Bartram CI, Williams CB: Carbon dioxide insufflation for more comfortable colonoscopy. *Gastrointest Endosc* 1984;**30**:68–70.

17 Williams CB: Who's for CO_2? *Gastrointest Endosc* 1986;**32**:365–367.

18 Mizobuchi S, Kuge K, Maeda H, et al.: Endoscopic clip application for closure of an esophagomediastinal-tracheal fistula after surgery for esophageal cancer. *Gastrointest Endosc* 2003;**57**:962–965.

24 Esophageal, Gastroduodenal and Colorectal Stenting

Peter D. Siersema

University Medical Center Utrecht, Utrecht, The Netherlands

Procedure(s) to be considered

Procedures that are required for stent placement in the gastrointestinal (GI) tract include endoscopy with a small (4–6 mm) or normal (8–10 mm) caliber gastroscope for strictures in the esophagus, a large (11.5–14 mm) caliber gastroscope or therapeutic duodenoscope (11–12.5 mm) for strictures in the distal stomach/duodenum, and a sigmoidoscope or colonoscope (12–14 mm) for strictures in the colorectum (Figure 24.1).

These endoscopic procedures are used for stent placement in the esophagus, distal stomach/duodenum and colorectum. These strictures are often malignant; however, benign strictures can also be stented, particularly in the esophagus. In addition, stents are placed for malignant esophagorespiratory fistulas and for benign esophageal leaks or ruptures.

Prerequisite level of expertise and skill for learning this

Basic prerequisites for learning to place stents include skill in upper endoscopy and colonoscopy, interpretation of fluoroscopic images, and experience in general stricture dilation techniques. Prior ERCP training is also very helpful.

There is a large variety in the degree of difficulty for stent placement. In general, esophageal stents are easiest to place, although the degree of difficulty may also vary. For example, stent placement of a midesophageal obstruction is usually straightforward, but proximal esophageal lesions are often more challenging to stent.

Gastroduodenal and colorectal stents are more difficult to place, which is due to the severity of these obstructions and the local anatomical situation. Endoscopists, who also perform more complex procedures, such as ERCP, should however be able to traverse complex gastroduodenal and colorectal strictures, to interpret difficult fluoroscopic images and to adequately place stents for malignant obstructions. In general, colorectal stent placement in the setting of an acute complete obstruction is difficult, since the patient is ill, bowel preparation inadequate, the anatomy angulated, and the lumen frequently not seen *en face*.

Another issue is the variety of stents and stent delivery systems that are currently available. It is difficult to master all of the specific characteristics of stents and their deployment systems. All currently available stents have their own degree of shortening in the GI tract.

Special considerations

The necessary skills for stent placement in the GI tract are best obtained in high volume tertiary referral centers. Patients requiring stent placement are often seen in centers with a high number of referrals for therapeutic endoscopy and/or a large GI oncology practice. The trainee must be supervised by a senior endoscopist (trainer) with expertise in stent placement for different types of strictures throughout the GI tract. The training is supported by instruction in dilation techniques for strictures. It is prerequisite that the trainee is familiar with indications for stent placement, knows contraindications for procedures, and is able to anticipate and to act upon complications that occur due to stenting [1].

Specific technical and cognitive skill sets

Stent placement requires sufficient cognitive skills with regard to the:
- indications for stenting malignant and benign strictures throughout the GI tract, benign esophageal ruptures and leaks, and esophagorespiratory fistulas;
- interpretation of noninvasive imaging results, such as computed tomography (CT) and contrast swallow;
- evaluation of clinical signs and symptoms following stent placement;
- available (endoscopic and nonendoscopic) management options for complications and recurrent obstruction;

Successful Training in Gastrointestinal Endoscopy, First Edition. Edited by Jonathan Cohen.
© 2011 Blackwell Publishing Ltd. Published 2011 by Blackwell Publishing Ltd.

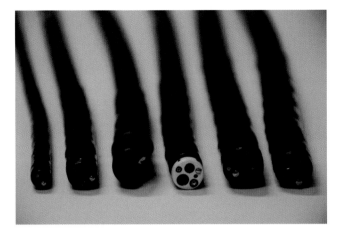

Figure 24.1 Endoscopes for stent placement in the gastrointestinal tract, from left to right: small caliber gastroscope, therapeutic duodenoscope, normal caliber gastroscope, large caliber gastroscope, sigmoidoscope and colonoscope.

- optimal timing for stent removal in benign indications; and
- placement of an additional (second) stent in case of stent dysfunction.

Necessary technical skills include therapeutic upper and lower endoscopy, guide wire placement, and biliary stent placement. As stent placement is sometimes indicated in extremely tight strictures, the trainee should also be able to dilate these strictures using balloon or Savary–Gilliard dilation. Training in dilation techniques is covered in a separate chapter in this volume. Moreover, as stent placement for benign indications is increasingly being performed, the trainee should have the skills to remove various types of stents.

The ability to manage procedure-related (e.g., perforation, hemorrhage) and long-term (e.g., fistula formation) complications and recurrent obstruction due to stent migration, tumoral or nontumoral tissue overgrowth, or food obstruction is essential.

It is important to note that the location of the stricture and its relation to surrounding organs is important to consider prior to stent placement. This is particularly true for obstructions in the proximal and midesophagus, benign esophageal ruptures and leaks, and gastric outlet obstruction.

Finally, it is important for trainees to develop skill in coordinating care with other providers such as oncologists, radiologists, general surgeons, and interventional bronchoscopists, in the event of proximal esophageal tumors that threaten upper airway compression.

Equipment

1 *Esophagus*
   a Small (4–6 mm) or normal (8–10) caliber gastroscope
   b Materials for marking the upper and lower tumor margin:
   - injection needle with lipid-soluble contrast agent such as lipiodol
   - external marker with tape to fixate
   c 0.018″–0.038″ stiff guide wire (preferably stiff)
   d Bougie or balloon dilation (max. 10–12 mm)
   e Partially- or fully-covered metal or nonmetal stent placed over-the-wire (OTW)
2 *Distal stomach/duodenum*
   a Large (11.5–14 mm) caliber gastroscope or therapeutic duodenoscope (11–12.5 mm)
   b ERCP catheter
   c Water-soluble contrast agent
   d 0.018″–0.038″ guide wire (flexible)
   e Balloon dilation (max. 10–12 mm)
   f Uncovered or covered metal stent placed through-the-scope (TTS)
3 *Colon/rectum*
   a Sigmoidoscope or colonoscope (12–14 mm)
   b Materials for marking the upper and lower tumor margin:
   - injection needle with lipid-soluble contrast agent
   c ERCP catheter
   d Water-soluble contrast agent
   e 0.018″–0.038″ guide wire (flexible)
   f Balloon dilation (max. 10–12 mm)
   g Uncovered or covered metal stent placed OTW (distal colon/rectum) or TTS
4 *Salvage accessories*
   a Hemostasis accessories—injection needle, epinephrine, endoclips, bipolar
   b Rat-toothed forceps—therapeutic size
   c Polypectomy snare

Key steps of proper technique

Esophagus

Stent placement for palliation of dysphagia or closure of esophagorespiratory fistulas is an alternative treatment option for patients who are otherwise not candidates for surgical resection. In addition, stents are increasingly used for (prolonged) dilation of benign esophageal strictures and for sealing benign esophageal ruptures or leaks [2].

Pre-esophageal stenting evaluation

Prior to esophageal stent placement, the endoscopist should evaluate the following items:

1 *Patient condition*

In malignant esophageal strictures, it is important to decide whether the patient is "fit enough" to benefit from stent placement. In patients with a WHO performance score of 4 (100% bedridden), the indication should be carefully evaluated.

2 *Tumor location*

Esophageal tumors can be located in the proximal, mid- or distal esophagus. For tumors in the proximal and midesophagus, there is a risk of coexisting tumor ingrowth into the trachea or bronchus or tumor compressing the airways. Placement of a tracheal stent should be considered prior to esophageal stent placement. Stents across the gastroesophageal junction are at an increased risk of migration. There is also a risk of gastroesophageal reflux.

Table 24.1 Characteristics of currently used partially- or fully-covered self-expanding esophageal stents.

Stent type	Covering	Length (cm)	Diameter (mm)	Release system	Radial force	Degree of shortening	Flexibility	Material	Stent Manufacturer
Ultraflex	Partial	10, 12, 15	18, 22	Proximal/distal	Low	30–40%	High	Nitinol/polyurethane	Boston Scientific, Natick, MA, USA
Polyflex	Full	9, 12, 15	16, 18, 21	Distal	High	0%	Low	Polyester/silicone	Boston Scientific, Natick, MA, USA
Wallflex	Partial	10, 12, 15	18, 23	Distal	High to strong	30–40%	Moderate	Nitinol/silicone	Boston Scientific, Natick, MA, USA
Evolution	Partial	8, 10, 12.5, 15	20	Distal	Moderate	10–20%	Moderate	Nitinol/silicone	Cook Medical, Limerick, Ireland
SX-Ella	Full	8.5, 11, 13.5	20	Distal	High	10–20%	Low	Nitinol/polyethylene	Ella, Hradec, Kralove, Czech Republic
Niti-S	Full	6, 8, 10 12, 15	18	Proximal/distal	Moderate	10%	Moderate	Nitinol/polyurethane	Taewoong, Seoul, South Korea
Alimaxx-E	Full to high	7, 10, 12	18, 22	Distal	Low	0%	Moderate	Nitinol/polyurethane	Merit, South Jordan UT, USA

Moreover, the distal stent end may damage the stomach wall at the level of the lesser curvature when the stent is placed too distally.

3 *Stent choice*

Partially- or fully-covered stents are now the predominantly used stent types in the esophagus (Table 24.1) (Figure 24.2). It has been shown that the functional result of uncovered esophageal stents is negatively affected by the high risk of tissue ingrowth through the uncovered stent mesh [3].

Recurrent dysphagia due to stent migration, tissue in- or overgrowth or food impaction is currently the most important cause of a poorly functioning stent. Stent designs have usually one or more items that may prevent recurrent dysphagia (Table 24.2). The optimal stent choice in a particular clinical situation is an important issue. In malignant esophageal strictures, partially-covered stents are a valuable option.

In benign strictures, fully-covered metal or plastic stents are preferable as the risk of nontumoral (hyperplastic) tissue ingrowth is reduced with these designs, making stent removal easier.

In benign esophageal ruptures or leaks without a stricture, large caliber covered stent devices are the stent type of choice. If a normal caliber stent is used, migration is a risk. Although fully-covered stents can easily be removed than partially-covered stents, many experts prefer a partially-covered stent in this situation, as the uncovered parts of the stent allow complete sealing.

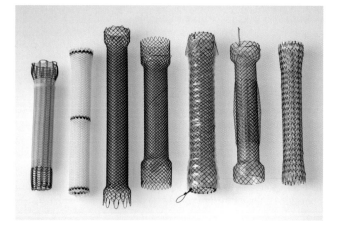

Figure 24.2 Currently available covered metal esophageal stents, from left to right: Ultraflex (Boston Scientific, Natick, MA, USA), Polyflex (Boston Scientific), Wallflex Esophageal (Boston Scientific), Evolution Esophageal (Cook, Limerick, Ireland), SX-Ella (Ella, Hradec Kralove, Czech Republic), Niti-S (Taewoong, Seoul, South Korea) and Alimaxx-E (Merit, South Jordan, UT, USA). As can be seen, some of these stents are fully covered, whereas others are only partially covered.

Table 24.2 Characteristics of currently used covered stents to minimize recurrent dysphagia.

- Tissue in- and overgrowth
  - Cover over entire stent length
  - Nonmetal/nonnitinol material
  - Expansion force that is intermediate between too high and too low
- Food obstruction
  - Larger diameter
  - Cover on luminal inside
- Migration
  - Resistance on outside of stent
  - Larger diameter
  - Shouldering of stent
  - Partial cover of stent (leaving proximal and distal stent parts uncovered allowing them to embed)

This is however a nonregistered indication of partially-covered stents.

It is generally believed that stents placed for a tumor causing extrinsic esophageal compression are at an increased risk of migration. Unfortunately, this is not based on comparative studies. Nevertheless, many experts place only partially-covered stents for extrinsic compression to reduce migration risk.

Stents are increasingly being used for strictures in the proximal esophagus, close to the upper esophageal sphincter (UES). Placement at this site requires careful positioning, as the upper stent end should not extend above the UES to prevent the risk of foreign body sensation. Other complications include stent-induced pain and tracheal compression. If the latter is the case, initial tracheal stent placement is advised. It is recommended that the endoscopist should be skilled and experienced in placing stents in the proximal esophagus. Finally, it is recommended to use only flexible stent designs, for example the Ultraflex stent (Boston Scientific, Natick, USA) to minimize the risk of complications. As all currently available stents have specific advantages but also drawbacks, we suggest to develop experience with a small selection of stents types, for example one partially-covered metal stent and one fully-covered metal or nonmetal (plastic) stent.

4 Coagulation parameters

Hemorrhage is not a very common procedure-related complication in esophageal stent placement; however, if occurring, it may have a dramatic outcome. Although routine evaluation of coagulation parameters is not indicated, it is recommended to control prothrombin time (PT) and activated partial thromboplastin time (APTT) when risk factors for abnomal results present, such as warfarin or heparin use or liver dysfunction.

Esophageal stent placement

In this section, the antegrade technique (Video 24.1) and the combined antegrade and retrograde (CAR) technique for esophageal stent placement are separately discussed.

Antegrade technique

For antegrade stent placement, the following steps need to be taken:

1 Stent placement is usually done with the patient under conscious sedation.

2 As a first step, the upper and lower margins of the tumor need to be identified (Figure 24.3(a)). If tumor obstruction does not allow passage of a standard gastroscope, the tumor can be dilated to 10–12 mm to measure stricture length and place a guide wire. However, dilation carries a risk of perforation. Therefore, it is preferable to use a small caliber gastroscope.

3 When stents are placed under fluoroscopic guidance, the proximal and distal margins of the stricture are demarcated by placing skin markers, clips or intramucosal injection of a

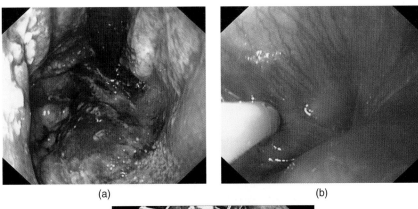

(a)   (b)

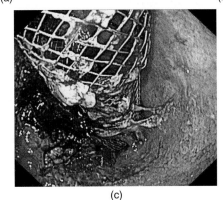

(c)

Figure 24.3 Steps to be taken in stent placement for esophageal cancer: (a) The first step is to identify the upper and lower margins of the tumor. (b) The proximal and distal margins of the tumor can be demarcated by the intramucosal injection of the lipid-soluble contrast agent lipiodol. (c) Stent expansion after placement can be confirmed endoscopically under direct vision.

radiopaque contrast agent (Figure 24.3(b)). It should be reminded that injecting lipid-soluble contrast agent will result in a persistent mark in the mucosa.

4 The next step is to place a stiff guide wire, for example a 0.038-inch Savary guide wire or 0.035-inch Amplatz guide wire, as distally as possible, preferably the duodenum. A stiff guide wire is preferred over a more flexible type as this reduces the risk of kinking. This is important as the stent is introduced over a guide wire, and not, as is the case with enteral stents, through the scope. A duodenal position of the guide wire is preferred, because some stent introduction systems have a tip that far extends the distal end of the stent.

5 The stent is then advanced over the guide wire. Most stents shorten during expansion (Table 24.1), which must be taken into account when positioning the introduction system. In order to prevent stent migration upon release from the introduction system, the system should not be advanced too distally. A stent that is no longer than 2–4 cm of the stricture length should be used to allow for a 1–2 cm extension above and below the proximal and distal tumor margins. For stents placed across the gastroesophageal junction (GEJ), stent length is guided by the rule that the distal stent end should not overlap the distal tumor margin by more than 1–2 cm to prevent laceration of the posterior stomach wall at the distal stent end and avoid kinking of the stent.

6 Stents can be placed under fluoroscopic and/or endoscopic control or using the markers on the stent introduction system as is the case with Ultraflex stents (Boston Scientific, Natick, USA) and SX Ella stents (Ella-CS, Hradec Kralove, Czech Republic). There is no objection to confirm endoscopically that the upper end of the stent is optimally placed. However, one should be careful to avoid stent dislodgement caused by friction between the still insufficiently deployed stent and the endoscope (Figure 24.3(c)). Stent expansion can also be confirmed fluoroscopically, or, afterwards, with a contrast swallow. A radiologic contrast study after esophageal stent placement is however not routinely indicated.

7 Stent placement is an outpatient procedure, which takes about 15–20 minutes. Patients should be reminded that the stent is a tube without peristaltic movement, which makes thorough chewing, small bites and effervescent fluids during meals important. Moreover, patient should be instructed not to rest in a supine position until 2–4 hours after a meal, especially when the stent is placed across the GEJ.

8 In most institutions it is preferred to prescribe high-dose proton pomp inhibitors (PPIs) when the distal stent end is placed across the GEJ to reduce reflux of acid fluid after the procedure. PPIs do not completely eliminate reflux of gastric contents. Alternatively, a stent with an antireflux mechanism can be used.

Combined antegrade and retrograde (CAR) technique

The vast majority of malignant or benign strictures can be endoscopically passed with a guide wire, followed by stent placement. Occasionally, it is very difficult to identify the true lumen of a stenotic esophagus, for instance in benign postradiation or caustic strictures in the proximal esophagus. In these circumstances, passing of a guide wire for dilation through antegrade endoscopy is unsuccessful. In order to reduce the risk of perforation, the CAR technique can be applied [4]. The following steps need to taken for this procedure:

1 A small caliber endoscope is passed retrogradely into the patient's esophagus through the gastric lumen through a mature gastrostomy or jejunostomy tract for access.

2 A guide wire is then passed via the endoscope and under fluoroscopic guidance through the distal margin of the stricture. In most cases, a 0.038″ flexible guide wire with floppy tip is sufficient; however, in extremely tight strictures, a 0.018″ guide wire is required.

3 If the lumen is also not detected on the distal side, it can be considered to puncture the stricture on the distal side using a guide wire with a rigid tip or a precut knife to provide a small access hole in the stricture. Both these procedures should be performed under fluoroscopic guidance and with a second gastroscope at the proximal side of the stricture.

4 The guide wire is antegradely picked up. Dilation up to 10 mm can be performed by Savary–Gilliard or balloon dilation. It is important to remember that in these tight strictures, it is worthwhile to consider dilating up to 13–16 mm in two or more dilation sessions using the "the rule of 3", meaning that per session 3 successive dilation steps of 1 mm are taken. It is recommend to place a feeding tube after the initial dilation to keep the tract open until the next dilation session. Dilation sessions should be repeated once to twice weekly until the intended diameter is achieved.

5 It should be kept in mind that stent size matters in the proximal esophagus, as the tracheal lumen can be compromised by using a stent that is too wide. Therefore, smaller diameter esophageal stents or combined placement of a tracheal stent is recommended. For esophageal stent placement, a 0.038″ stiff guide wire is used to guide stent placement.

6 For the following steps, see Section Antegrade technique starting at Step 5.

Post-esophageal stenting management

Stent removal for benign indications

For benign indications, it is not clear how long a stent should be left in the esophagus. Factors that influence stenting time include underlying cause, time since esophageal injury and stricture length. The following guidelines should be kept in mind in benign esophageal strictures [1]:

1 Strictures that are caused by ischemic injury, present within 6–12 months after the injury and are longer than 5 cm are stented for at least 8–16 weeks.

2 In all other cases, for example anastomotic strictures and caustic strictures, stents are inserted for a shorter period, usually 4 to 8 weeks.

3 When symptoms recur after stent removal, and recurrent stricture formation is noted, placement of a second stent can be considered.

4 In cases when partially-covered stents are used, endoscopy should be performed at 4-week intervals to visualize whether embedding and hyperplastic tissue ingrowth of the uncovered stent part in the esophageal mucosa has occurred. If this is the case, stent removal should be performed, and another, preferably fully-covered stent is placed.

5 As fully covered stents also carry a risk of (hyperplastic) tissue overgrowth, periodic endoscopy at 6-week intervals is recommended. When after stent removal the stricture is still present, it should be considered to continue stenting. This also depends on the time of occurrence of tissue overgrowth in a patient, with replacement of the stent at timeframes determined by this interval. In all cases, it is likely that the inflammation underlying the stricture will ultimately subside and the luminal diameter achieved at that time will remain, allowing the patient to eat a normal diet.

Management of complications
Procedure-related complications
Procedure-related complications are defined as being clinically evident within 1 week of stent placement. These complications are uncommon, occurring in less than 5% of cases.

• One of the most prominent is *perforation* due to dilation, passage of the endoscope, or stent placement itself. Stent placement is the treatment of choice for this complication; however, one should be prepared for infectious complications.

• *Hemorrhage* is another complication that results from manipulation of friable tumor tissue due to dilation, endoscope passage and stent placement. It is difficult to treat; sometimes, endoscopic haemostatic measures are effective, but in other cases, external beam radiation therapy in 5 fractions of 4 Gray can be helpful.

• *Chest pain* following stenting is commonly seen in patients that have been treated with prior radiation and/or chemotherapy. Treatment consists of the (temporary) use of analgesics, but in severe cases stent removal is needed.

• *Aspiration (pneumonia)* is a complication that usually occurs during or shortly after the stenting procedure when a patient is not positioned in the left-lateral position while sedated. Particularly tight strictures causing food obstruction in the esophagus and stents placed across the gastroesophageal junction predispose to this complication.

Long-term complications
Long-term complications are defined as being clinically evident at least 1 week after stent placement. These complications are more common, occurring in 20–30% of cases [5].

• *Hemorrhage* is the most severe long-term complication following stent placement. It is usually not related to stent placement however, caused by progressive tumor ingrowth into (larger) blood vessels surrounding the esophagus. External beam radiation therapy is mostly not effective. Symptomatic measures, such as repeat blood transfusions, can be considered, but the mortality of this complication is high.

• Another long-term complication of esophageal stent placement is *fistula formation*, most commonly at the proximal stent end as a consequence of pressure ulceration by the stent flange. It can be treated by placement of a second, partially overlapping stent.

• An important long-term complication of stent placement is recurrent dysphagia due to *stent migration* (Figure 24.4(a)), *tumoral* (in malignancy) (Figure 24.4(b)) or *nontumoral* (in malignant and benign causes) *tissue in-* or *overgrowth* (Figure 24.4(c)) or *food obstruction* (Figure 24.4(d)).

In case of *stent migration* into the stomach, the first step is to try repositioning the stent using a rat-toothed forceps or a snare, or, alternatively, remove the stent. It is preferable to use an overtube for stent removal. Removal should be performed by grasping the stent on one of its ends and pulling the stent along its long axis through the esophagus. Leaving the stent in the stomach carries a risk of complications (mostly pain). When repositioning of the migrated stent is not possible, another stent should be placed. It is advised to use another design stent in these cases, in order to reduce the risk of stent migration.

Additional stent placement is also the treatment of choice in patients with *tissue in-* or *overgrowth*.

Endoscopic stent cleansing is preferred in case of *food obstruction*. It is important to manipulate the stent carefully, because stent migration may occur while dislodging the food inside the stent.

Distal stomach/duodenum
Traditionally, surgical bypass (gastrojejunostomy) was the only treatment option for patients with malignant gastric outlet obstruction [6]. However, gastrojejunostomy requires general anesthesia and often carries significant morbidity due to the poor general health of patients. Stents that re-establish the luminal patency in patients with gastric outlet obstruction offer an alternative treatment option for patients who are otherwise no candidates for surgery.

Pre-gastroduodenal stenting evaluation
Before enteral stent placement in the distal stomach/duodenum, the following issues should be evaluated:

1 ***Patient condition:*** In more than 50% of patients with gastric outlet obstruction, this is caused by pancreatic cancer. It is important to realize that some of these patients may already have metastatic spread to the liver or peritoneal cavity when gastric outlet obstruction develops. This is in most cases associated with a poor medical condition, i.e., a WHO performance score of 4. It is unlikely that these patients will benefit from stent placement. Moreover, due to the presence of peritoneal metastases, additional obstructions may be present more distally in the jejunum/ileum. When this is the case, stent placement in the antral–pyloric or duodenal location will not resolve the symptoms.

2 ***Tumor location:*** An important issue to evaluate prior to stent placement is involvement of the CBD. There are three scenarios:

a When the CBD was already stented previously, the type of biliary stent, either plastic or metal, is important. If a plastic CBD stent is present, this should be removed and replaced by a metal stent in the CBD prior to gastroduodenal stent placement.

b Second, it may also be that the CBD and the distal stomach/duodenum are obstructed at the same time. In these cases, first a metal stent is placed in the CBD, followed by gastrodeuodenal stent placement.

c The CBD was not obstructed at the time of enteral stent placement, but becomes obstructed some time after stent placement. This will determine optimal duodenal stent position, i.e., preferably leaving the papilla free and not covering it.

3 ***Stent choice:*** Uncovered and covered enteral stents that are placed TTS are available for strictures in the distal stomach/

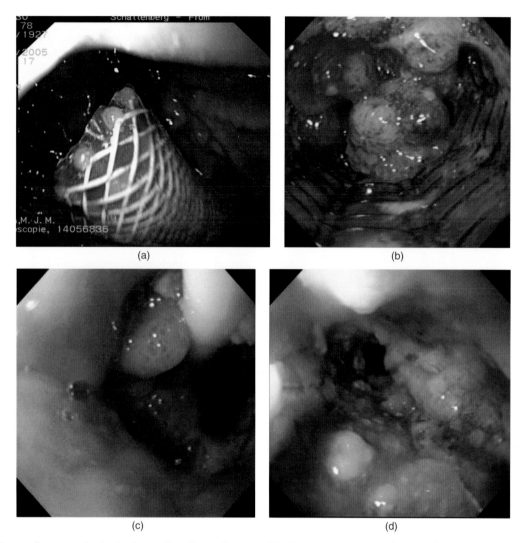

Figure 24.4 Causes of recurrent dysphagia after esophageal stent placement: (a) Migration of a stent into the stomach. (b) Tumor in- and overgrowth at the distal stent end. (c) Nontumoral (hyperplastic) tissue ingrowth at the proximal stent end. (d) Food obstruction inside a stent.

duodenum as well as in the colon/rectum (Table 24.3) (Figure 24.5). For many years, uncovered enteral stents were the predominantly used stent types. This is due to the following reasons:

a The diameter of covered enteral stents and introduction systems was initially too large to allow advancement through the working channel of a large caliber endoscope. Only recently, covered enteral stents for TTS use have become available, but these are not yet available in the United States (Table 24.3).

b It has been suggested that covered enteral stents have an increased risk of migration, although the latest generation covered stents have features that should prevent these stents from migrating.

c It has also been suggested that covered enteral stents in the duodenum may predispose to cholangitis and/or pancreatitis when placed across the papilla. Initial results with covered stents have shown favorable results. However, as covered stents have only recently been introduced, follow-up studies are needed to

establish whether covered enteral stents are indeed effective and safe. A disadvantage of uncovered enteral stents is the risk of tissue ingrowth, either by hyperplastic tissue or by malignant tissue ingrowth. Particularly in patients with prolonged survival, this may occur making placement of a secondary stent necessary [7].

Gastroduodenal stent placement

The following steps need to be taken for stenting gastric outlet obstruction (Video 24.2):

1 Gastroduodenal stent placement is usually performed under conscious sedation.

2 The next step is to identify the proximal and distal end of the tumor and its length. If the severity of the obstruction does not allow passage of a therapeutic gastroscope, an ERCP catheter with guide wire can be used to pass the stricture. Using contrast medium injected to the catheter the tumor length can be measured, tumor

Table 24.3 Characteristics of currently available enteral stents.

Stent type	Length (mm)	Diameter (mm)	Manufacturer	Over-the-wire (OTW)	Through-the-Scope (TTS)
Ultraflex precision colonic	57, 87, 117	Flair: 30; Body: 25	Boston Scientific, Natick, MA	OTW	
Wallstent colonic/duodenal	60, 90	20,22	Boston Scientific, Natick, MA		TTS
Wallflex colonic	60, 90, 120	Flair: 30, 27; Body: 25, 22	Boston Scientific, Natick, MA		TTS
Wallflex duodenal	60, 90, 120	Flair: 27; Body: 22	Boston Scientific, Natick, MA		TTS
Colonic Z	40, 60, 80, 100, 120	Flair: 35; Body: 25	Cook Medical, Winston-Salem, NC	OTW	
Evolution duodenal	60, 90, 120	Flair: 27; Body: 22	Cook Medical, Limerick, Ireland		TTS
Evolution colonic	60, 80, 100	Flair: 30; Body: 25	Cook Medical, Limerick, Ireland		TTS
Enteral (duodenal/colonic) D-type	40, 60, 80, 100, 120	Uncov. Body: 16, 18, 20, 22, 24 Covered (Comvi): Body: 18, 20, 22	Taewoong-Medical Co., Seoul, South Korea	OTW	TTS
Enteral (duodenal/colonic) (covered)	10, 30, 50, 70, 90	Flair: 24, 26, 28 Body: 16, 18, 20	Taewoong-Medical Co., Seoul, South Korea		TTS
Hanaro duodenal/pyloric	Cov: 60, 90, 110, 130; Uncov.: 80, 110, 140	Cov.. + Uncov.: 18	M.I. Tech Co., Seoul, South Korea		TTS
Hararostent colorectal	80, 110, 140	22	M.I. Tech Co., Seoul, South Korea		TTS
SX-Ella colorectal	70, 90, 80, 90, 110, 135	22, 25, 30	Ella-CS, Hradec Kralove, Czech Republic		TTS

characteristics can be delineated and the presence of more distally located strictures can be determined.

It is often not necessary to dilate a stricture in the distal stomach or duodenum, as visualization using an ERCP catheter gives enough information to guide stent placement. If still needed, it is advised dilating not further than 10–12 mm using balloon dilation.
3 Stents in the gastroduodenum can be placed with a large (11.5–14 mm) caliber gastroscope or therapeutic duodenoscope

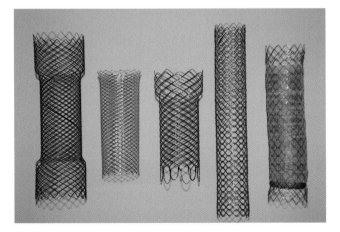

Figure 24.5 A selection from the currently available enteral stents for use in the distal stomach/duodenum, from left to right: Evolution Duodenal (Cook Medical, Limerick, Ireland), Wallstent Colonic/Duodenal (Boston Scientific, Natick, MA, USA), Wallflex Duodenal (Boston Scientific), D-type Duodenal (uncovered) (Taewoong, Seoul, South Korea), and D-type Duodenal (Comvi) (Taewoong).

(11–12.5 mm). Moreover, stents can also be placed in the distal duodenum or even proximal jejunum [8]. The use of a therapeutic gastroscope in this position can however be difficult, because of the reach of the endoscope and the risk of loop formation in the stomach due to the flexibility of the gastroscope. In these circumstances, one can use a colonoscope. A colonoscope is long enough to reach distally located strictures and offers better endoscopic stiffness than gastroscopes, which avoids looping in the stomach.
4 The next step is to place a flexible 0.038-inch guide wire with floppy tip through the stricture and advance it as distally as possible (Figure 24.6(a)). Correct positioning of the guide wire is done by using a combination of endoscopy and fluoroscopy. Fluoroscopy may aid in advancing the guide wire through the stricture and more distally.
5 The enteral stent is then carefully advanced through the endoscope inside the stricture (Figure 24.6(b)). Most enteral stents shorten during expansion (Table 24.3). This means that during deployment, the introduction device should be pulled back to correct for stent shortening (Figure 24.6(c)). If this is not done, this will result in the stent being positioned too distally and sometimes not bridging the stricture. Preventing enteral stent migration upon release is another reason why the stent should not be advanced too distally.

The position of the stent in relation to the papilla is an important issue to consider prior to gastroduodenal stent placement. It is important to keep the papilla uncovered if the stricture location allows this. This makes a future ERCP technically easier in case of CBD obstruction. If duodenal stent placement across the papilla is however indicated, it still may be technically possible to cannulate the CBD through the meshes of an

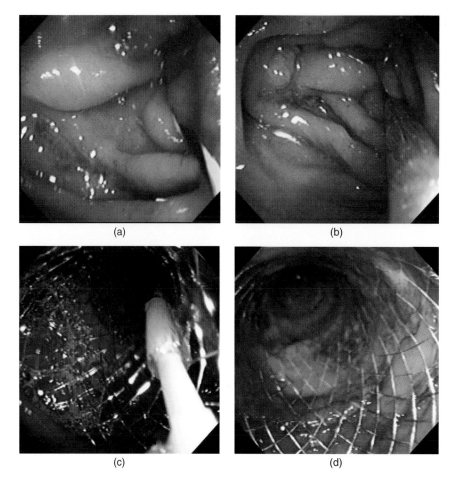

Figure 24.6 Steps to be taken in stent placement for gastric outlet obstruction: (a) The first step is to identify the margins of the tumor and to place a guide wire. (b) The next step is to advance the enteral stent inside the tumor. (c) Stent deployment can be followed endoscopically under direct vision. (d) Correct positioning of the stent can also be confirmed endoscopically (note the proximal tumor margin underneath the stent mesh).

uncovered enteral stent. Some authors have also reported that argon plasma coagulation can be used to make a "window" in the enteral stent for cannulation and placement of a biliary stent. If CBD stent placement by endoscopic means is not possible, this should be performed by radiologic means (percutaneous transhepatic cholangiography).

6 Enteral stents should be placed under combined fluoroscopic and endoscopic control. An enteral stent that is no longer than 2 cm of the stricture length, with the stent extending 1 cm on both sides, should be used. There is no objection to confirm endoscopically (Figure 24.6(d)) that the distal stent end is correctly positioned in relation to the proximal and distal tumor margin, and, if this is the case, the papilla. However, one should be careful to avoid stent dislodgement.

7 Stent placement is an outpatient procedure, taking about 15–30 minutes, when only an enteral stent is placed. In combination with CBD stent placement, the procedure may take more time. Due to the large storing capacity of the stomach, it is difficult to detect a poorly functioning enteral stent based on patient's symptoms only. It is therefore recommended to evaluate stent function endoscopically if stent dysfunction is suspected.

Post-gastroduodenal stenting evaluation

CBD obstruction

Patients should be instructed that (recurrent) CBD obstruction may occur some time after enteral stent placement. In case a CBD stent was already placed, this is, in most cases, caused by an obstructed CBD stent due to tumoral or nontumoral tissue in- or overgrowth. If a CBD stent was not previously placed, this may be due to tumor involvement of the CBD. In all cases, a primary/secondary CBD stent should be placed (see previous paragraph).

Management of complications

Procedure-related complications

Procedure-related complications are uncommon, occurring in 5–7% of cases [7].

• The most dramatic of these are *bleeding* and *perforation*. Endoscopic management is difficult, if not impossible.

• Other procedure-related complications include early *stent migration* and *stent dysfunction*. This can often be managed endoscopically by removing the stent, which is still possible at an early stage after stent placement, and replacing it by another enteral stent.

• Sedation-associated adverse events may also occur; in particular, given the fact that these patients present with some degree of obstruction, they carry a higher than average risk of aspiration. For this reason, consideration of preprocedure nasogastric suction and of airway protection during the procedure is sometimes warranted.

Long-term complications
Long-term complications are more common, but still occurring in less than 20% of cases [7]. The most frequently observed late complications are *stent migration* and stent occlusion by either *tumoral* or *nontumoral in-* or *overgrowth* or *food*. These complications can usually be managed endoscopically. *Stent migration* and *tumoral* or *nontumoral in-* or *overgrowth* are mostly managed by placing a second stent inside the obstructed stent. Stent occlusion by *food* can be managed by endoscopic cleansing of the stent. One should be careful not to dislodge the stent.

Colon/rectum

Approximately 10–30% of patients with primary colorectal cancer (CRC) present with obstruction. The indications for stent use have broadened from palliation to, nowadays, as bridge to surgery in patients with potentially operable acutely obstructing colon cancer [9]. Stent placement as a bridge to surgery permits bowel decompression, thorough bowel preparation, and a single-stage colon resection.

Pre-colorectal stenting evaluation

Prior to enteral stent placement in the colon/rectum, the following issues are important to consider:
1 Patient condition: It is not clear whether stent placement in a 50-year-old, otherwise healthy patient with acute total obstruction, in whom stenting is performed as a bridge to surgery is associated with a higher or lower risk of complications than the same procedure in an 80-year-old diabetic patient with subtotal obstruction and metastatic disease, in whom stent placement is a palliative measure. It is nowadays rare that combinations of patient-related risk factors are a reason not to perform stent placement. It is more likely that such a decision is determined by the expected risk of complications when an acute surgical procedure is performed for acute malignant obstruction and not initially a colorectal stent is placed as a bridge to surgery. On the other hand, in palliative patients, this decision is mainly based on the prognosis of patients' survival after stent placement.

Only recently it has been recognized that the use of chemotherapeutic agents, such as bevacizumab, is a separate, but important risk factor for complications in patients, in whom stenting is performed with a palliative intent. It has recently been reported that bevacizumab therapy nearly tripled the risk of perforation to almost 20% and shortened the mean time of delayed perforation to 22 days [10].
2 Tumor location: CRCs may be located in the right-sided colon, left-sided colon, or rectum. The difficulty of stent placement is highest with tumors located in the right-sided colon. Reported series have however shown similar efficacy and safety results for

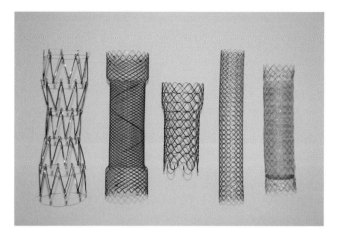

Figure 24.7 A selection from the currently available enteral stents for use in the colorectum, from left to right: Colonic Z (Cook Medical, Winston-Salem, NC, USA) Evolution Colonic (Cook Medical, Limerick, Ireland), Wallflex Colonic (Boston Scientific), D-type Colonic (uncovered) (Taewoong, Seoul, South Korea), and D-type Colonic (Comvi) (Taewoong).

stent placement in the right or left colon [11]. As a general rule, it can however be reminded that the more distally located CRCs are the easiest to stent.

It is important to note that stent placement in tumors within 10 cm of the anal sphincter is relatively contraindicated. Stents at this location are often associated with tenesmus and pain. Moreover, stents in the lower rectum are often expelled during defecation.

Stents in an angulated position have an increased risk of pressure ulceration on the colonic wall with hemorrhage and perforation as a result. Locations that are prone to this include the sigmoid, splenic flexure, and hepatic flexure.
3 Stent choice: As has been mentioned previously, both uncovered and covered enteral TTS stents are available for placement in the colon/rectum. In addition, colorectal stents are available that can be placed over a guide wire (Table 24.3) (Figure 24.7). These stents can be placed in left-sided tumors, occasionally as high as the proximal sigmoid and descending colon [12]. An advantage of guide wire-guided stents is that they are covered and have a larger diameter than colorectal TTS stents. This feature may reduce the risk of stent migration.

Colorectal stent placement

It is important to recognize the clinical situation for which colorectal stents are placed, either as a bridge to surgery or as palliative treatment. In general, colorectal stent placement as a bridge to surgery is technically more demanding than a palliative procedure, simply because these strictures are usually (sub)totally obstructed.

It is again stressed that dilation in the colorectum should be avoided if necessary. There is an increased risk of perforation and using an ERCP catheter and guide wire gives enough information to guide stent placement.

There is also an increased risk of perforation in an angulated sigmoid obstruction when the lumen is not clearly visible. In this situation, it can be challenging to pass a guide wire through the stricture. In order to overcome this, it can be considered to use a small (4–6 mm) caliber, flexible gastroscope to traverse the guide wire through the stricture and then backloading the larger caliber sigmoidscope or colonoscope over the guide wire to allow for placement of a TTS colorectal stent. Alternatively, it can be considered to use a highly flexible, hydrophilic, coated guide wire (Terumo, Somerset, NJ, USA) to get it across the stricture.

It is important to emphasize that it is important to rule out secondary sites of (malignant) obstruction with preprocedural radiological examinations. If these are present, one should consider additional stent placement, but, as often more metastatic sites are present, stent placement is no longer the preferred treatment option.

Colorectal stent placement using the TTS technique is not different from the gastroduodenal stent placement technique as previously prescribed (see Chapter 6). Similarly, stent placement using the guide wire technique is also not different from the esophageal stent placement technique as previously prescribed (see Chapter 6) (Video 24.3). These procedures will therefore not separately be discussed except for the following key technical troubleshooting maneuvers that are particular to stenting difficult colonic lesions.

Post-colorectal stenting evaluation

Management of complications
Procedure-related complications
These are not different from those previously described (see Chapter 6). In addition, tenesmus, pain, and fecal incontinence may occur after distal rectal stent placement. This can be managed with antispasmodic medication and laxatives; however, stent removal may be needed. In order to prevent stent obstruction, we recommend patients with a colorectal stent to use a soft diet, and the use of stool softeners and laxatives.

Long-term complications
These are not different from those previously described (see Chapter 6).

Setting and tools for training

Stent placement skills are taught to end of second and third year fellows during interventional endoscopy rotations or to advanced trainees (additional fourth year training). Even when fellows do not have exposure to more complicated stent placement procedures, some basic skills for stent placement are usually acquired during interventional endoscopy rotations. It is unknown how much training is required to gain proficiency in stent placement procedures. In the authors' opinion, at least ten esophageal stent placement procedures, and 10–15 gastroduodenal and/or colorectal stent placement procedures are required to gain a basic skill level. Continued experience may be important in maintaining one's skill level. Stent deployment can be readily practiced in *ex vivo* animal models. Access to such opportunities may be limited

and the benefit of such training for such procedures has not yet been validated.

Defining competency

Assessing competency may be problematic and depends on the volume of cases that is available to learn stent placement. The volume of stent procedures in a center is based upon center volume, especially for oncological cases, competing local expertise, and referral patterns for these procedures. There are currently no tools available to measure skill nor are there established parameters to establish competency. The authors' opinion is that key factors to look for in evaluating whether someone is competent in placing stents is the ability to accurately position a guide wire through different types of strictures, the technical skills to safely and effectively dilate complicated strictures, and the ability to place different types of stents. There is no benchmark of expert practices for these skills.

Maintaining skill level

Keeping skills may be difficult in centers with a relatively low volume of procedures, particularly for gastroduodenal and colorectal stent placement. It is unknown how much volume is needed to maintain skill level. Based on experience, we advice to perform at least one esophageal stent placement and one gastroduodenal or colorectal stent placement per month to maintain one's skill level.

Videos

Video 24.1 Esophageal stent placement procedure
Video 24.2 Duodenal stent placement procedure
Video 24.3 Through-the-scope colonic stent placement procdure

References

1 Siersema PD, de Wijkerslooth LRH: Dilation of refractory benign esophageal strictures. *Gastrointest Endosc* 2009;**70**:1000–1012.

2 Siersema PD: Treatment of esophageal perforations and anastomotic leaks: the endoscopist is stepping into the arena. *Gastrointest Endosc* 2005;**61**:897–900.

3 Vakil N, Morris AI, Marcon N, et al.: A prospective, randomized, controlled trial of covered expandable metal stents in the palliation of malignant esophageal obstruction at the gastroesophageal junction. *Am J Gastroenterol* 2001;**96**:1791–1796.

4 Mukherjee K, Cash MP, Burkey BB, et al.: Antegrade and retrograde endoscopy for treatment of esophageal stricture. *Am Surg* 2008;**74**:686–687.

5 Homs MYV, Steyerberg EW, Kuipers EJ, et al.: Causes and treatment for recurrent dysphagia after self-expanding metal stent placement for palliation of esophageal carcinoma. *Endoscopy* 2004;**36**:880–886.

6 Jeurnink SM, Steyerberg EW, van Hooft JE, et al.: Surgical gastrojejunostomy or endoscopic stent placement for the palliation of

malignant gastric outlet obstruction (SUSTENT study): a multicenter randomized trial. *Gastrointest Endosc.* (Epub ahead of print.)

7 Jeurnink SM, van Eijck CHJ, Steyerberg EW, et al.: Stent versus gastro-jejunostomy for the palliation of gastric outlet obstruction: a systematic review. *BMC Gastroenterol* 2007;**7**:18.

8 Jeurnink SM, Repici A, Luigiano C, et al.: Use of a colonoscope for distal duodenal stent placement in patients with malignant obstruction. *Surg Endosc* 2009;**23**:562–567.

9 Simmons DT, Baron TH: Technology insight: enteral stenting and new technology. *Nat Clin Pract Gastroenterol Hepatol* 2005;**2**:365–374.

10 Small AJ, Coelho-Prabhu N, Baron TH: Endoscopic placement of self-expandable metal stents for malignant colonic obstruction: long-term outcomes and complication factors. *Gastrointest Endosc* 2010;**71**:560–572.

11 Repici A, Adler DG, Gibbs CM, et al.: Stenting of the proximal colon in patients with malignant large bowel obstruction: techniques and outcomes. *Gastrointest Endosc* 2007;**66**:940–944.

12 Repici A, Fregonese D, Costamagna G, et al.: Ultraflex precision colonic stent placement for palliation of malignant colonic obstruction: a prospective multicenter study. *Gastrointest Endosc* 2007;**66**:920–927.

25 ERCP Management of Complicated Stone Disease of the Bile Duct and Pancreas

Nithin Karanth[1], Jonathan Cohen[2], & Gregory B. Haber[1]

[1]Lenox Hill Hospital, New York, NY, USA
[2]New York University School of Medicine, New York, NY, USA

Calculi of the biliary tract and pancreatic duct are a frequent problem encountered by the endoscopist. Indeed, while the majority of these stones can be removed via basic standard techniques of endoscopic retrograde cholangiopancreatography (ERCP), there remains those which will require a more advanced skill set. This chapter reviews the issues in stone disease of the pancreatobiliary tract that pose a challenge to the endoscopist, the tools available to deal with these problems, and the ideal ways in which competence in these techniques can be achieved and maintained.

A view adopted by the American Society for Gastrointestinal Endoscopy (ASGE) is that the inherent difficulty of an attempted ERCP procedure should be taken into account when using success rates (i.e., selective cannulation, clearance of stones from ducts) as a benchmark to gauge proficiency in a technique. It is therefore essential to be able to recognize potential factors that would make an ERCP fundamentally more difficult. There is a routinely used three-tier system assigning complexity to ERCPs. Standard, grade 1, include those stones ≤1 cm of the biliary tract that can be treated with standard endoscopic biliary sphincterotomy and removal via retrieval balloon or wire basket. Those classified as advanced, grade 2, involve removal of stones >1 cm. Tertiary, or grade 3 difficulty, encompass intrahepatic stones or any calculi removed via lithotripsy and all therapeutic pancreatic procedures. It is recommended that management of pancreatic duct stones, as well as any patients with Billroth II anatomy, be generally reserved for the advanced trainee [1,2]. Current recommendations are that those ERCP endoscopists with lower levels of expertise should not attempt cases with difficulty of grade 2 or 3 [3,4].

Proficiency in standard ERCP techniques such as selective cannulation and sphincterotomy should be attained before attempting to acquire the skills necessary for advanced procedures. Many reported series have shown that 85–95% of common bile duct stones and 50–75% of pancreatic stones can be successfully treated with basic approaches including sphincterotomy and retrieval of calculi with retrieval balloon and/or wire basket [3,5]. Training in

ERCP and stone removal using these standard techniques are covered in depth in a separate chapter in this textbook. Nevertheless, the presence of impacted or adherent stones, intrahepatic calculi, large stones (>10 mm), small diameter ducts, strictures, or aberrant anatomy can be confounding factors making removal of the pancreaticobiliary stones a very challenging proposition [3–5]. It is recommended that those trainees seeking to acquire the skills needed for treatment of complicated stone diseases of the pancreas and biliary system should pursue them in a formal training program.

As is the case in all aspects of endoscopy, it is essential that the trainee obtain technical competence in conjunction with the cognitive aspects of pancreaticobiliary stone disease. Comprehensive knowledge of the anatomy and physiology of the pancreaticobiliary system, as well as common anatomical variants, is vital. In addition, trainees should have a thorough understanding of the indications, limitations, contraindications, and complications of the various modalities used for complicated stone disease. During training, it is imperative that the trainees acquire knowledge of all the various catheters, guide wires, sphincterotomes, and devices at their disposal, and achieve proficiency in the handling of them [1–4]. As one technique or device does not work in all situations, trainees need to be exposed to and gain proficiency with a range of tools and techniques designed for the management of difficult stones. Physicians seeking advanced-tier ERCP training should do so in a high volume center with faculty accomplished in these techniques [6]. Numerous studies have shown that case volume is an independent predictor of ERCP-related complications and outcomes. Adverse outcomes are more likely for physicians performing less than 50 ERCPs annually and for centers performing less than 200 ERCPs annually [7]. Advanced therapeutic endoscopists should know the limitations of their skills, and recognize when involvement of surgery or interventional radiology is needed; thus, training in a center with these services readily available is key. In fact, perhaps the most important teaching to impress

Successful Training in Gastrointestinal Endoscopy, First Edition. Edited by Jonathan Cohen.
© 2011 Blackwell Publishing Ltd. Published 2011 by Blackwell Publishing Ltd.

upon the trainee is the ability to have a candid appraisal of their own abilities, recognizing when to consider stent placement as a temporizing measure and send selected patients elsewhere. This ability may possibly be the greatest safeguard in avoiding ERCP-related complications.

Mechanical lithotripsy

When standard techniques fail to clear stones from the biliary and/or pancreatic duct, mechanical lithotripsy can increase the success rate to greater than 90 to 95%. In cases where the biliary stone's diameter exceeds 10 mm, a mechanical lithotripter is often necessary. An endoscopic biliary sphincterotomy (as described in an earlier chapter) must be performed prior to attempting mechanical lithotripsy. The basic principle of mechanical lithotripsy is first to capture the stone securely, then to close the wires to the extent possible around it. Next, a metal sheath is advanced over the basket wires, sometimes after replacing the Teflon sheath of the basket with the firmer metal one. Then external pressure is applied to the basket wires in an attempt to crush the stone between the wires and the metal sheath. Various devices and methods are available to perform this basic operation and trainees should be familiar with all of them.

When possible, a first lesson is to try to anticipate when mechanical lithotripsy might be needed based on the size of the stone, the size of the duct, or the presence of any strictures. This begins with an accurate interpretation of preERCP radiologic information such as MRCP; in some circumstances, as in the case of stones above strictures and intrahepatic duct stones, this can provide information that may not be immediately obvious on the initial cholangiogram (Figure 25.1). In general, if there is a stone for which lithotripsy is anticipated, efforts to ensure a sufficiently

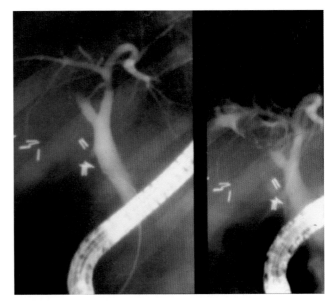

Figure 25.1 Initial cholangiogram fails to appreciate this large intrahepatic duct stone that might be anticipated on close examination of non-invasive pre-ERCP imaging such as an MRCP.

large sphincterotomy and maximal clearance of smaller stones distal to the larger stone using standard methods before attempting lithotripsy are advisable (Figure 25.2). Trainees should learn that lithotripsy occurs in two circumstances: first, when they are attempting to clear a stone using standard methods and the stone captured in the Dormia basket is found to be too large to be extracted in one piece. In this circumstance, if the stone cannot be dislodged from the basket, then it will need to be mechanically crushed. Second, when lithotripsy is clearly going to be required, a

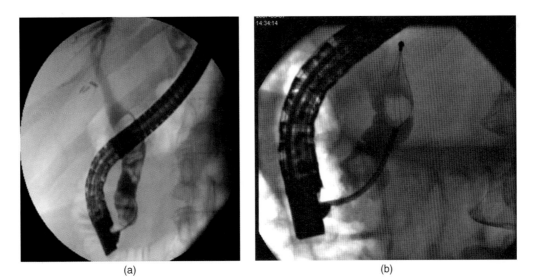

(a)   (b)

Figure 25.2 Trainees must learn to take steps to facilitate removal of large stones. (a) The cholangiogram in this case shows multiple small distal stones, which must be removed prior to attempting to extract the large proximal stone, and a sufficiently large sphincterotomy is required. (b) This image demonstrates a common error in grabbing a large proximal stone before addressing the large stone more distal first. Unless mechanical lithotripsy is planned, it will be quite difficult to extract the stone captured in the basket as shown.

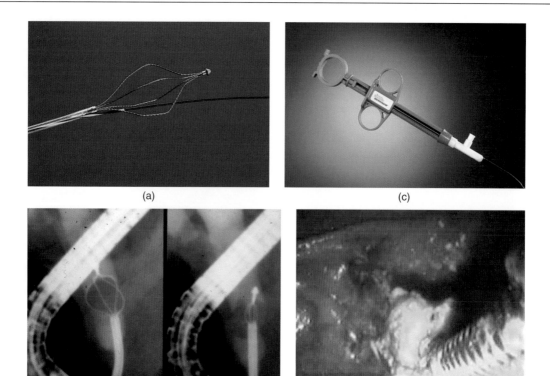

(a)

(c)

(b)

(d)

Figure 25.3 Through the scope mechanical lithotripsy using a Trapezoid basket (Boston Scientific Corp. Natick, MA, USA). (a) Basket monorailed over wire to facilitate access beyond a large stone. (b) Fluoroscopic image of stone once it has been captured and the basket has been closed on the left and then after crushing of the stone on the right. Note the position in the middle of the bile duct without angulation.

(c) Handle of basket can be closed manually or by placing it in a pneumatic dilation pump. (d) Endoscopic image of metal sheath and stone fragments. Following crushing the stone, the basket can be reopened for subsequent lithotripsy or used as a regular Dormia basket to remove fragments from the bile duct.

special basket designed to perform through the scope mechanical lithotripsy should be deployed initially to both capture and crush the stone. Commonly used devices for this include the Trapezoid baskets (Boston Scientific Corp., Natick, MA, USA) (Figure 25.3) and the LithoCrush V (Olympus America Inc., Center Valley, PA, USA) (Figure 25.4).

A Dormia basket, a reinforced basket with double length traction wire and a Teflon sheath, is used to capture the stone and then gently draw the stone towards the distal common bile duct (cbd). If the stone cannot be extracted, the handle and Teflon sheath can be removed from the device and replaced with a metal coil with an outer diameter of 6–9 Fr. A separate lithotripter handle with a knurled screw is then employed to draw the basket into the metal coil. The filaments of the basket cut through the stone as they are drawn into the metal coil. It is via this step by which mechanical fragmentation of the stone is achieved. In order to avoid impaction of stone fragments in the distal common bile duct, it is important to advance the basket (with the captured stone) into the middle of the duct prior to stone fragmentation. Once the stone is suc-

cessfully broken up, the duct can be cleared using basic ERCP techniques previously described [5,8,9].

Impaction of a "trapped" basket around a stone, fracture of the main operation wire, malfunction of the mechanical lithotripter crank handle, and ductal injury are the most frequently encountered complications of mechanical lithotripsy. These complications have been reported to occur with a varying frequency from 0.8 to 6%. Evaluations of reported complications and their treatments reveal that adverse events occurring during mechanical lithotripsy could be successfully managed endoscopically 94% of the time.

A captured stone that is hard and resists fragmentation can place a great deal of stress on all four branches of the basket, leading to fracture of the traction wire. The use of Dormia baskets with predetermined breaking points at either the base or tip of the lithotripter basket can reduce the risk of fracturing the traction wire. Despite these manufacturing modifications, traction wire fracture can still occur. An extension of the sphincterotomy and attempted dislodgement of the stone with changing of the basket is

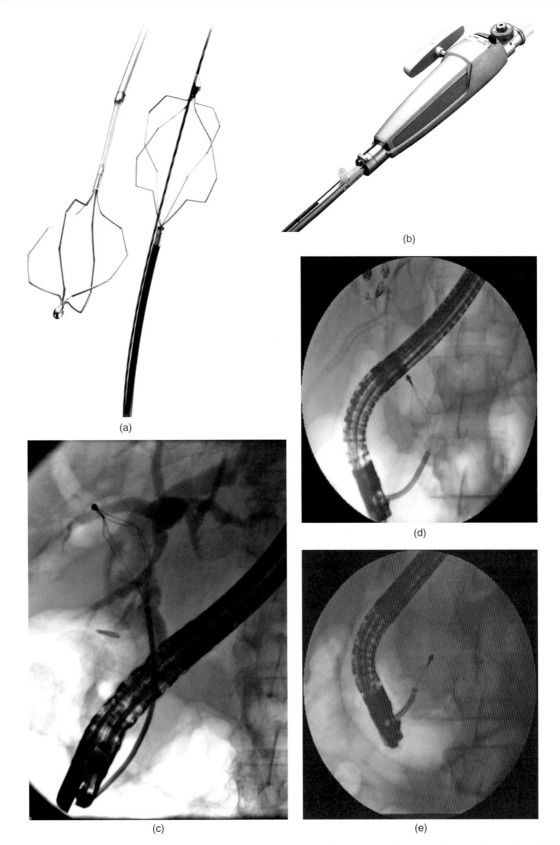

Figure 25.4 LithoCrush V Mechanical Lithotripsy (Olympus America Inc., Center Valley, PA, USA). (a) Image of open basket. (b) Reusable handle attaches to the disposable basket. Once stone is captured, the handle is turned to close basket on stone and pull the wires towards the metal sheath to crush the stone. (c) Open basket in bile duct. (d) Closure of the basket over the captured stone. (e) Fluoroscopic image of crushing of the stone.

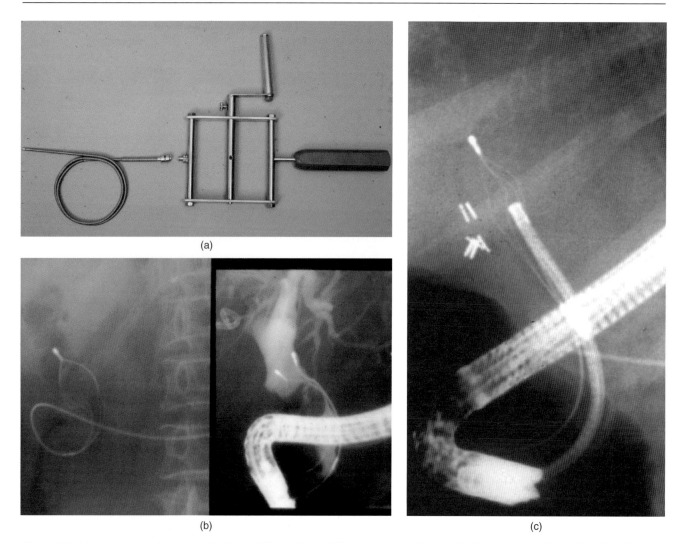

Figure 25.5 Salvage techniques for impacted baskets. (a) The Soehendra lithotripter crank and metal sheath that is deployed over the basket wires once the duodenoscope has been removed. If the basket traction wires fail, the basket and stone may be recaptured by a through the scope mechanical lithotripsy basket (b) and crushed together as shown in (c).

a frequently attempted solution. If the wire break point is outside the mouth, prompt exchange of the initial 80 cm metal sheath for one of a shorter length of 50–70 cm will often allow for seamless continuation of the lithotripsy procedure [5,8].

When a stone proves to be too hard to be crushed with the standard Dormia basket lithotripter, a Soehendra endotripter can be utilized (Figure 25.5). The shaft of the endotripter is shorter and thicker than the metal coil of the standard lithotripter, providing this with more force by which to break up durable stones. The duodenoscope is removed, and the endotripter is advanced over the basket under fluoroscopic guidance. The impacted stones are then either crushed or the wires of the trapped Dormia basket are fractured, in either case resolving the impaction (Video 25.1) [5,8,9]. It is essential that the trainee be well versed in this salvage method and the operations of the necessary equipment to do so, and it is equally important that the staff be similarly familiar with the technique.

One key to successful training in large stone management is the use of careful planning to avoid more cumbersome and lengthy salvage maneuvers by optimal initial therapeutic choices. Specifically, when the removal of a stone by standard techniques is questionable, initial attempts using a readily deflatable balloon may be favored over a Dormia basket if there is some likelihood that it will get stuck. Deflation followed by sphincterotomy extension or dilation may be easier than resorting to lithotripsy.

The other optimal strategy is to properly anticipate when lithotripsy is likely and in those cases begin directly with the through the scope lithotripsy basket of an appropriately large enough size to capture the stone. Trainees should learn which stones are likely to require lithotripsy, and understand how to operate the equipment, including putting the accessories together and performing the assistant's role in manipulation of the crushing handle. Even though it is essential for sufficient inservicing of ERCP assistants to remain familiar with this equipment, a trainee must learn to operate it as well in the event that the staff at hand is at all unclear about the equipment (Video 25.2).

Overall, the complication rate of mechanical lithotripsy in the pancreatic duct is nearly three times greater than that seen in the biliary tract. Pancreatic duct stones are harder than bile duct stones, making mechanical lithotripsy particularly difficult in this circumstance. Nevertheless, the most frequently encountered problems seen remain trapped or broken baskets and rupture of the traction wire. Management of these troublesome events is the same as described above for the common bile duct.

While large bile duct stone clearance should be possible in one or two sessions in most instances, trainees need to be aware of the most common reasons why mechanical lithotripsy may fail and when to consider other methods. Problems capturing the stone are often the most likely reason for mechanical lithotripsy failure. In some cases, there is too little room around the stone to pass the lithotripsy basket. A wire-guided technique may be used to help traverse the giant stone, open the basket and attempt capture on withdrawal. Another common problem is related to the presence of strictures. Stones larger than 2 cm or bigger than the diameter of the duct at the point of impaction are also particularly difficult to manage in this way, and the trainee should recognize that additional methods such as electrohydraulic lithotripsy (EHL) or laser lithotripsy may be required in these situations (Figure 25.6).

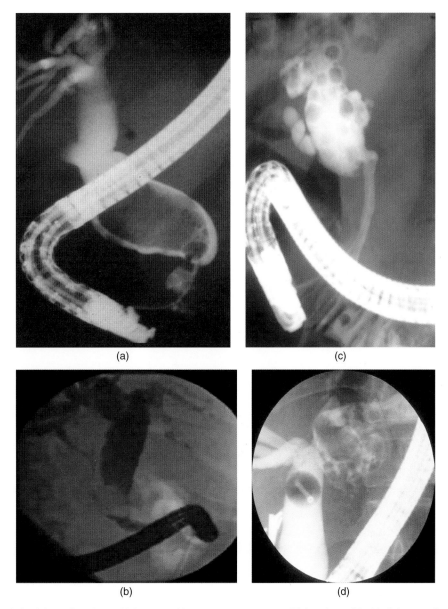

(a)

(c)

(b)

(d)

Figure 25.6 Stones at risk for failure of mechanical lithotripsy. (a) A giant stone >2 cm unlikely to be grabbed by lithotripsy basket. (b) Stones occupying the entire diameter of the bile duct making passage of lithotripsy basket alongside and above problematic. (c) Stones above biliary stricture. (d) Intrahepatic duct stones.

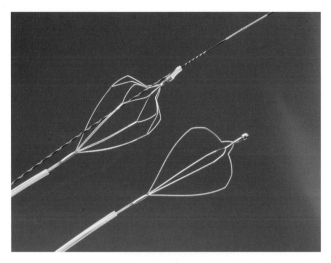

Figure 25.7 Photo of the open Flower basket (top) next to standard stone extraction 4-wire basket (below). The eight wires on the distal end of the Flower basket (Olympus America Inc., Center Valley, PA, USA) (top) are well suited to facilitate the retrieval of small stone fragments following lithotripsy.

Following successful mechanical lithotripsy of the large stones, trainees must learn to proceed to meticulously clear the duct of all fragments. This can be problematic in the very large diameter bile duct, often larger than the 15 mm balloons. On occasion, a special "Flower basket" (Olympus America Inc., Center Valley, PA, USA) with eight wires on the proximal half of the basket may be useful in retrieving small fragments (Figure 25.7). The trainee must be able to assess the fluoroscopic images and determine whether post-lithotripsy temporary placement of a pigtail biliary stent is necessary to ensure drainage in the event of unremoved residual fragments. Anyone learning to tackle large and challenging stone

management need to be well versed in the placement of biliary stents beforehand in the event of the need to place stents for this reason, or more importantly to ensure drainage in the event of a refractory large stone that will require additional methods at a later date.

Large diameter balloon sphincteroplasty

An alternative method to mechanical lithotripsy in the removal of large stones has been the use of large diameter dilation balloons, 12–18 mm in diameter, across the biliary sphincter with subsequent removal of large stones in one piece [10,11] (Figure 25.8). While case series have been reported using this technique, serious complications of bleeding and perforation have occurred, applicability may be limited, and the size of balloon utilized cannot be larger than the diameter of the distal duct. Trainees should be aware of this technique, but at present, it is best reserved for the most experienced endoscopists at tertiary centers with appropriate hospital backup in the event of severe adverse events.

Cholangiopancreatoscopy

Cholangiopancreatoscopy has been frequently used to assist in the removal of difficult pancreatic and bile duct stones. The major advantage of this endoscopic advancement is the ability to directly visualize large intraductal stones. The technique, various scopes, and accessories are reviewed extensively in another chapter. The 2.8 to 3.4 mm cholangioscopes with working lengths of 190 to 220 cm can be passed through a 4.2 mm working channel of a therapeutic duodenoscope. The larger cholangioscopes have a 1.2 mm working channel that allows the use of various other therapeutic accessories for management of stone disease as described

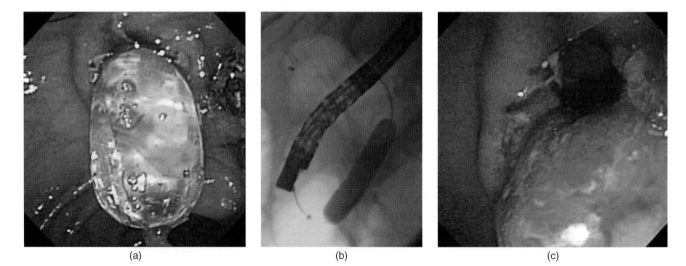

(a)   (b)   (c)

Figure 25.8 The use of large diameter papillary balloon dilation to extract large CBD stones is demonstrated. In this case, a small initial sphincterotomy has been made, perhaps lessening the risk of postdilation pancreatitis. (a) Endoscopic image of a 16-mm diameter balloon dilation being performed. (b) Fluoroscopic view with the inflated balloon revealing elimination of the waist; the diameter of the balloon was selected to be similar to that of the bile duct. (c) Endoscopic appearance following large diameter balloon dilation prior to attempting to extract the stone without lithotripsy.

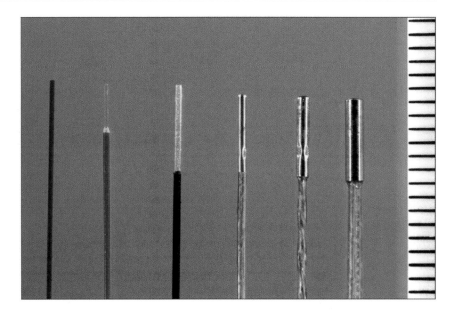

Figure 25.9 EHL and laser probes ranging in diameter from 1 to 4 Fr.

below [12,13,14]. Recently, the passage of ultrathin videogastroscopes directly into the bile duct for use in management of large stones has been described [15]. This may be achieved over a guide wire or using an anchoring balloon with a detachable handle.

Electrohydraulic lithotripsy

Electrohydraulic lithotripsy (EHL) provides the capability of focusing high-energy shock waves to a small area. This presents an effective means by which to treat difficult biliary and pancreatic stones, as well as mechanical basket impactions. Fragmentation of stones occurs by means of a series of spark charges created from a bipolar electrode placed at the surface of the stones while in an aqueous medium. The resultant high-amplitude hydraulic shock waves' energy is then transmitted to the stone, resulting in its destruction [14,16,17]. EHL offers a relatively lower cost technology in comparison to laser lithotripsy, and is available at most tertiary endoscopic centers. Endoscopists should attempt EHL only after having sufficient experience in advanced techniques of pancreatobiliary endoscopy. Furthermore, we recommend that comfort with EHL first be attained with biliary stones, given their softer nature, easier fragmentation, and better visualization prior to attempting treatment of pancreatic duct stones [18].

It is vital that the intensity of the shock waves produced be centered upon the target stones, otherwise ductal injury might ensue. As a result, it is recommended that EHL be only executed under direct visualization, using cholangiopancreatoscopy, since the use of a solely fluoroscopically-guided EHL probe might produce inadvertent tissue injury [14,16]. Current EHL probes measure 1.9 to 3.3 F, while the working channels of available cholangioscopes are 1.2 mm (Figure 25.9). Consequently, perifiber space is at best sparse, requiring great care when passing the EHL fiber through the working channel in order to avert kinking or breaking [17]. It is advised to straighten the cholangioscope when passing the EHL fiber, since the fiber is rigid and can easily damage the deflecting

joint of the scope. The accessory channel is commonly lubricated using silicone, olive oil, or cooking spray prior to advancing the EHL fiber to the tip, but not out of, the scope. The cholangioscope is subsequently loaded into the therapeutic duodenoscope, and used to cannulate the duct of interest. To facilitate cannulation, sphincterotomy of the selected duct should be performed if not previously done. Continuous irrigation of saline into the duct is then used to provide a fluid medium that amplifies the EHL power by tenfold, and allows the creation of the shock waves necessary for stone fragmentation. This is usually accomplished via a simple side arm device and water pump, or less preferably, pre-placement of a nasobiliary catheter (Figure 25.10). Pushing the miniendoscope into the long position will usually facilitate further advancement of the EHL fiber. The fiber should then be secured such that the probe protrudes no greater than 2 to 3 mm out of the scope. Subsequent maneuvering of the mother scope in conjunction with the operation of the daughter scope controls allows positioning of the fiber tip *en face* with the surface of the stone. The tip of the EHL

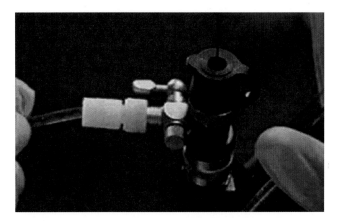

Figure 25.10 This photo illustrates the stopcock coaxial system that attaches to the accessory channel of the babyscope to facilitate the necessary continuous irrigation during EHL or laser lithotripsy.

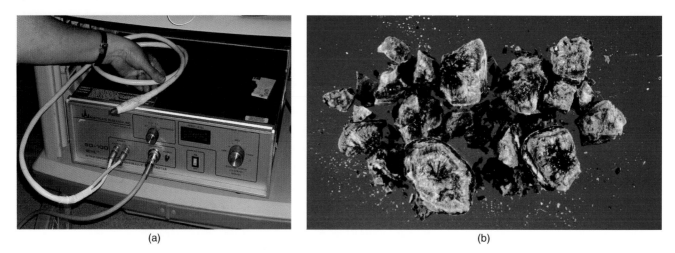

(a)   (b)

Figure 25.11 (a) Nortech AUTOLITH system (Northgaste Technologies Inc., Elgin, IL, USA) EHL generator. (b) EHL fractures the target stone in large pieces that can be retrieved using standard techniques.

fiber should be as close as to the stone as possible. Although the fiber can abut the stone if needed, such contact may reduce the functional lifespan of the EHL probe. As previously stated, it is essential that the ducts be continuously filled with saline during EHL. Not only does this provide the medium necessary for the functionality of EHL, but also allows the ducts to be flushed of stone debris after fragmentation.

Once ideal positioning of the fiber tip in relation to the stone is accomplished, the generator's foot pedal is depressed to deliver energy according to a preset power wattage usually in the range of 70 to 100 W (Figure 25.11). This is commonly provided at a frequency of 5 to 6 electrical impulses per second or as continuous pulsations. Usually, we start with a power setting of 70 W and increase by 10 W as necessary to a maximum of 100 W until fragmentation of the stone is accomplished. As the intraductal lithotripsy is performed, the transmitted energy can result in recoil of the EHL fiber back into the working channel or deflect the tip of the scope. It is essential to constantly monitor the position of the EHL fiber by endoscopic and fluoroscopic confirmation to help reduce potential injury to the duct or endoscope. Continuous saline flushing of the duct will assist in maintaining the visual field clear of debris [14,16,18]. After successful EHL, the fragmented stones are removed from the duct either by retrieval balloon and/or wire basket (Video 25.3). Antibiotics are administered at the physician's discretion based upon the case; however, routine prophylaxis is not necessary. Trainees need to be aware of current ASGE guidelines relating to indications for antibiotic prophylaxis, typically in ERCP reserved for procedures in patients with an obstructed bile duct.

Retrospective review of patients referred for EHL revealed success rates for stone fragmentation at 96%, making it a very effective weapon in dealing with difficult stone disease of the pancreatobiliary tree. Fragmentation failures are most often secondary to either hard stones or targeting problems. With calculi located in the left intrahepatic duct, it can often be difficult to navigate the acute angle with the daughter scope and obtain visualization of the

stone [16]. In some circumstances, achieving optimal access for stone targeting will require a percutaneous transhepatic cholangiogram and development of a tract with serial dilations to allow ultimate passage of a cholangioscope. Furthermore, failure to clear the ducts is increased in the setting of stones located above a stricture. Often, it is necessary to perform dilatation of the stricture prior to EHL in this circumstance. If performing EHL to treat a pancreatic duct stone, temporary placement of a pancreatic stent is advised with anticipation of its spontaneous passage during the recovery period.

The most commonly reported complications of EHL are hemobilia and ductal perforation attributed to inadvertent contact of the probe against the duct wall. The overall risk of these adverse events is estimated at 1%. Hemobilia can often be therapeutically addressed with local injection of epinephrine through the cholangioscope.

Perforation of the duct has been reported to be successfully managed endoscopically with placement of an overlying stent [16,18].

Laser lithotripsy

An alternative to EHL fragmentation of stones is laser lithotripsy. This technology works with the transmission of a laser beam by a flexible quartz fiber through the working channel of a cholangioscope. Repetitive pulses of focused laser light creates a power density in which electrons are torn away from their nuclei, transforming matter into a gaseous collection of ions and free electrons. This plasma created at the stone surface and surrounding fluid rapidly expands as it absorbs further laser energy, and then collapses, generating a spherical shock wave which results in stone fragmentation [19,20] Trainees will quickly notice that the laser pulverizes the stone into tiny fragments in contrast to the large fractured pieces that result from the deployment of the EHL fiber (Figure 25.12).

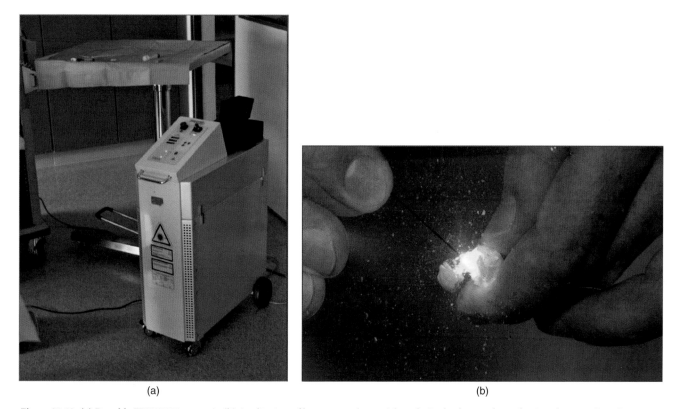

(a)   (b)

Figure 25.12 (a) Portable FREDDY Laser unit. (b) Application of laser to stone material results in shock wave that pulverizes the target into tiny fragments.

Prior to an institution adopting this technology, it is important for the physicians and staff to undergo training in laser safety, with regards to the biological effects and hazards of laser irradiation. As is standard practice with fluoroscopy, the procedure room door should be closed with a posted sign during active use of the laser. Use of laser eye protectors is recommended at all times during performance of laser lithotripsy. Widespread use of laser lithotripsy at endoscopic centers has been lacking primarily as a result of the great costs and limited availability of the necessary equipment [17].

Given the substantial power generated by the laser, it is reasonable to assume that inadvertent damage to the duct could occur. This has been verified in several in vitro and in vivo animal studies, which demonstrated that deep injury and perforation of the duct can occur with direct contact and perpendicular angulation of the laser fiber in relation to the duct wall. Moreover, injury was worsened with increasing pulse energies and exposure time. It is this finding that provided the basis for the development of a stone tissue detection system (STDS). This safety mechanism uses a small fraction of laser pulse energy, about 1 to 2%, to induce characteristic fluorescent radiation at the surface of the target. The created light is then transmitted back to the laser fiber where analysis of its intensity in a spectral range is performed. If the level is below a predefined threshold value, the laser pulse is automatically halted by a fast optical switch. As a result, a very small amount of laser pulse energy could be misapplied, limiting the amount of tissue absorption and injury [21,22].

The two types of laser technology available for lithotripsy are flashlamp-pumped pulsed dye lasers, such as rhodamine 6G dye, and pulsed solid-state lasers, such as Q-switched neodymium:YAG lasers. Versions of the STDS have been coupled to the rhodamine 6G dye laser and more recently to a frequency-doubled double pulse Q-switched neodymium:YAG laser (FREDDY) [21,22]. Like EHL, laser lithotripsy requires a specialized mother–daughter scope system permitting direct visualization of the stone in the duct. Nevertheless, with lasers coupled to STDS, fluoroscopic guidance alone of the laser fiber has been described, since the laser pulse would be terminated if contact with the stone were lost, preventing potential harm to the duct [21] (Video 25.4).

It is important to calibrate the output power and place the laser in off or standby mode prior to inserting the optical fiber into the working channel. The fiber should be secured to the endoscope to prevent accidental dislodgement. Rhodamine 6G dye laser is operated at pulse energies of up to 150 mJ, durations of 2.5 μs and repetition rates up to 10 Hz with the flexible quartz fiber in direct gentle contact with the surface of the stone [19,23]. Continuous ductal irrigation around the stone with saline is performed during laser lithotripsy similar to EHL. The fluid is essential in achieving effective propagation of the laser-induced shock waves. For laser systems with STDS, "blind fragmentation" of the stones can be performed without cholangioscopy. A 7 F metal marked catheter with a central laser fiber is advanced into the bile duct using a standard duodenoscope with fluoroscopy. The catheter is continuously perfused with a solution of 50% saline and 50% water-soluble nonionic contrast [21].

The application of laser lithotripsy to pancreatic duct stones is still evolving.

Extracorporeal shock wave lithotripsy and pancreatic duct stones

Endoscopic pancreatic sphincterotomy (EPS) is the initial step in preparing for pancreatic stone extraction. EPS is performed after deep cannulation of the main pancreatic duct is obtained with a standard pull-type sphincterotome advanced over a guide wire [24]. It is important that only a pure cutting current be employed in order to avoid damage to the pancreas and development of stenosis. Another EPS technique is to first place a pancreatic stent and then use a needle-knife to cut the pancreatic sphincter. Unfortunately, stent insertion in the setting of chronic pancreatitis is often difficult prior to stone removal, limiting the utility of this latter technique. If a dominant dorsal duct is encountered (i.e., pancreas divisum), EPS can be performed on the minor papilla using the same technique as that normally used on the major papilla. Complication rates of EPS in patients with chronic pancreatitis seem to be lower than for other indications, likely secondary to the accompanying periductal fibrosis and limited amount of adjacent acinar tissue. The endoscopic removal of pancreatic duct stones after EPS depends upon several factors: stones larger than 10 mm, more than three stones in the duct, location of stones in distal body or tail of pancreas, and strictures of the duct are all features negatively impacting successful outcome [24–27]. Such cases will often require additional steps to attain clearance of the duct (Video 25.5).

Prior to stone extraction, pancreatic duct strictures downstream from the calculi must be treated with dilation, using a 4–6 mm hydrostatic balloon catheter, and often subsequent stent placement. Given that larger bore stents have longer patency rates, the polyethylene stents employed are those with the largest diameter (8.5 or 10 F) that can traverse the stricture. Attempts at clearance of stones from the pancreatic duct can be subsequently attempted with basket or balloon. Nevertheless, having impacted, large and/or hard stones can result in the inability to achieve extraction of the calculi. Confounding the difficulty in confirming clearance of the duct is the fact that the pancreatic stones might be isodense with the injected contrast, preventing adequate fluoroscopic visualization [24–27].

Extracorporeal shock wave lithotripsy (ESWL) is a successful modality for the treatment of refractory biliary and pancreatic duct calculi [28–30]. Allowing the millimetric fragmentation of stones, the procedure facilitates subsequent endoscopic clearance of the pancreatobiliary tract. A commonly used application for ESWL is in the treatment of chronic calcified pancreatitis. Sufficient visualization of the pancreatic and neighboring anatomy is crucial prior to performing ESWL. This can usually be accomplished by obtaining plain films of the pancreatic region in left and right positions and an MRCP. Contraindications to the procedure are calcified aneurysms, lung tissue, or bone in the path

of the shock waves. In patients with a history of cardiac arrhythmias, ectopic ventricular beats can be seen during lithotripsy. As a result, in such patients shock waves should be delivered during the refractory period to steer clear of inducing possible ventricular arrhythmias.

Patients undergoing ESWL are placed in the prone position with minimal left lateral decubitus directionality to help separate the stone from the spine as the shock waves enter the body from the ventral aspect. Conscious or general anesthesia is provided, with the latter usually used in patients planned for ESWL and therapeutic ERCP during the same session [28–30]. As previously mentioned, the stones are identified in a focal area by using radiographic imaging prior to lithotripsy. The shock waves generated during the procedure occur in degassed water and are directed into the patient by means of a water cushion or basin. The deployment of several thousand shock waves to the stone in the predetermined focal area results in rapidly rising pressures in a concentrated field causing fragmentation of the calculi.

The stones located most downstream towards the pancreatic head should be targeted first, thus allowing drainage of debris through the papilla. Some endoscopic centers use the highest possible energy setting ($0.54 \ mJ/mm^2$) and deliver a total of 3000 to 5000 shock waves in one treatment session. If planning on performing therapeutic ERCP within a few hours after ESWL, it is recommended that the energy level be reduced to a maximum of approximately $0.33 \ mJ/mm^2$. Such a reduction in the power setting minimizes the amount of duodenal edema and erosions that might ensue, which might limit the subsequent endoscopic treatment [28]. ESWL treatment sessions usually require 45 min to 1 hour to perform. Following successful stone fragmentation, standard ERCP is performed to evaluate the duct and extract debris.

Overall morbidity from the ESWL and therapeutic ERCP is mainly attributed to complications stemming from the endoscopic portion of the therapy. The erosions seen in the gastric antrum and duodenum following ESWL is usually of minimal clinical consequence. It is important to warn the patient ahead of time that petechiae are commonly noted on the skin overlying the field penetrated by the shock waves. Again, this finding is of minimal long-term significance [28–30].

Difficult anatomy

There is a long and varied list of surgical procedures that result in altered anatomy often resulting in great lengths of bowel needing to be navigated by the endoscopist in order to gain biliary access. Such procedures include, but are not limited to, partial gastrectomy with a Billroth II gastrojejunostomy; Whipple resection with a Roux-en-Y limb of jejunum anastamosed to the pancreatobiliary ducts; and gastrojejunal bypass for obesity with a Roux limb of jejunum anastamosed to a small gastric pouch, just to name a few. It is important to have a discussion prior to the attempted ERCP with the surgeon in order to know what anatomical changes can be expected.

Various approaches to traverse the bowel include pediatric colonoscopes, push enteroscopes, spiral overtube assisted enteroscopes, and single or double balloon enteroscopes (DBE). The DBE system is particularly useful in cases with a long afferent limb. The details and techniques of small bowel enteroscopy are featured in a separate chapter of this textbook. It is important to ensure that the proper accessories are available, especially for DBE. The therapeutic DBE scope has a therapeutic channel of 2.8 mm and can therefore accommodate the diameter of most standard accessories. Nevertheless, needle knives, sphincterotomes, retrieval balloons, and baskets need to be specially ordered, since the standard version of these accessories would not be of sufficient length needed for the 2 m enteroscope.

Clearly, the use of a forward viewing endoscope lacking an elevator presents additional challenges in obtaining cannulation. In our opinion, papillary cannulation is best achieved with a straight dual lumen catheter with a hydrophilic tip guide wire and a separate channel for contrast. Once cannulation is accomplished, exchange of accessories can be performed over the wire in standard fashion. The easiest approach for sphincterotomy in these circumstances is placement of a stent followed by a needle knife cut over it. If a sufficiently long needle knife is not available, it is possible to adapt a snare by cutting off half of the snare loop and using the free end of the other half for the sphincterotomy. When performing stone extraction, it is prudent to be modest in the size of the sphincterotomy and use increased traction on the stone rather than make a larger cut with a greater potential for complications. If a larger stone is encountered, a balloon dilation after modest sphincterotomy is advisable [31].

Training modalities

A variety of novel training methods including the use of *ex vivo* simulators have been introduced to enhance instruction in therapeutic endoscopic techniques, and these are described in detail in other chapters of this book. Certainly, table top training can familiarize trainees with the accessories from setup to generator settings to communication steps with staff. Such simulator work provides excellent risk-free and pressure-free settings to transmit some of the technical skills and cognitive information detailed above in this chapter prior to and in parallel with the performance of real procedures with expert instruction. Large stone material can be placed in artificial tissue bile ducts attached via a Neo-papilla to the porcine *ex vivo* model to allow for simulation of mechanical lithotripsy [32]. Hands-on workshops on choledochoscopy (without stone therapy) via arterial tissue connected to the porcine duodenum have been conducted at the New York Society for Gastrointestinal Endoscopy (NYSGE) annual meeting in December 2009 and 2010. While this training appears to be a promising adjunct to education in this field, there is no data yet demonstrating any objective benefit from such experiences. Because at expert centers the stone clearance rate using standard methods alone or standard methods along with mechanical lithotripsy is so high, there are truly very few institutions with enough recalcitrant stones to generate a very high volume of EHL and/or laser cases on which to teach these techniques. This obstacle to training makes large bile duct stones

an ideal candidate for further development of simulator-based training once its benefit has been properly validated.

To supplement supervised formal training in management of large stones, there are excellent teaching videos available for purchase via the ASGE Learning Center or for free viewing and download from the Digital Atlas of Video Education (DAVE) Project [http://daveproject.org/]. Similarly, large stone cases are commonly presented at the various live endoscopy courses (Video 25.6). Such didactic learning is probably most helpful for experienced ERCPists looking for clinical pearls to refine existing technique and for advanced fellows concurrently immersed in performing real cases. It is well established that short courses and live demonstrations are no substitute for mentored, intensive instruction while performing real cases under the supervision of an expert.

Competency

How much supervised experience is needed to become competent to independently tackle these large bile duct stones and pancreatic duct stones? There is no data to suggest how many cases are typically performed before achieving the kinds of benchmark excellent stone clearance rates with low associated morbidity and adverse events that were described above. Mindful of reported outcome data from published series of large stone management, trainees and practicing ERCPists alike should track their own success rates both in terms of total stone clearance and the number of procedures required per patient to achieve this end.

Videos

Video 25.1 Mechanical lithotripsy
Video 25.2 Through-the-scope mechanical lithotripsy
Video 25.3 Importance of continuous irrigation and proper probe positioning in EHL and laser lithotripsy
Video 25.4 Laser lithotripsy with the Freddy laser
Video 25.5 Holmium laser lithotripsy of pancreatic duct stone
Video 25.6 Giant bile duct stone removal
Video 7.2 Wire guided cannulation following pre-cut sphincterotomy
Video 7.16 Billroth II cannulation with rotatable sphincterotome and guidewire
Video 7.17 Billroth II sphincterotomy utilizing a needle-knife over a common bile duct stent
Video 10.1 Spyglass: techniques in direct biliary visualization
Video 10.2 Electrohydraulic lithotripsy through a cholangioscope

References

1 ASGE Training Committee: ERCP Core Curriculum. *Gastrointest Endosc* 2006;**63**:361–376.
2 Johanson JF, Cooper G, Eisen GM, et al.: Quality assessment of ERCP. *Gastrointest Endosc* 2002;**56**:165–169.

3 ASGE Taskforce on Quality in Endoscopy: Quality Indicators for ERCP. *Gastrointest Endosc* 2006;**63**:S29–S34.

4 ASGE: Principles of training in gastrointestinal endoscopy. *Gastrointest Endosc* 1999;**49**:845-853.

5 Thomas M, Howell D, Carr-Locke D, et al.: Mechanical lithotripsy of pancreatic and biliary stones: complications and available treatment options collected from expert centers. *Am J Gastroenterol* 2007;**102**:1896–1902.

6 Williams EJ, Taylor S, Fairclough P, et al.: Are we meeting the standards set for endoscopy? Results of a large scale prospective study of endoscopic practice. *Gut* 2007;**56**:796–801.

7 Springer J, Enns R, Romagnuolo, et al.: Canadian credentialing guidelines for endoscopic retrograde cholangiopancreatography. *Can J Gastroenterol* 2008;**22**:547–551.

8 Ranjeev P, Goh K: Retrieval of an impacted Dormia basket and stone insitu using a novel method. *Gastrointest Endosc* 2000;**51**:504–506.

9 Hochberger J, Tex S, Maiss J, et al.: Management of difficult common bile duct stones. *Gastrointest Endosc Clin N Am* 2003;**13**:623–634.

10 Jeong S; Ki S-H, Lee DH, et al.: Endoscopic large-balloon sphincteroplasty for the removal of large bile duct stones: a preliminary study. *Gastrointest Endosc* 2009;**70**:915–922.

11 Attasaranya S, Cheon YK, Vittal H, et al.: Large-diameter biliary orifice balloon dilation to aid in endoscopic bile duct stone removal: a multicenter series. *Gastrointest Endosc* 2008;**67**:1046–1052.

12 Judah J, Draganov P: Intraductal biliary and pancreatic endoscopy: an expanding scope of possibility. *World J Gastroenterol* 2008;**14**:3129–3136.

13 ASGE Technology Committee: Cholangiopancreatoscopy. *Gastrointest Endosc* 2008;**68**:411–421.

14 Chen Y, Pleskow D: SpyGlass single-operator peroral cholangiopancreatoscopy system for the diagnosis and therapy of bile-duct disorders: a clinical feasibility study (with video). *Gastrointest Endosc* 2007;**65**:832–841.

15 Moon JH, Ko BM, Hong SJ, et al.: Intraductal balloon-guided direct peroral cholangioscope with an ultraslim upper endoscope (with videos). *Gastrointest Endosc* 2009;**70**:297–302.

16 Arya N, Nelles S, Haber G, et al.: Electrohydraulic lithotripsy in 111 patients: a safe and effective therapy for difficult bile duct stones. *Am J Gastroenterol* 2004;**99**:2330–2334.

17 DiSario J, Chuttani R, Croffie J, et al.: Biliary and pancreatic lithotripsy devices. *Gastrointest Endosc* 2007;**65**:750.

18 Howell D, Dy R, Hanson B, et al.: Endoscopic treatment of pancreatic duct stones using a 10F pancreatoscope and electrohydraulic lithotripsy. *Gastrointest Endosc* 1999;**50**:829–833.

19 Das AK, Chiura A, Conlin MJ, et al.: Treatment of biliary calculi using holmium:YAG laser. *Gastrointest Endosc* 1998;**48**:207.

20 Prat F, Fritsch J, Choury AD, et al.: Laser lithotripsy of difficult biliary stones. *Gastrointest Endosc* 1994;**40**:290.

21 Hochberger J, Bayer J, May A, et al.: Laser lithotripsy of difficult bile duct stones: results in 60 patients using a rhodamine 6G dye laser with optical stone tissue detection system. *Gut* 1998;**43**:829–833.

22 Wilkinson ML: Does laser lithotripsy hit the target? *Gut* 1998;**43**:740.

23 Prat F, Fritsch J, Choury AD, et al.: Laser lithotripsy of difficult biliary stones. *Gastrointest Endosc* 1994;**40**:290.

24 Elton E, Howell D, Parsons WG, et al.: Endoscopic pancreatic sphincterotomy: indications, outcome, and a safe stentless technique. *Gastrointest Endosc* 1998;**47**:240–249.

25 Delhaye M, Matos C, Deviere J: Endoscopic technique for the management of pancreatitis and its complications. *Best Prac & Res Clin Gastroenterol* 2004;**18**:155–181.

26 Neuhaus H: Therapeutic Pancreatic Endoscopy. *Endoscopy* 2004;**36**:8–16.

27 Dumonceau JM, Deviere J, Le Moine O, et al.: Endoscopic pancreatic drainage in chronic pancreatitis associated with ductal stones: long term results. *Gastrointest Endosc* 1996;**43**:547–555.

28 Sackmann M, Holl J, Sauter G, et al.: Extracorporeal shock wave lithotripsy for clearance of bile duct stones resistant to endoscopic extraction. *Gastrointest Endosc* 2001;**53**:27–32.

29 Costamagna G, Gabbrielli A, Mutignani M, et al.: Extracorporeal shock wave lithotripsy of pancreatic stones in chronic pancreatitis: Immediate and medium-term results. *Gastrointest Endosc* 1997;**46**:231.

30 Kozarek R, Brandabur JJ, Ball TJ et al.: Clinical outcomes in patients who undergo extracorporeal sock wave lithotripsy for chronic calcific pancreatitis. *Gastrointest Endosc* 2002;**56**:496.

31 Haber G: Double balloon endoscopy for pancreatic and biliary access in altered anatomy. *Gastrointest Endosc* 2007;**66**:S47–S50.

32 Matthes K, Cohen J: The Neo-Papilla: a new modification of porcine ex vivo simulators for ERCP training (with videos). *Gastrointest Endosc* 2006;**64**:570–576.

26 ERCP Management of Malignancy: Tissue Sampling, Metal Stent Placement and Ampullectomy

Douglas A. Howell

University of Vermont College of Medicine, Burlington, VT, USA;
Pancreaticobiliary Center, Maine Medical Center, Portland, ME, USA

Introduction

Endoscopic biliary stent placement to palliate jaundice has become the treatment of choice with self-expanding metal stents (SEMS) carrying significant patency and cost advantages [1]. Prior to metal stent placement, a secure pathologic diagnosis is almost always warranted.

Increasingly, endoscopic ultrasound (EUS)-guided fine needle aspiration can safely and reliably succeed in tissue sampling. A disadvantage may be the need for a second procedure, an added small risk, problems with availability, and added cost. Access to the hepatic hilum may also be difficult or unsuccessful.

Tissue sampling at ERCP has a long history, with one of the very first sphincterotomies done to introduce a biopsy forceps for bifurcation stricture biopsy in 1973.

Comprehensive tissue sampling to achieve a high yield comparable to EUS requires a special skill set, including training, thorough knowledge of available equipment, and experience [2].

Following tissue diagnosis, biliary stent placement is now routinely appropriate in most obstructive jaundice patients with both resectable and nonresectable malignancies. The choice of an SEMS compared to a temporary plastic stent, the training, equipment choices, and techniques are addressed later in this chapter.

Finally, the special challenge of managing ampullary neoplasms is covered in the last section of the chapter.

Tissue sampling at ERCP

To begin, specimens can be obtained from strictures of the biliary ducts and, rarely, from the pancreatic duct by aspirating bile or pancreatic juice, or performing brush cytology, ERCP-performed fine-needle aspiration (FNA), and forceps biopsy (Video 26.1). Tumors directly involving the duodenal wall, usually just above the papilla in the case of pancreatic cancer, can be similarly sampled.

We will discuss these techniques, the equipment and details of training individually.

Fluid aspiration

In the simplest but lowest yield technique, bile or pancreatic juice can be collected after deep cannulation. This older technique has declined in use and is now rarely reported due to higher yield techniques.

An important observation is that traumatizing the stricture prior to aspiration increases yield. Hard dilators or balloon dilation will disrupt the surface epithelium and permit malignant cells to enter the ducts. These procedures probably should not be employed to exclusively increase yield since better techniques are now more effective.

Brush cytology

Brush cytology remains the most popular technique at ERCP for tissue sampling. The technique and equipment are straightforward.

First, a guide wire is maneuvered through the stricture, usually of the CBD or biliary bifurcation. After an exchange to leave the guide wire in place, a device is placed for brushing.

Several devices are marketed to permit guide wire-assisted sampling:

1 **Geenen brush (Cook Endoscopy):** A guiding catheter is placed over the guide wire and maneuvered above the stricture. A sphincterotomy is not necessary. The guide wire must be removed and the Geenen brush is then advanced through the guiding catheter, advanced out through the end and the catheter is pulled below the stricture. The spring tip of the brush will maintain the position of the brush within the stricture during brushing. Both brush and catheter then are removed after the brush is pulled back into the catheter to prevent the loss of cells. The brush tip is subsequently cut off with wire cutters and placed immediately into transport media. The major disadvantage of this older technique is the loss of guide wire access requiring the replacement of the guide wire by recannulation.

Successful Training in Gastrointestinal Endoscopy, First Edition. Edited by Jonathan Cohen.
© 2011 Blackwell Publishing Ltd. Published 2011 by Blackwell Publishing Ltd.

2 *Monorail brush:* The above described equipment can be altered to maintain access by punching a small hole with a sharp 21-gauge needle about 1–2 cm inside the guiding catheter tip. The guide wire then enters the tip and exits the punched hole. The Geenen brush can then be preloaded prior to advancement over the in-place guide wire. The major difference is that the guide wire must be carefully pulled back to free the guide wire from the guiding catheter after it has been positioned well above the top of the stricture. This has been termed an "intraductal exchange". At no time should the guide wire tip be pulled back below the stricture. After this maneuver, the brush is extended and the stricture is sampled by brushing to and fro. The tip is then pulled back into the catheter and the device is removed leaving the original guide wire in place.

Several newer devices come preloaded and prepunctured for speed and ease (Fusion Cytology brush, Cook Endoscopy; RX Cytology brush, Boston Scientific Corp). These devices, like the monorail device, can be used with a short (260 cm) guide wire.

3 *Double lumen technique:* Two over-the-guide wire techniques using double lumen devices are in use. Preloaded 6 Fr and 8 Fr catheters have a guide wire lumen and a preloaded brush (Cytomax, Cook Endoscopy; RX Cytology Brush, Boston Scientific Corp). In their use, a long guide wire remains in place and the device is simply inserted and the stricture is brushed. The smaller 6 Fr device requires a 0.021 guide wire to be in place and the 8 Fr is compatible with the standard 0.035 guide wire. This larger device is rather stiff and certainly not optimal for pancreatic duct sampling.

4 An additional option for brushing includes a 10 Fr biliary introducer developed at our facility, for comprehensive tissue sampling as well as brushing (HBIN, Cook Endoscopy) (Figure 26.1).

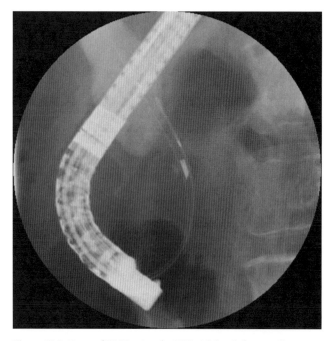

Figure 26.1 X-ray of ERCP using the HBI with brush for sampling.

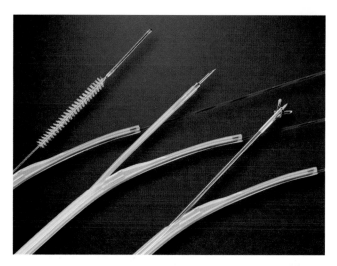

Figure 26.2 HBI and three tissue-sampling devices.

The HBIN device has a double lumen with a 0.035 lumen for the guide wire and a 5 Fr channel to introduce a variety of devices. Furthermore, the 5 Fr channel exits below a long dilating taper and is angled to direct the sampling devices toward the stricture rather than through its axis. Placement does not require sphincterotomy (Figure 26.2).

The device is used to dilate and traumatize the stricture prior to then advancing a flexible nosed brush, through the stricture. The device is advanced so the 5 Fr side port is above the stricture's top margin so the brush can be easily advanced into the dilated duct above. The unit is then pulled down placing considerable pressure on the brush to scrape away cells.

Several points about brushing need to be made at this point:
• Do not pull the brush out of any device as most of the cells will be lost. Always "park" the brush just inside the tip of the device, then remove the entire device being used.

• You must stent the pancreas after transtricture brush sampling of a pancreatic stricture. This explains the rare use of this technique as the management of that stent is then problematic. Therefore, we only use this technique when a pancreatic stent is warranted such as treating a pseudocyst or fistula above a suspected malignant stricture.

• Brush cytology has a low yield despite its popularity. Expect only an 8 to 30% true positive yield. Other techniques have a higher yield and when these are employed, brushing adds little. In our large series of forceps biopsy followed by ERCP FNA, brushing added no additional positives [3]. Our center no longer uses brush cytology as we will discuss later.

Fine needle aspiration

In an attempt to increase positive results compared to the disappointing ERCP brush cytology yield, a Chiba-type 22-gauge needle for FNA in the bile duct was introduced several years ago (HBAN 22, Cook) [4]. This device increased yield by sampling deeper than a brush. The technique of ERCP FNA using this device requires sphincterotomy and then free-hand placement. Technically, placement is moderately difficult due to needle length.

The device has a smooth, atraumatic ball-tip and is loaded with a retractable 22-gauge 7 mm long needle. The needle-containing catheter is precurved to assist in cannulation.

Placement requires placing the ball-tip on the lower edge of the sphincterotomy and sliding the device upwards while slightly advancing the endoscope tip. Placement can almost always be accomplished but does demand some hands-on training and experience.

The needle tip is then advanced into the undersurface of the stricture and forcefully thrust in deeply. After removal of the stylet, gentle aspiration with 10 cc dry syringe is performed, the needle is then withdrawn, and the content of the aspiration is expressed into transport media.

To ease needle catheter placement, a 3 Fr 22-gauge FNA needle was developed to fit down the biliary introducer (HBIN-35, Cook Endoscopy) that was discussed earlier. Placement involves inserting the 10 Fr introducer over the preplaced guide wire; the 3 Fr needle is preloaded in the 5 Fr channel. Care must be used in negotiating the acute retrograde angle to avoid tearing the wall of the HBI when advancing the 5 Fr needle around this sharp bend. When friction is felt, both devices are then advanced together carrying the needle up the duct. The HBI and needle are then pushed up to the lower edge of the CBD stricture and the needle is advanced into the lower aspect of the stricture. The FNA is then performed as described [5] (Video 26.2).

Forceps biopsy and cytology

In multiple studies, biopsy forceps have the highest yield in tissue sampling at ERCP [6]. Multiple forceps, which can be relatively easily introduced, are available, both reusable (ERCP forceps, Olympus; HBIF, Cook), and disposable (Cook and Boston Scientific Corp). In general, pediatric forceps are necessary as gastroscopy standard-size forceps are excessively stiff when advanced over the elevator.

Biopsies can be obtained from proximal strictures or distal biopsies (Figures 26.3 and 26.4).

Introduction requires sphincterotomy unless the biliary introducer (HBI) is used. This device accepts the 5 Fr HBIF (Cook Endoscopy) similar to the FNA needle described. Multiple biopsies are advised with a significant increase in yield by performing six biopsies rather than the standard three [7].

In summary, brush, FNA, and forceps can be employed individually at ERCP but true positive yields of each technique vary and are generally about 30–40%.

Triple sampling

To address these low yields of each of these techniques, centers have reported combining sampling procedures in a single setting. When using all three techniques, called "triple sampling", significantly higher yields are produced [6].

Triple sampling requires considerable effort, training and experience. At present, reports have been confined to only a few dedicated centers. Even so, true positive yields of tissue sampling have only approached 70%–80% for pancreatic cancer.

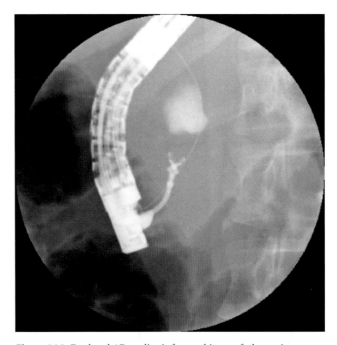

Figure 26.3 Freehand 6 Fr pediatric forceps biopsy of a low stricture at ERCP.

Intraprocedural ERCP tissue diagnosis

A major disadvantage of all techniques of ERCP tissue sampling has been the necessary delay in tissue processing before a definite diagnosis can be made. Although, a clinical diagnosis can at times still permit permanent stent placement, only a temporary plastic, or possibly, a potentially removable coated SEMS should generally be used without a tissue diagnosis.

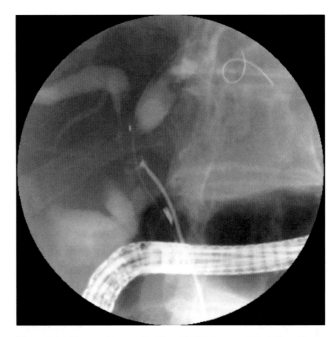

Figure 26.4 Forceps biopsy of a Bismuth IIIA tumor of the bifurcation using the HBI.

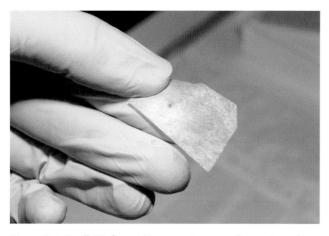

Figure 26.5 Small 6 Fr forceps biopsy specimen on saline moistened pad—appropriate for immediate SMASH prep.

To address this problem, we have developed a technique of intraprocedural diagnosis during a single ERCP, which permits appropriate stent placement. This forceps technique was patterned after the neurosurgical technique of intraoperative brain squash prep. In brief, the resection margins are biopsied and simply spread onto a glass slide for Papanicolaou staining during the operation. Rapid reading by a cytologist then guides further resection.

For sampling malignant appearing biliary strictures, a 5 Fr or 6 Fr forceps specimen is obtained from the lower aspect of the stricture and then forcefully smashed into a monolayer on a dry glass slide (Figures 26.5 and 26.6). An in-suite cytotech then immediately stains sequential specimens, which are examined by the cytopathologist. More specimens follow until a diagnosis is definitely made (Video 26.3).

Using this technique, cholangiocarcinomas can almost always be adequately sampled, often in just a few biopsies, but pancreatic cancer strictures are more difficult requiring 10 or 12 specimens at times. Overall, the intraprocedural diagnosis of pancreatic cancer causing a biliary stricture is about 75%. We then employ a comprehensive approach if 10–12 SMASH preps are negative by

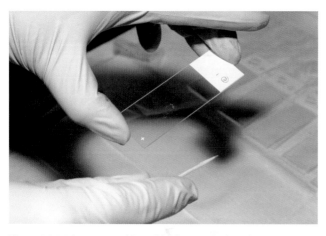

Figure 26.6 Vigorous smashing of the forceps specimen between two dry glass slides to form a monolayer before rapid Papanicolaou staining.

sending additional biopsies for histology and performing at least one ERCP FNA. This raises the yield to nearly 90% for pancreaticobiliary cancers [8].

Beware that metastatic disease producing biliary obstruction is much deeper and less infiltrative so the yield of ERCP tissue sampling, even by this comprehensive approach, is only 50%. Endoscopic ultrasound (EUS) is clearly the choice in this setting.

Metal stent placement

After a definite diagnosis of malignancy has been made most centers choose to place temporary plastic or permanent metal expandable stents. This permits clearance of jaundice, referral and further workup, and appropriate surgical or oncology consultation. A major recent development has been the practice of placing SEMS in both resectable and nonresectable patients [9,10]. This strategy can also facilitate neoadjuvant chemoradiation to downstage borderline resectable cases to then permit successful Whipple's resection, a strategy requiring some months of successful stenting [11].

Having a successful stent in place with preoperative clearance of jaundice also tends to simplify the surgery if, unfortunately, unresectability is discovered—a not infrequent event. Operating on an undrained patient places considerable pressure on the surgeon to perform an otherwise unnecessary and technically challenging biliary bypass.

Stent placement requires considerable knowledge, training and, experience as the consequences of stent misplacement can be very serious.

The first question facing the endoscopist is stent selection: plastic vs metal. If metal is indicated should the SEMS be coated or uncoated? What should be the overall length and diameter? Should the design be a foreshortening or nonforeshortening type? These decisions are greatly influenced by tissue diagnosis, as discussed above, and stricture location. The major types of SEMS are shown in Figure 26.7.

There are several scenarios for distal malignant obstruction that we can outline.

Tissue proven cancer, not resectable

Decision about stent type is based on life expectancy. A poor Karnofsky score with a low functional status suggests a short life span. For instance, metastatic disease to the liver of greater than 10% predicts short life expectancy. A 10 Fr or an 11.5 Fr plastic stent with a median patency of 90–120 days supports plastic stent selection in this setting. Be aware the 11.5 Fr diameter is more difficult to place and cannot be removed through the endoscope but probably does add some days or weeks of patency.

A good Karnofsky status, no or minimal metastatic spread supports SEMS as the cost-effective choice. If metal is indicated, the choice of SEMS should be based on comparative patency data, risk assessment, and cost.

As of this writing, coated biliary SEMS have not been shown to have better patency compared to uncoated SEMS [12]. However, several studies have noted that coated SEMS experienced increased

● **Foreshortening**

● **Non-foreshortening**

● **Coated SEMS**

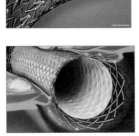

Figure 26.7 Major types of SEMS.

short-term complications, especially cholecystitis and migration of the stent with bleeding, perforation, and obstruction. A few have noted an increased pancreatitis risk, possibly due to compressive obstruction of the pancreatic orifice [13]. Coated SEMS, however, are much more removable should this feature need to be considered (Video 26.4).

A recent RCT comparing uncoated biliary SEMS in two diameters documented equivalent patency between two 10-mm diameter arms but much shorter patency at a diameter of 6 mm [14]. Currently, data supports a selection of uncoated 10 mm SEMS as the safest and most effective stent to palliate malignant jaundice.

Tissue proven cancer, resectable or borderline resectable

The routine use of SEMS in all malignant obstructions regardless of resectability demands further study. At present, if neoadjuvant therapy is planned, strong evidence supports using a short SEMS, keeping the upper margin below any potential line of resection to minimize the risk of recurrent obstruction during therapy [11]. The majority of centers continue to favor temporary plastic stents in operable candidates for extrahepatic obstruction.

No tissue diagnosis, resectable or nonresectable

Plastic stenting, or possibly potentially a removable coated SEMS should be chosen as rare tumor types are handled differently. Perhaps, the most frequently mistaken tumor for adenocarcinoma of the pancreas is gastrointestinal focal lymphoma, a disease which can be resolved with chemoradiation therapy. Metastatic breast and ovarian cancers can also be driven into remission leaving the patient with difficulties due to a nonremovable uncoated SEMS. Finally, benign lesions can mimic cancer, especially chronic pancreatitis and occasionally retroperitoneal fibrosis, and should not receive unremovable SEMS. Be aware that limited experience exists with coated, potentially removable, SEMS for benign disease. Recent reports have had mixed outcomes, and the tech-

nique not been compared to standard multiple plastic stent therapy. Finally, SEMS for benign biliary strictures have not been FDA approved [9].

Stent placement requires advanced skills of deep cannulation and guide wire insertion addressed earlier in this volume.

Extrahepatic SEMS placement

This discussion addresses CBD at least 1-2 cm below the bifurcation strictures. The discussion of hilar stricture stenting is addressed separately.

Upon guide wire passage through the biliary stricture, the approach then depends on the tissue diagnosis.

Stent placement for malignant disease should proceed as follows:

1 *Measure the stent length:* Measure the length of the stricture from the duodenal wall to the top of the stenosis. In general, the following rule is usually accurate (Figure 26.8):

a Periampullary = 5 cm length

b Top can be seen on fluoro below the edge of the ERCP scope = 7 cm length

c Top at upper edge of ERCP scope = 9 cm length

d Top involves the bifurcation; carefully measure as 12 cm may not be long enough.

Several methods of measure are in use. Many catheters have radiopaque markers, for instance every 5 cm (Figure 26.9). The tip of most hydrophilic guide wires is 5 cm long and this can be used as a movable measure if the outer catheter is pressed above the stricture to avoid losing access, or direct measurement can be calibrated from a spot radiograph using the 11 mm ERCP scope as the measuring unit.

The simplest procedure is to place a mark (tape or magic marker) on the cannulating catheter at the biopsy port when the

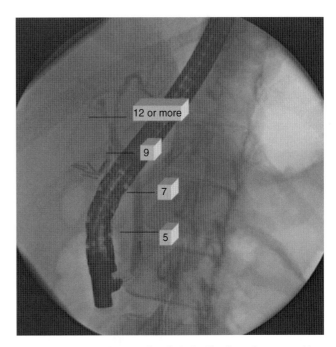

Figure 26.8 Appropriate stent lengths judged by the endoscope position.

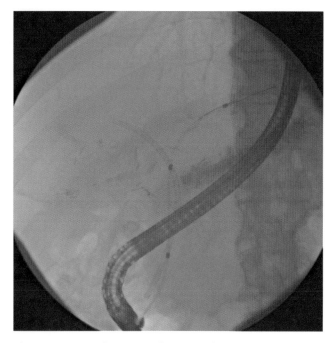

Figure 26.9 5 cm radiopaque markers on a catheter placed just at the top of a bifurcation stricture. Measured length from the duodenum is 12 cm.

radiopaque tip is just at the top of the stricture. Pull down, leaving the guide wire in place, until the tip is touching the papilla seen on the endoscope view—simply measure from the biopsy port to the mark. Remember that biliary stent length is measured between flaps—the actual length is long enough to extend above the stricture and project into the duodenum.

2 Sphincterotomy or not: Prior to actual stent placement, a decision regarding sphincterotomy is necessary. Two schools of thought exist. One favors sphincterotomy and one does not.

We favor performing sphincterotomy to facilitate biopsy, ease future access, and avoid compression of the pancreatic duct orifice. This may be most important in the unusual cases where the tumor has not obstructed the pancreatic duct. Others would prefer to avoid the recognized risks of sphincterotomy despite these advantages.

3 Position of the introducer: Once the guide wire has been traversed through the stricture, the appropriate type and length have been selected, and the sphincterotomy issue has been decided,

the stent and introducer can be advanced over the guide wire. The stent forward edge should be placed about 2 cm above the upper edge of the stricture. If a foreshortening SEMS was selected, an additional 1–2 cm should be advanced to accommodate the approximate 30% foreshortening. Careful placement should avoid leaving excess length in the duodenum as irritation of the opposite wall can result in bleeding or even perforation.

4 Deploy the stent: Once positioned, accurate deployment depends on good communication between the endoscopist and the assistant. As the stent is deployed by the assistant, it is critical that the endoscopist withdraws the outer catheter to prevent forward motion of the stent. Constant coaching of the assistant is necessary but the physician is responsible to withdraw the outer catheter at the same rate as deployment. This results in no forward motion of the stent and accurate placement is assured (Videos 26.5 and 26.6). In the event of malpositioning, prompt removal can generally be accomplished if the stent is too low using a snare. If too proximal, a second SEMS usually can be placed within it leaving the guide wire in position. One foreshortening type of SEMS (Wallflex, Boston Scientific Corp) can be reconstrained back into the introducer for repositioning, provided deployment has not progressed beyond the most distal radiopaque marker—the so called "point of no return."

Bifurcation SEMS placement

Managing malignant obstruction of the bifurcation is much more demanding and controversial. In general, these procedures should be performed at experienced centers.

Detailed understanding of liver and biliary anatomy and advanced techniques of selective guide wire placement is required to effectively approach these patients. Distribution of obstruction was classified by Bismuth and is depicted Figure 26.10.

Controversies in hilar stenting include differences in institutionally defined unresectability, choice of plastic vs metal stenting and, most contentious, attempting single vs multiple stent placement.

The main issue in bifurcation stenting is the increased risk of cholangitis since complete drainage can be accomplished in only a few anatomic situations. In addition, this unfortunate complication occurs more often when instrumentation of an obstructed duct is followed by failure to place a drainage stent successfully. In the past, this occurred most frequently when a second plastic

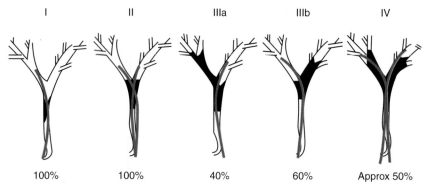

Figure 26.10 Anatomic distribution of the strictures was classified by Bismuth. Plastic stents to achieve optimal drainage are depicted in red.

stent or SEMS was attempted to be placed but proved not to be possible.

At present, SEMS appears to have a distinct patency advantage and a lower complication rate when a single stent is possible and efforts are made to avoid any contrast injection or guide wire placement on the side not planned to be drained. Pre-ERCP MRCP for planning and no contrast injection have been advocated by some authors [15].

Bilaterally SEMS placement has been advocated by many authors for advanced obstruction, especially when multiple lobes are isolated—classified as a Bismuth IV patient [16].

Several techniques have been reported including using long side-by-side stents to extend out into the duodenum, using usually Wallstents or WallFlexs (Boston Scientific) (Video 26.7). However, failure can still occur especially in the frequent circumstance when the distal CBD is small. Finally, the risk of pancreatitis seems a concern since most patients in this setting will have a normal pancreatic duct. At minimum, a sphincterotomy would appear advisable.

An alternate proposal has been to place the second SEMS through the sidewall of the first SEMS effectively draining both sides. This technique is technically difficult and may result in both failure of the second stent placement and early occlusion due to blocking the proximal position of the first stent. Finally, incomplete expansion of the second "thru" stent at the point of the sidewall passive may also result in short patency with difficult subsequent access.

To ease these problems with the stent-thru-a-stent, a South Korean paired stent has been developed (Bonastent Standard Sci Tech Inc., Seoul, South Korea) (Figure 26.11). The first stent has wider interstices in the region planned to be at the bifurcation. This has been reported to ease access to the opposite side. Long-term, intention to treat, mature data has yet to be presented.

A recent development has been the release of an uncoated SEMS mounted in a 6 Fr introducer (Zilver 635, Cook Endoscopy). This smaller introducer permits two 8 mm or 10 mm SEMS to be successfully placed in a side-by-side fashion following bilateral guide wire position, theoretically reducing the risk of cholangitis following a failed attempt at placing the second stent (Figures 26.12(a) and (b)). Experience to date is limited but the technique clearly eases the technical aspect compared to the previous described options, and will be discussed in more detail.

Prior to bilateral SEMS placement in all but the stent-thru-a-stent technique, placement of two guide wires into the desired ducts is required. Techniques of guide wire placement have been previously discussed. This remains challenging and needs special training and experience.

Two 6 Fr introducers are meant to be positioned prior to deployment by placing them down the biopsy channel simultaneously. Following the placement of two guide wires through the biliary obstructions to be drained, the stents are passed sequentially, and positioned to overlap the strictured areas with the bottoms carefully aligned within the duct. If possible, the ends can be positioned above the cystic duct takeoff to eliminate the possibility of postplacement cholecystectomy.

After positioning of both introducers, deployment can be accurately performed with the goal of leaving the bottoms precisely aligned to permit future access (Video 26.8). This feature is particularly important as clinical studies have reported up to a 40% reintervention rate in bifurcation cases, almost twice that of extrahepatic cases [14,15]. A major advantage of this newer option is minimizing the risk of being unable to pass the second stent after deployment of the first stent, a requirement of all other bilateral SEMS systems.

Further, experience is needed to determine the value of all of these bilateral SEMS placement techniques in these patients.

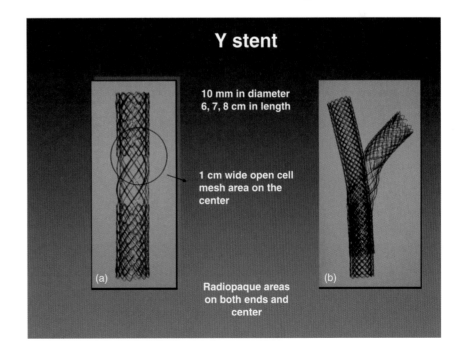

Figure 26.11 Stent-thru-a-stent system by a South Korean company can achieve bilateral drainage.

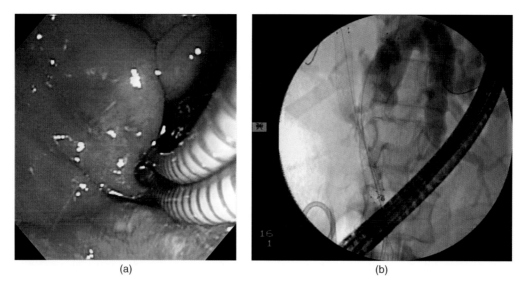

Figure 26.12 (a) Two 635 introducers are in position prior to deployment of either stent. (b) Optimal positioning in a Bismuth II patient leaving the bottoms of the stents aligned for future access.

These studies will be understandably complex as the outcome of patients depends on tumor types, tumor volume, and anatomic distribution (Bismuth type). Until these can be accomplished, the approach to bifurcation stenting should be aimed at minimizing short-term complications, especially infection of undrained lobes. Current experience has not supported proceeding with efforts at complete drainage using percutaneous techniques to access lobes left undrained after endoscopic best efforts [17].

Minimizing infection techniques include avoiding contrast injection, preprocedure prophylactic antibiotics, and possibly intraprocedural high dose antibiotic added to the radio-contrast. Our personal experience supports using tobramycin 10 mg/10 cc of contrast. This latter technique may be effective [18].

Management of ampullary neoplasms

Increasing reports have emphasized the role of endoscopy in evaluating and treating ampullary neoplasms as virtually all benign lesions of the ampulla can now be removed at ERCP [19].

Before undertaking removal, detection of complicating malignancy is desirable. Accurate examination can generally be done by direct endoscopic inspection and directed biopsy. Features of malignancy include ulceration, smooth induration, poor definition of margins, and malignant appearing strictures extending into the ducts (Figure 26.13). Using these criteria, all but six cases of malignancy involving 103 otherwise benign appearing ampullary adenomas were excluded from a multicentered series [19].

Some authors have advocated EUS to inspect ampullary polyps to add to detection of malignancy but, at present, there appears to be limited potential to improve accuracy especially when over-staging can occur due to inflammatory changes. The possibility that an occasional patient could have a nearby malignant lymph node due to metastatic disease without demonstrable malignancy in the primary ampullary tumor appears remote.

Once no features of malignancy are recognized in an ampullary neoplasm, generally by simple careful inspection, a decision about removal is required.

Asymptomatic, less than 1 cm, ampullary lesions detected at screening in familial adenomatous polyposis (FAP) patients should be left for continued endoscopic follow-up. The risks of rapid growth, severe symptoms, or degeneration to malignancy are very low and are likely lower then the risk of endoscopic removal.

Large or symptomatic benign lesions should be removed. Be aware that many pathologic tumor types have been reported but more than 90% will be tubular or tubulovillous adenomas. Hamartomas, carcinoids, gastric heterotopia, and gangliocytic paragangliomas are reported [20].

The techniques described for removal resemble colonic polypectomy, but with an important distinction. All studies include the early or final placement of a pancreatic stent to minimize the risk of pancreatitis. Debate as to the timing of stent placement and concerns whether early stent placement will interfere with the removal or pathologic interpretation of the resected specimen exists. Late placement after polyp removal may occur after pancreatic trauma has already occurred or might be unsuccessful due to failure to identify the orifice in the polypectomy bed. Both these events could result in pancreatitis. To date, most series reporting this technique report postampullectomy pancreatitis rates of 5–25%, some severe with a few fatal cases.

We prefer to identify and cannulate the pancreatic duct first, deeply advance a guide wire, perform pancreatic and biliary sphincterotomy, and place a pancreatic stent. In the vast majority

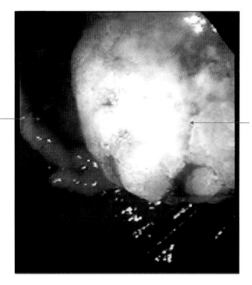

Benign ———————————— ———————————— Malignant

Figure 26.13 Benign and malignant features can be recognized in this large ampullary tumor.

of cases, sphincterotomies can be extended up onto the normal duodenal mucosa carrying the new orifices well above the polyp base. The polyp can then be removed using standard colonoscopic polypectomy technique. This approach reduces the risk of pancreatitis to that of routine ERCP with sphincterotomy and pancreatic stent placement [20] (Figure 26.14).

A major difference from colonoscopic removal is the need to use side-viewing ERCP endoscopes since the area cannot be accessed with front-viewing endoscopes. Standard snares, especially hemostatic clips, work poorly, or not at all, when angled retrograde over the elevator. Device placement is generally at 90° or greater which challenges these endoscopic devices designed for front-viewing endoscopes.

To respond to these problems, we advocate elevation of the lesion using a sclerotherapy needle and injecting dilute epinephrine and a small amount of methylene blue or indigo carmine dye to mark the submucosa. Epinephrine strength of 1:20,000–1:50,000 and a volume of 10–20 cc to visibly elevate the lesion and stain the submucosa should be used.

For removal, we recommend a 5 Fr pediatric snare or an EMR snare, either oval or hexagonal. Polyps less than 2 cm can often be removed as a single piece after sphincterotomy and pancreatic duct stent placement (Video 26.9). Piecemeal removal is generally needed for larger lesions. Collect all removed polyp fragments using a basket/net snare (Video 26.10).

Treating the edges with argon plasma coagulation (APC) may reduce the risk of recurrence or residual [19]. Care should be used around the new pancreatic orifice to minimize and avoid the later development of postcoagulation stenosis and the risk of pancreatitis from thermal injury, despite the use of a PD stent.

Finally, inspect the base carefully for potential bleeding sites, which may appear as end vessels or slow oozing areas. These can be treated with APC but we prefer to apply clips. The only currently available clip, which will work over the elevator, is the

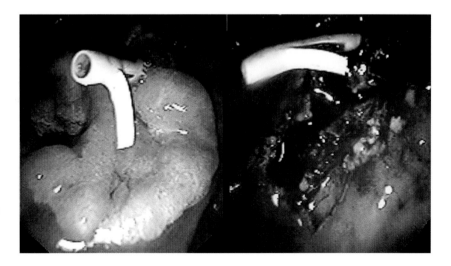

Figure 26.14 Here the sphincterotomies and the pancreatic stent have been placed (left). The entire polyp has now been recovered, avoiding loss of control of pancreatic drainage (right).

QuickClip (Olympus, Tokyo). For better performance, trimming the clear plastic outer sheath about 1.5 cm back will allow the elevator to directly contact the inner metal coil, which is more flexible. This then permits lifting of the clip and accurate application (Video 26.11).

After the initial ampullectomy session, we advise a repeat examination in about 4 weeks for biopsy, further ablation, cholangiopancreatography, and pancreatic stent removal. This greatly improves definitive ablation while minimizing risks. This approach has improved the outcome of attempting removal of large polyps [21].

To examine for intraductal polyp extension, some enthusiasm for intraductal endoscopy has developed with the recent approval of a semi-disposable 10-Fr system (Spy Glass, Boston Scientific Corp). However, we have found very distal visualization to be poor with this system. Reasonable assessment is possible with direct inspection, intraductal biopsy, and radio-contrast installation spot radiographs.

Extension of the polyp tissue into the ducts occurs in large lesions frequently, generally up the bile duct only. This has been reported as a major cause of failure, resulting in referral for surgery, but some recent reports do suggest that endoscopic ablation or complete removal can often still be successful [22] (Video 26.12).

Finally, long-term follow-up appears warranted since late recurrences have been noted in many series. Clearly, FAP patients are at a much higher risk of recurrence and often have extensive adenomas of the entire proximal small bowel. Remember that ampullary cancer is the second most common cancer after colon cancer in polyposis patients.

Thoughts on advanced endoscopy training

As a long-time Advanced Fellowship Director, the author of this chapter has an opinion regarding prerequisites for supervised training in these techniques.

Understanding that 3-year programs vary widely regarding hands-on-training, all gastroenterology 3-year fellows should be familiar with the indications, risks, and potential role of ERCP tissue aspiration, metal biliary stent placement, and ampullectomy. If their programs meet the ASGE training thresholds for competency in ERCP, clearly the tissue sampling technologies described in this chapter can be adapted due to their safety and close relationships to other endoscopic techniques even only if limited hands-on-experience was gained.

Likewise, the placement of SEMS below the hepatic bifurcation should be done under the general ASGE guidelines for competency which defines a limited minimum number of stent placements. The use of metal expandable stents for below the bifurcation obstruction requires similar skills to plastic stenting.

The higher risk procedures of bifurcation metal stenting and ampullectomy should be mastered in a supervised training setting. The potential for severe complications including severe bleeding, pancreatitis, sepsis, and perforation (some fatal), must be recognized. The subtleties of their avoidance require careful instruction and live demonstration. Most 3-year fellowships cannot provide sufficient training for these indications, justifying referral to expert centers or, at minimum, supervised mentoring by qualified senior group or institutional members.

The use of live conference demonstrations, archived videos and chapters, such as this one, should be valuable to reduce the number of such supervised procedures aimed at achieving competence but should not be a complete substitute for them.

Videos

Video 26.1 Three major techniques of ERCP tissue sampling
Video 26.2 Use of biliary introducer to facilitate triple sampling
Video 26.3 Forceps biopsies processed by SMASH technique during ERCP
Video 26.4 Placement and removal of a fully covered metal stent
Video 26.5 Standard uncoated transpapillary SEMS placement
Video 26.6 New ultraslim introducer with transpapillary SEMS
Video 26.7 Bilateral long SEMS placement of a bifurcation tumor (Wallflex, Boston, USA)
Video 26.8 Side-by-side internal SEMS placement using the ultraslim 635 introducer (Cook)
Video 26.9 Small ampullary adenoma removal
Video 26.10 Large ampullary adenoma removal
Video 26.11 Hemoclip control of postampullectomy bleeding (No audio)
Video 26.12 Removal of an intraductal ampullary adenoma

References

1 Gilbert DA, DiMarino AJ, Jr., Jensen DM, et al.: Status evaluation: biliary stents. American Society for Gastrointestinal Endoscopy. Technology Assessment Committee. *Gastrointest Endosc* 1992;**38**(6):750–752.

2 Ginsberg GG: *Clinical Gastrointestinal Endoscopy*. Philadelphia: Elsevier Saunders, 2005:874.

3 Bernadino KP: Intraprocedural histologic diagnosis during therapeutic ERCP: high yield of forceps squash prep. *Gastrointest Endosc* 2005;**61**(5):AB 198.

4 Howell DA, Beveridge RP, Bosco J, et al.: Endoscopic needle aspiration biopsy at ERCP in the diagnosis of biliary strictures. *Gastrointest Endosc* 1992;**38**(5):531–535.

5 Howell DA, Parsons WG, Jones MA, et al.: Complete tissue sampling of biliary strictures at ERCP using a new device. *Gastrointest Endosc* 1996;**43**(5):498–502.

6 de Bellis M, Sherman S, Fogel EL, et al.: Tissue sampling at ERCP in suspected malignant biliary strictures (Part 2). *Gastrointest Endosc* 2002;**56**(5):720–730.

7 Lawrence D, Howell DA, Lukens JN, et al.: ERCP tissue sampling to maximize yield: randomized study of two forceps types during triple sampling. *Gastrointes Endosc* 2004;**59**(5):P98.

8 Howell DA: Intraprocedural Tissue Diagnosis During ERCP Employing a New Cytology Preparation of Forceps Biopsy (Smash Protocol). *Am J Gastroenterol* 2011;**106**:294–299.

9 Kahaleh M, Brock A, Conaway MR, et al.: Covered self-expandable metal stents in pancreatic malignancy regardless of resectability: a new concept validated by a decision analysis. *Endoscopy* 2007;**39**(4):319–324.

10 Mullen JT, Lee JH, Gomez HF, et al.: Pancreaticoduodenectomy after placement of endobiliary metal stents. *J Gastrointest Surg* 2005;**9**(8):1094–1104; Discussion 1104–1105.

11 Sanders M: Placement of self-expanding metal biliary stents (SEMS) in patients with resectable pancreatic cancer. *Gastrointest Endosc* 2009;**69**(5):AB266.

12 Telford JJ, Carr-Locke DL, Baron TH, et al.: A randomized trial comparing the covered and uncovered wallstent in the palliation of malignant distal biliary obstruction: interim analysis. *Gastrointest Endosc* 2007;**65**(5):AB123.

13 Yousuke N, Hiroyuki I, Yutaka K, et al.: Efficacy and safety of the covered wallstent in patients with distal malignant biliary obstruction. *Gastrointest endosc* 2005;**62**(5):742–748.

14 Loew BJ, Howell DA, Sanders MK, et al.: Comparative performance of uncoated, self-expanding metal biliary stents of different designs in 2 diameters: final results of an international multicenter, randomized, controlled trial. *Gastrointest Endosc* 2009;**70**(3):445–453.

15 Freeman ML, Sielaff TD: A modern approach to malignant hilar biliary obstruction. *Rev Gastroenterol Disord* 2003;**3**(4):187–201.

16 Costamagna G, Tringali A, Petruzziello L, et al.: Hilar tumours. *Can J Gastroenterol* 2004;**18**(7):451–454.

17 Costamagna G.: ERCP and endoscopic sphincterotomy in Billroth II patients: a demanding technique for experts only? *Ital J Gastroenterol Hepatol* 1998;**30**(3):306–309.

18 Bernadino KP, Howell DA, Lawrence C, et al.: Near absence of septic complications following successful therapeutic ERCP justifies selective intravenous and intracontrast use of antibiotics. *Gastrointest Endosc* 2005;**61**(5):AB187.

19 Catalano MF, Linder JD, Chak A, et al.: Endoscopic management of adenoma of the major duodenal papilla. *Gastrointest Endosc* 2004;**59**(2):225–232.

20 Desilets DJ, Dy RM, Ku PM, et al.: Endoscopic management of tumors of the major duodenal papilla: refined techniques to improve outcome and avoid complications. *Gastrointest Endosc* 2001;**54**(2):202–208.

21 Eswaran SL, Sanders M, Bernadino KP, et al.: Success and complications of endoscopic removal of giant duodenal and ampullary polyps: a comparative series. *Gastrointest Endosc* 2006;**64**(6):925–932.

22 Bohnacker S, Soehendra N, Maguchi H, et al.: Endoscopic resection of benign tumors of the papilla of vater. *Endoscopy* 2006;**38**(5):521–525.

27 Sphincter of Oddi Manometry

Evan L. Fogel, Stuart Sherman & Glen A. Lehman

Indiana University School of Medicine, Indianapolis, IN, USA

The sphincter of Oddi (SO) is a complex smooth muscle structure surrounding the terminal common bile duct, main pancreatic duct, and the common channel, when present (Figure 27.1). The high-pressure zone generated by the sphincter varies from 4 to 10 mm in length. The SO regulates the flow of bile and pancreatic exocrine juice, and prevents duodenum-to-duct reflux (i.e., maintains a sterile intraductal environment). The SO possesses a basal pressure and phasic contractile activities; the former appears to be the predominant mechanism regulating flow of pancreatobiliary secretions. Although phasic SO contractions may aid in regulating bile and pancreatic juice flow, their primary role appears to be maintaining a sterile intraductal milieu.

Sphincter of Oddi dysfunction (SOD) refers to an abnormality of sphincter of Oddi contractility. It is a benign noncalculous obstruction to the flow of bile or pancreatic juice through the pancreatobiliary junction (i.e., the SO). This may cause pancreatobiliary pain, cholestasis and/or recurrent pancreatitis. The most definitive development in our understanding of the pressure dynamics of the SO came with the advent of sphincter of Oddi manometry (SOM). SOM is the only available method to measure SO motor activity directly [1,2]. SOM is considered by most authorities to be the most accurate means to evaluate patients for sphincter dysfunction [3,4]. Although SOM can be performed intraoperatively [5–7] and percutaneously [8], it is most commonly done in the ERCP setting. The use of manometry to detect motility disorders of the SO is similar to its use in other parts of the gastrointestinal tract. However, performance of SOM is more technically demanding and hazardous, with complication rates (in particular, pancreatitis) approaching 20% in several series. Its use, therefore, should be reserved for patients with clinically significant or disabling symptoms. One needs to appreciate, however, that SOM is not likely an independent risk factor for post-ERCP pancreatitis when the aspirating manometry catheter is used (see section Method of SOM). Questions remain as to whether the short-term observations (2–10 minute recordings per pull-through) reflect the "24-hour pathophysiology" of the sphincter [9–13]. Despite these problems, SOM is gaining more widespread clinical application. In this review, we will discuss the technique of SOM, with an emphasis on the technical and cognitive skill sets required.

Method of SOM

Sedation

SOM is usually performed at the time of ERCP. The initial step in performing SOM, therefore, is to administer adequate sedation, which will result in a comfortable, cooperative, motionless patient. All drugs that relax (anticholinergics, nitrates, calcium channel blockers, glucagon) or stimulate (narcotics, cholinergic agents) the sphincter should be avoided for at least 8–12 hours prior to manometry and during the manometric session. Early studies with midazolam and diazepam suggested that these benzodiazepines do not interfere with sphincter of Oddi manometric parameters, and therefore, are acceptable sedatives for SOM [14–18]. While one study did demonstrate a decrease in mean basal sphincter pressure in 4 of 18 patients (22%) receiving midazolam [19], these results have not been duplicated to date. Opioids had traditionally been avoided during SOM because of indirect evidence suggesting that these agents caused SO spasm [20–26]). However, two prospective studies [27,28] have demonstrated that meperidine, at a dose of ≤ 1 mg/kg, does not affect the basal sphincter pressure but does alter phasic wave characteristics. Since the basal sphincter pressure generally is the only manometric criterion used to diagnose SOD and determine therapy, meperidine may be used to facilitate conscious sedation for manometry. Recent preliminary data also suggests that a low dose of fentanyl, administered topically, does not affect the basal sphincter pressure [29]. Confirmatory data are awaited. Patients referred for SOM may take large doses of narcotics on a daily basis and frequently prove difficult to sedate at ERCP. Adjunctive agents for conscious sedation, therefore, have been sought. Our group demonstrated that droperidol did not significantly alter SOM results; concordance (normal vs abnormal basal sphincter pressure) was seen in 30 of 31 patients [30]. Wilcox and colleagues [31], on the other hand, suggested that droperidol did in fact influence SOM parameters. However, in their series of 41 patients, ERCP and SOM were carried out under general anaesthesia in all but seven patients. While it has been suggested that SO motor function is not influenced by general anaesthesia [1], the effects of newer anaesthetic agents are unknown, making interpretation

---

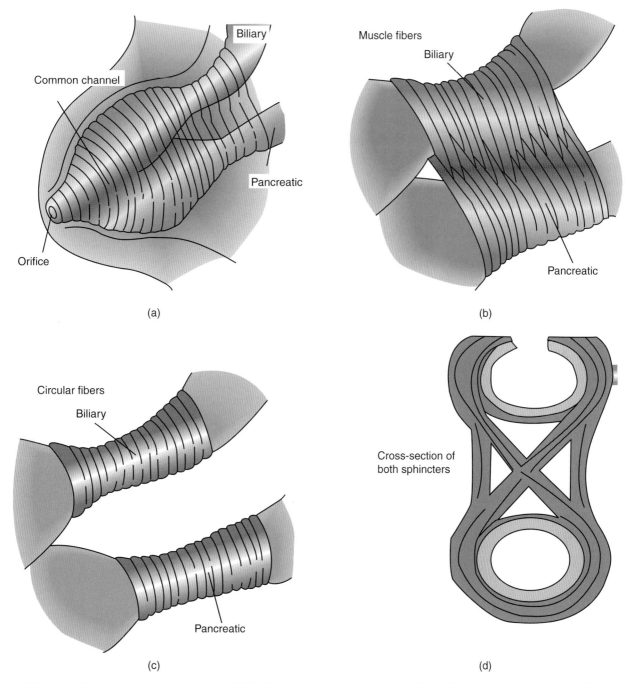

Figure 27.1 Schematic representation of (a) sphincter of Oddi, (b) demonstrating the circular smooth muscle that surrounds the common channel, (c) distal common bile duct and pancreatic duct, (d) cross-section of both sphincters.

of their results problematic. More recently, ketamine did not significantly alter SOM parameters, with concordance noted in 28/30 (93%) patients [32]. Limited experience with propofol suggests that this drug also does not affect the basal sphincter pressure [33,34], but further study is required before routine use of ketamine or propofol for SOM is recommended. If glucagon must be used to achieve cannulation, a 15-minute waiting period is required to restore the sphincter to its basal condition.

Equipment

Virtually all standards have been established with five French catheters; therefore, these should be used. Triple-lumen catheters are state of the art and are available from several manufacturers. Catheters with a long intraductal tip may help secure the catheter within the bile duct, but such a long nose is commonly a hindrance if pancreatic manometry is desired. A sleeve catheter is a perfused channel system that records pressure along its length,

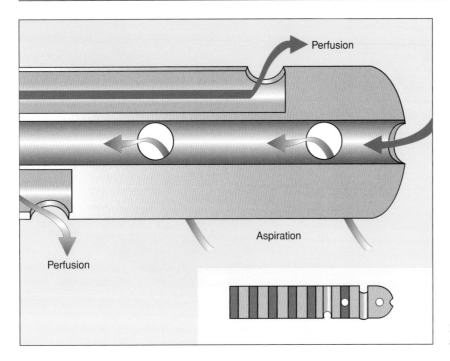

Figure 27.2 A modified triple-lumen aspirating catheter.

potentially limiting motion artifacts during performance of SOM [35]. Limited data from Australia suggests that this sleeve method is comparable to standard SOM with triple-lumen catheters [36], but more data are needed. Over the wire (monorail) catheters can be passed after first securing one's position within the duct with a guide wire. Whether this guide wire influences basal sphincter pressure has not been definitively elucidated (see section Technical performance of SOM). Some triple-lumen catheters will accommodate a 0.018 inch diameter guide wire passed through the entire length of the catheter and can be used to facilitate cannulation or maintain position in the duct. Guide wire-tipped catheters are also being evaluated. Early experience with performance of SOM using perfusion systems demonstrated unacceptably high post-procedure pancreatitis rates [37–40]. Presumably, overdistension of small caliber pancreatic ducts may lead to this complication. Aspiration catheters (Figure 27.2) in which one recording port is sacrificed to permit both end- and side-hole aspiration of intra-ductal juice and the perfusing fluid are therefore highly recommended for pancreatic manometry. These catheters have been shown to reduce the frequency of post-SOM pancreatitis while accurately recording sphincter pressures [39]. Most centers prefer to perfuse the catheters at 0.25 mL/channel/min using a low compliance pump. Lower perfusion rates will give accurate basal sphincter pressure measurements, but will not give accurate phasic wave information. The perfusate generally is distilled water, although physiologic saline needs further evaluation. The latter may crystallize in the capillary tubing of perfusion pumps and must be flushed out frequently. Solid state catheters [40,41] and microtransducer manometry systems [42] are also available and have been used by some investigators in an attempt to avoid volume loading of the biliopancreatic system during perfusion manometry [41]. Preliminary data from a few centers demon-

strate comparable SOM results to those achieved with perfusing catheters [40,42].

Technical performance of SOM (see accompanying Video 27.1)

SOM requires selective cannulation of the bile duct and/or pancreatic duct. Maximal efficiency is achieved by combining ERCP and SOM in a single session. It is preferable to perform cholangiography and/or pancreatography prior to performance of SOM, as certain findings (e.g., common bile duct stone) may obviate the need for SOM. This can simply be done by injecting contrast media through one of the perfusion ports. Alternatively, the duct entered can be identified by gently aspirating on any port (Figure 27.3). The appearance of yellow-colored fluid in the endoscopic view indicates entry into the bile duct. Clear aspirate indicates that the pancreatic duct has been entered. This technique may prove useful when attempting to access the bile duct following pancreatic SOM, as repeated pancreatic duct injections may increase post-ERCP pancreatitis rates [43]. If clear fluid is seen in the catheter, suggesting pancreatic duct entry, the catheter position is altered to achieve a more favorable angle for biliary cannulation. Blaut and colleagues [44] have shown that injection of contrast into the biliary tree prior to SOM does not significantly affect sphincter pressure characteristics. Similar evaluation of the pancreatic sphincter after contrast injection has not been reported. One must be certain that the catheter is not impacted against the wall of the duct in order to ensure accurate pressure measurements. On occasion, selective deep cannulation of the desired duct may only be achieved with a guide wire. However, a recent study in our unit

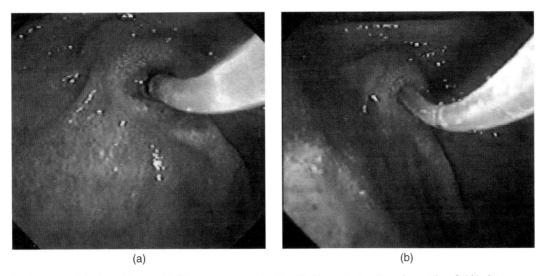

(a)   (b)

Figure 27.3 The duct entered during sphincter of Oddi manometry can be identified by aspirating the catheter. Clear fluid indicates pancreatic duct entry (a), whereas yellow fluid signifies entry into the bile duct (b).

found that stiffer shafted nitinol core guide wires used for this purpose commonly increase basal biliary sphincter pressure measured at ERCP by 50–100% [45]. Therefore, when wire-guided cannulation is performed, we recommend withdrawing the wire back into the catheter, outside of the duct and not traversing the sphincter, during performance of SOM. Alternatively, stiff guide wires need to be avoided or very soft-core guide wires must be used. Once deep cannulation is achieved and the patient acceptably sedated, the catheter is withdrawn across the sphincter at 1–2 mm intervals by standard station pull-through technique. Ideally, both the pancreatic and bile ducts should be studied. Current data indicate that an abnormal basal sphincter pressure may be confined to one side of the sphincter in 35–65% of patients with abnormal manometry [46–51], and thus, one sphincter segment may be dysfunctional and the other normal. Raddawi and colleagues [48] reported that an abnormal basal sphincter pressure was more likely to be confined to the pancreatic duct segment in patients with pancreatitis and to the bile duct segment in patients with biliary-type pain and elevated liver function tests.

Abnormalities of the basal sphincter pressure should ideally be observed for at least 30 seconds in each lead and be seen on two or more separate pull-throughs. From a practical clinical standpoint, we settle for one pull-through from each duct if the readings are clearly normal or abnormal. It is important that there be no kinking or impaction of the catheter to cause spurious pressure rises or artifacts which might impair interpretation of the manometry tracing. During the pull-through, it is necessary to establish good communication between the endoscopist and the manometrist who is reading the tracing as it rolls off the recorder or appears on the computer screen. This permits optimal positioning of the catheter in order to achieve interpretable tracings. Alternatively, electronic manometry systems with a television screen can be mounted near the endoscopic image screen to allow the endoscopist to view the manometry tracing during endoscopy. This can be particularly helpful when vigorous duo-

denal motility is present, necessitating constant attention be paid to catheter position in the duodenal lumen. Once the baseline study is completed, agents to relax or stimulate (e.g., cholecystokinin) the SO can be given and manometric and pain response monitored. The value of these provocative maneuvers for routine use needs further study before widespread application is recommended.

Interpretation criteria

Criteria for interpretation of a manometry tracing are relatively standard; however, they may vary somewhat from center to center. Some areas where there may be disagreement in interpretation include the required duration of basal sphincter pressure elevation, the number of leads in which basal pressure elevation is required, and the role of averaging pressures from the three (or two in an aspirating catheter) recording ports. Our recommended method for reading the manometry tracings is first to define the "zero" duodenal baseline before and after the pull-through. Alternatively, intraduodenal pressure can be continuously recorded from a separate intraduodenal catheter attached to the endoscope. The highest basal pressure (defined as the pressure above the zero duodenal baseline; Figure 27.4) that is sustained for at least 30 seconds is then identified. From the four lowest amplitude points in this zone, the mean of these readings is taken as the basal sphincter pressure for that lead for the pull-through. The basal sphincter pressure for all interpretable observations is then averaged; this is the final basal sphincter pressure. The amplitude of phasic wave contractions is measured from the beginning of the slope of the pressure increase from the basal pressure to the peak of the contraction wave. Four representative waves are taken for each lead and the mean pressure determined. The number of phasic waves per minute and the duration of phasic waves can also be determined. Most authorities use only the basal sphincter pressure as an indicator of

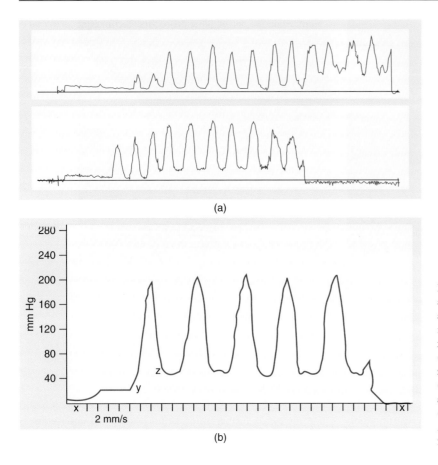

(a)

(b)

Figure 27.4 (a) An abnormal station pull-through at sphincter of Oddi manometry. The study has been abbreviated to fit onto one page. (b) Schematic representation of one lead of the above tracing. x: baseline duodenal 0 reference; y: intraductal (pancreatic) pressure of 20 mm Hg (abnormal); z: basal pancreatic sphincter pressure of 45 mm Hg (abnormal). Phasic waves are 155–175 mm Hg in amplitude and 6 seconds duration (normal). (Reproduced from Fogel EL, Sherman S: *Clin Perspect Gastroenterol* 2001;**5**:165, with permission from Elsevier.)

pathology of the sphincter of Oddi. However, data from Johns Hopkins University [52] suggest that intrabiliary pressure, which is easier to measure than SO pressure, correlates with basal sphincter pressure. In this study, intrabiliary pressure was significantly higher in patients with SOD than those with normal basal biliary sphincter pressure (20 vs. 10 mm Hg; p < 0.01). In a similar study, the Milwaukee group [53] found that increased pancreatic duct pressure correlated with increased pancreatic basal sphincter pressure (p < 0.001). Pancreatic duct pressure was significantly higher in SOD patients as compared with those with normal pressure (18 vs. 11 mm Hg; p < 0.0001). A pancreatic duct pressure greater than 20 mm Hg was 90% specific and 30% sensitive for the diagnosis of SOD. These studies await confirmation but support the theory that increased intrabiliary and/or intrapancreatic pressure is a cause of pain in SOD.

The best study establishing normal values for SOM was reported by Guelrud and associates [11]. Fifty asymptomatic control patients were evaluated and repeated on two occasions in ten subjects. This study established normal values for intraductal pressure, basal sphincter pressure, and phasic wave parameters (see Table 27.1). Moreover, the reproducibility of SOM was confirmed (see section Reproducibility of SOM). Various authorities interchangeably use 35 mm Hg or 40 mm Hg as the upper limit of normal for mean basal sphincter of Oddi pressure, for both pancreatic and biliary sphincter segments. Such upper limits of normal values are mean values plus three standard deviations. More studies

are needed to determine if 2 or 2.5 standard deviations above the mean would be more appropriate.

Interobserver variability for reading SOM is minimal when the observers are experienced in reading these tracings [54].

Table 27.1 Suggested Standard for Abnormal Values for Endoscopic Sphincter of Oddi Manometry Obtained from 50 Volunteers Without Abdominal Symptoms.

Basal sphincter pressure*	> 35 mm Hg
Basal ductal pressure	> 13 mm Hg
Phasic contractions	
Amplitude	> 220 mm Hg
Duration	> 8 s
Frequency	> 10/min

Source. Reproduced from Guelrud M, Mendoza S, Rossiter G, et al.: Sphincter of Oddi manometry in healthy volunteers. *Dig Dis Sci* 1990;35:38–46, with kind permission from Springer Science and Business Media.

Values were obtained by adding three standard deviations to the mean (mean obtained by averaging the results on 2–3 station pull-throughs). Data combine pancreatic and biliary studies.

*Basal pressures determined by: (1) reading the peak basal pressure (i.e., highest single lead as obtained using a triple-lumen catheter); and (2) obtaining the mean of these peak pressures from multiple station pull-throughs.

Reproducibility of SOM

It has been questioned whether the short-term pressure recording obtained during SOM reflect the "24-hour pathophysiology" of the sphincter, as patients with SOD may have intermittent, episodic symptoms [13]. If the basal sphincter pressure does vary over time, performance of SOM on two separate occasions may lead to different results and affect therapy. Three studies have demonstrated reproducibility of biliary SOM in 34 of 36 symptomatic patients overall [10,12], and 10 of 10 healthy volunteers [11]. However, reproducibility of pancreatic SOM was found in only 58% (7/12) and 40% (12/30) of persistently symptomatic patients with previously normal SOM at two large referral centers [9,13]. Other studies have also shown that SO basal pressures are not constant [55–57], perhaps due to the inherent physiological fluctuation of SO motor activity. Newer devices capable of portable, ambulatory, prolonged SOM would be of interest.

Complications of SOM

Several studies have indicated that pancreatitis is the most common major complication after SOM. Historically, using standard perfused catheters, pancreatitis rates of over 20% have been reported, especially following manometric evaluation of the pancreatic duct. Such high complication rates have limited more widespread use of SOM. While we now consider placement of a small diameter, protective, temporary pancreatic stent to be standard of care in these high-risk patients [58–60], a variety of other methods to decrease the incidence of postmanometry pancreatitis have been proposed. These include: (1) use of an aspiration catheter; (2) gravity drainage of the pancreatic duct after manometry; (3) decrease the perfusion rate to 0.05–0.10 mL/lumen/min; (4) limit pancreatic duct manometry time to less than 2 minutes (or avoid pancreatic manometry); and (5) use the microtransducer (nonperfused) system. In a prospective randomized study, Sherman and colleagues [39] found that the aspirating catheter (this catheter allows for aspiration of the perfused fluid from end and side holes while accurately recording pressure from the two remaining sideports) reduced the frequency of pancreatic duct manometry-induced pancreatitis from 31 to 4%. The reduction in pancreatitis with use of this catheter in the pancreatic duct and the very low incidence of pancreatitis after bile duct manometry lend support to the notion that increased pancreatic duct hydrostatic pressure is a major cause of this complication. Thus, we routinely aspirate pancreatic juice and perfusate when we study the pancreatic duct by SOM.

In summary, appropriate training is necessary for the physician who evaluates patients with ERCP and sphincter of Oddi manometry. At a minimum, the endoscopist must be skilled in diagnostic ERCP, since performance of SOM cannot be accomplished without selective cannulation of the pancreatic duct and bile duct. The physician must be aware of the limitations on sedation imposed by manometry, and be familiar with the equipment needed to perform the procedure. Technical skills in manometric pressure recording techniques must be acquired, limiting the maneuvers that may lead to recording artifacts. Appropriate training in interpretation of manometry tracings is essential for both the endoscopist and the manometrist. An expert panel has stated in their position paper that training should be obtained at a pancreatobiliary center that routinely performs SOM [2]. While there are no society guidelines recommending specific numbers of procedures that need to be performed during training, a minimum of 50 SOM studies performed during the course of a 3-year clinical GI fellowship or an advanced fourth year fellowship seems reasonable. There is no substitute for practice and experience.

Video

Video 27.1 Performance of Sphincter of Oddi manometry

References

1 Gandolfi L, Corazziari E: The international workshop on sphincter of Oddi manometry. *Gastrointest Endosc* 1986;**32**:46–49.

2 Hogan WJ, Sherman S, Pasricha P, et al.: Sphincter of Oddi manometry (position paper). *Gastrointest Endosc* 1997;**45**:342–348.

3 Lehman GA: Endoscopic sphincter of Oddi manometry: a clinical practice and research tool. *Gastrointest Endosc* 1991;**37**:490–492.

4 Lans JL, Parikh NP, Geenen JE: Application of sphincter of Oddi manometry in routine clinical investigations. *Endoscopy* 1991;**23**:139–143.

5 Sherman S, Hawes RH, Madura JA, et al.: Comparison of intraoperative and endoscopic manometry of the sphincter of Oddi. *Surg Gynecol Obstet* 1992;**175**:410–418.

6 Funch-Jensen P, Diederich P, Kragland K: Intraoperative sphincter of Oddi manometry in patients with gallstones. *Scand J Gastroenterol* 1984;**19**:931–936.

7 Oster MJ, Csendes A, Funch-Jensen P, et al.: Intraoperative pressure measurements of the choledochoduodenal junction, common bile duct, cysticocholedochal junction and gallbladder in humans. *Surg Gynecol Obstet* 1980;**150**:385–389.

8 Hong SJ, Lee MS, Joo JH, et al.: Long-term percutaneous transhepatic manometry of sphincter of Oddi during fasting and after feeding. *Korean J Gastroenterol* 1995;**27**:423–432.

9 Varadarajulu S, Hawes RH, Cotton PB: Determination of sphincter of Oddi dysfunction in patients with prior normal manometry. *Gastrointest Endosc* 2003;**58**:341–344.

10 Thune A, Scicchitano J, Roberts-Thomson I, et al.: Reproducibility of endoscopic sphincter of Oddi manometry. *Dig Dis Sci* 1991;**36**:1401–1405.

11 Guelrud M, Mendoza S, Rossiter G, et al.: Sphincter of Oddi manometry in healthy volunteers. *Dig Dis Sci* 1990;**35**:38–46.

12 Geenen JE, Hogan WJ, Dodds WJ, et al.: The efficacy of endoscopic sphincterotomy after cholecystectomy in patients with suspected sphincter of Oddi dysfunction. *N Engl J Med* 1989;**320**:82–87.

13 Khashab MA, Fogel EL, Sherman S, et al.: Frequency of sphincter of Oddi dysfunction in patients with previously normal sphincter of Oddi manometry studies. *Gastrointest Endosc* 2008;**67**:108.

14 Nebel OT: Manometric evaluation of the papilla of Vater. *Gastrointest Endosc* 1975;**21**:126–128.

15 Staritz M, Meyer Zum, Buschenfelde KH: Investigation of the effect of diazepam and other drugs on the sphincter of Oddi motility. *Ital J Gastroenterol* 1986;**18**:41–43.

16 Cuer JC, Dapoigny M, Bommelaer G: The effect of midazolam on motility of the sphincter of Oddi in human subjects. *Endoscopy* 1993;**25**:384–386.

17 Rolny P, Arleback A: Effect of midazolam on sphincter of Oddi motility. *Endoscopy* 1993;**25**:381–383.

18 Ponce Garcia J, Garrigues V, Sala T, et al.: Diazepam does not modify the motility of the sphincter of Oddi [letter]. *Endoscopy* 1988; **20**:87.

19 Fazel A, Burton FR: A controlled study of the effect of midazolam on abnormal sphincter of Oddi motility. *Gastrointest Endosc* 2002;**55**:637–640.

20 Economou G, Ward-McQuaid JN: A cross-over comparison of the effect of morphine, pethidine, pentazocine, and phenazocine on biliary pressure. *Gut* 1971;**12**:218–221.

21 Greenstein AJ, Kaynan A, Singer A, et al.: A comparative study of pentazocine and meperidine on the biliary passage pressure. *Am J Gastroenterol* 1972;**58**:417–427.

22 Radnay PA, Brodman E, Mankikar D, et al.: The effect of equianalgesic doses of fentanyl, morphine, meperidine and pentazocine on common bile duct pressure. *Anaesthesist* 1980;**29**:26–29.

23 McCammon RL, Stoelting R, Madura JA: Reversal of fentanyl-induced spasm of the sphincter of Oddi. *Surg Gynecol Obstet* 1983;**156**:329–334.

24 Joehl RJ, Koch KL, Nahrwold DL: Opioid drugs cause bile duct obstruction during hepatobiliary scans. *Am J Surg* 1984;**147**:134–138.

25 Helm JF, Venu RP, Geenen JE, et al.: Effects of morphine on the human sphincter of Oddi. *Gut* 1988;**29**:1402–1407.

26 Thune A, Baker RA, Saccone GTP, et al.: Differing effects of pethidine and morphine on human sphincter of Oddi motility. *Br J Surg* 1990;**77**:992–995.

27 Sherman S, Gottlieb K, Uzer MF, et al.: Effects of meperidine on the pancreatic and biliary sphincter. *Gastrointest Endosc* 1996;**44**:239–242.

28 Elta GH, Barnett JL: Meperidine need not be proscribed during sphincter of Oddi manometry. *Gastrointest Endosc* 1994;**40**:7–9.

29 Koo HC, Moon JH, Choi HJ, et al.: Effect of transdermal fentanyl patch on sphincter of Oddi – for application of pain management in pancreatitis. *Gastrointest Endosc* 2009;**69**:270.

30 Fogel EL, Sherman S, Bucksot L, et al.: Effects of droperidol on the pancreatic and biliary sphincters. *Gastrointest Endosc* 2003;**58**:488–492.

31 Wilcox CM, Linder J: Prospective evaluation of droperidol on sphincter of Oddi motility. *Gastrointest Endosc* 2003;**58**:483–487.

32 Varadarajulu S, Tamhane A, Wilcox CM: Prospective evaluation of adjunctive ketamine on sphincter of Oddi motility in humans. *J Gastro Hep* 2008;**23**:e405–e409.

33 Goff JS: Effect of propofol on human sphincter of Oddi. *Dig Dis Sci* 1995;**40**:2364–2367.

34 Schmitt T, Seifert H, Dietrich CF, et al.: Sedation with propofol during endoscopic sphincter of Oddi manometry. *Z Gastroenterol* 1999;**37**:219–227.

35 Craig AG, Omari T, Lingenfelser T, et al.: Development of a sleeve sensor for measurement of sphincter of Oddi motility. *Endoscopy* 2001;**33**:651–657.

36 Kawamoto M, Geenen J, Omari T, et al.: Sleeve sphincter of Oddi (SO) manometry: a new method for characterizing the motility

of the sphincter of Oddi. *J Hepato Bil Panc Surg* 2008;**15**:391–396.

37 Maldonado ME, Brady PG, Mamel JJ, et al.: Incidence of pancreatitis in patients undergoing sphincter of Oddi manometry. *Am J Gastroenterol* 1999;**94**:387–390.

38 Meshkinpour H, Kay L, Mollot M: The role of the flow-rate of the pneumohydraulic system on post-sphincter of Oddi manometry. *J Clin Gastroenterol* 1992;**14**:236–239.

39 Sherman S, Troiano FP, Hawes RH, et al.: Sphincter of Oddi manometry: decreased risk of clinical pancreatitis with use of a modified aspirating catheter. *Gastrointest Endosc* 1990:**36**:462–466.

40 Tanaka M, Ikeda S: Sphincter of Oddi manometry: comparison of microtransducer and perfusion methods. *Endoscopy* 1988;**20**:184–188.

41 Tanaka M, Ikeda S, Nakayama F: Nonoperative measurement of pancreatic and common bile duct pressures with a microtransducer catheter and effects of duodenoscopic sphincterotomy. *Dig Dis Sci* 1981;**26**:545–553.

42 Wehrmann T, Stergiou N, Schmitt T, et al.: Reduced risk for pancreatitis after endoscopic microtransducer manometry of the sphincter of Oddi: a randomized comparison with the perfusion manometry technique. *Endoscopy* 2003;**35**:472–477.

43 Freeman ML, DiSario JA, Nelson DB, et al.: Risk factors for post-ERCP pancreatitis: a prospective, multicenter study. *Gastrointest Endosc* 2001;**54**:425–434.

44 Blaut U, Sherman S, Fogel E, et al.: Influence of cholangiography on biliary sphincter of Oddi manometric parameters. *Gastrointest Endosc* 2000;**52**:624–629.

45 Blaut U, Sherman S, Fogel EL, et al.: The influence of variable stiffness guidewires on basal biliary sphincter pressure measured at ERCP. *Gastrointest Endosc* 2002:**55**:83.

46 Eversman D, Fogel EL, Rusche M, et al.: Frequency of abnormal pancreatic and biliary sphincter manometry compared with clinical suspicion of sphincter of Oddi dysfunction. *Gastrointest Endosc* 1999;**50**:637–641.

47 Aymerich RR, Prakash C. Aliperti G: Sphincter of Oddi manometry: is it necessary to measure both biliary and pancreatic sphincter pressure? *Gastrointest Endosc* 2000;**52**:183–186.

48 Raddawi HM, Geenen JE, Hogan WJ, et al.: Pressure measurements from biliary and pancreatic segments of sphincter of Oddi. Comparison between patients with functional abdominal pain, biliary or pancreatic disease. *Dig Dis Sci* 1991;**36**:71–74.

49 Rolny P, Arleback A, Funch-Jensen P, et al.: Clinical significance of manometric assessment of both pancreatic duct and bile duct sphincter in the same patient. *Scand J Gastroenterol* 1989;**24**:751–754.

50 Silverman WB, Ruffalo TA. Sherman S, et al.: Correlation of basal sphincter pressures measured from both the bile duct and pancreatic duct in patients with suspected sphincter of Oddi dysfunction. *Gastrointest Endosc* 1992;**38**:440–443.

51 Chan YK, Evans PR, Dowsett JF, et al.: Discordance of pressure recordings from biliary and pancreatic duct segments in patients with suspected sphincter of Oddi dysfunction. *Dig Dis Sci* 1997;**42**:1501–1506.

52 Kalloo AN, Tietjen TG, Pasricha PJ: Does intrabiliary pressure predict basal sphincter of Oddi pressure? A study in patients with and without gallbladders. *Gastrointest Endosc* 1996;**44**:696–699.

53 Fazel A, Catalano M, Quadri A, et al.: Pancreatic ductal pressures: a potential surrogate marker for pancreatic sphincter of Oddi dysfunction. *Gastrointest Endosc* 2002;**55**:92.

54 Smithline A, Hawes R, Lehman G: Sphincter of Oddi manometry: interobserver variability. *Gastrointest Endosc* 1993;**39**:486–491.

55 Guelrud M, Rossiter A, Souney PF, et al.: The effect of transcutaneous nerve stimulation on sphincter of Oddi pressure in patients with biliary dyskinesia. *Am J Gastroenterol* 1991;**86**:581–585.

56 Lee SK, Kim MH, Kim HJ, et al.: Electroacupuncture may relax the sphincter of Oddi in humans. *Gastrointest Endosc* 2001;**53**:211–216.

57 Torsoli A, Corazziari E, Habib FI, et al.: Frequencies and cyclical pattern of the human sphincter of Oddi phasic activity. *Gut* 1986;**27**:363–369.

58 Singh P, Das A, Isenberg G, et al.: Does prophylactic pancreatic stent placement reduce the risk of post-ERCP acute pancreatitis?

A meta-analysis of controlled trials. *Gastrointest Endosc* 2004;**60**:544–550.

59 Harewood GC, Pochron NL, Gostout CJ: Prospective, randomized, controlled trial of prophylactic pancreatic stent placement for endoscopic snare excision of the duodenal ampulla. *Gastrointest Endosc* 2005;**62**:367–370.

60 Saad AM, Fogel EL, McHenry L, et al.: Pancreatic duct stent placement prevents post-ERCP pancreatitis in patients with suspected sphincter of Oddi dysfunction but normal manometry results. *Gastrointest Endosc* 2008;**67**:255–261.

28 Pseudocyst Management

Michael J. Levy & Todd H. Baron
Mayo Clinic, Rochester, MN, USA

Procedure(s) to be considered

The procedures to be considered for pseudocyst drainage include upper endoscopy using a side-viewing endoscope, endoscopic retrograde cholangiopancreatography (ERCP), and endoscopic ultrasound (EUS). The procedures are used to obtain initial pseudocyst access and drainage, as well as to guide pancreatic duct interventions when necessary.

Prerequisite level of expertise and skill for learning this

Pseudocyst drainage is a technically challenging procedure. Performing endoscopists should have experience primarily with ERCP techniques, and when available, diagnostic and therapeutic EUS.

Special considerations

The necessary skills are best obtained in a high volume, tertiary referral center. The trainee must be trained by a trainer with particular expertise in pseudocyst access and drainage techniques, particularly ERCP and stent placement. Training is supported by instruction in related EUS disciplines as well.

Specific technical and cognitive skill sets

Pseudocyst management requires sufficient cognitive skills pertaining to clinical pancreatology, interpretation and use of noninvasive imaging (CT and MRI), and medical evaluation and follow-up of pseudocysts to properly guide use and performance of therapeutic intervention. Necessary technical skills include therapeutic ERCP with stent placement, balloon dilation, and guide wire management. Baseline EUS skills include EUS-guided fine needle aspiration (EUS-FNA). The ability to management procedure-related complications is critical.

It is important to note first and foremost that there are several types of pancreatic fluid collections that are often confused with pancreatic pseudocysts on imaging studies. These include acute fluid collections, pancreatic abscesses, and organized or walled-off pancreatic necrosis. This chapter addresses pancreatic pseudocysts and the methods used allow resolution of collections that are composed of liquid.

Acute fluid collections

Acute fluid collections arise early in the course of acute pancreatitis, are usually peripancreatic in location, and typically resolve without sequelae but may evolve into pancreatic pseudocysts. Acute fluid collections are liquefied and rarely require drainage [1].

Acute pancreatic pseudocyst

Acute pancreatic pseudocysts arise as a sequela of acute pancreatitis, require at least 4 weeks to form, and are devoid of significant solid debris. Acute pancreatic pseudocysts usually develop secondary to limited pancreatic necrosis that produces a pancreatic ductal leak (Figure 28.1). Alternatively, areas of pancreatic and peripancreatic fat necrosis may completely liquefy over time and become a pseudocyst [2]. Despite the requirement of at least 4 weeks for a pseudocyst to form, it is important to note that this time period in and of itself does not define the collection as a pancreatic pseudocyst. In patients with significant pancreatic necrosis ($\geq$ 30%), the early acute pancreatic and peripancreatic necrosis may resemble a pseudocyst radiographically, but instead represent organized or walled-off pancreatic necrosis (please see section Organized or walled-off pancreatic necrosis). By definition, if these collections contain significant solid debris (i.e., necrosis), they are not pseudocysts and endoscopic treatment of these collections by typical pseudocyst drainage methods must be avoided due to the risk of infectious complications resulting from inadequate removal of solid debris [3].

Chronic pancreatic pseudocyst

Chronic pancreatic pseudocysts arise as a sequela of chronic pancreatitis and form secondary to stricture and/or stones that lead to

Successful Training in Gastrointestinal Endoscopy, First Edition. Edited by Jonathan Cohen.
© 2011 Blackwell Publishing Ltd. Published 2011 by Blackwell Publishing Ltd.

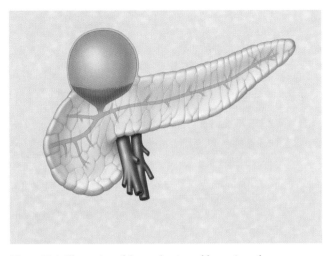

Figure 28.1 Illustration of the mechanism of formation of an acute pancreatic pseudocyst. Limited necrosis of the main pancreatic duct produces a ductal leak with accumulation of amylase-rich fluid.

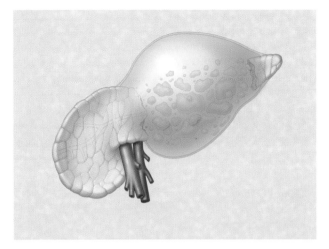

Figure 28.3 Illustration depicting organized pancreatic necrosis (walled-off necrosis). The collection is composed of liquid and solid, and is an expansion of the area.

main pancreatic duct obstruction. The resulting increased intraductal pressure leads to upstream ductal leak (Figure 28.2).

Pancreatic Abscess

Pancreatic abscesses have been defined in various ways. While some classification systems have suggested these are unique and rare entities that develop from limited pancreatic necrosis that becomes liquefied, it is probably most acceptable that an infected, liquefied collection of any type (e.g., infected pancreatic pseudocyst but not infected pancreatic necrosis) can be considered an abscess. Since these are liquefied they should resolve with endoscopic pseudocyst drainage techniques.

Organized or walled-off pancreatic necrosis

Over the ensuing several weeks after the onset of acute severe (necrotizing) pancreatitis, a collection may evolve to contain both liquid and solid necrotic debris (Figure 28.3). The resulting collection has been referred to as organized or walled-off pancreatic necrosis (WOPN) to differentiate this process from the early (acute phase) of pancreatic necrosis. The CT appearance often mimics an acute pseudocyst (Figure 28.4). Because the underlying solid debris is frequently not discernible by CT, its homogeneous appearance may lead one to embark on standard pseudocyst drainage methods which to not adequately remove the underlying solid material. This may result in serious infectious complications.

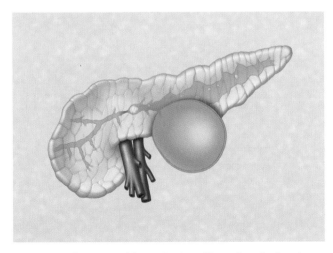

Figure 28.2 Illustration of the mechanism of formation of a chronic pancreatic pseudocyst. Obstruction of the main pancreatic duct by stones and/or stricture produces a duct blowout with accumulation of amylase-rich fluid.

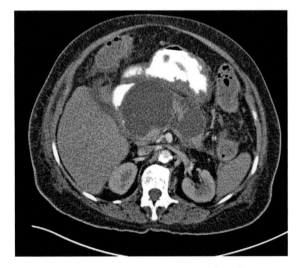

Figure 28.4 CT of organized pancreatic necrosis. This collection occurred after an episode of severe pancreatitis and could be confused with a pseudocyst.

CT features that may distinguish WOPN from pancreatic pseudocysts include larger size, extension to paracolic space, irregular wall definition, presence of fat attenuation debris within the collection, and pancreatic deformity or discontinuity [4]. Data suggest that MRI accurately distinguishes WOPN from a pancreatic pseudocyst [5]. Since these collections are composed of liquid and solid material they require more than pseudocyst drainage techniques to be successfully managed endoscopically.

Equipment

1 *Essential equipment*
- Linear array echoendoscope and/or side-viewing therapeutic endoscope (duodenoscope)
- Access device (e.g., dedicated needles, needle knife, cystenterotome)
- Electrosurgical generator—blended and coagulation
- Water-soluble contrast
- 0.018″–0.035″ guide wires (depending on needle used)
- 4, 6, 8, 10 mm dilating balloons
- 7 and 10 Fr double pigtail stents, array of lengths
- Array of straight pancreatic duct stents (5 Fr, 7 Fr, and 10 Fr diameters)

2 *Additional equipment (when employing EUS):*
- Linear array echoendoscope (ideally with high resolution Doppler and a therapeutic channel)
- 19-gauge EUS-FNA needle (22-gauge needle less often employed)
- 0.018″ and 0.035″ guide wires (depending on needle caliber used for puncture)

3 *Salvage accessories*
- Hemostasis accessories—injection needles, epinephrine, endoclips, bipolar electrocoagulation
- Rat-toothed forceps—therapeutic size
- Standard polypectomy snare

Key steps of proper technique

Pseudocyst drainage can be performed using a transmural (transgastric or transduodenal) and/or transpapillary approach. In turn, the transmural approach can be performed with a duodenoscope alone, using EUS for initial access, or achieving access and drainage both under EUS-guidance. These approaches will be discussed separately.

Prior to the procedure, there are several key aspects that must be considered.

Predrainage evaluation

Before embarking upon endoscopic drainage of a pancreatic fluid collection, the endoscopist must always ask the following questions:

1 Did the fluid collection arise secondary to pancreatic inflammation? There are many masqueraders of pancreatic pseudocysts, including: primary cystic pancreatic neoplasms (e.g., mucinous tumor or serous cystadenoma), extrapancreatic cystic lesions (e.g., duplication cyst, mesenteric cyst, or lymphoepithelial cyst), and

other lesions including a pseudoaneurysm, abutting gallbladder, etc. The endoscopist should always consider the possibility of these other cystic lesions, particularly in patients without a well-documented history of pancreatitis.

2 Could the patient have an underlying pancreatic neoplasia such as a carcinoma or an islet cell tumor? An elderly patient who presents with either "idiopathic pancreatitis" complicated by a fluid collection or someone who develops a documented pancreatic pseudocyst in the absence of clinical pancreatitis should be carefully evaluated to exclude an underlying pancreatic neoplasm causing pancreatic ductal obstruction and upstream ductal leak. Similarly, autoimmune pancreatitis may lead to pseudocyst formation [6]. Solid pancreatic tumors may undergo necrosis and cystic degeneration, and occasionally be mistaken for a pancreatic fluid collection.

Once the decision has been made to endoscopically manage a PFC, the following imaging and laboratory evaluation should be undertaken:

1 *Oral and intravenous contrast enhanced thin cut abdominal CT scan*: This allows the precise localization and proximity of the collection in relation to the stomach and duodenum in anticipation of possible transmural drainage. Additionally, the relationship of the collection to potential intervening vascular structures and to assess the potential presence of varices that may result from splenic vein or portal vein thrombosis. Pancreatic parenchymal and ductal features (e.g., presence of intraductal stones) may also be assessed. These parameters are used to guide therapy and also provide prognostic value.

Consideration should be given to performing the following imaging studies:

- *Endoscopic ultrasound (EUS)*: EUS may be performed prior to considering drainage of a pancreatic fluid collection for several reasons. First, if there is any diagnostic uncertainty then EUS evaluation of the cystic lesion, pancreas, and surrounding structures (e.g., lymph nodes or liver) often allows differentiation of a pseudocyst from noninflammatory cystic lesions. In the proper setting, this evaluation is often aided by EUS-guided cyst fluid analysis and tissue sampling of a solid component via fine needle aspiration and/or trucut biopsy. Second, EUS may be used to identify solid debris that often represents necrotic material, the presence of which may alter the management strategy. Finally, EUS examination of the intervening structures may provide useful information to guide the route and method of drainage. For instance, the presence of intervening vascular structures or solid organs may indicate the need for image-guided access. Thereafter, EUS may be used to guide transmural drainage (please see scetion Endoscopic drainage methods).
- MRI may be performed to identify solid debris that predicts the presence of necrosis.

2 *Coagulation parameters*: Given the high potential for bleeding complications, the laboratory examination must include platelet count and INR, and detailed history of anticoagulation medications taken is essential.

Types of endoscopic drainage

There are two approaches to drainage of pancreatic pseudocysts. The decision as to the approach is made based upon the size

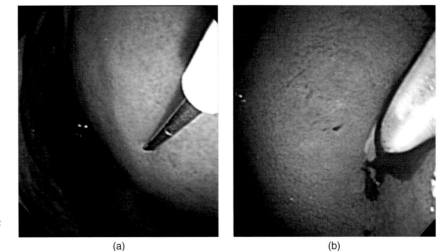

Figure 28.5 Endoscopic puncture of pancreatic pseudocyst. (a) Needle is seen exiting the endoscope but is not perpendicular to the gastric wall. (b) Puncture of pseudocyst after orienting needle.

(a) (b)

of the pseudocyst, the apposition or lack thereof to the gastric or duodenal wall, and presence or absence of pancreatic ductal communication. Thus, pancreatography can be performed prior to drainage if the approach has not been definitively determined based upon imaging. We believe that pancreatography should be performed in nearly all patients either at the initial drainage or during follow-up, particularly in patients with underlying chronic pancreatitis, since untreated ductal abnormalities (strictures and stones) may lead to recurrence after transgastric drainage. In addition, if the collection arose from severe acute pancreatitis there may be a major ductal disruption that needs to be addressed early to prevent ductal disconnection after the collection resolves with transmural drainage.

Transmural drainage

Transmural drainage of PFCs is achieved by passing a device through the gut (gastric or duodenal) wall into the fluid collection followed by dilatation of the tract from the gut wall into the fluid collection. One or more large-bore stents are placed through the gut wall into the fluid collection. As compared to transpapillary stenting alone, transmural drainage may be favored for fluid collections that are large, complex, or infected. Combined transpapillary and transmural drainage methods may also be performed.

NonEUS-guided transmural drainage

The nonEUS approach requires thorough familiarity with the anatomy as it relates to CT and MRI imaging. The entry point (stomach vs. duodenum) is usually selected prior to the procedure after careful review of the CT or MRI to determine the closest point of access that avoids traversal of critical structures.

Using a side-viewing endoscope (duodenoscope), a point of extraluminal compression (visible bulge) is identified and the puncture performed into the pseudocyst with or without cautery (Figures 28.5a and b, Video 28.1). If electrocautery is used, the initial identification of an adequate site of access can be achieved using a standard sclerotherapy needle, though the needle may not be long enough to allow transgastric puncture into the pseudocyst depending on the degree of edema and the pseudocyst

wall thickness. The tip of the duodenoscope is oriented to allow a perpendicular orientation to the puncture site (Figure 28.5b, Video 28.1). It is important to keep the duodenoscope close to the gastric or duodenal wall to maximize the mechanical advantage. With the assistance of the elevator the needle is rapidly advanced through the gut wall. Cyst access is confirmed by aspiration of fluid contents and/or injection of water-soluble contrast under fluoroscopy (Figure 28.6). If the entire procedure is done without electrocautery using the Seldinger technique, a needle is used that allows passage of a guide wire through the needle into the collection (Video 28.1). At the present time, no dedicated needles for this purpose are commercially available, though are expected to be released soon. We are using a commercially available sclerotherapy needle (Marcon–Haber, Cook Endoscopy) that accepts a 0.018″

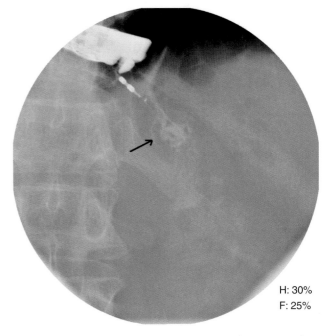

H: 30%
F: 25%

Figure 28.6 Contrast injection through needle passed transgastrically confirms entry into collection (arrow).

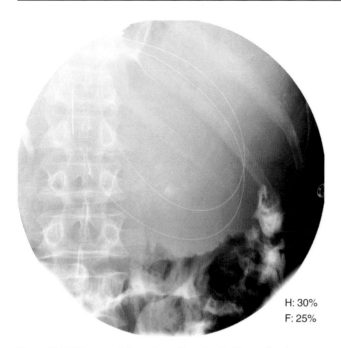

Figure 28.7 Wire passed through needle and coiled into collection.

guide wire. At least one large loop of wire is formed to help assure access during subsequent interventions (Figure 28.7, Video 28.1). If electrocautery is used, a wire-guided needle knife can be passed over the guide wire, which has been coiled into the collection. The needle knife is used to puncture into the cavity using either pure coagulation or a blended current.

Some endoscopists perform localization and entry into the collection using a needle without electrocautery using the Seldinger technique (Video 28.1). This method may be safer when EUS is not used because if the collection is not successfully entered with the needle (confirmed by aspiration of fluid and/or injection of radiopaque contrast), the needle is simply withdrawn without adverse sequelae. Similarly, if bleeding occurs upon needle entry, if gross blood is aspirated, or if a visible hematoma develops, the needle is withdrawn to allow the vessel to tamponade. Another transmural entry site may be chosen during the same endoscopic session. The disadvantage to this approach is that it can be difficult to pass a dilating balloon over the needle-created tract when a transgastric approach is chosen.

Once the collection has been successfully entered, the needle knife or puncture needle is withdrawn leaving the guide wire coiled in the collection (Video 28.1). The transmural tract is balloon dilated to 8–10 mm using standard biliary dilating balloons (4 cm length) (Figure 28.8a and b, Video 28.1) to allow placement of one or more double pigtail 10 Fr stents (Figure 28.9a and b, Video 28.1). Some endoscopists dilate to 18 mm, whereas others avoid this approach given the potential heightened risk of bleeding or perforation. There are insufficient data to determine the relative benefit and risk of aggressive dilation and we generally only do so during therapy of WOPN due to the need to pass a forward-viewing endoscope directly into the cavity to debride the necrotic material. The balloon is inflated with contrast to allow visualization of a waist. Half-strength contrast is preferred since it is less viscous and allows more rapid balloon deflation, especially when balloons of 10 mm or larger are used. When deflating the balloon a large amount of fluid may rapidly flow from the collection (Video 28.1), which creates two problems. The first is

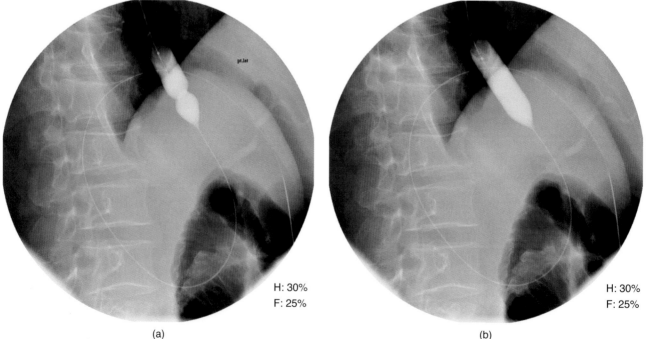

(a)   (b)

Figure 28.8 Balloon dilation of gastric wall. (a) Waist seen in balloon. (b) After effacement of waist.

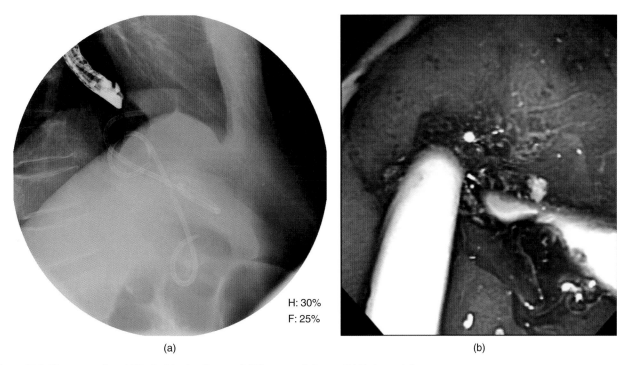

H: 30%
F: 25%

(a)   (b)

Figure 28.9 Placement of two 10 Fr double pigtail stents. (a) Fluoroscopic image. (b) Endoscopic image.

the potential for aspiration and the second is loss of endoscopic view. This situation can often be avoided by slowly deflating the balloon, thereby allowing the fluid to be adequately aspirated via the endoscope. Some endoscopists place a nasogastric tube prior to performing the drainage procedure to allow any fluid to be suctioned. However, the presence of a balloon within the accessory channel may prohibit adequate suction. If necessary, the balloon may be rapidly deflated and quickly withdrawn to maximize suction capacity. During this time the endoscope should be kept in close proximity to the access point and continuous suction applied to the endoscope to optimize fluid removal until the view improves and the fluid egress slows. Finally, one can consider endotracheal intubation as a preventative measure.

Prior to stent placement, some endoscopists prefer to pass a second guide wire in anticipation of a second stent. This can achieved in one of several ways: a "freehand" passage can be performed where the wire is passed without a catheter; a standard catheter can be passed into the collection with a wire alongside the first wire; or a large catheter (10 Fr Soehendra dilator [7]) or double-lumen catheter preloaded with a second wire can be passed over the existing wire [8].

The final step is placement of transmural stents. The length varies but short (5 cm long) double pigtail stents are adequate in nearly all cases. Traditional straight stents should be avoided for transmural drainage because of the propensity to migrate and the increased risk of delayed bleeding which may occur when the cavity collapses and abuts the distal end of the stent [9]. Assuming a therapeutic channel endoscope is used, 10 Fr stents are placed. Some stents are available with endoscopically and fluoroscopically visible markers to help assure proper placement. If not, an indelible marker is used to place a mark at the midpoint of the stent

(Video 28.1). Again, it is important to keep the endoscope as close as possible to the gastric or duodenal wall during the initial passage of the stent. The stent is passed into the cavity until the midpoint is identified. The endoscope is then withdrawn away from the wall while advancing the remaining portion of the stent out of the endoscope (Video 28.1). This last maneuver is important so as to not place the entire stent within the collection. If a second guide wire was not already secured, one can be passed alongside the initial stent (Video 28.1). A second wire can be placed using the guide wire and pusher tube of the just-deployed stent as a catheter to "recannulate" (reenter) the cyst cavity. It is important to ensure that the second guide wire has entered the cavity and not passed between the transmural site and the luminal wall (outside the cavity). The wire should be seen to coil within the cavity, which by this point should be air-filled and allow an outline to be seen. The second stent is then placed alongside the first as previously described.

EUS-guided transmural drainage

During the EUS exam, an initial inspection of the PFC and surrounding structures may provide key information to help guide subsequent interventions. Initial imaging allows one to determine the presence of viscous contents verus nonviscous fluid, and/or necrosis that may impact the decision to perform drainage. It is also used to exclude the presence of intervening structures such as gastric varices or adjacent organs that may contraindicate drainage or modify the point of access. After identifying a needle trajectory that minimizes the distance from the gut wall to the cyst wall, an FNA needle is inserted under EUS guidance into the pseudocyst (Figure 28.10). We prefer large caliber (19-gauge) needles that accommodate a 0.035″ guide wire, which provides greater

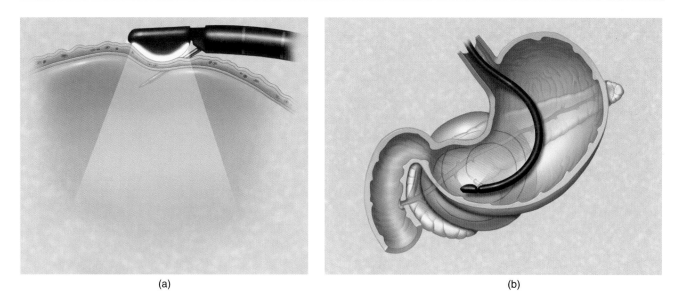

(a)   (b)

Figure 28.10 EUS-guided drainage. (a) Illustration of EUS-guided puncture. (b) Illustration of guide wire passed through EUS needle.

stiffness and facilitates subsequent interventions. The guide wire is coiled within the pseudocyst cavity to help maintain access during subsequent interventions. Although EUS imaging assures that the cyst was entered, radiopaque contrast may be injected and/or cyst fluid aspirated for additional confirmation. The outer catheter of the needle can be advanced into the cyst to provide an initial dilatation that may facilitate subsequent passage of the dilating balloon.

Once accessed, the FNA needle is withdrawn and the entire tract is balloon-dilated and the remainder of the procedure follows what was outlined for nonEUS guidance.

Transpapillary drainage

If the collection communicates with the main pancreatic duct, placement of a pancreatic stent with or without pancreatic sphinc-

terotomy is an approach that is useful, especially for collections measuring < 5–6 cm that are not otherwise approachable transmurally [10]. The proximal end of the stent (toward the pancreatic tail) may directly enter the collection or bridge the area of leak into the pancreatic duct upstream from the leak (Figure 28.11a and b). Data suggest that complete bridging of the duct leak results in the greatest success rate [11]. The diameter of pancreatic stent used is dependent on the pancreatic ductal diameter, but is usually 7 Fr. In patients with chronic pancreatitis there are often strictures and/or stones downstream from the leak site. These must be traversed with a guide wire in order for successful stent placement (Figure 28.11c, Figure 28.12). We find that hydrophilic wires are particularly useful for this. In addition, strictures may need to be dilated in order to allow stent passage. If possible, the obstructing stone(s) should be removed, though this can be attempted

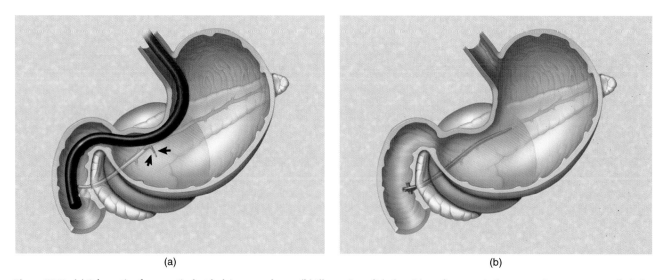

(a)   (b)

Figure 28.11 (a) Schematic of pancreatic duct leak into pseudocyst. (b) Illustration of ideal position of pancreatic duct stent placement across a leak site.

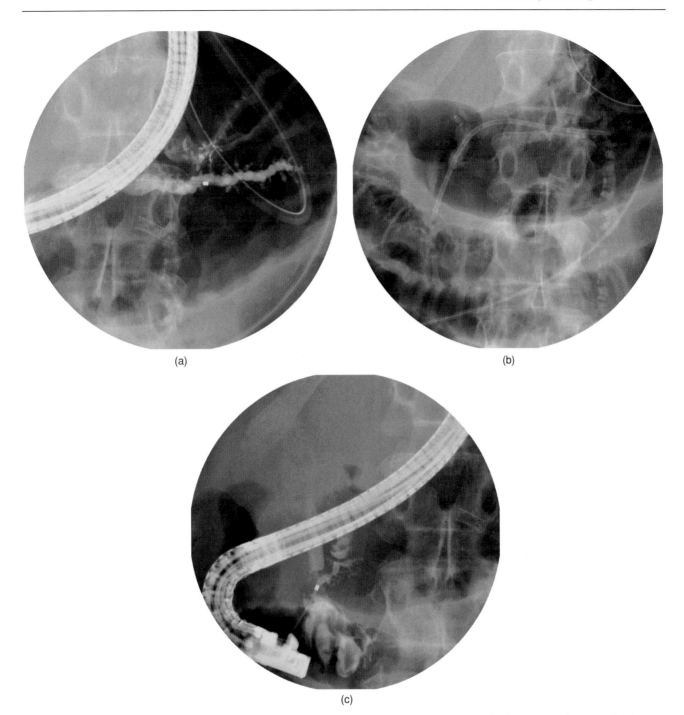

(a)

(b)

(c)

Figure 28.12 Pancreatic duct leak in setting of chronic pancreatitis. (a) Pancreatogram showing leak superiorly. (b) Pancreatic duct stent placed across leak site. (c) Stricture at head responsible for downstream obstruction.

once the pseudocyst has resolved. Pancreatic duct stone removal is often more complicated than bile duct stone removal because the stones are much harder, are frequently impacted in strictures and side branches, and have sharp facets that result in rupture of stone-removal balloons. Extracorporeal shock wave lithotripsy is employed to remove stones when endoscopic techniques fail [12].

The advantage of the transpapillary approach over the transmural approach is the avoidance of bleeding or perforation that may occur with transmural drainage. The disadvantage of transpapillary drainage is that pancreatic stents may induce scarring of the main pancreatic duct in patients whose pancreatic duct is otherwise normal (i.e., patients with acute pseudocysts and small side branch disruption) [13,14].

Setting and tools for training

At the present time, pseudocyst drainage skills are taught to upper-level fellows (third year) during ERCP rotations or to advanced trainees (additional fourth year training). If such fellows do not have exposure to pseudocyst drainage, some basic skills for performing the procedure are acquired during EUS and ERCP rotations.

It is unknown how much training is required to gain proficiency in pseudocyst drainage. One study involving 175 patients who underwent pancreatic fluid collection drainage by an experienced therapeutic endoscopist demonstrated a significant improvement in pseudocyst resolution rates after the first 20 procedures versus subsequent procedures (45% vs. 93%). In the authors' opinion, at least 10 drainage procedures are required to gain a basic skill level. It is unknown whether the time period over which these cases were performed is also important but presumably a shorter duration of exposure would also result in greater competency. In addition, continued experience is important in learning and maintaining one's skill level. We also believe that one cannot learn such skills adequately with currently available simulator-based training. Theoretically, an animal model could be used for training. One such model has been described in canines [15], though the cost of this would likely be prohibitive. Given the relatively low volume of cases at many centers, realistic adaptation of ex-vivo EUS simulators to allow for repetitive practice of these skills would be an attractive complement to real case experience mentored by experts. Developments along these lines are already underway.

Defining competency

Assessing competency may be problematic unless an adequate volume of cases is available for one to learn the techniques. In some centers, endoscopic drainage is performed commonly based upon center volume, competing local expertise, and referral patterns. There are no tools that are available to measure skill nor are there established parameters in which to gauge competency. Our opinion is that key factors to look for in evaluating whether someone has been successfully trained is ability to accurately puncture during FNA (nonpseudocyst) and ERCP skills such as maintaining guide wire access and endoscope positioning. There is no benchmark of expert practice for this particular skill.

Maintaining skill level

Keeping skills well honed may be difficult for these relatively low volume procedures. It is unknown how much volume is needed to maintain skill level. We suggest that at least one drainage procedure per month is necessary.

Video

Video 28.1 Pancreatic pseudocyst drainage

References

1 Adkisson KW, Baron TH, Morgan DE: Pancreatic fluid collections: diagnosis and endoscopic management. *Seminars in Gastrointestinal Disease* 1998;**9**:61–72.

2 Kloppel G: Pathology of severe acute pancreatitis. In: Bradley EL, III (ed), *Acute Pancreatitis: Diagnosis and Therapy.* New York: Raven Press, 1994:35–46.

3 Hariri M, Slivka A, Carr-Locke DL, et al.: Pseudocyst drainage predisposes to infection when pancreatic necrosis is unrecognized. *Am J Gastroenterol* 1994;**89**:1781–1784.

4 Takahashi N, Papachristou GI, Schmit GD, et al.: CT findings of walled-off pancreatic necrosis (WOPN): differentiation from pseudocyst and prediction of outcome after endoscopic therapy. *Eur Radiol* 2008;**18**:2522–2529.

5 Morgan DE, Baron TH, Smith JK, et al.: Pancreatic fluid collections prior to intervention: evaluation with MR imaging compared with CT and US. *Radiology* 1997;**203**:773–778.

6 Welsch T, Kleeff J, Esposito I, et al.: Autoimmune pancreatitis associated with a large pancreatic pseudocyst. *World J Gastroenterol* 2006 Sep 28;**12**(36):5904–5906.

7 Ang TL, Teo EK, Fock KM: EUS-guided drainage of infected pancreatic pseudocyst: use of a 10F Soehendra dilator to facilitate a double-wire technique for initial transgastric access (with videos). *Gastrointest Endosc* 2008;**68**:192–194.

8 Seewald S, Thonke F, Ang TL, et al.: One-step, simultaneous double-wire technique facilitates pancreatic pseudocyst and abscess drainage (with videos). *Gastrointest Endosc* 2006;**64**:805–808.

9 Cahen D, Rauws E, Fockens P, et al.: Endoscopic drainage of pancreatic pseudocysts: long-term outcome and procedural factors associated with safe and successful treatment. *Endoscopy* 2005;**37**:977–983.

10 Barthet M, Lamblin G, Gasmi M, et al.: Clinical usefulness of a treatment algorithm for pancreatic pseudocysts. *Gastrointest Endosc* 2008;**67**:245–252.

11 Telford JJ, Farrell JJ, Saltzman JR, et al.: Pancreatic stent placement for duct disruption. *Gastrointest Endosc* 2002;**56**:18–24.

12 Guda NM, Partington S, Freeman ML: Extracorporeal shock wave lithotripsy in the management of chronic calcific pancreatitis: a meta-analysis. *JOP* 2005;**6**:6–12.

13 Kozarek RA: Pancreatic stents can induce ductal changes consistent with chronic pancreatitis. *Gastrointest Endosc* 1990;**36**:93–95.

14 Smith MT, Sherman S, Ikenberry SO, et al.: Alterations in pancreatic ductal morphology following polyethylene pancreatic stent therapy. *Gastrointest Endosc* 1996;**44**:268–275.

15 Salinas A, Triebling A, Toth L, et al.: The pathogenesis of pancreatic pseudocysts–a canine experimental model. *Am J Gastroenterol* 1985 Feb;**80**(2):126–131.

Enteral Access Techniques: Percutaneous Endoscopic Gastrostomy and Jejunostomy

James A. DiSario

University of Utah Health Sciences Center, Salt Lake City, UT, USA

Introduction

Endoscopic procedures for percutaneous enteral access include percutaneous endoscopic gastrostomy (PEG), percutaneous endoscopic gastrostomy with jejunal extension (PEG-J), and direct percutaneous endoscopic jejunostomy (DPEJ) [1]. These procedures have specific indications, and many common and unique techniques that must be imparted to the trainee. Fundamental principles are those of standard esophagogastroduodenoscopy (EGD), guide wire techniques, push enteroscopy and fluoroscopy. PEGs are the mainstay for long-term provision of enteral nutrition. Jejunal access is required for persons with intolerance to gastric feeds, regurgitation of gastric contents, aspiration pneumonia, and severe acute and/or chronic pancreatitis [2]. The instruction process involves a stepwise progression in procedural training from PEG to PEG-J, and ultimately to DPEJ. The trainee should be taught both the endoscopic and abdominal wall maneuvers required for these procedures. Additionally, the beginner must be taught about replacement and removal of these tubes, stoma management, and complications [3–5].

Prerequisite expertise and skill

Most enteral nutritional access procedures are Level 1, which means that they are appropriate for the routine practice of gastroenterology [3–7]. The trainee should understand that these procedures are a mainstream part of the practice of gastroenterology, can be performed in a safe and efficient manner with proper techniques, and are effective in the short and long terms. Trainees must understand the principles of gut anatomy and physiology. They should be skilled in EGD prior to attempting PEG, and guide wire manipulation, push enteroscopy, and basic fluoroscopy as prerequisites for jejunal access procedures. The trainee must also understand principles of sterile surgical technique, and

wound and stoma care. Because of the difficulty in maneuvering the endoscope in the jejunum, and the need for an assertive trocar puncture into the jejunum, DPEJ is most appropriately taught only after the trainee has developed significant PEG and enteroscopy skills [5–7].

Success in DPEJ placement depends in part on the patient's body habitus as abdominal wall and omental fat may limit the ability to transilluminate adequately. Jejunostomy placement is generally easier in patients with previous abdominal surgery because of adhesions that may cause small bowel adherence to the abdominal wall and limit motion. This type of patient is good for initial training for the novice [2–5].

Setting

Training should be done in accredited training programs with trainers who are experts in endoscopy and teaching [3,6,7]. Training in most enteral access procedures can be done in appropriately accredited standard ambulatory or inpatient units. Jejunal access procedures may require fluoroscopy and the requisite facilities. Requirements for trainees are generally those of EGD; however, jejunal access procedures may require more experience with the technique being performed [8].

Equipment

There are numerous commercially available products for enteral nutritional access. It is not necessary for the trainees to know all about the numerous products but they must be made familiar with one or two types of devices for each technique. PEG, PEG-J, and DPEJ gastrostomy devices are often made of silicone or polyurethane, are 12 to 24 Fr, contain an internal fixation apparatus that may have a balloon or molded mushroom shape, and have an external bolster and a coupling device. Generally, they come in kits that contain all necessary supplies including: topical

Successful Training in Gastrointestinal Endoscopy, First Edition. Edited by Jonathan Cohen.
© 2011 Blackwell Publishing Ltd. Published 2011 by Blackwell Publishing Ltd.

disinfectants, syringes and needles, injectable anesthetics, a scalpel, an endoscopic snare, a guide wire, antibiotic ointment, dressing materials, and instruction booklets for the providers and patient. PEG-J jejunal extension tubes range from 9 to 12 Fr, are about 60 cm long, and may come with or without a central lumen for passage over a wire. Other systems may also contain T-fasteners, a sequential dilation apparatus for the track, and a peel-away sheath. PEG-J kits may have a separate jejunal tube that passes through the PEG with a coupling device. DPEJ insertion may be done with a standard PEG kit. Replacement tubes are available in various diameters with an adjustable external fixation bolster and an inflatable internal fixation balloon. There are also tubes with a mushroom-shaped internal fixation tip that can be stretched straight with the enclosed stylet. The mushroom shape will return when the stylet is removed. These tubes come in preset lengths for the stoma track and require a measuring device. Endoscopic clips may be useful for J-tube fixation [8].

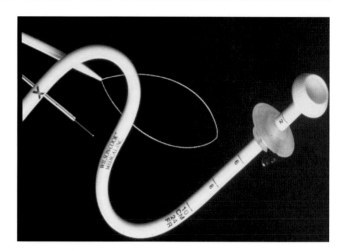

Figure 29.1 The pull-PEG apparatus. The image shows a 24-Fr polyurethane PEG tube with a mushroom-type internal fixation design and a moveable external bolster over the tube.

Key steps for proper technique

Percutaneous Endoscopic Gastrostomy (PEG) insertion, replacement and removal

Pull- or push-type PEG insertion

Pull-type PEGs are systems where the PEG tube is attached to a loop in the wire passed through the abdominal wall and out through the mouth. The wire is pulled from outside the abdomen to retract the PEG tube through the mouth, esophagus, and out the stoma. A pull-PEG apparatus is shown in Figure 29.1, a commercial kit in Figure 29.2, and the procedure is demonstrated in Figure 29.3. The push-type employs a guide wire pulled through the abdominal wall and out through the mouth. The PEG tube

is inserted over the guide wire and pushed through the mouth, esophagus, stomach and abdominal wall where it is grasped and pulled through [2,9]. The push-PEG procedure is shown in Figure 29.4. The following steps should be taught to the trainee:

1 *Prophylactic antibiotics:* Give antibiotics if the patient is not already on treatment.

2 Position the patient supine.

3 *Abdominal preparation and draping:* Use sterile technique prepping from the presumed PEG site outward in a spiral fashion. Cover the entire abdomen with sterile drapes. This may be done after transillumination and digital indentation is assured.

4 *Sterile attire:* The person doing the abdominal maneuvers should wear a sterile gown and gloves.

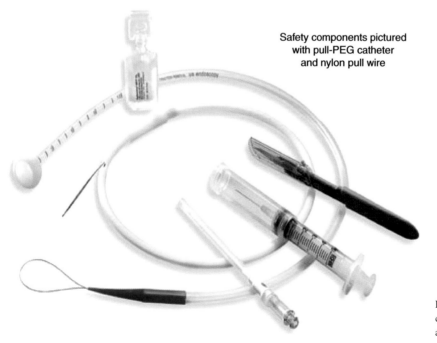

Safety components pictured
with pull-PEG catheter
and nylon pull wire

Figure 29.2 A commercial pull-PEG kit. The kit contains a silicone PEG tube, guide wire, local anesthetic, scalpel, syringe, and trocar.

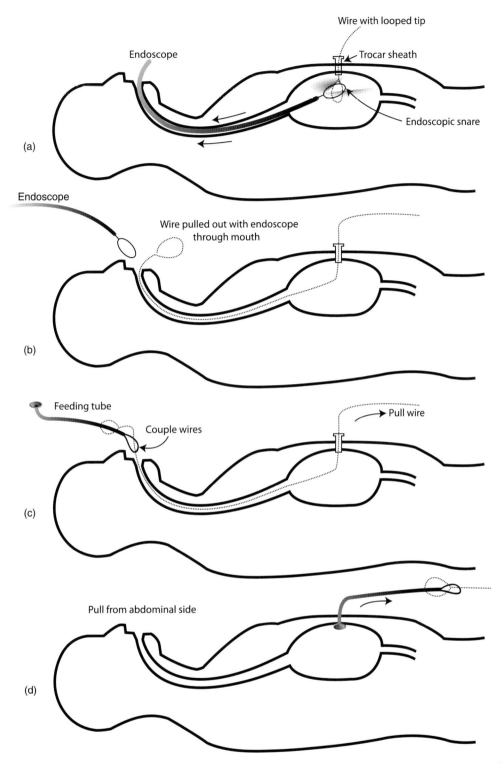

Figure 29.3 The pull-PEG. (a) The endoscope is positioned in the stomach, a loop-tipped guide wire is passed through the transabdominal trocar sheath and ensnared in an endoscopic snare, and the endoscope is retracted. (b) The endoscope is pulled out through the mouth and the transabdominal wire is released. (c) The pull-PEG feeding tube is coupled with the transendoscopic wire which is retracted from the abdominal side. (d) The transendoscopic wire and pull-PEG feeding tube are pulled through the abdominal wall, the trocar sheath is removed, and retraction is continued until the internal retention bumper is felt to abut the gastric and abdominal walls.

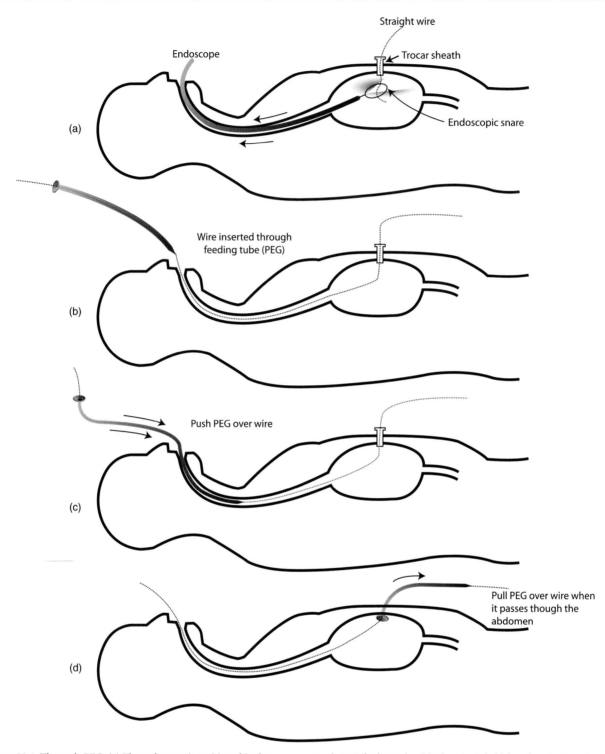

Figure 29.4 The push-PEG. (a) The endoscope is positioned in the stomach, a straight-tipped guide wire is inserted through the transabdominal trocar sheath and ensnared in the endoscopic snare, and the endoscope is retracted out through the mouth. (b) The transabdominal wire is released from the snare and inserted through the push-PEG feeding tube. (c) The wire is held firm from both ends and the push-PEG is pushed over the wire. (d) The trocar sheath is removed, the tip of the feeding tube is grasped when it passes through the abdominal wall and the feeding tube is then pulled until the internal retention bumper is felt to abut against the gastric and abdominal walls.

5 *Sedation and analgesia:* Administer standard mild to moderate sedation and analgesia.

6 *Perform EGD:* Endoscopists frequently find lesions that change clinical management. Esophageal intubation in the supine position is facilitated by flexing the neck. Carefully observe and suction the oropharynx to prevent aspiration in the supine patient.

7 *Abdominal site selection:* The optimal site is in the left upper quadrant at least 2 cm inferior to the costal margin. This will minimize the potential for the ribs to touch the PEG tube and cause pain when the patient sits upright. Other sites can also be used, including through a scar or prior PEG site. Site selection is dependent on transillumination and digital palpation.

8 *Gastric insufflation:* This causes the anterior gastric wall to abut the abdominal wall, and allows for transillumination.

9 *Gastric site selection:* The anterior aspect of the gastric body is generally best. Position the PEG in the proximal body, which directs the axis of the PEG tube toward the pylorus. This is useful if the PEG is ever to be converted to a PEG-J. Distally-placed PEG tubes are angled more superiorly. This would require a jejunal extension tube to make an acute angle toward the pylorus. PEG-J conversion would then be difficult or impossible, and jejunal extension tubes unstable and prone to displacement.

10 *Transillumination:* Position the tip of the endoscope close to the anterior gastric wall to direct the light through the abdominal wall. Darken the endoscopy room and use the transillumination mode on the endoscopic processing unit for a brighter light to facilitate this maneuver if necessary.

11 *Digital abdominal pressure (Video 29.1):* Apply digital abdominal wall pressure at the brightest transillumination site. Assure that there is direct indentation on the gastric view. Digital abdominal pressure may be used to help locate the transillumination site when it is not clearly seen in the standard fashion.

12 *Mark the spot:* Mark the site of maximal transillumination and digital indentation with a sterile marker or other device.

13 *Anesthetize the site:* Use a small caliber (25 gauge) needle for injection of the local anesthetic.

14 *The safe track (Video 29.2)* [10]: Attach fluid filled syringe with a medium gauge needle of adequate length to enter the stomach through the selected site. Aspirate back on the plunger as it is inserted. The needle should be endoscopically seen to enter the stomach at the same time that air is seen to enter the syringe. This helps to assure that there is not a loop of bowel interposed between the stomach and the abdominal wall. If air is seen in the syringe before the needle enters the stomach, there is likely to be interposed bowel. In this circumstance, the entire PEG process must be redone at a different site or the procedure aborted. For efficiency, use the syringe with the local anesthetic for the safe track and anesthetize the peritoneum and abdominal wall as the needle is withdrawn.

15 *Position the endoscopic snare:* Pass a snare through the endoscope and position it near the safe track site in the gastric mucosa.

16 *Trocar insertion (Video 29.3):* Insert the trocar through the safe track and endoscopically visualize it in the stomach. Gently ensnare the trocar and remove the obturator. Put a finger on the open trocar sheath to minimize air (and insufflation) loss, which could change the position of the stomach.

17 *Insert the guide wire (Video 29.4):* Pass the guide wire through the trocar sheath and grasp it with a snare a few centimeters from the tip. Pull the tip of the snare with ensnared guide wire slightly inside the working channel of the endoscope.

18 *Retract the endoscope and guide wire:* Unlock the knobs on the endoscope and gently retract it through the mouth while the person doing the abdominal maneuvers advances the wire to avoid tension. Leave the trocar sheath in place to prevent trauma to the puncture site. Clamp a hemostat on the abdominal end of the wire to avoid inadvertent retraction into the stomach or out through the mouth.

19 *Incision:* Make a 1 cm long incision at the puncture site adjacent to the wire. Orient the incision on the horizontal axis for a better cosmetic outcome in the event that the PEG is removed.

20 *Pass the gastrostomy tube (Video 29.5):* Secure the tube to the oral end of the wire (or pass it over the wire for push-type kits), liberally apply sterile lubrication, and pull (or push) it through the mouth and out through the abdominal incision site. If repeat gastroscopy is desired, facilitate esophageal reintubation by ensnaring the internal fixation bolster (mushroom tip) of the PEG tube with the snare extended slightly from the endoscope. Gently follow the tube through the pharynx and into the stomach.

21 *Secure and dress the PEG tube (Video 29.6):* Remove the wire and trim the external aspect of the tube from 15 to 20 cm from the skin. Gently retract the tube until the internal bolster abuts the abdominal wall. Slide the external fixation bolster onto the tube and push it down from 10 to 15 mm from the skin. Attach the coupling hubs to the tip of the tube and open it to gravity drainage for at least 2 hours. Antibiotic ointment and a dressing may be applied.

Peel-away sheath type PEG insertion [2,5]

This technique is demonstrated in Figure 29.5. The following steps should be taught to the trainee:

1 Position, preparation, and site selection as per steps 1 through 13 above.

2 *T-fasteners:* Insert three T-fasteners and secure the external discs that lock the sutures several centimeters apart in an equilateral triangle around the selected gastrostomy site. Perform a safe track maneuver by aspirating with a syringe on each T-fastener introducer needle [10].

3 Anesthetize the site. Use a small caliber (25 gauge) needle for injection of the local anesthetic.

4 Insert the introducer needle. Insert the introducer needle at the selected site in the center of the T-fastener triangle.

5 Pass the guide wire. Insert the guide wire through the introducer needle. The wire can be positioned free in the stomach. Remove the introducer needle, leaving the guide wire in place.

6 *Incision:* Make a 1 cm incision at the puncture site.

7 Dilate track and insert sheath. Lubricate the incision with water-soluble lubricant. Advance the serial dilator and peel-away sheath apparatus over the wire. Sequentially dilate the track by inserting the telescoping catheters with torquing motions.

8 Insert the peel-away sheath. Disengage the dilators from the sheath, lubricate the sheath and advance it over the dilators and

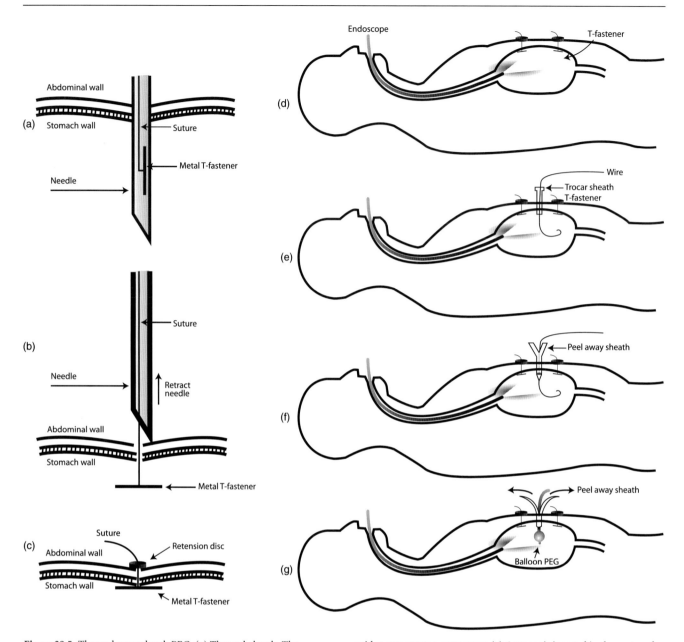

Figure 29.5 The peel-away sheath PEG. (a) The peel-sheath. The T-fastener apparatus is a hollow needle containing a small metal T-fastener with a suture connected to the center. The needle is inserted through the abdominal wall and into the insufflated stomach under endoscopic guidance. (b) The needle is retracted leaving the T-fastener connected to the suture in the stomach. (c) The T-fastener is pulled to appose the stomach against the abdominal wall, an external retention disc is attached, and the suture trimmed. (d) Three T-fasteners are positioned on the abdominal wall and deployed under endoscopic guidance to create a gastropexy. (e) A trocar is inserted in the center of the T-fastener triangle, a guide wire is inserted through the trocar sheath, and the sheath is removed. (f) An apparatus comprised of telescoping sequentially tapered dilators within a peel-away sheath is inserted over the guide wire and into the stomach. The dilators are removed leaving the peel-away sheath in place. (g) A feeding tube with an internal retention balloon is inserted through the peel-away sheath, the balloon inflated, the sheath peeled away, the balloon inflated, and the tube pulled until the balloon is felt to abut the gastric and abdominal wall.

into the stomach. Remove the dilators and guide wire leaving the peel-away sheath in place.

9 Insert the gastrostomy tube. Select an appropriate long or low-profile gastrostomy tube. Peel the sheath to about half of its length. Lubricate and insert the balloon-tipped gastrostomy tube through the sheath. Inflate the balloon according to manufacturers' instructions.

10 Peel away the sheath. Peel off sheath leaving the gastrostomy tube in place.

11 Remove the endoscope.

	Yes	No
Pre-procedure Appropriate indication Antibiotics		
Procedure Complete EGD		
PEG Maneuvers Insufflation Appropriate abdominal site Appropriate stomach site Transillumination Digital indentation Safe track Incision Tube insertion Tube trimming, assembly, & stoma dressing		
Subjective assessment Procedure successful Facile with procedure Competent		
Morbidity at 30 days Complication: Treatment: Outcome:		

Trainee:

Trainer:

Date:

Procedure number:

Duration:

Figure 29.6 PEG assessment form.

12 Secure and dress the PEG tube. Gently retract the tube until it abuts the abdominal wall. Advance the external fixation bolster over the tube from 10 to 15 mm from the skin. Open the tube to gravity drainage for at least 2 hours. Antibiotic ointment and a dressing may be applied.

PEG replacement and removal

It is important that the trainee understands that before replacement or removal of a PEG, the gastrostomy track must have developed mature fibrosis to prevent the stomach from separating from the abdominal wall. This would result in peritonitis from extravasation of gastric contents. Track maturation may occur within 3 weeks in a healthy, well-nourished person and up to 12 weeks in sick and malnourished persons. The removal technique is dependent on the device. Most commercially available endoscopic gastrostomy tubes are shaped with a flared mushroom-like internal retention bolster. The tube is simply pulled out with moderate traction. This can be done in virtually any setting. Complications and management must be understood. The following steps should be taught to the trainee [2,5]:

A *PEG replacement:*
  1 Position the patient supine
  2 *Abdominal preparation and draping:* Sedation is generally not required. Anesthetize the track with topical lidocaine gel. Securely cover PEG tube and stoma with a towel or drape to prevent spattering with removal.
  3 Remove the PEG tube. Support the abdominal wall with one hand and pull the tube with moderate force with the other. The tube will stretch and pop out.
  4 Insert the replacement gastrostomy tube. Lubricate and insert a balloon-tipped gastrostomy tube and inflate the balloon according to the manufacturers' instructions. For stretch-type tubes, measure the tract with a measuring device and choose a tube of appropriate length. Insert the stylet into the tube and

push until the tube stretches straight. Insert the lubricated tube through the stoma and remove the stylet.

5 Secure the PEG tube. Gently retract a balloon tube until it abuts the abdominal wall. Position the external fixation bolster to 10 mm from the skin. A dressing is not usually required.

6 Verify position. Irrigate the PEG with 50 mL of water. Verify that gastric contents can be aspirated into the syringe.

B *PEG removal:* This maneuver is the same as PEG replacement, with the exception that the stoma is dressed with gauze to prevent leakage of gastric contents. The stoma should close within 24 to 48 hours.

Percutaneous endoscopic gastrostomy with jejunal (or duodenal) extension (PEG-J) and direct percutaneous endoscopic jejunostomy (DPEG) insertion, replacement and removal

There are several techniques of PEG-J insertion that all begin with PEG placement as listed above. J-tube (extension tube) insertion may be achieved with a drag and pull technique or various wire-guided techniques. It is easier to place the tubes in the duodenum, but they are more prone to displacement than jejunal tubes. Fluoroscopy is helpful. The trainee should be taught the following steps [2,5]:

A *PEG-J insertion:* PEG-J tubes may be placed at the time of gastrostomy or through an existing gastrostomy. These devices have both jejunal and gastric ports for concomitant enteral feeding and gastric decompression.

I *De novo PEG-J insertion drag and pull technique:*

1 Select appropriate equipment. Use a commercially available PEG-J kit with a PEG tube and a compatible J-tube extension or use separately packaged compatible devices.

2 Select an appropriate endoscope. A gastroscope is best if the J-tube only needs to be placed into the distal duodenum. A pediatric colonoscope or enteroscope may be required for deep jejunal placement.

3 Insert the PEG as outlined above, but maintain the endoscope in the stomach.

4 Insert the J-tube. Lubricate the interior of the J-tube to minimize binding of the stylet and maintain the stylet in the J-tube. Insert the lubricated J-tube (extension tube) with a suture fixed to the tip through the PEG. Achieve an airtight seal between the PEG and J-tube with a commercial device or copious lubricating gel. Air leakage around the J-tube makes endoscopy very difficult.

5 Grasp the J-tube. Pass grasping forceps through the endoscope and grasp the suture on the J-tube. Grasping forceps are preferable to biopsy forceps, which may cut the suture.

6 Position the J-tube. Advance the endoscope dragging the J-tube into the desired area of small bowel. It is safer and easier to maneuver the endosocpe with the forceps slightly inside the working channel. Advance the forceps to push the J-tube farther into the small bowel and maintain its position, and simultaneously withdraw the endoscope as far as possible. The person working the abdominal aspects of the procedure may apply gently forward pressure on the J-tube to help maintain its position.

7 Remove the endoscope. Release the suture and retract the forceps to the tip of the endoscope. Grasp the side of the J-tube

with the forceps and push it distally to maintain position while further retracting the endoscope. Continue with gentle pressure from outside the patient. Repeat as required until the endoscope is removed. Great care must be taken as J-tubes notoriously fall back into the stomach due to friction from the endoscope [1,2,11].

8 Secure the J-tube. Remove the stylet and couple the J-tube with the PEG.

II *Wire-guided insertion technique:* The Trainee should be taught the following steps:

1 Select appropriate equipment and endoscope, and insert the PEG as outlined in steps 1 through 3 above.

2 Grasp the guide wire. Reinsert the endoscope and pass an endoscopic grasping forceps through the PEG tube from inside the stomach to outside the patient. Grasp the guide wire and retract it into the stomach.

3 Maintain an air lock. Use an air lock device or lubricating gel to prevent air loss and maintain insufflation.

4 Position the guide wire. Advance the endoscope into the small intestine while holding the guide wire. Securely hold the guide wire in the forceps. Withdraw the endoscope as far as possible while pushing forward on the forceps to maintain the position in the small bowel and tension of the guide wire.

5 Insert the J-tube. Introduce the lubricated J-tube over the guide wire and into the small bowel as far as possible. Open the forceps, release the guide wire, and withdraw the forceps to the endoscope.

6 Remove the endoscope. Grasp the side of the J-tube with the forceps and push forward to maintain its position while retracting the endoscope. Repeat as required until the endoscope is removed.

7 Secure the J-tube. Couple the J-tube with the PEG and remove the guide wire.

III *Transabdominal endoscopic insertion technique:* This approach is simplified, efficient, and effective using a small caliber (≤ 5 mm) gastroscope passed through the PEG stoma [2,12]. The trainee should be taught the following steps:

1 Select appropriate equipment and endoscope, and insert a 24 Fr PEG as listed in steps 1 through 3 above. Use a PEG that is of sufficient size to accommodate passage of the small caliber gastroscope.

2 Insert the transabdominal endoscope. Insert the small caliber gastroscope through the PEG tube and advance it through the stomach and into the small bowel.

3 Insert the guide wire. Pass the guide wire through the working channel of the endoscope deeply into the small intestine. Stiff, shaft wires with an atraumatic tip give better results.

4 Remove the transabdominal endoscope. Remove the small caliber gastroscope while advancing the guide wire with equivalent motions to maintain position in the small bowel.

5 Insert the J-tube. Direct the J-tube over the guide wire and into the small intestine.

6 Remove the guide wire.

7 Secure the J-tube. Couple the J-tube with the PEG.

IV *PEG-J insertion technique through an existing PEG:* These techniques are much the same as insertion through a de novo PEG with some caveats. A jejunal extension tube can be coupled with an appropriately sized indwelling or replacement PEG. There are one piece PEG-J replacement tubes that can be inserted through a mature stoma after removing the indwelling PEG tube. It may be challenging to maintain an air lock for drag and pull, and wire-guided techniques. Transabdominal endoscopy works very well in this setting [2,12].

B *DPEJ insertion:* The trainee should appreciate that DPEJ is performed much like PEG, only in the jejunum, using a colonoscope or enteroscope. DPEJ is technically more difficult due to the lack of fixed anatomy and frequent motion. PEG kits may be used, but DEPJ requires small tubes. Transillumination is more challenging and there is no standard site on the abdominal wall for insertion. The stoma may be placed anywhere on the abdominal wall or flanks if necessary. The stoma tracks are not as robust as in the stomach, and tube replacement or removal may need to be done with endoscopic assistance. Many of the steps described for PEG placement are the same for DPEJ with maneuvers unique to DPEJ outlined below [2,5,13–15]. The trainee should be instructed in the following steps:

1 Provide antibiotic prophylaxis; patient position, abdominal preparation and drapes, sterile attire; and perform EGD as for PEG.

2 *Jejunal transillumination:* Observe for jejunal transillumination on insertion and withdrawal. It may be beneficial to darken the endoscopy room and use the transillumination mode for brighter light to facilitate this maneuver. Be prepared to initiate DPEJ placement whenever good transillumination is seen in an appropriate jejunal location.

3 *DPEJ site selection:* The optimal site is dependent on transillumination and position in the jejunum. Sites that are away from the belt line are preferable. Upper abdominal sites at least 2 cm inferior to the costal margins are good. This will minimize the potential for pain when the ribs contact the J-tube as the patient sits upright. Other sites can also be used, including through a scar, prior feeding tube sites, and even on the flanks if absolutely necessary.

4 *Insufflation:* This causes the anterior aspect of the jejunum to abut the abdominal wall.

5 *Jejunal site selection:* Any segment of the jejunum where there is good transillumination and digital imprint is acceptable. For pancreatitis patients, it may be optimal to go at least 30 cm beyond the ligament of Trietz to minimize pancreatic stimulation with feeds.

6 *The safe track:* Perform the safe track as described for PEG [10].

7 Secure the position. Quickly ensnare the safe track needle to secure the position and prevent loss of juxtaposition of the jejunum to the abdominal wall.

8 *Trocar insertion:* Insert the trocar immediately adjacent to the safe track needle and endoscopically visualize it in the jejunum. Efficiently remove the snare from the safe track needle, gently ensnare the trocar, and remove the obturator. Put a finger on the open trocar sheath to minimize air (and insufflation) loss, which could change the position of the jejunum.

9 Perform guide wire passage, endoscope retraction, and abdominal incision as per PEG.

10 Pass the DPEJ tube. Secure the tube to the oral end of the wire (or pass it over the wire for push-type kits), liberally apply sterile lubrication, and pull (or push) it through the mouth and out through the abdominal incision site. If repeat enteroscopy is desired, facilitate esophageal reintubation and jejunal insertion by ensnaring the internal fixation bolster (mushroom tip) with the snare protruding from the working channel. Gently follow the tube through the pharynx to the jejunostomy site.

11 Secure and dress the DPEJ tube as described for PEG.

Setting and tools for training

Most training in enteral access procedures is done in the endoscopy suite. Ancillary resources include textbooks, instructional videos prepared by professional societies and industry, and a variety of online resources. An experienced mentor is key to learning these procedures. This is not only true for the technical aspects, but also for understanding the indications, contraindications, and ethical and legal issues associated with enteral feeding. This is particularly important for situations involving neurologically impaired patients. When and whether to do these procedures is as important as how to do them, and the role of the mentor in these aspects ought to be stressed. Imparting skill in communicating with patients and their families regarding all aspects of these procedures is of fundamental importance.

According to the American Multisociety Core Curriculum in Gastroenterology, a threshold of 130 EGD procedures are required for basic competency and 15 gastric components of PEG procedures are necessary [3]. However, a recent multisociety position statement emphasizes that threshold numbers for competency are not always applicable due to an individual's experience and skills set, and the type and frequency of the procedure [7]. There are plastic animal stomach/intestinal models that can be used for demonstrations and hands-on training. These are often available at meetings and sponsored by national societies and/or industry for exposure to their products. One randomized study showed no advantage from simulators for training in PEG, but trainees scored better for control of GI bleeding, polypectomy, and esophageal dilation. The authors speculated that the two-person nature of PEG may have resulted in performance improvement despite the lack of prior training [16].

Defining competency

There are no specific data on how to define competency in enteral access procedures, or standardized factors that determine successful training [3,5–7]. However, generally accepted indicators for training and quality can be applied including documentation of appropriate indications, informed consent, patient risk assessment (ASA class), risk reduction (prophylactic antibiotics, discontinued anticoagulants), appropriate procedure duration (PEG 20 to 30 minutes), and endoscopic landmarks as required for EGD [2,3,5,7]. Credentialing indicators such as number of procedures performed, and rates of procedure success and morbidity can also be applied [17–20]. A sample PEG assessment form is shown in Figure 29.4. Ultimately, the training program director must provide documentation of a trainee's competency largely based on direct observation [3,7].

Other than for PEG, there are no data on the number of procedures that are generally required for competence in trainees skilled in EGD. Competence in PEG placement must first be achieved. Thereafter, it is this author's opinion that about ten PEG-Js and ten DEPJs are adequate for most trainees. However, it must be stressed that numbers alone do not define competence. Comprehensive understandings of the procedures, facility with the technical aspects, and direct observation by a trainer with objective and subjective attestation to competency are also required.

Maintenance of skills

There are no specific recommendations on indicators for maintenance of skills, especially for lower volume procedures such as PEG-J and DPEJ, and it is appropriate to apply general principals used for other procedures. A retrospective cohort study in a surgery residency program spanning the decade from 1987 through 1997 showed that the overall mean was five PEGs per resident per year, with 13 per resident in the final year. There was a 97% PEG success rate and 88% for PEG-J. The authors concluded that surgical residents should become competent in PEG placement by performing adequate numbers of procedures with fully trained staff [21]. In the absence of data, each institution must establish its own policies for required numbers of procedures performed. It is this author's opinion that a minimum total of ten procedures (PEGs, PEG-Js, and/or DPEJs) each year are required for most active endoscopists to maintain competence. However, assessment of competence should not be based on numbers alone. This should be part of continuing quality improvement and recredentialing programs [17–23].

Videos

Video 29.1 Abdominal wall site selection with digital pressure
Video 29.2 The safe track
Video 29.3 Abdominal wall incision
Video 29.4 Guide wire insertion
Video 29.5 Pull PEG maneuver
Video 29.6 PEG completion
Video 29.7 PEG placement in ex-vivo simulator

References

1 DiSario JA, Baskin WN, Brown RD, et al.: Endoscopic approaches to enteral nutritional support. *Gastrointest Endosc* 2002;**55**:901–908.

2 DiSario JA: Endoscopic approaches to enteral nutrition. *Best Pract Res Clin Gastroenterol* 2006;**20**:605–630.

3 American Association for the Study of Liver Diseases, American College of Gastroenterology, AGA Institute, American Society for Gastrointestinal Endoscopy: A journey toward excellence: training future gastroenterologists – the gastroenterology core curriculum, third edition. *Gastrointest Endosc* 2007;**65**:875–881.

4 Esophagogastrduodenoscopy (EGD): Core Curriculum June 2004. Available: www.asge.org (accessed 09 January 2011)

5 Endoscopic Approaches to Enteral Feeding: Core Curriculum 2002. Available: www.asge.org (accessed 09 January 2011)

6 American Society for Gastrointestinal Endoscopy (ASGE): Principles of training in gastrointestinal endoscopy. *Gastrointest Endosc* 1999;**49**:845–853.

7 Report of the Multisociety Task Force on GI training. Gastrointest Endosc 2009;**70**:823–827.

8 ASGE Technology Committee, Kwon RS, Banerjee S, Desilets D, et al.: Enteral nutritional access devices. *Gastrointest Endosc* 2010;**72**:236–248.

9 Baron TH, Dominitz JA, Faigel DO, et al.: Role of endoscopy in enteral feeding. *Gastrointest Endosc* 2002;**55**:794–797.

10 Foutch PG, Talbert GA, Waring JP, et al.: Percutaneous endoscopic gastrostomy in patients with prior abdominal surgery: virtues of the safe tract. *Am J Gastroenterol* 1988;**83**:147–150.

11 DiSario JA, Foutch PG, Sanowski RA: Poor results with percutaneous endoscopic gastrojejunostomy. *Gastrointest Endosc* 1990;**36**:257–260.

12 Alder DG, Gostout CJ, Barron TH: Percutaneous transgastric placement of jejunal feeding tubes with an ultrathin endoscope. *Gastrointest Endosc* 2002;**55**:106–110.

13 Shike M, Latkany L, Gerdes H, et al.: Direct percutaneous endoscopic jejunostomies for enteral feeding. *Gastrointestl Endosc* 1996;**44**:536–540.

14 Bueno JT, Schattner MA, Barrera R, et al. Endoscopic placement of direct percutaneous jejunostomy tubes in patients with complications after esophagectomy. *Gastrointest Endosc* 2003;**57**:536–540.

15 Rumalla A, Baron TH: Results of direct percutaneous endoscopic jejunostomy, an alternative method for providing jejunal feeding. *Mayo Clin Proc* 2000;**75**:807–810.

16 Haycook AV, Youd P, Bassett P, et al.: Simulator training improves practical skills in therapeutic GI endoscopy: results from a randomized, blinded, controlled study. *Gastrointest Endosc* 2009: **70**:835–845.

17 The ASGE/ACG Taskforce on Quality in Endoscopy: Ensuring competence in endoscopy. Available: www.asge.org (accessed 09 January 2011)

18 Bjorkman DJ, Popp JW Jr: Measuring the quality of endoscopy. *Gastrointest Endosc* 2006 Apr;**63**(Suppl 4): S1–S2.

19 Faigel DO, Pike IM, Baron TH, et al.: Quality indicators for gastrointestinal endoscopic procedures: an introduction. *Gastrointest Endosc* 2006 Apr;**63**(Suppl 4): S3–S9.

20 Cohen J, Safdi MA, Deal SE, et al.: Quality indicators for esophagogastroduodenoscopy. *Gastrointest Endosc* 2006;**63**(Suppl 4): S5–S10.

21 Lowe JB, Page CP, Schwesinger WH, et al.: Percutaneous endoscopic gastrostomy tube placement in a surgical training program. *Am J Surg* 1997;**174**:624–627.

22 Eisen GM, Baron TH, Dominitz JA, Faigel DO, et al.: Methods of granting hospital privileges to perform gastrointestinal endoscopy. *Gastrointest Endosc* 2002;**55**:780–783.

23 Standards of Practice Committee, Dominitz JA, Ikenberry SO, Anderson MA, et al.: Renewal of and proctoring for endoscopic privileges. *Gastrointest Endosc* 2008;**67**:10–16.

30 The Endoscopic Management of Immediate Complications of Therapeutic Endoscopy

David A. Greenwald[1,2] & Martin L. Freeman[3]

[1] Montefiore Medical Center, New York, NY, USA
[2] Albert Einstein College of Medicine, New York, NY, USA
[3] University of Minnesota, Minneapolis, MN, USA

Introduction

Endoscopy is no longer merely diagnostic; therapeutic maneuvers are integral parts of most procedures. With increasingly complex therapy possible during gastrointestinal endoscopy comes an increased risk for complications. These complications, including bleeding, perforation, pancreatitis, infection, airway issues, and hypotension, must be immediately recognized and appropriately managed. The skills to assess and manage risk preprocedure, to recognize and manage serious problems that occur during endoscopy, and finally the ability to manage these issues successfully are an important part of training for endoscopy today. Other chapters in this volume have looked at training in the various procedures in gastrointestinal endoscopy such as upper endoscopy, colonoscopy, ERCP, and EUS as well as training in associated techniques such as electrosurgery. This chapter focuses solely on training to recognize and manage immediate complications of therapeutic endoscopy (Table 30.1).

Assessing risk prior to procedure

Patients being considered for therapeutic endoscopy need to be assessed preprocedure for risks that can be anticipated, and then steps can be taken to minimize or mitigate those risks. Issues to be addressed preprocedure include a number of factors related to the cardiopulmonary risk of sedation, analgesia, or anesthesia; and risks related to the specific procedure such as bleeding for polypectomy, EMR, or sphincterotomy; or pancreatic risks related to ERCP. Sometimes, the set of risk factors for these aspects overlap, but often the set of risk factors is completely different. For example, cardiopulmonary risk is generally higher in older, sicker patients, while post-ERCP pancreatitis risk is higher in younger,

healthier patients; bleeding risk is generally related to parameters related to coagulation status of the patient, and the type of procedure done.

Cardiovascular complications of endoscopy related to sedation and analgesia are common, accounting for nearly half of the reported complications in one ASGE survey [1,2]. Cardiovascular complications may be more likely to occur in a subset of patients including those who are obese, older, have pulmonary disease such as COPD and sleep apnea, have a history of cardiac disease, have certain body features such as short necks, or have a history of substance abuse. Those who have been difficult to sedate in the past are also of concern. Cardiovascular complications range from minor, such as transient and asymptomatic rhythm changes, to more severe, such as myocardial infarction and shock/hypotension. Respiratory conditions range from subtle hypoxemia to severe respiratory depression. Adequate training in sedation and monitoring allows for such problems to be anticipated and avoided wherever possible. Training may include standard courses in BLS and ACLS, which describe common scenarios in cardiopulmonary complications, and helps to teach and train about proper management [3,4]. Knowledge of the use of appropriate resuscitation equipment is also of paramount importance. Careful use of sedating agents along with the use of standard monitoring equipment helps to limit the number and severity of cardiopulmonary complications.

Use of mock airway drills to practice in the event of a compromised airway should be part of training for therapeutic endoscopy. Similarly, a working knowledge of the medications and techniques necessary to recognize and manage common cardiovascular complications such as brady and tachy arrhythmias, hypotension and cardiac arrest is necessary, as well as adequate training in the use of reversal agents for medications given for sedation for therapeutic endoscopy.

Assessment before the procedure may also reveal an increased risk for bleeding either because of medication use or an underlying

Successful Training in Gastrointestinal Endoscopy, First Edition. Edited by Jonathan Cohen.
© 2011 Blackwell Publishing Ltd. Published 2011 by Blackwell Publishing Ltd.

Table 30.1 Check list for mastery in training to recognize and manage complications.

1. Know your limits.
2. Know when to ask for assistance.
3. Team training.
4. Excellent communication between all members of team.

coagulopathy. Training should include familiarity with guidelines for the management of anticoagulants and antiplatelet agents in endoscopy [5].

Intraprocedure recognition of complications

Risks of therapeutic endoscopy

Perforation of the upper GI tract during diagnostic endoscopy is very uncommon, with rates of 0.03% in an ASGE survey [1]; risk factors including the presence of a Zenker's diverticulum, anterior cervical osteophytes, esophageal strictures, and malignancies. Perforation is more common with therapeutic maneuvers including dilation of benign and malignant strictures, stent placement, and dilation of achalasia. Training to minimize complications in dilation includes knowledge of the different dilating options and then making appropriate decisions. In one series comparing dilating systems, perforations were substantially more common with blind passage of Maloney type dilators than with the use of balloon-based systems or wire-guided dilators. In achalasia, avoiding higher inflation pressures (greater than 11 psi) or by limiting dilations to less than 15 mm diameter may be associated with a decreased likelihood of perforation [6,7]. In malignant strictures, dilation of a stricture with or without previous radiation treatment to that area did not influence perforation rates [8]. Perforations may occur after dilation for gastric outlet obstruction as well.

Training in the recognition and management of perforations includes understanding that the most common sign of perforation is pain; other symptoms of note are fever, crepitus, chest pain (often pleuritic), and pleural effusion. Diagnosis may be seen with air radiographs of the neck. If a perforation is suspected, recognition may be confirmed by the use of a water soluble contrast media initially, or CT scan, depending on site and extent of perforation.

Bleeding may occur during therapeutic endoscopy in many situations, including during the treatment of ulcers, dilation of strictures, stent placements, and management of variceal hemorrhage. Induction of bleeding during nonvariceal hemostasis is reasonably common, occurring in up to 5% of procedures [9]. Fortunately, it is usually easy to control during the procedure. Bleeding has also been reported in up to 6% of patients after endoscopic variceal sclerotherapy and band ligation, as a consequence of the resultant ulcers [10]. Practice in the management of acutely bleeding lesions, whether on porcine models or via the use of simulators, may be useful in training to manage bleeding complications in the upper GI tract.

Other risks of therapeutic upper endoscopy that may be seen immediately following the procedure include aspiration, stent migration, and mucosal injury following foreign body removal. Proper training in the equipment used for foreign body removal, including use of overtubes, latex hoods, and a variety of graspers is crucial to minimizing complications, which have been reported in about 8% of foreign body removals [11]. Esophageal overtube placement and use has been associated with bleeding and perforation, often due to pinching of the overtube into the esophageal mucosa. Latex hoods fitted over the end of the endoscope may protect the GI mucosa from trauma as the foreign body is retrieved. In the case of foreign body removal, training should include extracorporeal simulation of the removal of the foreign body to assess for efficacy and safety of the planned technique prior to its attempt inside the GI tract (Video 30.5).

Risks of therapeutic colonoscopy

Complications as a result of diagnostic colonoscopy are very rare, with perforation rates estimated to be 0.35% [1,12]. Therapeutic colonoscopy, however, has an increased rate of complications, with major complications reported to occur 0.2–0.3% of the time. Complications include bleeding, perforation, and cardiovascular and cerebrovascular events [13]. Risk factors for developing complications during therapeutic colonoscopy include the concomitant use of antiplatelet agents or anticoagulants. Postpolypectomy bleeding rates decrease with increased experience of the endoscopist [14]. While the rate of perforation does not clearly seem to be related to the size of the polyp being removed, right colon polyps seem to be associated with the highest risk of perforation due to the thinness of the wall in that section of the colon [15].

Training should include learning techniques to help avoid complications. For example, proper technique in closing the snare during polypectomy is important to prevent entrapment of normal mucosa along with the polyp. Too rapid closure of the snare and guillotining of a polyp before cautery effect has occurred can be associated with increased bleeding. Use of saline or epinephrine injected under flat polyps, particularly in the right colon, seems to be effective in decreasing perforation associated with polypectomy in that area.

Perforation during colonoscopy can occur for a variety of reasons, including barotrauma, direct bowing, and force against the colon wall, or as a result of therapeutic procedures [16]. Management of perforation begins with recognition, and early recognition and prompt intervention may decrease patient morbidity and mortality. Signs of colon perforation include persistent abdominal pain and often prolonged abdominal distension. Fever and leukocytosis may follow. Evaluation for perforation typically includes the use of radiography; plain X-ray or CT may show free air. Management of perforations typically includes surgical consultation, although nonsurgical management may be appropriate in selected situations. Patients with so-called "mini-perforations" may be managed with bowel rest, intravenous antibiotics, and frequent observations looking for clinical worsening.

Some perforations may be managed endoscopically with clips (Videos 23.1, 23.2 and 30.2). Practice with clips to close perforations on *ex vivo* models may help endoscopists gain expertise in this technique prior to using it during an actual perforation (Video 30.2). The "ideal" situation for clipping to close a colonic perforation would appear to be a small, linear tear that is recognized immediately in a well-prepped colon in a relatively fit patient. Trainees can also learn and practice on modified animal tissue models the technique of using an angiocath to release air in the event of a pneumoperitoneum. The topic of training to perform closure of tissue defects is covered in more detail in a separate chapter in this book.

Postpolypectomy hemorrhage can occur immediately or be delayed, occurring at rates reported between 0.3 and 6.1%, with a large ASGE survey reporting a 1.7% rate of postpolypectomy bleeding in over 600 patients [1]. Immediate postpolypectomy bleeding is often obvious at the time of the therapeutic maneuver, and can be managed through the use of a variety of techniques, including injection, thermocoagulation, endoloops, and endoscopic clips [17] (Figures 30.1a–d) or a combination of techniques, as well as nonendoscopic modalities such as embolization and surgery (Video 30.4). Training in the use of cautery, loops, and clips may be obtained through the use of *ex vivo* models and

hands-on training sessions, which allow the participant to become familiar with a wide variety of devices and their application. Since the devices and techniques vary in their complexity, and since endoscopists vary in their ability, it is unclear at this point how much training is required for any given individual to become skilled in the endoscopic management of postpolypectomy bleeding.

Risks of therapeutic ERCP/EUS

Complications of therapeutic ERCP include pancreatitis, hemorrhage, perforation, and cardiopulmonary complications [18]. While post-ERCP pancreatitis is clinically important and occurs with a rate of 1–7% [19], and post-EUS/FNA pancreatitis may occur about 2% of the time, it falls outside the scope of this chapter on endoscopic management of immediate complications of therapeutic endoscopy, and so will not be discussed further here. However, it is critical that ERCP trainees learn to recognize risk factors for post-ERCP pancreatitis in their preprocedure evaluation and receive instruction on ways to minimize the risk of this complication (Table 30.2). Instructors should emphasize the best way to avoid post-ERCP pancreatitis is to avoid doing

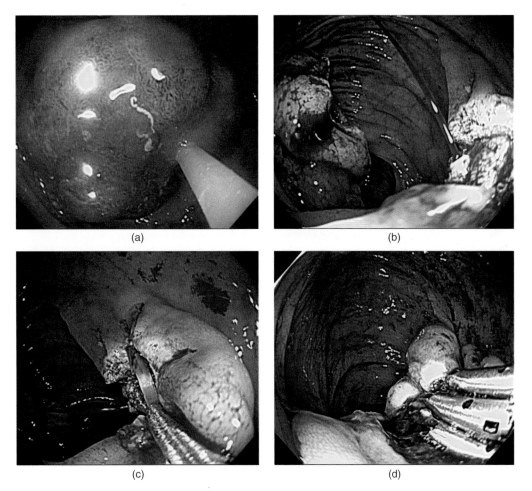

(a)

(b)

(c)

(d)

Figure 30.1 (a) 3-cm sigmoid polyp undergoing snare polypectomy. (b) Spurting arterial hemorrhage immediately postpolypectomy. (c) Positioning of endoscopic clip around base of artery. (d) Control of hemorrhage with clips.

Table 30.2 Risk factors for post-ERCP pancreatitis in multivariate analyses.

Yes*	Maybe†	No‡
Female sex	CBD stone absent	Small CBD diameter
Younger age	Normal serum bilirubin	Periampullary diverticulum
Suspected SOD	Chronic pancreatitis absent	Pancreas divisum
Prior post-ERCP pancreatitis	Pancreatic brush cytology	Allergy to contrast media
Recurrent pancreatitis	Pain during ERCP	Prior failed ERCP
Pancreatic duct injection	Pancreatic acinarization	Therapeutic versus diagnostic
Pancreatic sphincterotomy (minor papillotomy)	Low endoscopist volume	Intramural contrast injection
Balloon dilation (of intact biliary sphincter)	Trainee participation	Biliary sphincterotomy
Difficult or failed cannulation		Sphincter of Oddi manometry (using aspirated catheter)
Precut (access) sphincterotomy		

Prospective series of >500 cases.
SOD, sphincter of Oddi dysfunction.
*Significant by multivariate analysis in most studies or by meta-analysis.
†Significant by univariate analysis only in most studies, or by single multivariate analysis.
‡Inconsistent significance by univariate analysis, not significant by multivariate analysis.

the procedure when it is not indicated. Also, it is important to use good judgment when a procedure is not proceeding well and should be stopped. While participation by fellows has generally been shown not to correlate with ERCP complications, this probably reflects case selection bias. One study (Sherman et al.), did show independent risk for post-ERCP pancreatitis with participation by a fellow [20]. Currently, placement of pancreatic stents is considered standard of care for prevention of post-ERCP pancreatitis among individuals thought to be at higher risk for developing this complication. Fellows need specific instruction in techniques of guide wire placement and effective pancreatic stent placement [21].

Hemorrhage as a result of sphincterotomy has been reported to occur from 0.76–2% of the time, although perhaps half of this occurs in a delayed fashion [22–24]. Severe hemorrhage, defined as requiring two or more units of blood, surgery, or angiography, occurs in 0.1–0.5% [22,23]. Clinically significant bleeding after EUS/FNA or other therapeutic maneuvers associated with EUS has rarely been reported. Postsphincterotomy hemorrhage is associated with underlying coagulopathy and use of anticoagulants within 72 hours of the sphincterotomy, use of precut sphincterotomy, and with sphincterotomy performed by an endoscopist with a low case volume (less than 1 per week). Length of the sphincterotomy does not appear to be an independent risk factor for postsphincterotomy bleeding. Management of postsphincterotomy hemorrhage includes use of many of the same techniques described for postpolypectomy bleeding above. Treatment of bleeding following sphincterotomy through a duodenoscope requires specific knowledge of not only use of a duodenoscope but also the devices that can fit and function past an elevator. For example, hemostatic clips can be extremely difficult to place and deploy because of the bend in the elevator. Only special injection needles work reliably in this setting. For similar reasons, generally only a 7F thermal probe will fit through a therapeutic duodeno-

scope. A technique unique to management of postsphincterotomy bleeding is the use of a controlled radial expansion balloon placed in the bile duct through a bleeding sphincterotomy to provide tamponnade. Thus, training for the treatment of ERCP complications requires the ability to perform hemostasis through a duodenoscope, and practice with the devices outside a patient in a model or a simulated situation is advisable (Video 30.3).

Perforation during therapeutic ERCP is usually the result of either guide wire manipulations, periampullary perforation during sphincterotomy or perforation away from the ampulla. Rates have been reported as 0.3–0.6% [22,24]. Perforation during EUS appears to occur at a similar rate as for standard upper endoscopy [25]. Training in the management of ERCP-associated periampullary perforation complications includes prompt recognition followed by treatment with aggressive biliary and duodenal drainage (Video 30.1). When this is done appropriately, along with the use of broad-spectrum antibiotics, nonoperative treatment results in clinical resolution in approximately 85% of patients [26]. As for bleeding, endoscopic clips may play a role, with the caveat that placement of clips through a duodenoscope requires specific techniques and poses certain limitations. Perforations remote from the papilla are often not recognized until sometime after the procedure, may present with persistent abdominal pain or distension, are diagnosed radiographically by the presence of free air, and are usually managed surgically.

Avoiding complications

Since the potential for significant complications when doing therapeutic endoscopy is clearly present, a few general principles are critical. First and foremost, each therapeutic endoscopist, trainee, and GI associate must know their own limits and not take on clinical challenges for which they are not prepared. This applies equally to endoscopists and associates assisting with the procedure, both of whom may be unfamiliar with the equipment or the proposed techniques. Knowing when to ask for assistance is crucial, and knowing other alternatives, including nonendoscopic alternatives, is part of successful training for performance of therapeutic endoscopy. Lastly, the concept of teamwork cannot be overemphasized. All members of the team should be trained in a given therapeutic technique (i.e., the concept of "team training"). Communication between members of the team is also vital, with input from nurses, technicians, and endoscopists all valued throughout the procedure.

Training to manage complications

Simulations to anticipate complications are an effective tool in learning their management. Mock airway management drills, mock perforations managed on *ex vivo* simulators (Videos 1.3, 7.10, 23.1, 23.2, 23.3, 23.4), and mock refractory bleeding, again on models, are valuable training tools. Simulations are valuable because learning to manage complications during actual procedures is limited by pressures to safely and rapidly complete the procedure once a problem has occurred, as well as by the relative infrequency of complications in the first place. Simulators and mock drills allow for nearly unlimited repetition to learn and then practice skills and techniques. Opportunities for such simulator-based training are now possible at both regional and national courses through the use of portable simulators and animal tissue. Training is available on a limited basis at the local level using the same tools.

Having appropriate equipment readily available to get out of a jam is also important in training to avoid and manage complications. For example, having an array of devices available for removal of foreign bodies, and being familiar beforehand with their use, is invaluable when it comes time for the "real thing." A specific example may be experience with wire cutters, which may be needed in selected cases where a device has become stuck and removal is impossible, and their use may mitigate the need for an operative intervention. Again, both the cognitive skills about when to use such a tool and the technical skill to know what to do with it are critical elements in training prior to beginning complicated endoscopic therapeutic maneuvers.

Postprocedure Follow-Up

All endoscopic complications should be reviewed afterwards in a systematic process through quality assurance and performance improvement to assess strategies for better outcomes in subsequent procedures. By using such a process, alterations in techniques or plans can be formulated and implemented, and common issues can be studied.

Videos

Video 30.1 Ampullectomy
Video 30.2 Perforation
Video 30.3 ES bleed
Video 30.4 Management of immediate bleeding during cap EMR

Video 30.5 Detection and endoscopic management of mucosal tear complicating upper endoscopy
Video 1.3 Use of simulator to teach what not to do: improper submucosal lift in EMR leads to perforation on purpose
Video 7.10 Use of Neopapilla to allow for training in management in postsphincterotomy bleeding
Video 14.5 Narrow band imaging [NBI] combined with probe confocal laser endoscopy [pCLE] of low grade dysplasia in Barrett's esophagus with targeted band endoscopic mucosal resection [EMR]
Video 23.1 Graphic demonstration of closure of a linear and circular perforation
Video 23.2 Closure of defect
Video 23.3 Use of clips to close esophageal perforation
Video 23.4 Closure of gastrointestinal perforations
Video 26.10 Large ampullary adenoma removal

References

1 Silvis SE, Nebel O, Rogers G, et al. Endoscopic complications: results of the 1974 American Society for Gastrointestinal Endoscopy Survey. *JAMA* 1976;**235**:928–930.
2 Benjamin SB. Complications of conscious sedation. *Gastrointest Endosc Clin N Am* 1996;**6**:277–286.
3 ASGE. Training in patient monitoring and sedation and analgesia. *Gastrointest Endosc* 2007;**66**:7–10.
4 ASGE. Monitoring equipment for endoscopy. *Gastrointest Endosc* 1995;**42**:615–617.
5 ASGE, Anderson MA, Ben-Menachem T, Gan SI, et al.: Management of antithrombotic agents for endoscopic procedures. *Gastrointest Endosc* 2009;**70**:1061–1070.
6 Nair LA, Reynolds JC, Parkman, HP, et al. Complications during pneumatic dilation for achalasia or diffuse esophageal spasm: analysis of risk factors, early clinical characteristics, and outcome. *Dig Dis Sci* 1993;**38**:1893–1904.
7 Kozarek RA, Botoman VA, Patterson DJ. Long term follow up in patients who have undergone balloon dilation for gastric outlet obstruction. *Gastrointest Endosc* 1990;**36**:558–661.
8 Ng TM, Spencer GM, Sargeant IR, et al. Management of strictures after radiotherapy for esophageal cancer. *Gastrointest Endosc* 1996;**43**:584–590.
9 ASGE. Complications of upper GI endoscopy. *Gastrointest Endosc* 2002;**55**:784–793.
10 Piai G, Cipolletta L, Claar M, et al. Prophylactic sclerotherapy of high risk esophageal varices: Results of a multicentric prospective controlled trial. *Hepatology* 1988;**8**:1495–1507.
11 Berggreen PJ, Harrison ME, Sanowski RA, et al. Techniques and complications of esophageal foreign body extraction in children and adults. *Gastrointest Endosc* 1993;**33**:626–630.
12 Nelson DB, McQuaid KR, Bond JH, et al. Procedural success and complications of large scale screening colonoscopy. *Gastrointest Endosc* 2002;**55**:307–314.
13 Lieberman DA, Weiss DG, Bond JH, et al. Use of colonoscopy to screen asymptomatic adults for colorectal cancer. Veterans Administration Cooperative Study Group 380. *N Engl J Med* 2000;**343**:169–174.
14 Rodgers B, Silvis S, Nebel O, et al. Complications of flexible fiberoptic colonoscopy and polypectomy. *Gastrointest Endosc* 1975;**22**:73–77.

15 Waddas D, Sanowski R. Complications of the hot biopsy forceps technique. *Gastrointest Endosc* 1988;**34**:32–37.

16 ASGE. Complications of colonoscopy. *Gastrointest Endosc* 2003;**57**: 441–444.

17 Parra-Blanco A, Kaminaga N, Kojima T, et al. Hemoclipping for post-polypectomy and postbiopsy colonic bleeding. Descriptive analysis. *Gastrointest Endosc* 2000;**51**:37–41.

18 ASGE. Complications of ERCP. *Gastrointest Endosc* 2003;**57**:633–638.

19 Freeman ML, DiSario JA, Nelson, DB, et al. Risk factors for post ERCP pancreatitis: a prospective multicenter study. *Gastrointest Endosc* 2001;**54**:425–434.

20 Cheng CL, Sherman S, Watkins JL, et al., Risk factors for post-ERCP pancreatitis: a prospective multicenter study. *Am J Gastroenterol* 2006;**101**:139–147.

21 Freeman ML. Pancreatic stents for prevention of post-ERCP pancreatitis: for everyday practice or for experts only? *Gastrointest Endosc* 2010;**71**:940–944.

22 Freeman ML, Nelson DB, Sherman S, et al. Complications of endoscopic biliary sphincterotomy. *N Engl J Med* 1996;**335**:909–918.

23 Loperfido S, Angelini G, Benedetti G, et al. Major early complications from diagnostic and therapeutic ERCP: a prospective multicenter study. *Am J Gastroenterol* 1998;**48**:1–10.

24 Masci E, Toti G, Mariani A, et al. Complications of diagnostic and therapeutic ERCP: a prospective multicenter study. *Am J Gastroenterol* 2001;**96**:417–423.

25 ASGE. Complications of EUS. *Gastrointest Endosc* 2005;**61**:8–12.

26 Enns R, Eloubeidi MA, Mergener K, et al. ERCP related perforations: risk factors and management. *Endoscopy* 2002;**34**:293–298.

IV Challenges for the Future

31 Assessing Manpower Needs in Gastroenterology and Digestive Endoscopy: Lessons from the Past and Implications for the Future of Endoscopic Training

Girish Mishra[1] & Alan Barkun[2]

[1] Wake Forest University School of Medicine, Winston-Salem, NC, USA
[2] McGill University, McGill University Health Centre, Montreal, QC, Canada

The practice of medicine has always greatly been influenced by evolving technologies that not only assist physicians in delivering optimal patient care but also often directly contribute to shaping subsequent diagnosis and therapy. This is no truer than for gastroenterology and, more particularly, gastrointestinal endoscopy in which there have been great and rapid evolutions from diagnostic into therapeutic endoscopic techniques amidst the emergence of competing technologies. Such converging dynamics have indeed brought our specialty to a critical crossroad. An understanding of both the contributing factors leading to this and of the processes involved in predicting future patterns of health care delivery are now required as a matter of survival for our specialty. This chapter attempts to focus on the latter.

Modeling manpower

Before one can properly assess manpower needs specifically as they relate to endoscopic training, one must turn to the basic tenets of economics—the law of supply and demand. Unfortunately, projections based exclusively on supply and demand can be woefully erroneous as will be pointed out in the upcoming paragraphs. In economic theory, the notion of "manpower" is seemingly synonymous with human capital. Human capital, when broken down to its core, denotes a stock of knowledge and skills that represents the ability to perform labor, and thus create economic value. The current concept of human capital was introduced by Jacob Mincer (1958), and applied by Gary Becker (1962) [1,2]. In its current view, human capital is thought of as a "physical means of production" (e.g., factories). Therefore, similar to making investments in a factory, individuals can make investments in human capital (e.g.,

training, education, medical treatment). The effectiveness of the human capital is determined by the "rate of return," which is often expressed as the amount of economic value produced in relation to the corresponding investments made in human capital.

An alternative approach to assessing manpower relates to its characterization in the context of labor economics. The fundamentals of labor economics can be traced back to the Roy model that is based on "'self selection" [3]. A more practical interpretation of this theory is that rational beings make optimizing decisions about what markets to participate in. These decisions apply to all aspects of life, including employment, location, education, and marriage. Through his discourse on "Thoughts on the Distribution of Earnings," Roy describes the following factors as affecting occupational choice: (1) The fundamental distribution of skills and abilities; (2) Correlations among these skills in the population; (3) Technologies for applying these skills; and (4) Consumer tastes that impact on the demand for different types of outputs.

Econometrics is a discipline that develops and applies quantitative or statistical methods to the study and elucidation of economic principles. So what do these economic theories have to do with manpower issues in endoscopic training? Roy was the first to posit that workers have skills in each occupation, but they can only use one skill or the other. The original Roy model is based on the assumption that skills are distributed in a logarithmic rather than normal fashion and that the pursuit of comparative advantage in a free market reduces earnings inequality compared to the earnings distribution that would result if workers were randomly assigned to sectors. Noted econometrician, Heckman points out in "The empirical content of the Roy model" through complex hierarchical and regression analysis that earning densities need to be factored into the "self selection" and geographical

Successful Training in Gastrointestinal Endoscopy, First Edition. Edited by Jonathan Cohen.
© 2011 Blackwell Publishing Ltd. Published 2011 by Blackwell Publishing Ltd.

preferences for earnings [3]. So if we analyze manpower issues in endoscopic training from a very theoretical and economic-based approach, earning potential has to be factored into the discussion and equation. The request for training more endoscopists will only be met if there exists a clear need for their services. The next several paragraphs thus address physician needs.

Physician workforce estimates

The ability to correctly predict future demands of professional services bears obvious and significant implications for both the prospective employer and the student contemplating a future career. Predictions are often just that—estimates based on a perspective, or a mathematically derived model. It is instructive to review the very recent past during which forecasting had suggested both a physician and a gastroenterologist surplus that would overwhelm the medical workplace. Such a review will allow us to factor in many nuances that can lead to a better determination of actual manpower needs in endoscopic training. In 1976, the Graduate Medical Education National Advisory Committee (GMENAC) undertook a study of physician supply. It predicted that by 1990 there would be a surplus of 70, 000 active physicians (a 13% surplus) doubling to nearly 145,000 by 2000 [4]. In an extremely analytical and somewhat controversial essay in the mid-1990s, Cooper suggested that "in terms of physicians alone, there is no evidence of major impending national surplus."[5]. He assessed physician supply and demand for the period extending to 2020 from three perspectives: physician utilization in group- and staff-model health maintenance organizations, physician distribution, and the future supply of nonphysician clinicians. Cooper postulated that physician supply would initially increase more rapidly than its demand, resulting in a surplus of 31,000 physicians in the year 2000, increasing to 62,000 physicians in 2010, after which the gap would narrow.

In response to the growing perception of "physician glut" that abounded in the mid-1990s, two studies approached this question using different methodologies to achieve a more accurate means of calculating physician estimates, including the need for specialists. T.P. Weil used four methodologies in parallel to assess whether a predetermined population base had an inadequate, sufficient, or excess number of physicians. Using physician–population ratios per 100,000 persons, he supplied the number of physicians needed for 28 clinical disciplines, adopting a managed care perspective for most analyses. Although the data reported are outdated, his conclusions based on varying inputs and models remain pertinent today. A first table provides a comparison by clinical specialty of the number of physicians for a service area population of 100,000. The number of specialists needed is reportedly based on (a) the then available numbers in the United States; (b) the estimates of need reported in the GMENAC study; (c) the staffing of a large HMO with 2.4 million subscribers; (d) the staffing in the Minneapolis region with its high HMO penetration; and (e) the staffing in Wichita, Kansas where there was low managed care penetration. Not surprisingly, the number of full-time equivalents (FTEs) varied from as low as 1.3–19, further highlighting the inexact science for predicting physician requirements, including those of subspecialists.

He then proposed the following guidelines be used to determine physician needs: (1) Determine the composition, utilization patterns, and cost per case (adjusted by case mix intensity) of each member of the hospital's existing medical staff, clinical department, and sections; (2) Individually interview all key members of the hospital's medical staff and governing board officers; (3) Administer physician questionnaires to gauge needs; (4) Perform physician–population ratio calculations using various models (as shown above) and; (5) A composite summary projecting that specialties should be open or closed to meet community, hospital, or subscriber needs. Using this methodology, he calculated the existing FTE equivalent of three gastroenterologists needed per 100,000 persons to be decreased by a factor 0.04 in a community hospital—not an intuitive means of quantifying the number of gastroenterologists needed.

An alternative approach has also been described to determine an adequate supply of physicians in the United States. Also performed in the late 1990s, Greenberg and Cultice appropriately placed the context of their work by claiming that "observers of the health care scene in the United States increasingly support the proposition that there are too many specialist physicians and not enough generalists and that, as a consequence, the nation is suffering in two respects: excessive health care costs for all and inadequate access for some"[6]. These investigators based their projections on the Health Resources and Services Administration's Bureau of Health Professions (BHPr) model. The BHPr physician requirement model divides patient care in three domains: Population, physician specialty, and care setting. Secondary data were analyzed and put into matrices for use in the mainframe computer-based model. This model produced a projected number of physicians, by specialty, required to handle the demand of health care in each of various projection years.

This model is unique in that it allows for changes in the demographic composition of the United States, as well as assumptions about the percentage of patient's insured by the differing options-fee-for-service, HMOs, and so on versus those who are uninsured, utilization rates, and physician productivity. Despite these permutations, the results of this methodology consistently confirmed that the number of physicians required would decline. Thus, the authors contended that the "Bureau's demographic utilization model represents improvements over the data-driven methodologies that rely on staffing ratios and similar supply-determined bases for estimating requirements. The model's distinct utility rests in offering national-level physician specialty requirements forecasts."

How have these models fared when tasked with estimating requirements for medical specialists? Anderson and colleagues compared three methods for estimating the requirements for otolaryngologists [7]. They identified three basic methods based on (1) the utilization and/or staffing patterns of managed care organizations, (2) current utilization patterns and anticipated changes in demographic and insurance coverage as well as estimates of physician productivity to predict demand for physician services, and (3) a modified Delphi technique that asks a group of physicians in their specialty to suggest the number of individuals with that disease who should see a physician in their specialty, and to estimate the time required to treat the patient. Anderson and colleagues computed national requirements for otolaryngologists in 1994 and 2010 by each of these three methods. The estimates were compared to the number of active otolaryngologists actually (or anticipated to be) providing patient care in that year. The estimated number of otolaryngologists required varied significantly depending on the method used. Wide variations occurred depending on the assumptions used across models. Furthermore, the models were very sensitive to minor alterations in assumptions with disparate resultant conclusions showing surpluses or shortages. They concluded the managed care model had the greatest potential to yield reliable estimates because it reflects actual staffing patterns in institutions that are attempting to use physicians efficiently. The following paragraphs will focus specifically on modeling in gastroenterology and, more specifically, the endoscopic workforce that needs to be trained.

Gastroenterology workforce modeling

The landmark study commissioned by the Gastroenterology Leadership Council (GLC) was the first analyzing the gastroenterology physician workforce [8]. This study compared US gastroenterologist-to-population ratios with those of other countries and of major health maintenance organizations (HMOs). Importantly, investigators projected the growth of the supply of gastroenterologists under various scenarios.

Authors abstracted data that examined the current distribution and scope of practice in gastroenterology from two large national data sets: (1) the Health Care Financing Administration (HCFA) Medicare Part B file and (2) the Area Resource File (ARF).

Future supply of gastroenterologists was determined by first obtaining from BHPr the age and sex-specific physician death rates and retirement/exit rates. They projected their model over a 50-year period to illustrate the time it would take for some policy options to achieve a steady-state workforce. Survey of the American Gastroenterology Association (AGA) training programs and the National Study of Internal Medicine Manpower (NaSIMM) was used to determine the training stream, number of positions offered and matched. They chose to use the NaSIMM estimate of fellowship graduates ($n = 490$) in the final model. Mathematically, the investigators used the following formula:

$$\text{Supply}_{N+1} = \text{Supply}_N - \text{Retirements}_{N+1}$$

$$-\text{Deaths}_{N+1} + \text{Graduates}_{N+1}$$

A Markov model to determine future supply using a decision tree analysis yielded similar results as those obtained by the methodology described above. Finally, the investigators modeled future supply while adopting five different scenarios: current training levels, or assuming, respectively, 25%, 50%, two-third reductions in these, or outright elimination of gastroenterology training.

ARF data pointed out that the number of practicing gastroenterologists increased by 500% between 1974 and 1994 while the size of the general population increased by 20%. The percentage of gastroenterologists representing the physician pool increased from 0.8% in 1985 to 1.25% in 1992. The investigators also pointed out that 59% of the approximately 7,500 practicing gastroenterologists were younger than 45 years of age, while only 3% were 65 or older. Taken together, these statistics suggested the existing pool of gastroenterologists in 1996 would remain in practice for the foreseeable future. The period from 1977 to 1994 saw an increase in the number of graduates from 398 to 490. During the same timeframe, the number of 3-year programs increased from 7 to 45%.

This study also elucidated the breakdown of consultative versus procedural services offered by gastroenterologists and nongastroenterologists. Meyer and colleagues found that 60% of the bills generated by gastroenterologists were for office-based cognitive and consultative services, while only 22% were for procedural services—yet these produced 49% of the income generated by gastroenterologists. Their study also shed further light on the number of "GI" procedures performed by the nongastroenterologists. They found that 21% of the esophageal procedures (1992 Medicare data) were billed by generalists—general practitioners, general pediatricians, family practitioners, and general internists—and a similar percentage was performed by surgeons. Approximately 40% of the colonoscopies were performed by nongastroenterologists. Shockingly, 16% of ERCPs were performed by nongastroenterologists. For all procedures, gastroenterologists performed a higher proportion of therapeutic than diagnostic procedures. These authors also argued that by volume alone, the generalist saw more patients with GI disorders (based on ICD codes) and, hence, the supply for gastroenterologists should be further reduced. The authors then projected the future supply of gastroenterologists in the United States corrected for population growth until 2042. They report that if the current number of training positions remains unaltered, the number of gastroenterologists will double in approximately 28 years; if all fellowship training programs were eliminated, the number of gastroenterologists would decrease by 20% (Figure 31.1). According to the AGA position paper on training and education published in 1989, the suggested need was for 9,000 to 10,000 gastroenterologists [9]. Using Meyer's model, that workforce would be achieved in the year 2002 if training positions were cut by 25%. Based on this model, the GLC recommended that gastroenterology trainee numbers be reduced by 50% over the ensuing 5 years, with an immediate 25% reduction. There was also voluntary downsizing underway so that in 1996 the number of filled positions was 223 compared to 375 in 1993 representing a 41% reduction in positions filled and a 25% reduction in positions offered (based on 1997 National Resident Matching Program data).

Finally, the authors offered some suggestions as to how to achieve a reduction in fellowship graduates. They offered that accelerating the transition from 2-year to 3-year programs while holding the number of fellows constant would cause a modest reduction. The need for an additional year was felt justified so that the trainees could embark on meaningful research and obtain skills in interventional endoscopy and hepatology. Therefore, an additional year of training was mandated: starting in the summer of 1996, 3 rather than 2 years of training were required to be board eligible. The following statement: "if the current practice

Supply of Gastroenterologists Needed per 100,000
Corrected for Population Growth Until 2042
(Assuming a Fixed Demand of 3.0 Gastroenterologists per 100,000, as present in 1992)

Change in Training Positions	Year			
	2002	2012	2022	2042
No reduction	4.0	4.6	5.1	5.6
25% reduction	3.5	3.8	4.0	4.1
50% reduction	3.1	3.0	2.8	2.8
Complete elimination	2.2	1.3	0.5	-

Figure 31.1 Projection of the number of gastroenterologists corrected for population growth until 2042. Population projections were obtained from the Bureau of the Census. [15].

and training of gastroenterologists remains unchanged in the face of an evolving health care system that favors the staffing pattern of large managed care organizations, an increasing oversupply of gastroenterologists will persist in the physician workforce" was also endorsed by the leaders of several GI societies in the United States.

Future projections in gastroenterology: lessons from the past

The precipitous fall in the number of applicants for gastroenterology fellowships in the mid-1990s had as much to do with the changing sociopolitical climate in the first half of the 1990s that centered on Clinton's health care reform proposal as the release of any of the aforementioned manpower calculations. The time period from 1995 to 1998 saw a drastic reduction in the number of gastroenterology trainees by 35% as medical residents were leery of becoming a gastroenterologist when the overriding message was that primary care medicine would supersede demands for specialists. In 1996, there were fewer applicants for GI fellowship positions than there were positions offered in the Match, which was subsequently abolished in 1999 [10]. A highly critical appraisal of its workforce by the GLC that claimed an excess of gastroenterologists in practice, a highly uneasy group of internal medicine residents fearful of the future, and the closing of training programs with further extension to three years had all led to a drastic decline in trainees, at the dawn of an era that would require an unending demand for GI endoscopists to perform screening colonoscopies.

Endoscopic demands for screening colonoscopy

Medicare had not routinely provided reimbursement for colon cancer screening, other than patients identified as high risk, until a policy change in 2001 allowing for coverage of screening colonoscopies in all individuals. Gross and colleagues were able to determine the use of colonoscopy and stage at colon cancer diagnosis across three time points using the surveillance, epidemiology, and end results (SEER) and Medicare-linked databases for individuals aged 67 years or older with a primary diagnosis of colon cancer between 1992 and 2002, compared to a group of Medicare beneficiaries who lived in SEER areas but who were not diagnosed with cancer [11]. The three periods corresponded to different Medicare coverages: Period 1—1992–1997 (no screening coverage); period 2—January 1998 to June 2001 (limited screening coverage); and period 3—July 2001 to December 2002 (universal screening coverage). Comparison was made between the use of flexible sigmoidoscopy and colonoscopy during these time periods. Colonoscopy used increased from an average of 285/100,000 per quarter in period 1; to 889/100,000 per quarter in period 2; to 1,919/100,000 people per quarter in period 3 ($p < 0.001$ for all comparisons). A concomitant finding of detecting more cancers in earlier stages across these time periods was also found.

Seeff and colleagues estimated the number of average-risk persons aged 50 years or older not screened for CRC, and the number of procedures required for this population, and the endoscopic capacity to deliver this unmet need [12]. Approximately 42 million average-risk people aged 50 years or older had not been screened for CRC in 2004. The only means to screen the unscreened population within 1 year was to use a fecal occult testing followed by a diagnostic colonoscopy for positive tests. The capacity available in 2002 had been for 6.7 million flexible sigmoidoscopies and 8.2 million colonoscopies [13]. Thus, in 2004, Seeff and colleagues suggested that depending on the proportion of available capacity used for CRC screening, it could take up to 10 years to screen the unscreened population using flexible sigmoidoscopy or colonoscopy.

Globally, most countries appear to be far less equipped than the United States to tackle the burden of screening all those eligible. In the United Kingdom, the concern of inadequate capacity to screen for CRC was soon overshadowed by the stark realization of inadequate training in many centers performing colonoscopies. A survey of 9,223 colonoscopy procedures carried out during 4 months in three of the countries' National Health Service (NHS) regions found a wide variation in practice, unacceptable complication rate, and lack of standardization in training [14]. Only 40% of the 234 colonoscopists had received formal training, and only 17% of these clinicians had received supervised training for their first 100 colonoscopies. The authors concluded that "unless there is a dramatic increase in manpower and resources available [to do colonoscopies], the introduction of a national screening program would rapidly overburden already inadequate facilities." Issues in Canada remain largely unsettled as the country aims to decide whether a future program should be targeted at the mass, average-risk population, or just the high-risk individuals [15]. This has evolved and population-based screening programs have now been initiated in many provinces.

Detailed modeling techniques have consistently suggested that the available manpower would be insufficient to screen the United States population. Vijan and colleagues estimated that the annual demand for colonoscopy ranged from 2.21 to 7.96 million [16]. If one used a conservative estimate of a single screening colonoscopy at age 65, an additional 1,360 to 4,160 gastroenterologists would be needed representing an overall increase in approximately 13–40% of the working force depending on the sensitivity analyses. If, however, the most effective but most resource intensive strategy was used (100% subjects screened, beginning at age 50, followed by a colonoscopy every 10 years), the pool of gastroenterologists would have to increase fourfold. Such realizations fuelled the development of competing diagnostic imaging technologies, such as CT colonography (CTC) especially as a tool adapted for mass screening given its low complication rate, patient tolerability and presumed (at least upfront) lower costs.

CTC, commonly referred to as "virtual colonoscopy," has been received with mixed results—the radiology community has expressed its exuberance claiming this test to be the ideal screening method, while the gastroenterology community has maligned this technology for its inferior sensitivity when compared to conventional colonoscopy. Wide acceptance of emerging technology is often largely dependant on coverage by either the government or third-party payers. Then, it stands to reason that CTC would be similarly received and adopted. However, the Centers for Medicare and Medicaid Services (CMS) recently issued a memorandum stating that it would not approve monetary reimbursement for Medicare-eligible individuals who undergo a virtual colonoscopy noting that "the evidence is inadequate to conclude that CT colonography is an appropriate colorectal cancer screening test . . . CT colonography for colorectal cancer screening remains noncovered" [17].

Endoscopic training for the surgeon

Increasing endoscopic exposure with a concomitant increase in procedural competency has been mandated by the Residency Review Committee for Surgery (RRC-S) and therefore all surgical training programs. Despite the 293% increase in required flexible gastroenterology experience for general surgery residents, flexible

endoscopy exposure for the residents remains variable [18]. The national average case volumes abstracted from the American Council of Graduate Medical Education (ACGME) database suggests that residents fall short by nearly 50% in achieving their required numbers [19]. Asfaha, et al. found that the general residents are finishing training without performing enough upper endoscopies and colonoscopies to meet the American Society for Gastrointestinal Endoscopy (ASGE) training guidelines [20]. This data lend further credence to the argument raised by many gastroenterologists that question the current "double standard" that exists in the number of colonoscopies required for credentialing surgeons versus those for gastroenterologist A recent review of 24,509 adult outpatient GI endoscopies performed at six Winnipeg hospitals over 2 years revealed that the complication rate was the highest for endoscopists performing fewer than 200 procedures each year [21]. The authors reported a very modest completion rate of only 65% (72% for gastroenterologists vs. 59% for general surgeons, $p < 0.005$). The overall colonoscopy completion rate was 69% (78% for gastroenterologists, 62% for general surgeons, $p = 0.03$). There was a slightly increased perforation rate for colonoscopies without additional procedures performed by general surgeons (0.1%) and family physicians (0.3%) compared with the gastroenterologists (0.02%) ($p = 0.03$).

In response to the growing concern regarding quality, complications and the need to enhance the endoscopic training for surgical residents, general surgery programs are now mandated by the RRC-S in association with the ACGME to train surgical residents in endoscopy. In February 2006, the RRC-S increased the required experience in flexible sigmoidoscopy during general surgery residency training—2009 graduates must complete 85 total gastrointestinal endoscopy cases, including 35 upper endoscopic procedures and 50 colonoscopies [18]. These requirements are less stringent than those of the American Society of Gastrointestinal Endoscopy (ASGE) requiring 130 EGDs and 140 colonoscopies before procedural competence may even be assessed, volumes shown to be associated in most trainees with a 90% success rate in intubating the esophagus and the pylorus or the splenic flexure and cecum, respectively [22].

The surgical viewpoint has consistently maintained that endoscopic skill acquisition is greatly skewed to the left for surgeons when compared to gastroenterologists and surgical data have challenged threshold competency numbers. Wexner, et al. prospectively analyzed 13,580 colonoscopies performed by surgeons and found that the complication rate was not significantly associated with either the level of experience or the number of prior annual colonoscopies [23]. Prior colonoscopic experience did have an impact on completion rate ($p < 0.001$) and was inversely proportional to the time to completion ($p < 0.001$), however, a minimum of 50 prior colonoscopies and 100 annual colonoscopies were associated with a significant improvement in the rate of completion. They argued, thus, that no minimum number of cases can be mandated for credentialing to perform "safe" colonoscopies. These findings are supported by a recent performance study determining the standard of care rendered by surgeon endoscopists in a Veterans Affair (VA) medical center evaluating the indications for colonoscopy and outcome performance measures according to established quality indicators for colonoscopy [24]. Using CRC quality indicators from the Society of American Gastrointestinal and Endoscopic Surgeons (SAGES), the American Cancer Society (ACS) guidelines for postcancer resection surveillance, and the ASGE quality indicators for colonoscopy, the authors found that 99% of the colonoscopies were performed in accordance with established criteria; cecal intubation rates were 97% and adenoma detection rates were 26%.

Colorectal surgeons spend considerable amount of their training acquiring colonoscopic skills, and, as such contribute to the overall manpower available for performing colonoscopy. Results from a survey probing the importance of colonoscopy in colorectal surgeons' practices found that colonoscopy plays a major role in the practices of colorectal surgeons across the world, accounting for approximately one-quarter of clinical time and total charges [25]. Existing data also suggest general surgeons perform colonoscopies with as low a morbidity rate and as high a completion rate as their colorectal surgery and gastroenterology colleagues suggesting they too have an important role to play in providing endoscopic services [26]. The imperative set forth by the RRC-S and the ACGME for increased endoscopy training for general surgery trainees has necessitated changes in scheduling and the overall design of surgery residency programs [18,27,28]. Although the discrepancies in the number of procedures required for credentialing GI trainees differ from those of general surgery residents, future manpower calculations for endoscopic training needs to account for an increasingly more experienced surgeon to assist in coping with the increased need for colonoscopists. However, "in the end, it is not just about procedure numbers. It is about properly preparing trainees for the environment in which they will practice and the use of validated measurements of procedural competence to know if they are ready to do so in a safe and effective manner" [29].

Asfaha, et al. discovered that surgeons in Calgary, Canada who work in smaller communities, of <100,000 population, have doubled their procedure volume in EGDs and quadrupled their colonoscopy volume [20]. Practice patterns for the rural US surgeon are strikingly similar. Thompson, et al. conducted a study characterizing the general surgery workforce in rural America [30]. Only 10.6% of the nation's general surgeons are female. Furthermore, the overall size of the rural general surgical workforce has remained static over the last decade, but based on demographic data, this number will decline considerably in the near future. When this information is combined with the knowledge that rural surgeons perform more procedures than their urban counterparts, nearly double the laparoscopic procedures and triple the number of endoscopies, the implicit deduction is a glaring disconnect between supply and demand—most pronounced in the rural sectors of America [31]. A SAGES 2007 rural surgery survey found that the nearest gastroenterologist resides more than 20 miles away in 50% of rural surgery practices [32]. The rural surgeon is the first physician of choice in 65% of rural surgery environments when it comes to performing a screening colonoscopy and second in 32%.

Future demands for endoscopy

The realization that the actual current demand for gastroenterologists significantly exceeds GI society forecasts from the mid-

1990s should serve as an invaluable lesson since the current and upcoming scenario for gastroenterology workforce is now appearing eerily similar.

Experts gathered at a recent consensus meeting that assessed the impact of future technologies on gastroenterology practice scrutinized the services offered by gastroenterologist, both cognitive and technical [33]. Acknowledging that endoscopy comprises a large portion of the current daily practice of a gastroenterologist both in private practice and at academic centers, these thought leaders suggested the emergence of new technologies (endoscopic and competing alike) may lead to a substantial change in rates and types of endoscopies. Additional factors include declining reimbursement and the demands brought on by an aging and increasing obese population as the authors cite is undeniable. The Future Trends Committee (FTC) of the AGA Institute convened to address these concerns and to probe the question "if endoscopy disappears, then what?" in April 2006. They identified obesity treatment as an area of huge opportunity for gastroenterologist [34]. The panel thus recommended the AGA Institute should conduct educational programs on obesity treatment, especially in relation to surgical and in the future, endoscopic treatments. Gastroenterologists today are also reminded that screening colonoscopies will likely wane in the future owing to the advent of competing diagnostic modalities, including CTC and wireless endoscopy. Conversely, it is likely that over the next 5 years, conventional diagnostic endoscopic procedures will decrease considerably but that sophisticated diagnostic and therapeutic procedures will likely increase.

Demand for training in gastroenterology

After considerable debate, the GI Match was reintroduced in 2007 [35,36]. The total number applicants has remained stable at 914 and 879 for the academic years 2007 and 2008, respectively [37]. With nearly identical number of applications in this last academic year, the National Residency Matching Program (NRMP) reported the number of matched GI positions to be 345 with 6% being International Medical Graduates (IMG)-US Foreign and 21% being International Medical Graduates Foreign [38]. An alternative surrogate way of analyzing the competitiveness for GI training positions utilizes the average number of applications per applicant for both US Medical Graduates (USG) and IMGs. Based on this criterion, gastroenterology positions ranked number 1 at 36.5 applications per applicant for USGs, slightly ahead of cardiology at 33.7 in 2007; similar results were noted in 2008 according to ERAS. It would thus appear that interest in gastroenterology remains quite high for the foreseeable future, and this issue no longer seems to be a limiting factor when addressing manpower concerns. A recent report further suggests that the United States will need 1,050 more gastroenterologists by 2020 to meet the demands for colonoscopy [39]. If screening rates increase by 10%, 1,550 more gastroenterologists will be needed according to this same report.

The creation of more training spots to accommodate changing demand based on community needs and on applicant interest is unfortunately not so rapidly accomplished. Fellowship positions are expensive to offer, and teaching institutions rely heavily on government support to do so. This presents both financial and bureaucratic obstacles to rapid adjustment of supply of endoscopists in response to changing needs. Perhaps if those in the community had the opportunity to subsidize the training of additional endoscopists to help them find individuals to hire to keep up with case workload, supply could be made more dynamic and corrections to errors in manpower predictions would be far easier to make.

Conclusions

Manpower estimates are clearly an inexact science despite sophisticated modeling programs and algorithms replete with useful data. Basic economic theories and more sophisticated econometric techniques lead to an obvious and logical realization that as long as there are acceptable returns in gastroenterology, trainees will continue to gravitate to this field and in turn, endoscopy, which constitutes a significant portion of a gastroenterologist's practice. It is hoped that the detailed lessons learned from the past—specifically recognizing limitations in forecasting supply and needs—prove useful as we attempt to predict future needs in endoscopic training in 2010 and beyond. Competing technologies such as CTC will undoubtedly impact the need for colonoscopies but the current lack of Medicare coverage limit its penetration. Gastroenterologists will be asked to perform increasingly challenging therapeutic maneuvers as a significant part of their daily work, the extent to which can only be hypothesized at present. The surgeon endoscopist will assume an increasing presence in endoscopy units throughout the country. Gastroenterologists need to dismiss major misgivings regarding the discrepancies in training number for surgeons and appreciate that the majority of endoscopies in rural America continue to be provided by the rural surgeon. Areas of endoscopic opportunity for gastroenterologists will include the management of obesity. To paraphrase one of the greatest visionaries on endoscopic training, we can conclude with Peter Cotton that "after all that has happened in the world of digestive endoscopy, it is tempting to assume that the golden days are over. That would be wrong; the future is bright [...] I cannot predict how important endoscopy may be in that distant day, but suggest that we keep our focus on the patient's best interests and cling to the important attribute that got us started—flexibility" [40].

Acknowledgements

I would like to thank Dr. Manish Tripathi, Assistant Professor of Marketing at Emory University Goizueta Business School for helping with the economic theories described in this chapter. Dr. Barkun is a Research Scholar from the Fonds de la recherché en Santé du Québec.

References

1 Mincer J. Investment in human capital and personal income distribution. *J Polit Econ* 1958;**66**(4):281–302.

2 Becker G. Investment in human capital: a theoretical analysis. *J Polit Econ* 1962;**70**(55):S9–S49.

3 Heckman JJ, Honore BE. The empirical content of the Roy model. *Econometrica* 1990;**58**(5):1121–1149.

4 Tarlov AR. Shattuck lecture–the increasing supply of physicians, the changing structure of the health-services system, and the future practice of medicine. *N Engl J Med* 1983 May 19;**308**(20): 1235–1244.

5 Cooper RA. Perspectives on the physician workforce to the year 2020. *JAMA* 1995 Nov 15;**274**(19):1534–1543.

6 Greenberg L, Cultice JM. Forecasting the need for physicians in the United States: the Health Resources and Services Administration's physician requirements model. *Health Serv Res* 1997;**31**(6):723–737.

7 Anderson GF, Han KC, Miller RH, Johns ME. A comparison of three methods for estimating the requirements for medical specialists: the case of otolaryngologists. *Health Serv Res* 1997;**32**(2):139–153.

8 Meyer GS, Jacoby I, Krakauer H, Powell DW, Aurand J, McCardle P. Gastroenterology workforce modeling. *JAMA* 1996;**276**(9): 689–694.

9 Modlin IM, Sabesin SM, Shape WJ Jr, Rubin W. Manpower in gastroenterology in the United States: a position paper of the Training and Education Committee of the AGA. *Gastroenterology* 1989;**96**(3):956–958.

10 Niederle M, Roth AE. The gastroenterology fellowship Match: how it failed and why it could succeed once again. *Gastroenterology* 2004;**127**(2):658–666.

11 Gross CP, Andersen MS, Krumholz HM, McAvay GJ, Proctor D, Tinetti ME. Relation between Medicare screening reimbursement and stage at diagnosis for older patients with colon cancer. *JAMA* 2006;**296**(23):2815–2822.

12 Seeff LC, Manninen DL, Dong FB et al. Is there endoscopic capacity to provide colorectal cancer screening to the unscreened population in the United States? *Gastroenterology* 2004;**127**(6):1661–1669.

13 Seeff LC, Richards TB, Shapiro JA et al. How many endoscopies are performed for colorectal cancer screening? Results from CDC's survey of endoscopic capacity. *Gastroenterology* 2004;**127**(6):1670–1677.

14 Bowles CJ, Leicester R, Romaya C, Swarbrick E, Williams CB, Epstein O. A prospective study of colonoscopy practice in the UK today: are we adequately prepared for national colorectal cancer screening tomorrow? *Gut* 2004;**53**(2):277–283.

15 Twombly R. Recommendations raise workload issues for colon cancer screening. *J Natl Cancer Inst* 20043;**96**(5):348–350.

16 Vijan S, Inadomi J, Hayward RA, Hofer TP, Fendrick AM. Projections of demand and capacity for colonoscopy related to increasing rates of colorectal cancer screening in the United States. *Aliment Pharmacol Ther* 2004;**20**(5):507–515.

17 Yoest P. Colon scans not covered. *Wall St J* May 13, 2009.

18 Bittner JGt, Marks JM, Dunkin BJ, Richards WO, Onders RP, Mellinger JD. Resident training in flexible gastrointestinal endoscopy: a review of current issues and options. *J Surg Educ* 2007;**64**(6):399–409.

19 Accreditation Council for Graduate Medical Education. Case entry for general surgery. 2007. Available: http://www.acgme.net/ residentdatacollection/documentation/Manuals/Case_Entry_440.pdf (accessed March 26, 2007).

20 Asfaha S, Alqahtani S, Hilsden RJ, MacLean AR, Beck PL. Assessment of endoscopic training of general surgery residents in a North American health region. *Gastrointest Endosc* 2008;**68**(6):1056–1062.

21 Singh H, Penfold RB, DeCoster C et al. Colonoscopy and its complications across a Canadian regional health authority. *Gastrointest Endosc* 2009;**69**(Suppl. 3):665–671.

22 Cass OW, Freeman ML, Cohen J et al. Acquisition of competence in endsocopic skills (ACES) during training: early results of a multicenter study. *Gastrointest Endosc.* 1995;**41**(4):317. [meeting abstract].

23 Wexner SD, Garbus JE, Singh JJ. A prospective analysis of 13,580 colonoscopies. Reevaluation of credentialing guidelines. *Surg Endosc* 2001;**15**(3):251–261.

24 Tran Cao HS, Cosman BC, Devaraj B et al. Performance measures of surgeon-performed colonoscopy in a Veterans Affairs medical center. *Surg Endosc* 2009;**23**(10):2364–2368.

25 Kann BR, Margolin DA, Brill SA et al. The importance of colonoscopy in colorectal surgeons' practices: Results of a survey. *Dis Colon Rectum* 2006;**49**(11):1763–1767.

26 Mehran A, Jaffe P, Efron J, Vernava A, Liberman MA. Colonoscopy: why are general surgeons being excluded? *Surg Endosc* 2003;**17**(12): 1971–1973.

27 Morales MP, Mancini GJ, Miedema BW et al. Integrated flexible endoscopy training during surgical residency. *Surg Endosc* 2008;**22**(9):2013–2017.

28 Bittner JGt, Coverdill JE, Imam T, Deladisma AM, Edwards MA, Mellinger JD. Do increased training requirements in gastrointestinal endoscopy and advanced laparoscopy necessitate a paradigm shift? A survey of program directors in surgery. *J Surg Educ* 2008;**65**(6): 418–430.

29 Dunkin BJ, Vargo JJ. Measuring procedural competence in endoscopy: what do the numbers really tell us? *Gastrointest Endosc* 2008;**68**(6):1063–1065.

30 Thompson MJ, Lynge DC, Larson EH, Tachawachira P, Hart LG. Characterizing the general surgery workforce in rural America. *Arch Surg* 2005;**140**(1):74–79.

31 Ritchie WP Jr, Rhodes RS, Biester TW. Work loads and practice patterns of general surgeons in the United States,1995–1997: a report from the American Board of Surgery. *Ann Surg* 1999;**230**(4):533–542. [discussion 42-3].

32 Broughan TA. SAGES 2007 rural surgery panel. *Surg Endosc* 2008;**22**(7):1579–1581.

33 Regueiro CR. Will screening colonoscopy disappear and transform gastroenterology practice? Threats to clinical practice and recommendations to reduce their impact: report of a consensus conference conducted by the AGA Institute Future Trends Committee. *Gastroenterology* 2006;**131**(4):1287–1312.

34 Sharaf RN, Weinshel EH, Bini EJ, Rosenberg J, Sherman A, Ren CJ. Endoscopy plays an important preoperative role in bariatric surgery. *Obes Surg* 2004;**14**(10):1367–1372.

35 Richter JE. Should the national GI Fellowship Matching Program be restored? Pro: gastroenterology match: good for all the players. *Am J Gastroenterol* 2004;**99**(1):6–7.

36 Niederle M. Restarting the gastroenterology match. *Am J Gastroenterol* 2005;**100**(5):1202–1203.

37 ERAS 2004-2008 statistics for fellowship specialties. Available: http://wwwaamcorg/programs/eras/programs/statistics/fellowship/p/gastro_imhtm. 2009. [serial on the Internet.]

38 NRMP information. National Resident Matching Program (NRMP). Leavwood, Kan. Available: https://servicesnrmporg/r3/reports/matchres_statscfm. 2009. [serial on the Internet.]

39 Growing Shortage of Gastroenterologistss to Affect Screening Capacity for #2 Cancer Killer. 2009.

40 Cotton PB. Digestive endoscopy in five decades. *Clin Med* 2005;**5**(6): 614–620.

32 Providing Resources and Opportunities for Retraining for Practicing Endoscopists

John Petrini

Sansum Clinic, Santa Barbara, CA, USA

Significant variation exists in endoscopic training programs throughout the world and within the United States. Even more significant is the lack of training availability for endoscopists once they are finished with their fellowship training. Training in endoscopy is optimally obtained in conjunction with a thorough education program in digestive diseases. The ability to physically perform the procedure cannot be isolated from the understanding of the visual image. Training programs that certify competence in endoscopy are also certifying that the trainee is knowledgeable in the indications, contraindications, normal and abnormal anatomy, therapy, and complications, as well their treatment, for each procedure. This education cannot be obtained without an extensive training program in gastrointestinal medicine. Once obtained, however, these skills need to be continuously practiced and improved. The ability to acquire new skills in endoscopy beyond training is dependent upon many factors. The most important are the knowledge base that is present prior to the new technique being attempted and the availability of exposure to the technique prior to adoption. This chapter explores the possibility of training beyond fellowship as the field of gastrointestinal endoscopy evolves.

The current practice of endoscopy is based upon the direct visualization of the gastrointestinal tract and recognition of the normal and abnormal anatomy, as well as its ramifications. All standard endoscopic procedures are variations on the basic principle of visualizing the gastrointestinal tract and extending therapeutic devices out of the instrument into the digestive system. The ability to manipulate the instrument throughout the gastrointestinal tract is but a part of the procedure. Biopsy, polypectomy, control of bleeding, and injection are extensions of the procedure and usually learned during training. However, each advance, such as sclerotherapy, injection polypectomy and endoscopic mucosal resection builds upon the basic technique of injection. If a device such as the argon plasma coagulator becomes available, the major learning steps are specific to the device and its application. For instance, the depth of burn, settings for power delivery, flow of argon gas, distance from the surface for proper application, are all specific to the argon plasma coagulator and need to be learned prior to application of the probe. The use of this instrument is merely an extension of other thermal energy applicators.

The only truly new development over the last six decades has been the use of endoscopic ultrasonography (EUS) to extend the gaze of the endoscopist beyond the lumen and into adjacent structures. This development has created the first major division in endoscopic practice, as individuals not trained in endoscopic ultrasonography have severe limitations in their ability to become facile in the technique. The demands of clinical practice, be it private practice or academic medicine, create time barriers to on-the-job training for endoscopists. It is nearly impossible for a busy practicing gastroenterologist to be able to devote enough time to learn the technique of endoscopic ultrasonography and become trained in the anatomy, pathology and implications of findings obtained at ultrasonography, as well as the manipulation of the instrument to obtain the necessary images and biopsy or aspiration of suspect lesions. The expenses associated with time away from the practice and the limited availability of training centers makes adoption of EUS quite challenging outside of a fellowship setting. Hands-on experience in the presence of an expert in the procedure, which has been the hallmark of effective endoscopic training, requires a relative long training period and limits dissemination of this technique outside of a formal endoscopic training program, and even then, only during an advanced endoscopic training fellowship.

As new developments in endoscopic science occur, rapid applicability depends upon creating a cadre of well-trained and equipped endoscopists. How to effectively establish this training is not well defined, however, and may create one of the two scenarios: either the new procedure will be available only at referral centers where the technique(s) has been developed or adoption by less well-trained endoscopists will create discrepancies in care delivered. In this age of physicians and patients keeping score

Successful Training in Gastrointestinal Endoscopy, First Edition. Edited by Jonathan Cohen.
© 2011 Blackwell Publishing Ltd. Published 2011 by Blackwell Publishing Ltd.

on quality measures and benchmarking, it will be increasingly difficult to justify developing competency on the go on real patients as long as fully trained and competent individuals are available to provide the same services.

Some lessons can be learned from the recent major shift in surgical techniques from open procedures to laparoscopy. When larparoscopic cholecystectomy was first reported in 1987, the technique was widely recognized as a significant advance in the field of surgery, if not by surgeons, by many demanding patients [1]. Many conscientious surgeons realized that there was a gradual learning curve for competence in the technique, and substantial training was going to be required before widespread adoption was accomplished. Yet some surgeons felt that the technique was merely an extension of their previous laparoscopic experience, including work in the pelvis (primarily gynecologic), and that previous experience with this technique allowed them to extend the laparoscope into the new territory of the gallbladder fossa. Some surgeons desiring early adoption attended university or academic society recognized didactic courses that included work in an animal lab, while other training programs offered relatively little exposure to hands-on training with a live animal model. In either case, supervision in patients was unusual. The surgeons were then granted privileges at their local hospitals and began to train/supervise and credential other members of the surgical staff. Some surgeons attended 3-, 2-, or even 1-day training sessions that were of variable quality with little or no animal model experience, and then began to use the technique on patients. Others simply watched videotape demonstrations and then began operating on patients. It was not until 1990 that the Society of American Gastrointestinal Endoscopic Surgeons (SAGES) came out with a guideline outlining formal training and competency determination [2]. There is some redemption in laparoscopy, since most difficulties that arose during early experience with laparoscopy could be dealt with through conversion to an open procedure, an option that will likely not be available to endoscopists. Advancing from cholecystecomy to appendectomy, bowel resection, gastric bypass, fundoplication, as well as a variety of other surgical procedures, was seen as an extension of the original laparoscopic procedure. Surgeons currently coming out of current surgical training programs are already familiar with laparoscopic techniques and have adopted laparoscopy as an integral part of the surgical armamentarium.

One of the major problems, however, was that in the early years of laparoscopy, there was often nothing to prohibit surgeons from adopting laparoscopy without any formal training. Hospitals that wanted to provide the latest and greatest surgical procedures as a marketing tool would be less likely to argue against a competent general surgeon who has had some laparoscopic experience but had never done a specific laparoscopic surgery, such as cholecystectomy. In its most extreme form, surgeons with no formal training in laparoscopic cholecytectomy would adopt the familiar "see one, do one, teach one" strategy of advancing medical procedures and observe a colleague initially to gain familiarity with the technique. Not surprisingly, complications, particularly biliary leaks and injuries, from early laparoscopic cholecystectomy were higher than those of open cholecystectomy [3].

As endoscopy has advanced and new techniques have evolved, most endoscopists, rightly or wrongly, felt that these techniques were extensions of their prior training. Many endoscopists, often without any formal training, have adopted techniques such as injection sclerotherapy, variceal band ligation, endoscopic mucosal resection, and saline-assisted polypectomy. As endoscopy expands and evolves, however, the ability of endoscopists to simply adopt a technique without dedicated training will likely be reduced. While the current trend progressing towards more minimally invasive surgery, including Natural Orifice TransEndoscopic Surgery (NOTES®), will likely be outside the realm of the practicing gastroenterologist, some gastroenterologists in academic centers may wish to work closely with general surgeons and become facile in the techniques.

However, as new developments in endoscopy are introduced, there will be some techniques that can be adopted by endoscopists who have already completed their fellowships. Capsule endoscopy was one such development. Aided by previous familiarity with visualization of the normal and abnormal anatomy of the digestive tract, as well as computer-assisted review, many endoscopists participated in hands-on training courses and review of several early cases to become proficient in the technique. If chromoendoscopy, high-resolution endoscopy, narrow band imaging, autofluorescence imaging, confocal fluorescence/laser microscopy, optical coherence tomography, or other technical developments find their way into clinical practice, there will certainly be some practicing physicians who will desire advanced training in one or more of these techniques. One group of investigators recently demonstrated that as few as 35 examples of confocal microscopy findings could be used to train experienced endoscopists in the technique to approach the level of the expert endomicroscopists [4]. Similarly, another group showed that a lecture series showing narrow band imaging (NBI) photos would help to allow endoscopists to better categorize diminutive colorectal polyps [5]. Thus, it seems likely that experienced endoscopists can adopt these skills with additional intensive hands on training. Clearly the endoscopists will need to fully understand the science behind these new technologies, as well as the indications and appropriate application. These new techniques and developments, however, continue to be extensions of skill sets that are already mastered by trained endoscopists.

The primary limitations on training endoscopic procedures after fellowship are a lack of suitable models, small numbers of available trainers, time constraints due to demands of clinical practice, and the inability of training facilities to provide appropriate educational material for large numbers of trainees.

The lack of suitable models for training in endoscopy has been seen as a major impediment, which is manifest in the need to perform procedures on patients during the training process. There are as of this writing no completely acceptable mechanical or computer models for endoscopic training. Numerous candidate models have been developed but none have been found to be as realistic as human patients. In addition, there is little impetus to develop the same kind of quality simulators as those used in the aviation industry. The simulators employed to prepare commercial and military pilots are prohibitively expensive (average

$8,000,000), but are developed due to the extremely high consequences of pilot error [6]. Losing a jumbo jet with 250 passengers and crew through inadequate training is an unacceptable outcome for poor preparation. Developing a multimillion dollar simulated endoscopic ultrasound trainer to benefit a limited number of private practitioners is not likely to occur.

Endoscopic simulators have nevertheless evolved over time. Initial models were static devices that attempted to improve hand–eye coordination. Most have been largely forgotten as newer models were developed, although a few of the rubber colon models are still lying around in some endoscopy centers. Joseph Leung has produced a fairly sophisticated static model to teach ERCP and sphincterotomy techniques. The basic concepts are easily and effectively demonstrated, and there is some transference of the training to patients [7]. However, the simulator cannot capture the real life situation, with a desperate need to perform the procedure safely and effectively, complete with medical and legal overlay.

More sophisticated models utilizing mannequins and computer modeling have been developed. There are two such models in wide spread use: the Accutouch simulator and the Simbionics simulator. Both have their advantages and disadvantages but are being used to improve the introductory skills of trainees prior to exposure to patients. The ASGE has produced a technical review of these simulators [8]. Demonstration of the utility of these devices in reducing time needed to achieve technological expertise is still unavailable.

One of the more durable of the recent simulators has been the *ex vivo* Erlangen model and subsequent compactEASIE model. These devices use porcine esophagus and stomach to create a natural tissue feel for training in endoscopic therapy. Addition of the duodenum and part of the liver allows for a rudimentary ERCP training as well. These preparations are very useful to demonstrate therapeutic techniques, including banding, polypectomy, endoscopic clip placement, cautery devices, argon plasma coagulation, injection techniques, and foreign body removal. The Erlangen model was initially set up with simulated blood vessels that could "bleed" red colored fluid to provide a somewhat more realistic training experience. These models have been extremely valuable in teaching beginning therapeutic skills at the ASGE's First Year Fellows Courses. However, they are not yet proven adequate for teaching basic endoscopy skills.

The use of endoscopic simulators for training has been the focus of a recent review in Gastrointestinal Endoscopic Clinics of North America (July, 2006; Volume 16 Number 3). While a number of devices and simulators are available, none have been able to clearly demonstrate improvement in time to achieve expert status, although they have been able to reliably differentiate experts from novices.

Another major impediment to training endoscopic skills is the lack of available experienced trainers. When endoscopy was in its infancy, many "experts" were simply early investigators in the field, developing the skills on the job as the new instruments were manufactured. The ability to bring direct vision to the inside of the gastrointestinal tract was novel and exciting, but early endoscopists could hardly have been called experts. It took decades for endoscopic skills to develop to their current state. Even when the current population of gastroenterologists arrived in training programs, many training centers were staffed with endoscopists that had little formal training in high-quality endoscopic work.

Most gastroenterology training programs recognize the need for experienced endoscopists to provide hands-on training for new fellows. Yet these educators are also facing competing demands to bolster clinical work and increase the financial well-being of the department. There is no question that the number of procedures a faculty member can complete in any given period of time will be greatly reduced by the addition of hands-on training of fellows in GI training programs. The available pool of clinical adjuncts is also in peril, as the clinical volunteer faculty is also facing the impact of being away from their practices. The need to maintain clinical services will be impacted by the cost of providing training to the next generation of endoscopists.

Given the current financial pressures, it is very difficult to imagine a program being able to devote several months to training a practicing gastroenterologist who wants to pick up a new skill. While programs will continue to provide extensive training in basic endoscopy, including therapy, the fellows will likely not be able to learn the advanced skills of ERCP and EUS within the standard fellowship. There are currently 49 institutions offering advanced fellowship training in these two procedures and the number of available slots is between 61 and 64 [9]. There are some concerns that even within these narrow fellowship goals, there are advanced fellows who do not get enough experience with advanced procedures [10]. Thus, the ability of a practicing gastroenterologist to pick up advanced training within the current structure will be very unlikely. A new paradigm in advanced endoscopic training will be required for practicing endoscopists to acquire these skills.

It will be necessary to develop a program to train practitioners in advanced endoscopic skills using a combination of computer-based cognitive training and advanced simulators, live animal models, or cadavers. The two major components of training in endoscopy are the technical skills necessary to perform the procedure and the cognitive skills required to know the indications, normal and abnormal anatomy, potential complications, and their treatment and the requirements for treatment and follow-up based upon the findings. Since endoscopic procedures are now performed in a digital format, it should be relatively easy to develop a standard procedural map during each procedure. These movements, as well as deviations from the appropriate and necessary movements, can be computerized and an ideal procedure defined. The trainee needs only to duplicate the same movements as the expert who initially performed the procedure to complete the task successfully. Deviation from the original procedure movements can be identified and codified in a manner that allows the trainee to see the effects of the movements that he or she makes. In this manner, a set of programmed movements based upon normal and abnormal anatomy that will guide the trainee can be created. These movements would need to be set into a simulator, once again creating the need for capital investment, but should be far less complicated than the all-encompassing flight simulators used in aviation.

Since the basics of the anatomy, including both normal and pathologic states, can be learned in advance, a training manual,

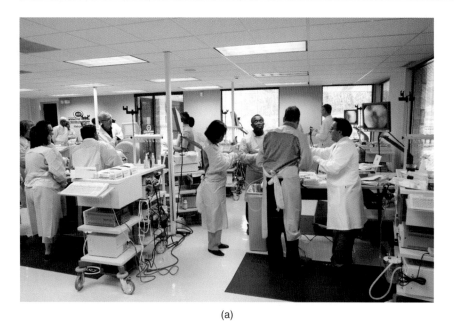

(a)

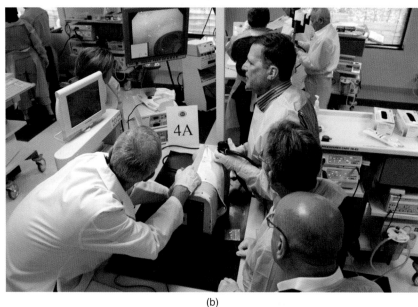

(b)

Figure 32.1 (a) View of interior of current ASGE ITT Center showing several workstations and the ability to provide hands-on training in small groups. (b) Close-up of a single workstation at the current ASGE ITT Center, utilizing a colon model and Olympus UDP system for training in proper colonoscopy technique.

perhaps in an online version, that individuals who wish to learn an advanced endoscopic skill can complete at their own pace would be ideal. This would eliminate the need for classes and training sessions that would require time away from the trainee's practice. Only after the trainee was able to demonstrate successful completion of the initial cognitive training would the trainee to be allowed to have hands-on experience with either a model or a patient.

The ITT Center in Oak Brook, IL provides a novel example of how trainees can be brought together from around the country to learn a specific endoscopic skill. The programs offered include capsule endoscopy, treatment of Barrett's epithelium, sedation, advanced colonoscopy, and a number of other training programs (Figure 32.1). It is also the site of the First Year Fellows' Courses

held each year for introductory training in endoscopy. The major limitations of the current ITT center are due to the relatively small size of the facility, the lack of live animal or cadaver models, and the lack of radiology equipment. Some of these shortcomings will be addressed once the new ASGE training facility in nearby Downer's Grove, IL is completed. This building is planned to include the capability to offer live animal and cadaver models that can provide training that more closely simulates live patients. Plans for this facility are currently under development (Figure 32.2).

There is, of course, a cost associated with the development of this type of training. It is unlikely that universities and academic centers will want to invest the capital in these simulators and online training manuals, and there are far too little resources available outside of industry. It seems most likely that the instrument

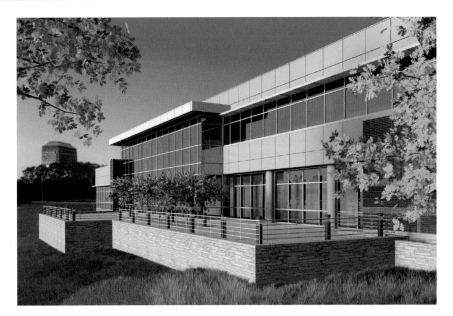

Figure 32.2 Artist's rendering of the new ASGE ITT Center. The new facility, as currently planned, will have fluoroscopy capability as well as the ability to incorporate live animal and cadaver models. Plans to make the laboratory activities available via live transmission are in consideration.

manufacturers who wish to sell more of their equipment would be the ones to benefit from this expanded training and are therefore the most likely source for the funds necessary to create these training programs. If the training is directed towards competent and adequately trained endoscopists who have already mastered the basic endoscopic skills, there is a reasonable expectation that this type of training could be used to develop advanced endoscopic training for practitioners.

The development of new endoscopic procedures and techniques will undoubtedly continue. While some techniques are extensions of previously learned skills, there will be some that are so novel and unique that a new set of skills will be required to proficiently perform the procedure. It is hoped that with adequate investment in training programs for those endoscopists already in practice that these new procedures can enjoy more rapid dissemination to the benefit of the larger patient population [see Figure 32.1].

References

1 Reddick EJ, Olsen D, Daniell J, Saye W, McKernan B, Miller W, Hoback M. Laparoscopic laser cholecystectomy. *Laser Med Surg News Adv* 1989;30–40.

2 SAGES. Granting privileges for laparoscopic (peritoneoscopic) general surgery. Society of American Gastrointestinal Endoscopic Surgeons, Los Angeles, 1990.

3 MacFadyen BV Jr, Vecchio R, Ricardo AE, Mathis CR. Bile duct injury after laparoscopic cholecystectomy. The United States experience. *Surg Endosc* 1998;**12**:315–321.

4 Buchner AM, Gomez V, Gill KR et al. The learning curve for *in vivo* probe based confocal laser microscopy (pCLE) for prediction of colorectal neoplasia. *Gastrointest Endosc* 2009;**69**:AB364–AB365.

5 Higashi R, Uraoka T, Kato J et al. Does intensive training improve the diagnositc accuracy of narrow band imaging (NBI) in differntiuating neoplastic from non-neoplastic colorecal diminutive polyps? *Gastrointest Endosc* 2009;**69**:AB223.

6 Cohen J, Nuckolls L, Mourant RR. Endoscopic simulators: lessons from the aviation and automobile industries. *Gastrointest Endosc Clin N Am* 2006;**16**:407–423.

7 Leung JW, Liao WC, Wand HP et al. A RCT of mechanical simulator practice and usual training vs. usual training on novice trainee clinical ERCP performance. *Gastrointest Endosc* 2009;**69**:AB141.

8 American Society for Gastrointestinal Endoscopy. Technology status evaluation report. Endoscopy simulators. *Gastrointest Endosc* 1999;**50**:935–937.

9 Advanced Endoscopy. Fellowship Programs July 2009. *Gastrointest Endosc* 2009;**70**:34A–39A.

10 Azad JS, Verma D, Kapadia AS, Adler DG. Can U.S. GI fellowship programs meet American Society for Gastrointestinal Endoscopy recommendations for training in EUS? A survey of U.S. GI fellowship program directors. *Gastrointest Endosc* 2006;**64**:235–241.

33 Evolving Role of GI Societies and Industry in Training Endoscopists to Perform New Techniques: Supporting the Process and Setting the Standards

John A. Martin[1] & Christopher J. Gostout[2]

[1] Northwestern University Feinberg School of Medicine, Chicago, IL, USA
[2] Mayo Clinic, Rochester, MN, USA

Background

Historical perspective

Over the course of the past decade, there has been an enthusiasm and resultant evolution in endoscopic training not witnessed in the antecedent three decades since the inception of formal endoscopic training. The traditional "see one, do one, teach one" method long espoused in medical and surgical training had been adopted by and adapted to training in the new field of endoscopy at its nascence [1,2]. However, since the mid- to late-1990s, endoscopic training has undergone a renaissance at all levels, from the fundamental to the cutting edge. Multiple coincident trends not only in endoscopy but also in medical education and in health care delivery at large have helped drive this. These include the burgeoning appearance of new technologies and techniques, increased emphasis on relevance and accountability in medical education and training, pressures from within and outside of the medical community to deliver higher quality, cost-effective care [3,4], and the advent of awareness, concern, and interest in the application of new paradigms in procedural training [5–7].

An unprecedented number of new technologies are being introduced by the endoscopic industry, from completely novel imaging and tissue-acquisition technologies such as endoscopic ultrasound (EUS), to image enhancement technologies such as high-definition video endoscopy, to extended anatomical capabilities represented by deep enteroscopy and capsule endoscopy technologies, to a seemingly limitlessly expanding array of interventional devices involving endoluminal stenting, closure, hemostasis, excision, and ablation. This technological abundance has not only created an increasing need for greater time and effort directed towards endoscopy training during fellowship but has also driven a demand for courses and other venues designed to impart new skills to update already fully trained, busy, practicing endoscopists in time-efficient formats. At the same time, in medical education and training at large, pedagogical initiatives are being directed towards improving the entire learning experience by increasing clinical relevance from the first day of medical school forward, through earlier and better correlation of science to clinical medicine, through the introduction of clinical material earlier in medical education, and by applying novel teaching methods, procedures, and technologies. Such methods were often adapted from other disciplines, professions, and occupations, such as case studies, procedural simulations on live animals and animal parts, and enhanced computer haptics.

The advent of using *ex vivo* animal organs as models created a high-fidelity, economical format for demonstration and training of gastrointestinal flexible endoscopic therapies on a large scale. These explant animal models offer a hands-on experience comparable to the live-animal model to vastly more trainees as a result of their low cost, easy availability, and overwhelmingly simplified logistical deployment [8,9].

Making it all possible: novel simulator platforms in endoscopic training

Simulators have been applied to training in gastrointestinal endoscopy for over three decades. All types of simulators provide the trainee with hands-on experience in endoscopic techniques in settings that replicate intraluminal gastrointestinal conditions with varying fidelity without exposing patients to trainee operators. As therapeutic intervention has expanded, the role of simulators in all phases of training have gained in importance and garnered intense interest. Endoscopic simulators can be grouped simply into five basic types: completely synthetic models (plastic mannequins and rubber or latex models of the upper GI tract and colon), three-dimensional models, computer or video

Successful Training in Gastrointestinal Endoscopy, First Edition. Edited by Jonathan Cohen.
© 2011 Blackwell Publishing Ltd. Published 2011 by Blackwell Publishing Ltd.

simulators, live sedated or anesthetized animals, and explanted animal organs attached to and supported by synthetic frames configured to mimic human gastrointestinal anatomy [10,11]. Progress in computer technology and increased experience with *ex vivo* animal models has created realistic characteristics that more closely reproduce the visual appearance and tactile sensation of actual clinical settings and circumstances. Gastroenterology and surgical training programs increasingly are integrating these models into their curricula [12–14].

Live, anesthetized animals represented the initial iteration of hands-on simulator training in gastrointestinal endoscopy and were good models because of their high fidelity in terms of appearance, tactile sensation, and tissue response to endoscopic manipulation [7], but share protean and substantial limitations. Prominent among these is that the investment required in terms of facilities for appropriate procurement, care, sedation, analgesia, perioperative, and postoperative management is cost-prohibitive in many endoscopic training settings, particularly those whereby a single simulation or demonstration render the model unusable for repetitive use. For example, once a sphincterotomy has been performed on the porcine papilla, the animal is no longer usable for another sphincterotomy. Live animal training can expose the sponsoring institution to criticism from animal-rights activists and organizations [15].

Computer-based simulators have evolved over their nearly three decades of development. While haptics, visual fidelities, and clinical scenario reproduction have improved markedly over the past decade, substantial limitations still exist with respect to the overall ability to faithfully reproduce tactile feedback response on tissue manipulation and recreation of the overall clinical experience. While most systems are compact and require little active maintenance, initial entry investment remains high, with each individual unit costing upwards of $100,000 if a number of simulation modules are included [16].

A more practicable application for using real tissue in endoscopic training involves acquiring selected sections of the gut of animals slaughtered for food (chiefly pigs), and using these organs ex vivo in a configuration mimicking the human gastrointestinal tract. The overall cost of explant organ simulation is minuscule compared to live-animal simulations. The porcine upper gastrointestinal tract was the first of such simulators to appear. Originally, specially trained butchers selectively dissected these specimens, but this can readily be performed in any abattoir under specific direction [17]. The liver, gallbladder, and bile ducts can also be included if pertinent to the simulation, and may be modified by the addition of other animal tissue to enhance reproduction of biliary anatomy specifically pertinent to endoscopic retrograde cholangiopancreatography (ERCP) [18]. Luminal contents are removed by lavage, and then the organs are inspected for compliance with food hygiene regulations before being approved for use, and may be preserved at $-18°C$ before use [19]. The fresh or thawed specimen then is attached to a supporting frame structure, commonly a tray-like plastic mold that conforms the organ(s) to a normal configuration. This type of model was first described in 1995 employing needles to pin the tissue to a cork plate for upper gastrointestinal endoscopy [20]. The Erlanger Active Simulator

for Interventional Endoscopy (EASIE) or Erlanger Endo-Trainer was originally designed for surgical applications, and refined and downsized specifically for endoscopic application as the compactEASIE; both were designed for use with porcine specimens [19,21].

The characteristics of the porcine gastrointestinal tract prepared and oriented in the anatomic mold permit further manipulation and modification of the tissues to simulate pathology applicable to endoscopic therapy [22]. Initial outlays for the equipment used for mounting the organ components are comparatively low (approximately $3,000 for a molded anatomic tray); costs for purchasing organs and technician time for harvesting, preparation, and disposal are approximately $150–200 per simulation [16]. Compared to computer simulation, however, this simulator platform, much as the live animal platform, requires high faculty-to-trainee ratios and staff support. Nonetheless, the advantages of the explant model are many, and the smaller, more portable tray models allow mobility with options for training at more than a fixed location. Of course, dedicated endoscopy simulator training centers with permanently installed fixtures, complete amenities, and fully stocked resources allow for tightly controlled conditions, predictability, and flexibility to accommodate special needs as they might arise in real time.

The pioneering work of Juergen Hochberger marked a major advance in endoscopic training; his innovation in developing this essential *ex vivo* training tool, by expanding it's applicability and integrating its use into rigorous and validated training programs had unprecedented impact on simulation in hands-on endoscopic training. The details of the development of various simulators and their validation for various techniques are covered in detail in other chapters in this text. After initial use primarily in the research setting with sporadic demonstrations at endoscopic meetings, intensive hands-on workshops based on the *ex vivo* tabletop animal tissue models gained popularity in the late 1990s, primarily at regional GI meetings such as the New York Society for Gastrointestinal Endoscopy (NYSGE). This explant model, with its efficiency, economy, fidelity, and flexibility, acted as the catalyst making possible the archetypal dedicated hands-on endoscopy training facility of the American Society for Gastrointestinal Endoscopy (ASGE), the Interactive Training & Technology Center (IT&T Center) located in Westmont, IL, a suburb of Chicago [23]. This facility was designed specifically to provide hands-on training in endoscopy using models similar to the Erlangen compactEASIE endoscopy simulator, with 10 endoscopic simulator stations in a large room with an open configuration. The center is operated and managed by full-time nursing and technical staff, and overseen by both ASGE executive and educational management and a physician board of directors. Expert faculty are chosen by education and training committees on a course-by-course basis from ASGE membership, and active faculty and staff supervision and instruction are provided for the entire duration of every course held at the center, with each faculty member supervising and instructing a small group of trainees at each station. In 2009, 15 interactive and hands-on CME courses were held on-site at the ASGE IT&T Center, in addition to six fellows' courses and two nursing courses (Table 33.1). Both the number of courses

Table 33.1 ASGE IT&T Center Interactive
and Hands-On Courses in 2009

First-year fellows' course (5)
Advanced fellows' video editing course
Basic capsule endoscopy (2)
Quality (3)
Advanced capsule endoscopy
Enteral nutrition
Small bowel
Esophageal
Colonoscopy
Enteroscopy
Sedation
Bariatrics
Managing IBD
ERCP boot camp
Nursing course (2)

Does not include ASGE interactive and hands-on
courses offered off-site.
The number inside brackets shows the number of
times course offered.

offered and overall course attendance have increased dramatically
year to year, with new courses and novel formats added each year
and recurring courses continuously refined. The attendance at the
IT&T Center has doubled over the last 3 years, to over 1,100 in
2009.

Evolving role of industry

The role of the device and endoscope industry in training endoscopists has been necessarily intensive, multifaceted, and integrated into the practical curriculum throughout the history of
endoscopic training. As such, it continues to incorporate new
aspects and features as procedural training evolves, particularly
in the hands-on training realm. Industry's contribution to endoscopic training has always entailed considerable investment in
providing instruments and devices, including not only durable
capital equipment such as endoscopes and processors, electrosurgical generators, and platforms to accommodate and integrate
these components, but also a continuous supply of consumables,
mainly in the form of disposable or limited-reuse endoscopic
accessory devices [8]. Industry has also traditionally provided generous levels of support for courses held by GI societies, academic
institutions, and other endoscopy groups, and is an important
and necessary source of funding particularly for hands-on venues,
which are much more resource-intensive than didactics-only presentations. Additionally, industry is also called upon to provide
on-site support and expertise in the form of technical representatives to help assemble, organize, deploy, and, in some cases, assist
in demonstrating their new and often complex technologies. In
the case of computer-based and synthetic simulation models, it is
industry that produces and conveys these items for their ultimate

application in simulator-based learning stations, which, as their
fidelity improves, are being increasingly recognized to be a useful
complement to more traditional methods of medical education
and training [24]. Although the support from industry is vital,
maintaining a balanced training opportunity is equally vital in an
environment of intense continuing medical education scrutiny.

In supporting hands-on endoscopy learning experiences for
the primary education of trainees as well as for skill enhancement training of fully fledged endoscopists, industry benefits
in multiple ways. First, they benefit from a unique interface
with their customers in an environment where industry and
academia/education are visibly symbiotic. Second, such settings
represent an opportunity for industry participants to provide necessary product, place it directly into the hands of the trainees and
help them utilize these items properly by providing expert technical assistance to the eager learners, many of whom are performing
these techniques for the first time. The positive impact such experiences have on participants has the potential to be prominent
and longstanding. In the case of practicing gastroenterologists
attending focused training workshops, these sessions may serve
as a unique opportunity for manufacturers to gain valuable feedback about their products from individuals most representative
of their main customers. Such practical return on investment has
been a major driver of industry support for training. Of course,
the relationship this paradigm establishes between industry and
education generates an aspect of ambivalence held by many educators involved in hands-on endoscopic training: while they wish to
present clinical material in an unbiased manner, they often cannot
offer the optimal experience, particularly in a resource-intensive
hands-on context, without substantial financial and logistical support from industry.

Not to be overlooked is industry's primary role in the creation of prototypical hands-on training facilities in the surgical
realm, which have had substantial impact in serving as inspiration, example, and, to a substantial extent, a blueprint for future
analogous endeavors in endoscopic training. The Ethicon Endo-
Surgery Institute, on the grounds of the Ethicon Endo-Surgery,
Inc. world headquarters in Cincinnati, OH, opened in 1992, followed by similar facilities in Germany and Japan [25]. Integrating
multiple operating suites with research and lecture space into one
facility, each such site provides an environment for training in
basic and advanced surgical techniques taught by surgical faculty,
as well as for research on surgical procedures and products. The
outstanding features of this endoscopic surgical learning facility
inspired one noted American academic medical educator to refine
his original ideas to create a simulation learning facility for gastrointestinal endoscopists in a way that would incorporate many
of the best and most applicable features of the Ethicon Endo-
Surgery Institute. While this facility would possess the manifold
advantages of being supported by industry, in contradistinction,
it would be designed, operated, and managed by a prominent
nonprofit GI endoscopy Society—and thus represent a neutral
field for education, training, and research, independent from
any particular industry source or academic institution. The next
section details the outcome of this historical, paradigm-altering
endeavor.

Evolving role of GI societies

A prototypical example of an organization advancing the role of GI Societies in training endoscopists to perform new techniques is the American Society of Gastrointestinal Endoscopy (ASGE). While the ASGE, from its inception in 1941, was dedicated to advancing endoscopic education, training, research, standards, and practice, its Interactive Technology & Training (IT&T) Center was a completely new venture into an education and training format which would transcend the traditional didactics- and passive visual-based formats that had longdominated endoscopic learning. The development of this unique concept and facility provides an interesting and highly pertinent case study in this very young genre of endoscopic training. It is also extremely useful to understand how a concept that began as an idea inspired by industry's foray into a new type of surgical hands-on training facility—witnessed and experienced firsthand with awe, intrigue, and delight by an insightful endoscopic academician with a zeal for teaching, a vision for the future of training, and a personal mission to carve out a niche for the GI organization that he was to lead—chanced upon the great fortune of an industry sponsor looking for a substantial educational effort to fund at that very point in time. The collision of these two formidable forces and the fusion that resulted led to the creation of a never-before seen type of facility dedicated to hands-on endoscopic training on a never-before-dreamed-of scale. This effort created a unique niche for the organization yet to be even remotely mimicked—much less replicated—by any similar GI organization, and in doing so has crafted a brand for that organization.

IT&T center initiative

Dedicated and opened in November 2003, the ASGE IT&T Center was the brainchild of then-President-elect of the ASGE, Christopher J. Gostout, of the Mayo Clinic in Rochester, MN. As he thought about a strategy for what he wanted to accomplish during his year as ASGE president, Gostout focused on two key items for which to garner undivided ASGE Governing Board and leadership support: A hands-on course dedicated to training first-year gastroenterology fellows early in their academic year, with didactic and technical education and training provided by expert endoscopy faculty culled from the ASGE, and a new hands-on training facility built, funded, and operated by the ASGE with substantial support from industry. This entity would become the IT&T Center. While he and his Developmental Endoscopy Unit (DEU) nursing director already had experience in building and running their own institutional endoscopy training facility at the Mayo Clinic, Gostout's concept for the ASGE IT&T Center was spawned by visits to an industry-developed training site, the Ethicon/Johnson & Johnson surgical training lab in Cincinnati, OH [25], and to the Medical Education and Research Institute (MERI), a 501 (c) (3) nonprofit hands-on medical teaching and training facility dedicated primarily to surgical procedural instruction in Memphis, Tennessee, inspired by a neurosurgeon in 1992 and opened in an old post office building in 1994 [26]. Gostout felt that, during his tenure as president and beyond, the

ASGE should take a leadership position in directing hands-on education and training in gastrointestinal endoscopic methods. In addition, he felt that the society should become the focal point for the introduction of new techniques and technologies in endoscopy, thus becoming the "go-to" source and location for institutions, industry, and practices seeking a "neutral" procedural training ground—and perhaps even credentialing—opportunity. The ASGE could, in turn, provide the exact faculty selections to meet such needs without difficulty, without bias, and with transparency—an important issue that could sometimes be tricky for industry alone to effect. Of course, the realization of an undertaking on this large of a scale would require substantial funding—not only in terms of equipment, instruments, and initial investment—but also directed towards a long-term operating budget to pay for staffing, faculty honoraria, and other recurring expenses, and—in the case of the First-Year Fellows' Course—funding to pay for the attendees' expenses.

To make this dream a reality, Gostout went to Patricia V. Blake, CAE, ASGE executive director, explaining to her that an affordable, animal-parts model of the human digestive tract utilizing an *ex vivo* pig stomach had recently been perfected, and that this would deliver a high-fidelity hands-on endoscopic experience replicating life-like handling of human tissue at minimal cost and with manageable logistics, without the need for live animals [20]. Together, Gostout, Blake, and Lori Herman, RN, Gostout's DEU unit nurse director, drew up plans and a business model, and, with the help of Vanessa Kizart, ASGE Meeting Services Director, found a suitable location near the ASGE Headquarters in Oak Brook, IL, a suburb of Chicago, jetting from concept to reality within less than a year. Blake saw the potential this project represented for the ASGE, as she recalled in an interview for the October 2007 issue of the Forum, the journal of the Association Forum of Chicagoland: "[Gostout] asked me, 'What do you think about setting something up here to teach people?' My immediate reaction was that this is something we can own and we can control. This is our brand" [27].

None of this could have happened without a serious financial commitment from industry. Industry has played a requisite fully integrated, lynchpin role since the nascence of the ASGE IT&T Center from the standpoint of both capital investment and recurring costs. In the case of the IT&T Center, in what amounted to serendipitous good fortune, Gostout was contacted at just the right time by the Olympus Corporation, the world's largest manufacturer of gastrointestinal endoscopes and a leading supplier of endoscopic instruments and accessories. They happened to be experiencing a very successful year and offered to assist Gostout with funding for any endoscopic education and training initiatives he would foresee for his year of ASGE Presidency. Gostout subsequently wrote a letter to Olympus outlining his strategy for the IT&T center with a line-item request for the necessary resources to assemble the facility, and Olympus pledged to support the center, supply it with endoscopes, and commit to covering four years of operating costs, while agreeing to Gostout's requirement that the IT&T Center be an even playing field, and thus still provide an opportunity for other endoscope and instrument manufacturers to contribute to the venture. Other industry supporters soon followed, joining the cause to turn this concept for learning into reality. The IT&T Center was born, and, just a few months later, hosted the inaugural First-Year Fellows' Hands-On Endoscopy Course in the summer of 2004.

Expanding course offerings and brand extension

The First-Year Fellows' Course expanded quickly, from three regional courses offered in 2004 to five regional courses in 2005, all hosted at the IT&T Center. All five courses were filled to capacity based on registration information. The financial resources required to meet these demands were expectedly substantial. These expenses have been covered through generous financial support from industry sponsors, who also donated endoscopic devices and provided technical support personnel. An endeavor of this magnitude would clearly be impossible without such corporate assistance.

Clearly, the nascence of the IT&T Center education and training model required the coalescence of need identification and conceptualization on the part of the ASGE society-physicians involved, business-model formulation and execution along with facility planning and logistical expertise on the part of ASGE executive and administrative staff, and resource allocation on the part of industry. However, the initial success and growth in the execution and application of this model would not have been possible without the benefit of the talent, skill, knowledge, and effort of a dedicated GI nurse expert. Terri Herzog, RN, CGRN, a certified endoscopy nurse at a local university hospital endoscopy unit with experience in hands-on endoscopy training, was recruited to the ASGE as the Assistant Director of Training and Technology, in order to set up and operate the IT&T Center with its various simulation models. Her initial mandate included the recruitment, training, and management of a staff of nurses and technicians to assist her in the day-to-day operations of the facility. Her role in the organization has evolved rapidly to include not only supervision of the IT&T facility but also assistance and oversight of education and training committees for the ASGE, critical participation in the conceptualization and execution of all new hands-on courses introduced at the IT&T Center as well as for off-site hands-on training endeavors of the organization, and the identification and deployment of new simulation formats. The clinical pertinence of her role is enhanced by her continued active practice as an endoscopy nurse at her university medical center's tertiary care endoscopy unit 2 days a week.

The First-Year Fellows' Course also represented a major innovation as a prototypical "living course"—one wherein a professional and academic society designs a specific, modular, complete introductory course replete with learning objectives and standardized material that is then successively enhanced and updated by faculty year by year. In the past, multiple GI societies have collaborated to publish documents—embodied in the GI Core Curriculum—to provide guidance as to specific topics all gastroenterology trainees should be taught during fellowship, and minimum core procedural competencies they should develop in the course of training. For new fellows, various introductory courses had been conducted for many years, with notable collaborative efforts by regional societies such as the New York Society for Gastrointestinal Endoscopy

(NYSGE), which was founded as a response to the recognition and forethought of luminary pioneers such as Jerome Waye and Sidney Winawer who understood the profound value and importance to the greater community of patients in disseminating good colonoscopic technique by creating training opportunities for endoscopists throughout greater New York.

The ASGE First-Year Fellows' Course was not only broad in its aspiration to reach all US trainees but also innovative in its effort to cull the training essentials from successful forerunner regional introductory courses such as those sponsored by the NYSGE, the Mayo Clinic, and others, into a standard template, and integrate interactive video-based discussion and, of course, the essential intensive hands-on *ex vivo* model training in several basic skill sets. The hands-on part was crafted based on lessons from the NYSGE workshops with the simulators and then tailored to the capabilities and logistics of the newly opened IT&T Center. One key challenge to overcome was how to greatly increase the scale of the endeavor in order to train a large number of fellows, while still maintaining high faculty-to-trainee ratios and sufficient scope time per skill station per fellow to allow for a meaningful learning experience. In sum, the national society possessed the necessary foresight and gathered the resources and commitment to offer a unique hands-on experience for fellows and to create an integrated and comprehensive introductory endoscopy curriculum to complement and reinforce the varying introductions to endoscopy available to trainees at their home institutions.

The early success surrounding the First-Year Fellow's Course was to represent only the beginning of what was originally conceived as a fixed-location center primarily committed to providing entry-level endoscopic training; the IT&T Center has since rapidly expanded to include a constantly changing catalog of sophisticated, increasingly complex, advanced, and highly focused hands-on courses devised to meet the needs of the fully-trained and even expert endoscopist seeking to learn the latest endoscopic techniques using cutting-edge novel technologies under the tutelage of focused, authoritative national and international faculty. In addition to courses held at the Westmont, IL, facility itself, hands-on courses of nearly every type held at the IT&T Center have been replicated at off-site locations, often as part of a large national meeting such as Digestive Diseases Week (DDW) or the Natural Orifice Surgery Consortium for Assessment and Research (NOSCAR). Large, "modular" endoscopy meetings are already planned by the ASGE, exemplified by EndoFest 2010, which will combine multiple didactic and hands-on course venues occurring simultaneously at an off-site location, so that attendees can customize exactly which combination of didactic offerings and hands-on training sessions they will attend to best meet their needs and goals during the multiday event (Video 33.1).

Taking this concept a step further are ongoing discussions regarding the potential use of the IT&T name to brand all interactive learning formats offered by the ASGE: interactive web-based learning, webinars, on-site and off-site hands-on course offerings, on-site and off-site didactic course offerings, hands-on and other interactive course sponsorships and endorsements, interactive durable learning materials, and other novel course formats. The potential utility of the IT&T Center beyond instructive applications has garnered great interest since before the facility ever came on line. It is well recognized that sophisticated simulation devices were in use in other professions and occupations long before they found application in medicine. In these other professions, simulators were also initially applied mainly to basic training. However, over time, as haptics improved and the fidelity of models and their sophistication grew, they became applicable to advanced training, new technology development, and, ultimately, for assessing continued competence of already-expert operators: witness the airline industry and its use of flight simulators for certification and recertification [28]. Gostout realized early on that that the ASGE IT&T center might evolve in this direction: Initially to introduce freshly minted first-year fellows to basic therapeutic endoscopic techniques hands-on early in their training—hopefully before they had taken too much call—then quickly to expand course offerings in the direction of opportunities for fully trained, experienced operators. Such experiences would be designed to enhance their already-acquired skills, to learn new skills and be introduced to new procedures, techniques, and technologies. This would all occur in a controlled environment free of the constraints of the active patient-care setting, earning CME credit in the process.

The logical next step would be to find ways to incorporate such a simulation facility into certification, credentialing, recertification, and recredentialing applications as the sophistication of simulator-based modeling and the capabilities of the facility grow. Another idea that Gostout had was for the IT&T Center to serve as an incubator for new ideas, for both new technology and new techniques, and for the development of new methods of delivering training. To accomplish this, he conceived of assembling teams of endoscopists with expert skills in the various procedures, and having these "teams" then be connected with industry, payers, etc., through the IT&T Center, to identify new concepts, provide feedback on emerging techniques and technologies, and educate the payers regarding what these procedures really do, what they are, and what they represent in terms of clinical application and outcomes. In the spirit of accurately representing this substantially expanded educational role the IT&T Center of today occupies, and that which the IT&T Center of the future is projected to build upon, the original name of the IT&T Center was changed from "Interactive Training and Technology" to "Institute for Training and Technology."

While the ASGE IT&T Center presently exists in its original leased physical location for its seventh year, land has already been purchased and architectural drawings completed for a new, combined IT&T Center, ASGE Conference Center, and ASGE Corporate Headquarters all on one campus owned by the ASGE and purpose-built from the ground-up. This integrated expansion and multifaceted facility enhancement was enthusiastically spearheaded by ASGE Past President John L. Petrini. This was done in large part out of his recognition of the growing importance the ASGE must take in providing opportunity and guidance for endoscopists in practice seeking to maintain their skills and retool for the future as technology and the demands for endoscopic services evolve and expand. The goal for this free-standing facility, one of Gostout's original goals, is to be able to accommodate live animals

and cadaver models in addition to the *ex vivo* animal parts models and computer simulators. This facility could also serve as a research center to facilitate ASGE-sponsored research and provide an investigative facility for those who may not have access to one at their home institution. Gostout even dreamed about creating ASGE sabbaticals during which an endoscopist could do his or her work at the IT&T Center.

Future directions and challenges

GI society role in navigation and standardization of new technology evaluation and adoption

The development of new endoscopic technology is a landscape that is far from flat. There are the obvious successes and failures, from the durability and continuous improvement of the charge-coupled device-driven videoendoscope to the fleeting appearance and momentary disappearance of many an endoscopic antigastroesophageal reflux technology. However, looking beyond these pinnacles and abysses, there are a great many more endoscopic technologies that have dotted this horizon which were first introduced with great enthusiasm and fanfare, sometimes at considerable cost, only to flounder ultimately because of failure to fulfill a robust clinical need, inability to achieve success at obtaining reimbursement, insufficient or inadequate data to demonstrate effectiveness, or because of inordinate skill or time required on the part of the endoscopist utilizing the device. That endoscopic technology development has been a largely haphazard and unorganized process is at once highlighted and lamented in a recent editorial by Kaltenbach, Soetikno, Rex, Fennerty, and Sharma, who go on to propose an organized, programmatic approach to new endoscopic technology development facilitated or directed by one or more professional gastroenterology societies [29]. The authors cite that one of the reasons so few novel endoscopic technologies ultimately demonstrate high clinical impact or durable marketplace success is that present-day device development in endoscopy is largely a result of happenstance, or of technology being developed by individuals or groups without sufficient clinical background or input to be able, first, to identify the most important clinical need, and then to follow through by developing technology to meet this specific clinical void. Instead, technology is developed with limited clinical input as to the most important unsolved endoscopic issues of the day, and then brought to market with inadequate study and trial, leading to the proverbial "technology looking for a clinical application." Neither serving a pressing clinical need nor possessing rigorous efficacy or cost-effectiveness data, many such technologies die in development, shortly after introduction, or following unsuccessful bids to obtain reimbursement. The authors proposed putting into the hands of one or more professional GI societies, with their interdisciplinary panel of experts, the charge of identifying key clinical needs in endoscopy, establishing performance thresholds for new technologies to meet such identified clinical needs, formulating appropriately rigorous studies and trials to assess such technologies, evaluating and setting performance thresholds for their use in the clinical setting, generating technology assessment and standards of practice documents to support use of such devices, and working to seek appropriate reimbursement therein.

This initiative came to fruition in 2010 as the ASGE PIVI Program (the Preservation and Incorporation of Valuable endoscopic Innovations that improve digestive health program), currently underway with three PIVI initiatives developed and introduced effective summer 2010: "Accuracy Thresholds for Differentiating Colonic Polyps so that One Could Either Ignore or Potentially Discard Resected Lesions Found During Colonoscopy," "Thresholds for Endoscopic Ablation and Releasing from Surveillance Patients with Non-Dysplastic Barrett's Esophagus," and "Efficacy Thresholds for Bariatric Procedures." Any group or individual may identify a clinical need in endoscopy not adequately addressed by existing technology, and submit a PIVI proposal to the ASGE Standards of Practice or Technology Committee for consideration. If such a proposal is accepted by these ASGE committees, a multidisciplinary expert task force is organized to determine a performance threshold that the new technology must attain in order to meet the identified unmet clinical endoscopic need. Then, once a technology is appropriately studied by investigators and demonstrated to exceed the PIVI performance threshold, it is supported by the ASGE through the Standards of Practice and Technology committees, which formulate and publish a joint assessment document supporting not only the utilization of the technology in clinical practice but also supporting its reimbursement by payors [30]. The IT&T Center itself and its concept is proposed to occupy a critical role in the subsequent deployment of such a comprehensive endoscopic technology development pipeline.

In the future, it is envisioned that the innovation process will begin with the identification of clinical needs. Next, potential technological solutions for such problems would be initiated, fostered, and executed. Once this has occurred, the assessment of the product of such development will be undertaken and disseminated amongst participating research institutions, and ultimately supported through clinical deployment, acceptance as a newly documented standard of care, and through lobbying of government and third-party payers to establish appropriate reimbursement. Once a technology is successfully supported through this development paradigm by the ASGE, the Education and Institute for Training and Technology Committees will subsequently develop education and training materials and courses directed towards training physicians in the proper use of the new technology. In this way, the IT&T Center will serve as the perfect platform for the dissemination of education and training efforts specific to each new PIVI-supported technology. Through this process, the IT&T Center promises to be an ideal environment in which to work out the best ways to train endoscopists in a new technology or technique, and perhaps even to conduct trials to validate such training programs as they are developed. This novel notion that the development of reliable training programs are essential to the process of innovation and acceptance of technological advance will ensure an ever-important role for IT&T in the coming years.

With paradigm-changing initiatives such as these, the lines between technology development and training in new technology will be less clearly drawn. As gastrointestinal endoscopists are increasingly dependent on industry and initiatives by the ASGE to support the effort to train and retrain their ranks, the great potential this offers to add efficiency to the development and acceptance of innovation into clinical practice represents an enormous value to justify that ongoing and increasing support. Further, it will serve to solidify the growing acceptance of the principle that the development of validated training programs and the support of opportunities to provide that training are integral components of the process of new technology development going forward.

Video

Video 33.1 Endofest 2010

References

1 Bloom MB, Rawn CL, Salzberg AD, Krummel TM. Virtual reality applied to procedural testing: the next era. *Ann Surg* 2003;**237**:442–448.

2 Gerson LB, Van Dam J. The future of simulators in GI endoscopy: an unlikely possibility or a virtual reality? *Gastrointest Endosc* 2002;**55**: 608–611.

3 Institute of Medicine. *To Err Is Human: Building A Safer Health System.* National Academy of Sciences Press, Washindton, DC, 1999.

4 Institute of Medicine. *Crossing the Quality Chasm: A New Health System for the 21st Century.* National Academy of Sciences Press, Washington, DC, 2001.

5 Alinier G. A typology of educationally focused medical simulation tools. *Med Teach* 2007;**29**:e243–e250.

6 Greenwald D, Cohen J. Evolution of endoscopy simulators and their application. *Gastrointest Endosc Clin North Am* 2006;**16**:389–406.

7 Hochberger J, Maiss J, Magdeburg B, Cohen J, Hahn EG. Training simulators and education in gastrointestinal endoscopy: current status and perspectives in 2001. *Endoscopy* 2001;**33**:541–549.

8 Cisler JJ, Martin JA. Logistical considerations for endoscopy simulators. *Gastrointest Endosc Clin North Am* 2006;**16**:565–575.

9 Matthes K, Cohen J, Kochman ML, Cerulli MA, Vora KC, Hochberger J. Efficacy and costs of a one-day hands-on EASIE endoscopy simulator train-the-trainer workshop. *Gastrointest Endosc* 2005;**62**:921–927.

10 Gerson LB, Van Dam J. Technology review: the use of simulators for training in GI endoscopy. *Gastrointest Endosc* 2004;**60**:992–1001.

11 Bar-Meir S. Endoscopy simulators: the state of the art, 2000. *Gastrointest Endosc* 2000;**52**:701–703.

12 Clark JA, Volchok JA, Hazey JW, Sadighy PJ, Fanelli RD. Initial experience using an endoscopic simulator to train surgical residents in flexible endoscopy in a community medical center residency program. *Curr Surg* 2005;**62**:59–63.

13 Sedlack RE. Endoscopic simulation: where we have been and where we are going. *Gastrointest Endosc* 2005;**61**:216–218.

14 Hochberger J, Matthes K, Maiss J, Koebnick C, Hahn EG, Cohen J. Training with the CompactEASIE biologic endoscopy simulator significantly improves hemostatic technical skill of gastroenterology fellows: a randomized controlled comparison with clinical endoscopy training alone. *Gastrointest Endosc* 2005;**61**:204–215.

15 American College of Surgeons insists on using cruel animal labs. PETA home page. 11 Nov 2005. Available: http://www.stopanimaltests.com/ (accessed November 21, 2009).

16 Sedlack R, Petersen B, Binmoeller K, Kolars J. A Direct comparison of ERCP teaching models. *Gastrointest Endosc* 2003;**57**:886–890.

17 Neumann M, Mayer G, Ell C, Felzmann T, Reingruber B, Horbach T, Hohenberger W. The Erlangen Endo-Trainer: life-like simulation for diagnostic and interventional endoscopic retrograde cholangiography. *Endoscopy* 2000;**32**:906–910.

18 Matthes K, Cohen J. The Neo-Papilla: a new modification of porcine *ex vivo* simulators for ERCP training. *Gastrointest Endosc* 2006;**64**: 570–576.

19 Hochberger J, Euler K, Naegel A, Hahn EG, Maiss J. The Compact Erlangen Active Simulator for Interventional Endoscopy: a prospective comparison in structured team-training courses on 'endoscopic hemostasis' for doctors and nurses to the 'endo-trainer' model. *Scand J Gastroenterol* 2004;**39**:895–902.

20 Freys SM, Heimbucher J, Fuchs KH. Teaching upper gastrointestinal endoscopy: the pig stomach. *Endoscopy* 1995;**27**:73–76.

21 Neumann M, Hochberger J, Felzmann T, Ell C, Hohenberger W. Part I. The Erlanger Endo-Trainer. *Endoscopy* 2001;**33**:887–890.

22 Gerson LB, Van Dam J. Technology review: the use of simulators for training in GI endoscopy. *Gastrointest Endosc* 2004;**60**:992–1001.

23 American Society for Gastrointestinal Endoscopy home page. http://www.asge.org (accessed November 21, 2009).

24 Huang GC, Gordon JA, Schwartzstein RM. Millennium conference 2005 on medical simulation: A summary report. *Simul Healthc* 2007;**2**: 88–95.

25 Ethicon Endo-Surgery home page. http://www.ethiconendo.com (accessed November 21, 2009).

26 MERI home page. http://www.meri.org (accessed November 21, 2009).

27 Digital Forum, October 2007: Association Forum of Chicagoland. http://www.associationforum.org/ (accessed November 21, 2009).

28 Cohen J, Nuckolls L, Mourant RR. Endoscopy simulators: lessons from the aviation and automobile industries. *Gastrointest Endoscopy Clin N Am* 2006;**16**:407–423.

29 Kaltenbach T, Soetikno R, Rex DK, Fennerty MB, Sharma P. Polyp imaging as a template for moving endoscopic innovation forward to answer key clinical questions. *Gastrointest Endosc* 2010;**71**:142–146.

30 Fennerty MB. ASGE News 2010;17(July/August):1. http://www. asgenews-digital.com/asgenews/asge20100708?pg=5#pg1 (accessed September 5, 2010).

34 The Importance of Skills Assessment and Recording Personal Outcomes in the Future of Training

Peter B. Cotton[1] & Roland M. Valori[2]

[1]Medical University of South Carolina, Charleston, SC, USA
[2]Gloucestershire Hospitals NHS Foundation Trust, Gloucestershire, UK

Endoscopy is now a major part of most gastroenterologists' professional lives. Interest in assessing and documenting the skill levels of endoscopists has increased substantially in recent years for many reasons. Patients and potential patients have become more aware of the fact that endoscopic expertise varies, and that outcomes can be compromised by poor performance. Their awareness has risen partly because the profession has (rather belatedly) started to expose some dirty linen, and to publish papers showing imperfect performance.

While cognitive elements play an important role in determining outcomes, research has focused on technical aspects, which are (somewhat) easier to measure. In the past, most published series came from expert centers extolling their skills, while those less skilled neither measured their outcomes, nor publicized them for obvious reasons. Colonoscopy provides an excellent example. Many studies by experts published cecal intubation rates of close to 98% [1]. Then a British multicenter audit showed only 77% adjusted cecal intubation, [2] and a study in the USA showed that less than half of 104 endoscopists were reaching the cecum in 90% of cases [3]. These technical deficiencies were then emphasized by reports of "miss-rates" from back-to-back colonoscopies [4], missed colorectal cancers, and huge variations in adenoma detection rate [5]. The advent of CT colonography provided additional evidence and reasons for lesions missed at optical colonoscopy [6]. One leading authority editorialized that "Colonoscopy is not as good as gold" [7] even when done by experts, and likened the difficulties (and importance) in choosing a colonoscopist to selecting a roofing contractor [8].

ERCP is another procedure of significant interest in this context. It is technically challenging, and carries substantial risks, which are increased by technical failure. Experts claim very high technical success rates [9], but the less experienced rarely present their data. A comprehensive audit from Britain showed that only 77% of trained endoscopists achieved a cannulation rate of > 80%, and the rate averaged only 66% for senior trainees with > 200 cases [10].

The wish to understand and document performance is driven also by medico–legal and employment issues. In the USA, insurance payments may eventually be linked to outcomes, and patients with high deductible plans are shopping around for value.

These facts clearly show that there are substantial quality challenges in endoscopy, and that it behooves us as professionals to study and understand the problems, and to put in place mechanisms to document and to enhance performance. This process begins in the training environment, which has been largely unstructured until recently. Trainees were apprenticed to various mentors, who might or might not (often not) have much interest in teaching, or have any training in how to teach. Trainees varied in their dedication to self-study, and were not motivated by any sort of formal assessment process. Competency was assumed when the allotted training years had passed.

One of the first attempts to provide guidance about a training end point came from the American Society for Gastrointestinal Endoscopy (ASGE) in 1986 [11]. The committee pulled some numbers out of the air (e.g., 100 ERCPs), and added the word "threshold" to them. This was intended to mean that trainees must achieve certain numbers before asking their supervisors for some sort of assessment, and guidance about their progress, but the subtlety was lost, especially when other disciplines recommended lower numbers. The blinders were taken from our eyes, at least for ERCP, with the seminal study from Duke University, which assessed trainees prospectively, and showed that trainees were only approaching 80% competency at 180–200 cases [12].

It is self-evident that being involved in a certain number of cases is no guarantee of competence. Trainers vary in their practice spectra, skills, and enthusiasm, and trainees vary in their learning rates. Furthermore, there has been no definition of a "case", i.e., how much of a procedure had to be done for it to count.

The only way to assess skill levels is by sequential, rigorous, and objective assessment based on clear criteria or objectives.

The initial training period

Competency means that the practitioner should be allowed to practice the specific procedure without supervision, but there are levels of complexity. Thus, the first step is to set the stage appropriately, by defining clearly the overall goal of the training period. The ERCP community recognizes three "grades of difficulty" (Table 34.1) [13]. Grade 1 procedures are those (mainly biliary) contexts and techniques that anyone offering ERCP should be able to address to a reasonable level, but grades 2 and 3 procedures require extra training and experience. Most standard training programs, like GI fellowship in the USA, aim only to reach competence in grade 1 cases. Extra training (including 4th year programs in the USA) is needed to address more complex cases, during which success rates in grade 1 cases should improve also. Similar grading schemes are being developed for upper endoscopy, colonoscopy, and EUS.

Secondly, the training path should be dissected into constituent parts that can be addressed individually. This means designing a curriculum for the specific needs of the trainee, to include all relevant aspects. Cognitive aspects are important but often overlooked in the rush to learn technical skills. Practitioners must have an appropriate knowledge base of the conditions they may encounter, the risks of endoscopy (and how they are minimized and man-

Table 34.1 Grades of difficulty for ERCP. (Adjusted from Schutz SM, Abbott RM: Grading ERCPs by degree of difficulty: a new concept to produce more meaningful outcome data. Gastrointest Endosc 2000;51:535–539, with permission from Elsevier.)

Grade 1	Biliary and pancreatic cannulation Biopsy, cytology Biliary sphincterotomy Bile duct stones < 10 mm Stents for bile leaks Stents for non-hilar tumors Prophylactic pancreatic stents
Grade 2	Cannulation in Billroth II cases Minor papilla cannulation Bile duct stones > 10 mm Stents for hilar tumors
Grade 3	Sphincter manometry Direct ductoscopy ERCP after Whipple/Roux Y diversion Therapy in Billroth II cases Intrahepatic stones All pancreatic therapies Ampullectomy Pseudocyst drainage

aged), their limitations, and potential alternatives. The technical elements can be dissected similarly, and addressed sequentially.

Thirdly, all of these elements should be tested. The cognitive aspects can be assessed with standard tests, and are addressed to a certain extent in specialty examinations like the GI boards in the USA. Assessing technical skills during training is more difficult, but made easier if the constituent steps to proficiency are defined and tested to a predetermined competency framework.

The preferred approach for assessing the technical aspects of procedures is Direct Observation of Procedural Skills (DOPS) [14], otherwise known as Objectively Structured Assessment of Technical Skills (OSATS) [15]. DOPS and OSATS provide a competency framework that utilizes graded descriptors to assess progress acquiring the various competencies. During the training period DOPS assessment is used formatively, i.e., to aid the training process by defining the gaps and setting objectives for improvement.

None of this can happen unless each trainee has a primary mentor who is responsible for overseeing these processes and who ensures that individual trainers assess their trainees on a regular basis.

Progress along these lines is being made in several countries. Trainees in Australia are required to complete and submit a log of all their procedures to a central "Conjoint committee". The log has to be signed off after every 20 procedures by their supervisor. At the point of credentialing the supervisor has to provide a report confirming that the trainee is competent for independent practice (http://www.conjoint.org.au). In Britain, an "e-portfolio" project is being rolled out (www.thejag.org.uk).

Credentialing

Credentialing is the process for determining whether a practitioner is ready to perform specific procedures independently (www.jets.nhs.uk). Hitherto, and in most places still, this has been done very casually, with only (perhaps) a letter of recommendation from someone in the training program. That person often has had little personal knowledge of the trainee, and no hard data, and assumes that the trainee is fit to fly in the absence of any negative comments from supervisors.

In the USA, most trainees enter private practice, and do their procedures in independent endoscopy units that vary in their stringency in the process of allowing use of the facilities. Hospitals have privileging committees, which can be influenced by the wish to increase business, or to reduce competition. Granting privileges too easily to someone who turns out to be incompetent can result in legal action [16].

It is self-evident that credentialing should be much more rigorous. The applicant must provide evidence of appropriate medical or surgical training, and data on prior experience, with specific outcomes of each type of procedure. There should be a legally binding letter of recommendation from the endoscopy training program director.

To determine competence accurately on the basis of procedural outcomes, such as completion rates for colonoscopy or cannulation rates for ERCP, or patient outcomes, such as missed rates of cancer or adverse events such as pancreatitis, requires very large numbers of cases. Trainees will achieve competence for solo practice long before such numbers are achieved. Thus, an alternative method for determining competence is necessary. As has been argued earlier, actual numbers of procedures is a poor guide to competence. Data on technical outcomes, such as completion rates for colonoscopy or cannulation rates for ERCP, do provide some guidance, but results may be different when trainees leave the mother ship.

DOPS can be used summatively to credential individuals for independent practice. In the United Kingdom, it is recommended that for a summative assessment there should be two assessors performing DOPS on a minimum number of cases (www.thejag.org.uk). This credentialing process can usually be completed during one endoscopy list and for trainees is usually done in the center that they are currently working in. As trainees rotate through several centers during their training it is not considered necessary for the assessment to be carried out in an independent center (which would be much more complicated, time consuming, and costly).

Recredentialing established endoscopists is a different situation, and more difficult one. It should probably be done in an independent center. There is a good example of this special credentialing process ongoing in Britain for colonoscopists wishing to participate in the bowel cancer screening program. Applicants must submit a summary of their lifetime experience of colonoscopy, provide a more detailed audit of the previous year's performance, complete a knowledge-based multiple-choice questions and then be assessed using a summative DOPS technique by two examiners, while performing two colonoscopies. More than 200 colonoscopists have been through this process (with significant numbers failing). The test performs well, and early data from the screening program from more than 40,000 colonoscopies indicates that this cohort of colonoscopists is achieving the required minimum performance, and in most cases exceeding it by a comfortable margin. For example, more than half the cohort have unadjusted completion rates of > 95%, adenoma detection rates exceed those in the screening pilot, and there have been no perforations unrelated to therapy (Rutter M, personal communication).

Competence in practice

The true test of competence is how individuals perform in independent practice. Despite earlier pleas [17], the idea of continuing to document performance after "graduation" is only now creeping into the mainstream [18]. Most individuals have viewed continuous assessment and "report cards" as a bureaucratic invasion, but the tide is turning, for many reasons. Firstly, properly trained and competent gastroenterologists are seeing their business threatened by others with less training. Without data, their claim to the high ground is slippery at best. Secondly, payers, patients (and indeed plaintiff lawyers) are all increasingly interested in data. Professionals, comfortable with their performance, can only benefit from being able to provide documentation.

A key challenge is to determine what data should be collected, and there is no shortage of individuals and organizations wishing to offer suggestions [19–22]. All agree that the data points should be relatively few, easy to collect, and clinically relevant. For colonoscopy, withdrawal times seemed to be a good quality metric, but too easy to game. Connected and more relevant is the adenoma detection rate, but this is difficult to collect since it involves collating delayed data from pathology. The debate continues.

Defining the relevant data and wanting to collect it is only the start. Providing the methods and infrastructure to do so is equally challenging. The increasing popularity of electronic endoscopy reporting systems should facilitate the process, since most of the key data points are already entered in generating the report. However, attempts to extract these data directly from reporting systems have proven difficult to date. Usually, auditing performance means entering quality data separately on paper, or to a central website. This is time-consuming and expensive. Equally important, and difficult, is arranging to aggregate and to analyze the resulting data in a meaningful way. Hanging over all such projects is the question of data quality, for everything is self-reported. Being able to extract the data from reporting systems would help, since the reports are legally binding documents. It is worth remembering that, when the only purpose of collecting data is to allow practitioners to compare themselves with others (i.e., there are no published league tables), the only person deceived by inaccurate data is the one who enters it.

A good example of what can be done has been published recently from a single practice group in the USA, who responded to a challenge to collect community data from the joint ASGE/ACG Task Force on Quality. Thirteen physicians collected data from their ERCP procedures at eight community hospitals for a year, including a 30-day call for delayed events [23]. The results of the group were reassuring, but were not broken down by individual.

There are two broader pilot projects in progress in the USA, intended to allow practitioners to compare themselves with their peers and with published standards. Pike in Virginia has spearheaded a pilot project in colonoscopy, sponsored by his regional hospital system [18]. Endoscopists can volunteer to upload data on each procedure, including pathology results and delayed adverse events. They receive reports of their own performance, comparison with others, and suggested benchmarks. More than 20,000 cases have been logged. The range of cecal intubation rates is shown in Figure 34.1. A similar project for ERCP (the ERCP Quality Network) was launched by Cotton in 2007 with sponsorship from Olympus America (although it is open to contributors worldwide). Eighty-five participants have entered more than 13,000 cases. Participants can access summaries of their own ERCP practice and performance immediately from a central website, and can compare them with all others in the system, without individual identifiers. The range of reported biliary cannulation rates is shown in Figure 34.2. In the future they will be able to compare themselves with specific peer groups, for example those in the same country, practice setting or level of experience. Although personal benchmarking is the main goal, downloaded data can be analyzed in detail, for instance to look at performance by experience 24].

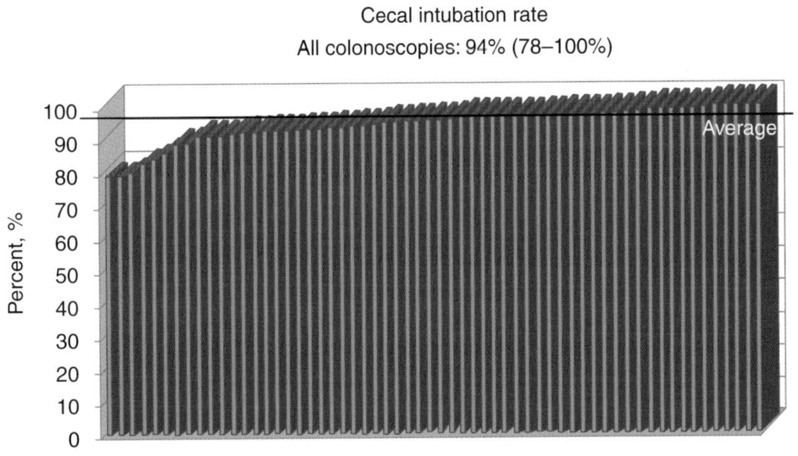

Cecal intubation rate
All colonoscopies: 94% (78–100%)

Figure 34.1 Benchmarking in colonoscopy. Individual and average cecal intubation rates in the Colonoscopy Quality Improvement Project. (Reproduced from Pike IM, Vicari J: Incorporating quality measurement and improvement into a gastroentrerology practice. Am J Gstroenterol 2010, withe permission from Nature.)

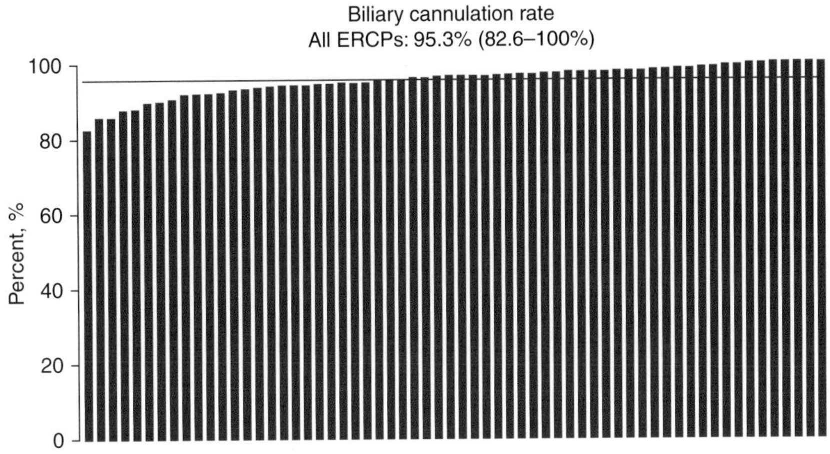

Biliary cannulation rate
All ERCPs: 95.3% (82.6–100%)

Figure 34.2 Benchmarking in ERCP. Individual and average biliary cannulation rates in the ERCP Quality Network. (Reproduced from Garrow DA, Romagnuolo J, Cotton PB: Comparing ERCP practice and outcomes by level of experience. GIE 2009;69:AB 231, with permission from Elsevier.)

The ASGE and ACG have recently initiated a joint national project which eventually will allow members to upload their data to a central website, hopefully directly from their report writers, and thereby to obtain "practice summaries" and benchmarking. This will start with colonoscopy, and will be entirely voluntary. However, it is hoped that peer pressure, and the value of having the data, will persuade most people to collaborate. Work still needs to be done in refining the most relevant data points.

Impact of practice measurements on the training process

The objective assessment of endoscopists beyond the training period should in turn improve future training, by highlighting common areas of deficiency in practice that need remediation. Learning is a lifelong process.

Conclusion

Patients deserve competent endoscopists, and it is currently the responsibility of the profession to ensure that appropriate quality assessment and documentation processes are in place. We have

been complacent, and only now, through review of objective data, can we see that much needs to be done. If we fail to act vigorously, others will take over. Who would knowingly fly with a pilot who had not been assessed rigorously, and recently? Of course, pilots have a strong personal incentive to perform well, since any adverse outcomes will also affect them severely. We should care just as much.

References

1 Leiberman DA, Weiss DG, Bone JH, et al.: Use of colonoscopy to screen asymptomatic adults for colorectal cancer. *N Engl J Med* 2000;**343**:162–168.
2 Bowles CJ, Leicester R, Romaya C, et al.: A prospective study of colonoscopy practice in the UK today: are we adequately prepared for national colorectal cancer screening tomorrow? *Gut* 2004;**53**:277–283.
3 Cotton PB, Connor P, McGee D et al.: Colonoscopy practice variation among 69 hospital-based endoscopists. *GIE* 2003;**57**:352–357.
4 Rex DK, Cutler CS, Lemmel GT, etal.: Colonoscopic miss rates of adenomas determined by back-to-back colonoscopies. *Gastroenterology* 1997;**112**(1):24–28.
5 Barclay RL, Vicari JJ, Doughty AS, et al.: Colonoscopic withdrawal times and adenoma defection during screening colonoscopy. *N Engl J Med* 2006;**355**(24):2533–2541.

6 Pickhardt PJ, Nugent PA, Mysliwiec PA, et al.: Location of adenomas missed by optical colonoscopy. *Ann Intern Med* 2004;**141**(5): 352–359.

7 Lieberman D: Colonoscopy: as good as gold? *Ann Intern Med* 2004;**141**:401–403.

8 Lieberman D: Home repair and colonoscopy: quality counts. *GIE* 2006;**64**:563–564.

9 Cotton PB: ERCP training, competence and assessment. In: Cotton PB, Leung JWC (eds), *Advanced Digestive Endoscopy: ERCP*. Massachusetts: Blackwells Scientific Publications, 2006;9–16.

10 Williams EJ, Taylor S, Fairclough P, et al.: Are we meeting the standards set for endoscopy? *Gut* 2007;**56**:821–829.

11 Report of Multi-society Task Force on GI Training. *GIE* 2009;**70**: 823–827

12 Jowell PS, Baillie J, Branch MS, et al.: Quantitative assessment of procedural competence; a prospective study of training in endoscopic retrograde cholangiopancreatography. *Ann Intern Med* 1996;**125**:983–989.

13 Schutz SM, Abbott RM: Grading ERCPs by degree of difficulty: a new concept to produce more meaningful outcome data. *Gastrointest Endosc* 2000;**51**:535–539.

14 Wilkinson JR, Crossley JGM, Wragg A, et al.: Implementing workplace-based assessment across the medical specialties in the United Kingdom. *Med Educ* 2008;**42**(4):364–373.

15 Swift SE, Carter JF: Institution and validation of an observed structured assessment of technical skills (OSATS) for obstetrics and gynecology residents and faculty. *Am J of Obstet & Gynecol* 2006;**195**(2):617–621.

16 Faigel DO, Baron TH, Lewis B, et al.: Ensuring competence in endoscopy. Available: www.asge.org (accessed May 2008).

17 Cotton PB: How many times have you done this procedure, doctor? *Am J Gastroenterol* 2002;**97**:522–523.

18 Pike IM, Vicari J: Incorporating quality measurement and improvement into a gastroentrerology practice. *Am J Gstroenterol* 2010. (In press)

19 Cotton PB: Outcomes of endoscopy procedures. *GIE* 1994;**40**:514–518.

20 Cotton PB, Hawes RH, Barkun A, et al.: Excellence in endoscopy: toward practical metrics. *GIE* 2006;**63**:286–291.

21 Rex DK, Petrini JL, Baron TH, et al.: Quality indicators for colonoscopy. *Gastrointest Endosc* 2006;**63**(Suppl 4):S16–S28.

22 Bjorkman DJ, Popp JW: Measuring the quality of endoscopy. *Am J Gastroenterol* 2006;**101**:864–865.

23 Colton JB, Curran CC: Quality indicators, including complications, of ERCP in a community setting: a prospective study. *GIE* 2009 Sep;**70**(3):457–467.

24 Garrow DA, Romagnuolo J, Cotton PB: Comparing ERCP practice and outcomes by level of experience. *GIE* 2009;**69**:AB 231.

Index

Note: Page numbers with *f* and *t* refer to figures and tables, respectively.

Successful Training in Gastrointestinal Endoscopy, First Edition. Edited by Jonathan Cohen.
© 2011 Blackwell Publishing Ltd. Published 2011 by Blackwell Publishing Ltd.

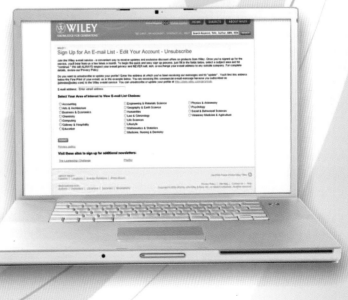